Introduction to Molecular Vaccinology

Matthias Giese

Introduction to Molecular Vaccinology

Springer

Matthias Giese
Institute for Molecular Vaccines
Heidelberg
Germany

ISBN 978-3-319-25830-0 ISBN 978-3-319-25832-4 (eBook)
DOI 10.1007/978-3-319-25832-4

Library of Congress Control Number: 2016934043

Springer Cham Heidelberg New York Dordrecht London

Printed on acid-free paper

Springer International Publishing AG Switzerland is part of Springer Science+Business Media (www.springer.com)

Rerum cognoscere causas.

To my brothers Bernhard and Thomas. Both died of cancer some months apart.
Nothing is so difficult but that it may be found out by seeking…
I am sure.

Foreword

Vaccine research and development is a growing field. The recombinant DNA and nanotechnology did much enlarge the repertoire on vaccines and improved also the quality of the products. Nevertheless, there are still areas of classical unmet needs: infectious diseases, such as HIV, hepatitis C, malaria in humans, or *Clostridia* and other bacteria in animals, or unmet need in the elderly. New effective vaccines for older adults are strongly recommended but how to circumvent the merciless immunosenescence?

Together with the rapid progress in genomics, proteomics, and bioinformatics, new areas for vaccines arose in the last decade: therapeutical immunizations against cancer diseases or against noninfectious and noncancer diseases (NINC) as described in this book. The immune therapy will expand, and concomitant vaccine targets will dramatically diversify. The antibiotic administration will decrease. The only adequate alternatives are antibacterial vaccines. Thereby the specific adjuvant system will have a fundamental impact on the success of these new therapeutical vaccine strategies. Precancerous cells need a niche in which they can thrive and prosper to cancer cells. This niche is the tumor microenvironment and protects the malignant cells against the immune systems. Adjuvant agents can alter the microenvironment around the tumor to boost the effectiveness of anticancer vaccines, e.g., by resulting in CTL infiltration into tumors.

Vaccinology is more than a simple combination of antigens with a proper adjuvant. Vaccinology means to go deeper and understand, in a more holistic approach, biological systems as series of more or less dependent subsystems like the immune system and the nervous system influencing each other by dynamic functions. There is also a need to learn more about the regulations of immune genes by microRNAs (miRNAs); miRNAs turn a gene on or off. What is the signal for this switch, and could a vaccine also turn a target gene on or off?

Also new trends in vaccine productions are discussed here: transgenic plants fulfill all criteria for a successful production of animal or human antigen proteins. Plant-expressed eukaryotic proteins are properly folded, posttranslationally modified, and assembled in a biologically active form. They are naturally free of human or animal microbial toxins and pyrogens and recognized as safe. During the recent Ebola virus epidemic in West Africa, a cocktail of tobacco-produced monoclonal antibodies, called ZMapp, was first used experimentally to treat some people with the Ebola virus disease.

The author of this textbook, Matthias Giese, is a professional vaccine developer for 25 years who was extensively trained in several international pharmaceutical companies, with a fruitful combination of human and animal vaccines. I met him in the late 1990s, when he just had developed a therapeutical DNA vaccine against equine arteritis virus (EAV). With this vaccine we could completely cure chronically EAV-infected stallions.

But the most important lesson we learnt from our long-term activities was that professional vaccinology is still a stepchild in most countries. The global list of chairs in universities for vaccinology is very short, and there is also no chair for vaccinology in Germany. Vaccines still seem to be a minor matter, but only vaccines can prevent global outbreaks of dangerous infectious diseases.

Leipzig, Germany
October 2015

Gerald Fritz Schusser, Dipl. ECEIM
Prof. Dr. Dipl. ECEIM
University of Leipzig/Germany
Faculty for Veterinary Medicine
Department of Large Animals Medicine

Preface

In 2013, Springer Publishing globally presented my books *Molecular Vaccines: From Prophylaxis to Therapy*, Volume 1 and 2. Neither the publisher nor I had a premonition of the amazing success these books would have within a short time only. Obviously, not only me but thousands of colleagues all over the world were confronted with the same old problem I also had before, problems with the standard vaccine literature: too many diverse books and often with an oscillating quality. *Molecular Vaccines: From Prophylaxis to Therapy* closed a gap. It was the first compendium of its sort and presented most of all scientific aspects of modern vaccinology in two volumes, with contributions of 150 experts from 21 nations and 5 continents.

This new textbook is based on the successful concept of my first books and was inspired in numberless lectures by my critical students and colleagues. The book is structured in three main parts, Vaccine Science, Vaccine Design, and Therapeutical Vaccines, subdivided in 13 descriptive chapters, with lots of new subjects, and 208 mostly colored figures and 55 tables. Each chapter combines theory and practice: it begins with a more general overview of the presented topic, and following this, the research is explained based on practical approaches. Thereby, selected and adapted studies chosen from *Molecular Vaccines: From Prophylaxis to Therapy* are incorporated into this new book in a condensed version and with particular reference to the original article in Volume 1 or 2.

New chapters such as "Formulation" are now included and explain the long way from an antigen to an active ingredient to a final formulated vaccine, which is monitored by stress and potency tests and operated over the entire life cycle of the product. Other chapters such as "Cancer Vaccines" are now much more extended to take into account the rapid progress in this field. Neoantigens, a new class of mutated and patient-specific antigens, present in tumor cells but not in normal cells, and the lack of central tolerance against them is discussed as well as the combination of immune checkpoint modifiers with cancer vaccines offering a new strategy to treat cancer diseases.

Also in "Introduction to Molecular Vaccines," veterinary vaccine approaches are discussed. DNA vaccines, i.e., can pave the way to products for human health. The first veterinary DNA vaccine was registered already in 2005. This vaccine is effective and biologically absolutely safe.

Finally yet importantly, I would like to thank my son Sebastian, University of Freiburg, for his fruitful discussions and ideas. Special thanks go again to Raphael Lekscha, Heidelberg, for his excellent technical preparations of my illustrations for this new book. This time we had long, long sessions together, but the new figures are fantastic. I am grateful to Springer Publishing and particularly to Claudia Panuschka and Silvia Herold, Vienna, who made this textbook possible, and Claus-Dieter Bachem, Heidelberg, for his technical support.

Heidelberg, Germany
October 2015

Matthias Giese

Contents

Part III Therapeutical Vaccines

Part I

Vaccine Science

From Pasteur to Personalized Vaccines

1

Contents

In science credit goes to the man who convinces the world, not the man to whom the idea first occurs. Francis Galton

1.1 History of Vaccination

Anno domini 1881: Louis Pasteur (1822–1895) was on track to become the first leading vaccinologist at the time and to win the race against the development of the first artificial attenuated vaccine to his rival, the veterinarian Henry Toussaint. One year ago, he developed a vaccine against avian cholera (fowl cholera). Pasteur isolated the causative agent of this zoonotic disease, *Pasteurella multocida* (a gram-negative, nonmotile *coccobacillus*). The economic losses caused by avian cholera were enormously at this time and also today.

Cholera Vaccine. Emile Roux (1853–1933), Pasteur's assistant, came up with the idea to develop a series of immunization experiments with different aged cultures of *Pasteurella*:

(A) Immunization of 12 chickens with fresh cultivated *Pasteurella*
(B) Immunization of 12 chickens with aged cultures of *Pasteurella*
(C) Immunization with old cultures of *Pasteurella*

Eight days later, 12/12 chickens of group A died, but 4/12 chickens of group B survived, and surprisingly 11/12 chickens of group C survived. In the following challenge experiment, 8/11 immunized chickens survived. This was the confirmation that an old culture of *Pasteurella* could be used as vaccine to protect against avian cholera. Today it's known that this vaccine developed serious side effects and was not able to reduce the shedding, and the duration of immunity was very short.

M. Giese, *Introduction to Molecular Vaccinology*, DOI 10.1007/978-3-319-25832-4_1

1.1.1 Pasteur and Oxygen

Pasteur concluded that the virulence of *Pasteurella* could be manipulated by the conditions of cultivation. The interruption or complete stopping of the process of cultivation resulted in a still living but weakened form of *Pasteurella*. Pasteur believed that only the exposure of the bacilli to oxygen was the reason for this attenuation.

The big difference between Jenner's smallpox vaccination and Pasteur's cholera vaccine was the source of the weakened form of the agent. It was known that a microorganism, e.g., smallpox, could exist in a virulent and in an avirulent natural form. And Edward Jenner (1749–1823) applied the avirulent natural form. Pasteur isolated the pathogen and attenuated this pathogen by special laboratory conditions. For the first time, he generated an artificially weakened vaccine against an infectious disease.

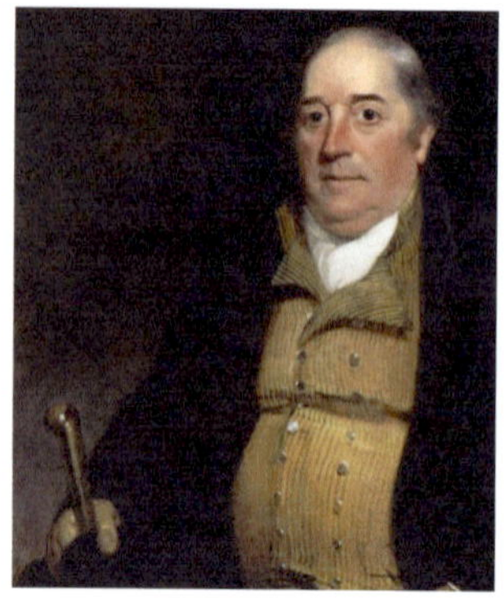

Fig. 1.2 Benjamin Jesty (1736–1816) (Image – credit: Wellcome Library, London/UK)

1.1.2 Jenner and Jesty

Jenner (Fig. 1.1) could build his empiric experiments on long tradition. In earlier times when the people were closer to their animals, farmers had the reputation of being healers for animals and man. They have used serous fluids from sick animals to protect their herds via inoculation under the skin – a usual practice to protect flocks against sheep pox.

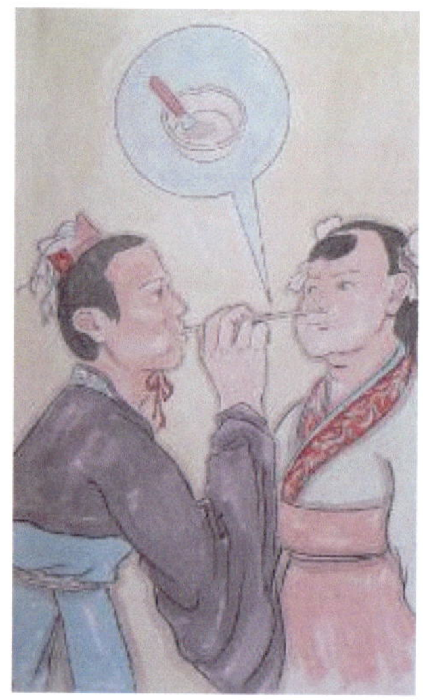

Fig. 1.3 Smallpox powder inoculation into the nose, China, tenth century

Already in 1774, Benjamin Jesty (Fig. 1.2), a dairy farmer in Dorset, England, became aware that those people infected with cowpox were subsequently protected against smallpox what was not an uncommon observation with peasantry in the late eighteenth century. Owing to his courage and ingenuity, he inoculated his wife and two sons with matter from cowpox lesion on one of his cows by scratching the skin.

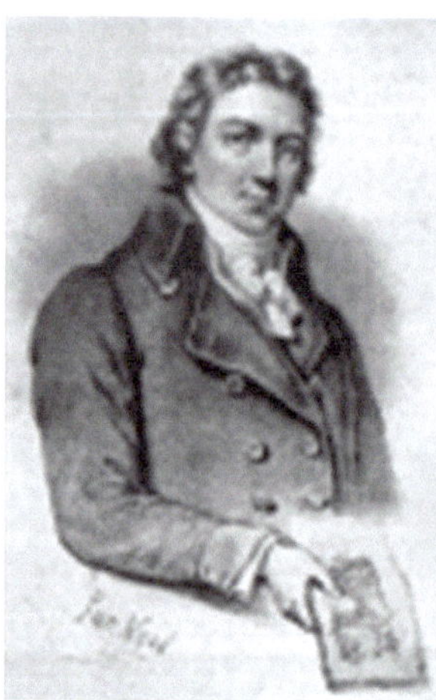

Fig. 1.1 Edward Jenner (1749–1823)

Benjamin Jesty made his immunization experiments 22 years earlier than Edward Jenner. The farmer Benjamin Jesty is rightly one of the pioneers for vaccination.

The origin of smallpox inoculation (vaccination) dated around the tenth century. The inoculation of dried and pulverized pustules against smallpox did not become widely known in China and was reserved to the upper class (Fig. 1.3).

But the oldest conveyed vaccination probably took place in Rome by Gaius Plinius Secundus, Pliny the Elder (AD 23–AD 79). He used serous fluids of dogs suffering from rabies to vaccinate people against rabies disease.

Back to Pasteur and his times: Also Henri Toussaint (1847–1890) was elaborating on vaccines, but in contrast to Pasteur who believed that only a live vaccine would be the appropriate stimulus for the immune system, Toussaint used

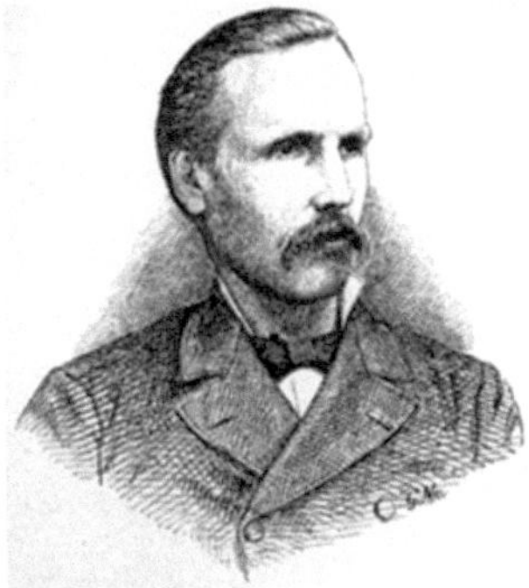

Fig. 1.4 Henri Toussaint (1847–1890)

the antiseptic phenol to inactivate his anthrax vaccine and later potassium dichromate for the cholera vaccine (Fig. 1.4).

Who would be the first scientist introducing the proof of concept of an artificially generated vaccine, demonstrating its feasibility and the potential of being used in the field?

In the small village Pouilly-le-Fort in June 1881, Pasteur was invited to give the first public demonstration of a lab-generated vaccine for sheep against anthrax. Group A with 25 sheep was immunized and group B with 25 sheep as control group. Both groups were subsequently challenged. The results were impressive: 24/25 vaccinated sheep have survived but 23/25 unvaccinated animals have died. The real scandal followed immediately. Pasteur refused to open his lab protocols, to display all details of the development of this vaccine – with good reason.

1.1.3 Toussaint's Protocol

Pasteur thievishly used Toussaint's inactivation protocol, heat combined with potassium dichromate treatment and not his own oxygen-based procedure – how the public and scientific community were convinced at this time. Pasteur's own studies were unsuccessful because oxygen was not able to kill the anthrax' spores. Pasteur won the competition with Toussaint. He never gave credit to Toussaint, the real inventor of this inactivation principle. Glory and publicity for Pasteur, and a deep fall into oblivion for Toussaint. *The winner takes it all…* The medical historian Gerald L. Geison interpreted Pasteur's copy and paste behavior as fair scientific swindle (Gerald L. Geison: The Private Science of Louis Pasteur, Princeton University Press, 1997, USA).

1.1.4 First Rabies Vaccine in 1885

Pasteur's worldwide breakthrough took place in 1885. Inspired again by Emile Roux's experiments with rabies,

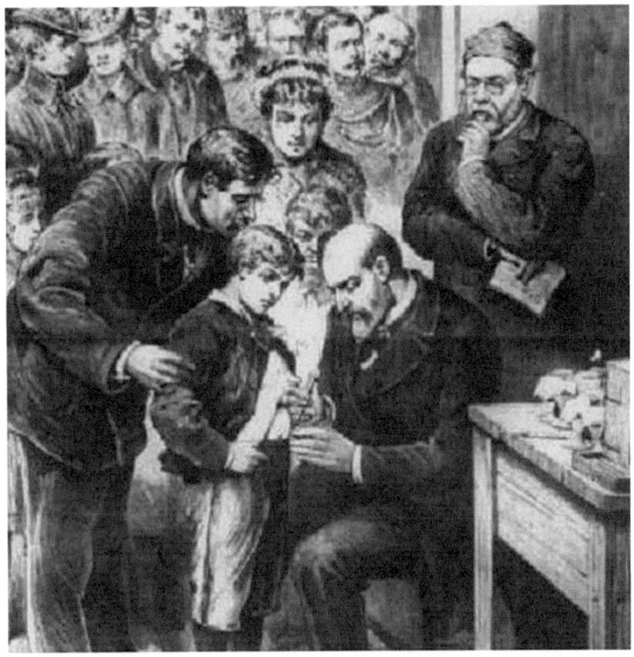

Fig. 1.5 Pasteur (1822–1895) injected the first inactivated rabies vaccine to the 9-year-old Joseph Meister in 1885

Pasteur developed a killed vaccine produced of emulsified and air-dried spinal cords of infected rabbits. The existence of any virus was unknown at this time. Well known was the zoonotic character of this disease and the neurological symptoms so that the doctors made the educated guess of affected sickened nerve tissue.

Joseph Meister was a 9-year-old boy when he was bitten by a rabid dog. The boy got 13 injections in which Pasteur used stepwise more fresh isolated nerve tissue with more virulent pathogens (Fig. 1.5). On October 26, 1885, Pasteur announced Joseph Meister's healing. Pasteur was hailed as a hero. Whether this series of immunizations was the reason for the healing is as yet not proven because the risk of contracting rabies after such an exposure is estimated at around 10 %. Marginal to notice that Pasteur tested the rabies vaccine as prophylactic treatment in only 11 dogs, and only one therapeutic immunization of an infected rabbit was passed before Joseph Meister was vaccinated. Also, a first treatment of a rabies-infected girl, the 11-year-old Antoinette Poughon, shortly before Meister, failed. Girl and rabbit died.

Nonetheless, this was the first documented therapeutic vaccination in human medicine worldwide (Hervé Bazin: L'Histoire des vaccinations, John Libby Eurotext, 2008, France; Pasteur Vallery-Radot (ed): Œuvres de Pasteur. Volume 6: Maladies virulentes, virus-vaccins et prophylaxie de la rage – Méthode pour prévenir la rage après morsure, Masson, Paris 1933, France). Table 1.1 summarizes major milestones in the history of vaccines.

Table 1.1 Scientific quantum jumps in the history of vaccines

430 BC	The Greek Thucydides observed that those patients who survived smallpox did not become re-infected.	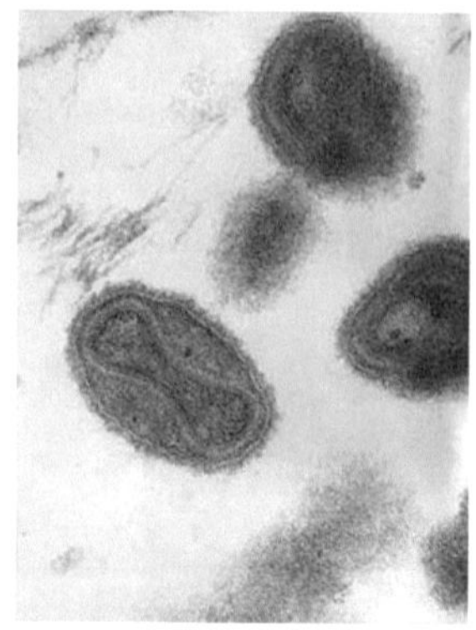
1st century AD	In China: **smallpox inoculation** (vaccination) dated around the 10th century.	
1674	Antoni van Leeuwenhoek (1632-1723) made **microscopes** consisting of a single, high-quality lens and began to observe bacteria and protozoa.	
1774	The first recorded smallpox vaccination: The farmer Benjamin Jesty (1736-1816) made his immunization experiments with cowpox against smallpox infection.	Smallpox is believed to have emerged in human populations about 10,000 BC.
1796	Edward Jenner's (1749-1823) first **smallpox vaccination** based on empiric data.	
1802	The Royal Prussian Smallpox Vaccination Institute in Berlin/ Germany–the **first vaccination institute worldwide**.	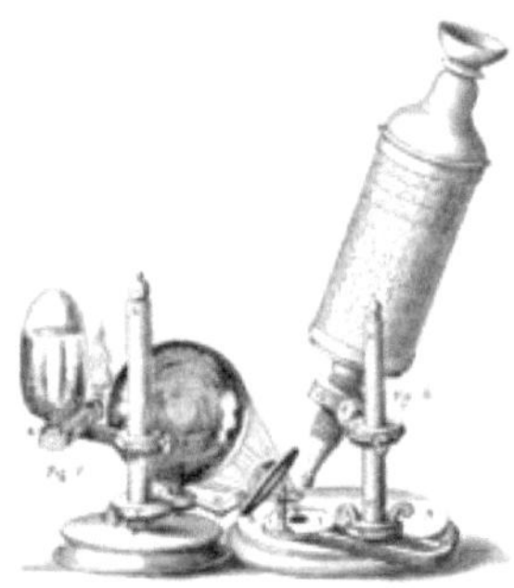
1807	In Bavaria/ Germany: the **first compulsory vaccination law** against smallpox.	
1885	Louis Pasteur (1822-1895): The **first artificially attenuated (rabies) vaccine** in humans. ...... The **first tissue culture (chicken)** by Wilhelm Roux.	1665 – microscope by R. Hook ten years before van Leeuwenhoek.
1890	**Koch's postulates** (Robert Koch, 1843-1910)are four criteria that were established to identify the causative relationship between a microbe and adisease.	

Table 1.1 (continued)

1890s	Already in the 1890s William B. Coley injected streptococcal organisms in patients with solid tumors **("Coley's Toxins")** to activate the immune system.	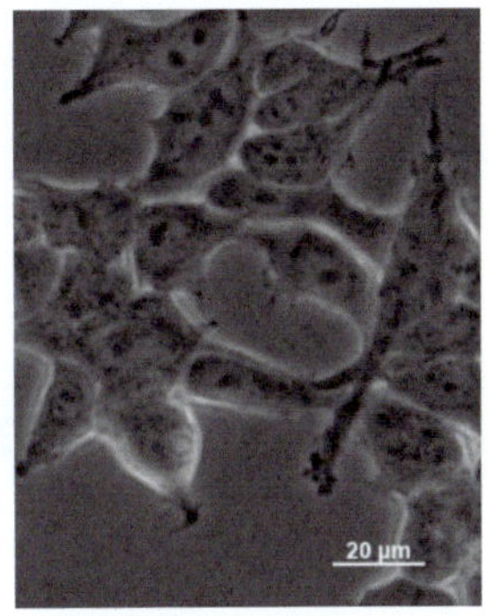
1901	Emil von Behring (1854-1917) together with Japanese bacteriologist Shibasaburo Kitasato(1852-1931) discovered the **antibodies**. Behring received the first Nobel Prize for medicine in 1901.	The first tissue culture in 1885. (Photo: 293-TK cells by S.Giese, Germany)
1921	**BCG vaccine**: The oldest in wide use across the world. The bacille Calmette-Guérin (BCG) vaccination is 90 years old, first used in humans in 1921.	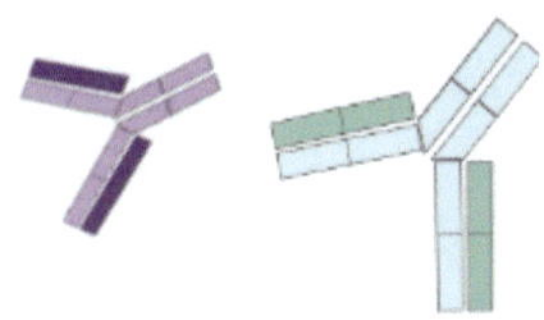
1953	Discovery of the **DNA** by **Watson and Crick** based on the landmark experiments of the Swiss chemist **Friedrich Miescher** who first identified what he called "nuclein" inside the nuclei of human white blood cells (1869).	Monoclonal antibodies produced by hybridoma technology in 1975.
1954	Jonas Salk developed the first effective **polio vaccine**. The results were published in *The Journal of the American Medical Association.* What a benefit for mankind but NO Nobel Prize for this brilliant development.	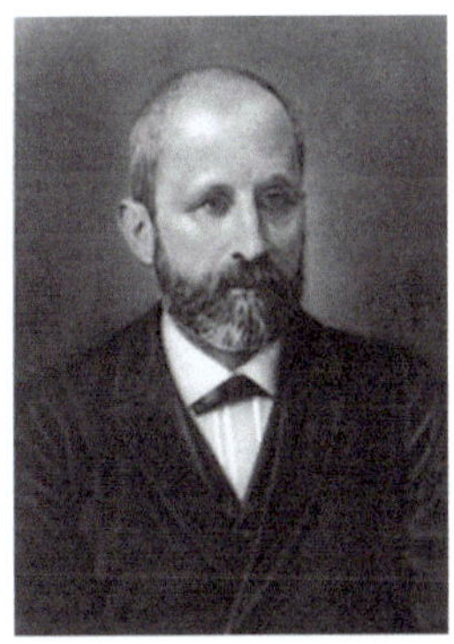 Firedrich Miescher (1844-1895).

Table 1.1 (continued)

1964	The first scientific report on an autologous (personalized) cancer vaccine (whole tumor homogenate, mixed with Freund's adjuvant and 3x injected intramuscularly in patient)	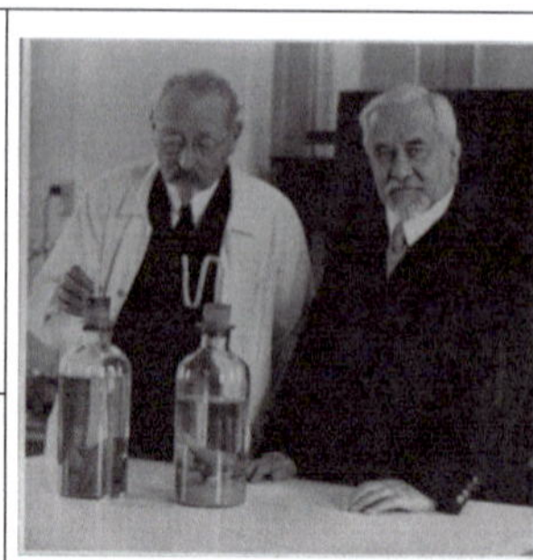
1980	The WHO declared **smallpox eradicated** – the first infection eradicated by vaccination.	
1984	**Hepatitis B vaccine.** First recombinant vaccineby using genetic engineering. Production since 1986.	Camille Guerin (1863-1933) and Albert Calmette (1872-1961) developed the BCG vaccine against tuberculosis: *Today, the oldest registered vaccine in wide use across the world.*
1995	Christiane Nüßlein-Volhard, Edward B.Lewis and Eric F. Wieschauswere awarded the Nobel Prize for their discovery of the Toll gene in Drosophila , the basis for all **Toll Like Receptors** (1997: first TLR in human).	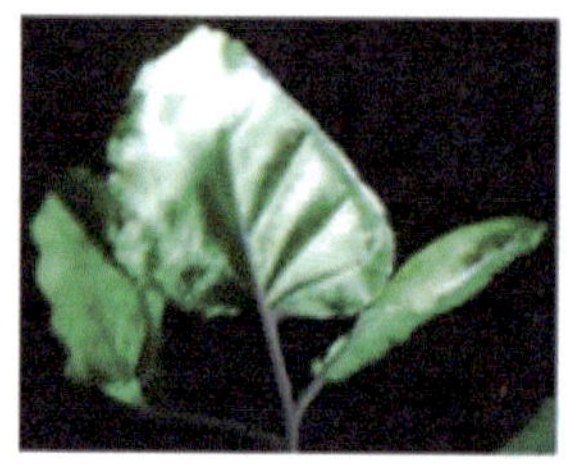
2010	FDA's approval for the first dendritic cell (DC) vaccine - a therapeutical autologous whole cell cancer vaccine –56 years after the first approach with autologous cancer cells.	
2014	Ebola crisis in Africa: For the first time (tabaco) plant-derived monoclonal antibodies without FDA/ EMA approval were used as emergency therapy for passive immunization.	Bioprocessing of monoclonal antibodies and vaccines in transgenic plants.

1.2 Systems Vaccinology

Isolation of a pathogen, inactivation or attenuation, and injection – the basic rules for the development of any vaccine. *Pasteur vaccines* are with us since a century. Estimated 95 % of all global licensed vaccines for animal health are still Pasteur vaccines. The development is cheap and simple. The situation for human vaccines is quite different.

Without any doubt, these classical vaccines have dramatically improved our life. And in almost the same manner but mostly unnoticed by the public, the huge progress in molecular sciences completely changed the vaccine research and development.

Systems vaccinology focuses on studying prediction of immunogenicity and efficacy of vaccines. The goals are to identify and quantify immune response-related genes of the innate and adaptive system, proteins and their roles in various networks, to understand the interactions of immunocompetent cells and organs, to integrate adjuvant-derived in vivo data and mechanistic animal studies (e.g., transgenic or knockout models), and finally to implement mathematical models and algorithms required for simulation and theoretical predictions on the system level.

Rational vaccine design integrates the understanding of the biology of the targeted pathogen. Each pathogen has a molecular bar code, referred to as pathogen-associated molecular patterns, or PAMPs, and displayed on the pathogen surface. PAMPs are recognized by various types of pattern recognition receptors (PRRs) (see Chap. 2).

The development of Pasteur vaccines is essentially trial and error and has not been accompanied by a fundamental understanding of precisely how protection arises. Thanks to the progress in molecular sciences and system approaches, vaccine developments will open new indications, speed up, and improve the manufacturing of vaccines. Systems vaccinology enables rational vaccine design. Table 1.2 illustrates the differences between classical and modern vaccinology.

Reverse Genetics Versus Forward Genetics. Established in the 1990s, reverse genetics starts the functional analysis of a gene first by gene sequencing. Once decoded, this sequence is well directed (targeted) altered by using various techniques, and the effect on the organism is studied. Therefore, the causal relation between a targeted mutagenesis and the resulting new phenotype is stringent, precisely and reproducibly.

The opposite direction is given by the classical so-called forward genetics. Starting with a given phenotype, the genetic basis for this phenotype is investigated. The first pathogen altered by reverse genetics techniques was influenza virus [1, 2]. Since then, site-specific mutations allow the engineering of viruses with defined biological properties.

More complex organisms as bacteria can also be studied for vaccine development by reverse genetics.

African Meningitis Belt. *Neisseria meningitidis*, a gram-negative *diplococcus* and often referred to as meningococcus, is an encapsulated bacterium that colonize the nasopharynx and occasionally causes invasive disease. It infects only humans, no animal reservoir is known. The classification of the 13 serogroups is according the polysaccharide capsule surrounding the bacterium, but only six groups, namely, A, B, C, W-135, X, and Y are associated with severe, invasive disease and can cause epidemics [3]. The WHO reports that the major disease burden is in the Third World and every year 400 million people living in the "African meningitis belt" (21 countries, from Senegal to Ethiopia, Fig. 1.6) suffer on bacterial meningitis caused by *Neisseria*, with a case-fatality ratio (CFR) of 10.6 % in 2010 (GHO: Meningococcal meningitis, http://www.who.int/gho/epidemic_diseases/ meningitis/en/index.html, WHO 2013).

Meningococcus. Meningococcal disease is a global health problem and sporadically occurs throughout the world. Mainly meningococcus serogroup A and recently also groups W-135 and Y are the causative agents in Africa, whereas serogroups B, C, and Y (in the Unites States) are predominantly in industrialized countries. Several vaccines are on the market. In 2010, the WHO prequalified the first serogroup A meningococcal conjugate vaccine (PsA-TT) developed solely for Africa (MenAfriVac, Serum Institute of India, Ltd.). Meanwhile, some quadrivalent meningococcal conjugate vaccines against serogroups A, C, W-135, and Y are licensed

Table 1.2 Differences between classical and modern vaccine approaches

Key points	Classical Pasteur vaccinology	Systems vaccinology
Lab experiments	**Wet**	**In silico prediction with bioinformatic analysis followed by wet experiments for confirmation**
Antigen	Isolation, inactivation/attenuation, application of (whole) pathogen	Isolation, characterization, modification of single antigens
Epitopes	No focus for development	Focus on T and B cell epitopes
Immune response	Serum antibody response (as correlate of protection)	Understanding of the complex network of immune mechanisms
Adjuvant	Standard adjuvants	Development of new specific adjuvants
Application route	Mostly intramuscular application	Mucosa immunization as new application route
Vector systems	None	Natural and artificial vector systems
Nanomedicine	None	Natural and artificial nanoparticles as carrier
Biomarkers	Seldom	Search for highly specific biomarkers
Animal models	Try and error	Mechanistic models (transgenic/knockout)
Indications	Infectious diseases	New indications (cancer, autoimmunity, drug addiction, obesity, etc.)
Production	Simple	Recombinant expression
Costs	Cheap	High
Basic principle	Empiric vaccine design	Rational vaccine design

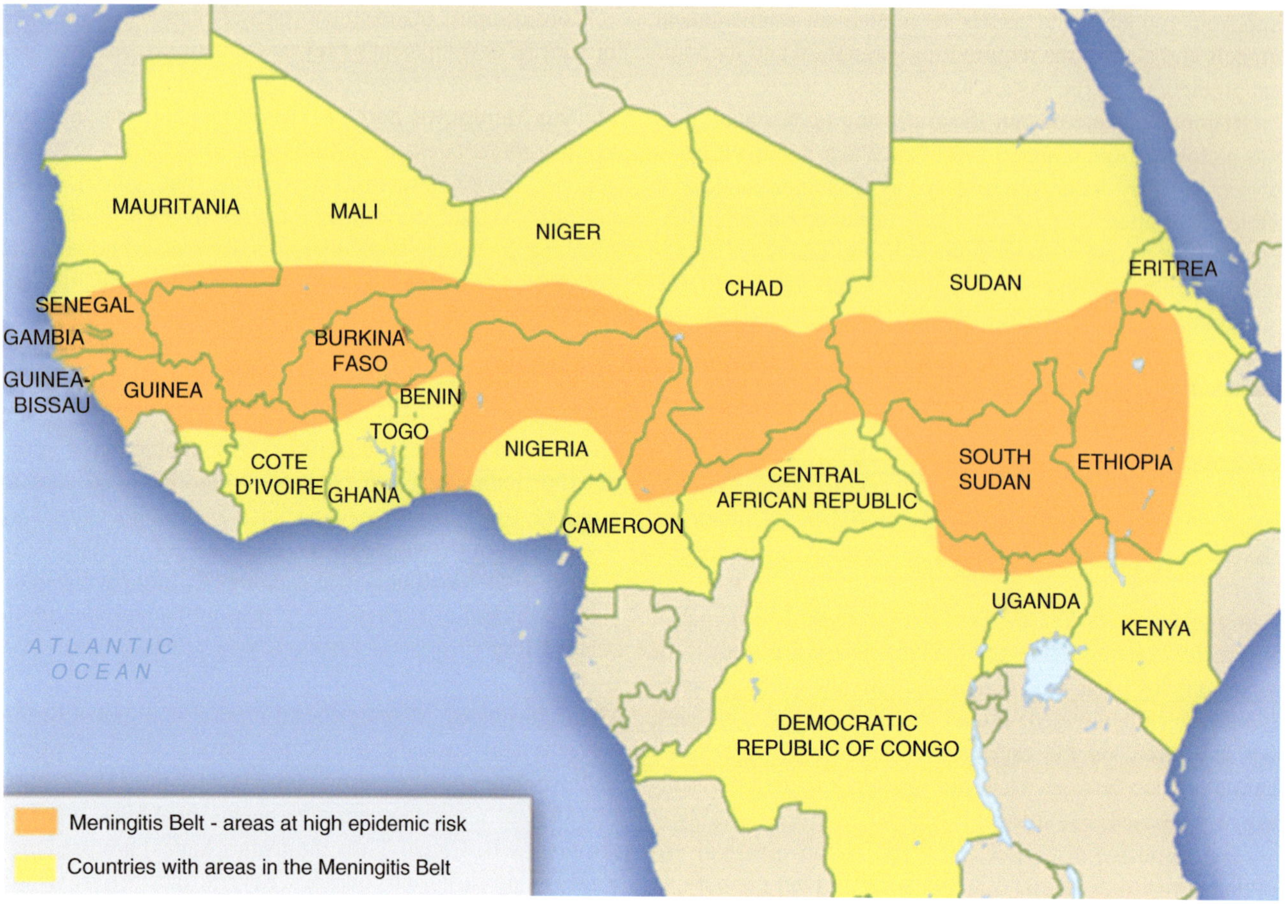

Fig. 1.6 African meningitis belt: Areas with epidemics of meningococcal meningitis (World Health Organization. International Travel and Health. Geneva, Switzerland: 2012)

in Europe, North America, and Asia for persons 2–55 years. These conjugate vaccines replaced the former polysaccharide vaccine based on capsule polysaccharides which are poorly immunogenic in infants. Because this type of vaccine is T cell independent, no memory response is measurable and the induced immunity is short lived (see Chap. 2).

Hepatitis B Recombinant Versus Plasma Vaccine. The first registered human recombinant vaccine was against hepatitis B virus infection. In 1984, the cDNA of the surface antigen (HBsAg) was cloned into a vector for transfection of yeast cells as production system [4–6]. This recombinant product replaced the former hepatitis B vaccine, a so-called plasma vaccine: HBsAg particles were isolated from the blood of chronically infected patients, purified and inactivated. Preclinical and clinical studies demonstrated the safety, efficacy, and economy of the first recombinant vaccine. The stringent enhancements and consistent applications of molecular biology turned out to be the right way in biomedical research both in drug and in vaccine development.

1.2.1 Reverse Vaccinology

The bottleneck is the meningococcus serogroup B (MenB). This pathogen causes 50 % of the meningococcal meningitis worldwide. A vaccine development based on the main capsule polysaccharide has been impeded. The antigenic structure of this bacterial carbohydrate molecule is identical to fetal brain-cell adhesion molecules [7]. Additionally, the sequences of the most surface proteins are highly variable. But the major concern about possible autoimmunity led to vaccine development with the use of noncapsular structures. Following the routes of reverse genetics demonstrated on a virus and the first publication of the entire genome of a bacterium [8], the genome of the virulent MenB strain MC58 was completely sequenced for identifying vaccine candidates [9]. Later on, this approach will be called *Reverse Vaccinology* including immunological and biochemical studies [10].

Neisseria Meningococcus Neisseria meningococcus serogroup B, strain MC58: single singular chromosome, 2,2 megabase pairs in size, 2,272,360 nucleotides, 2225 genes

(2063 for proteins). All genes were sequenced. Five hundred seventy open reading frames (ORFs) for gene prediction were identified, from these 350 ORFs could be successfully expressed in *E. coli*. From these potential vaccine candidates, among them lipoproteins, outer and inner membrane proteins, transmembrane, and unknown proteins, 28 novel proteins were found to generate neutralizing antibodies against MenB in mice and showed bactericidal activities. Only seven recombinant proteins were positive in several tests and selected for further studies. Finally, five candidates were combined in a vaccine formulation named rMenB (Novartis) [11]. Clinical trials with this vaccine are ongoing.

The exclusive goal of reverse vaccinology is to discover novel antigens and to predict epitopes for B and T cell responses. This approach focuses on isolated parts of microbial organisms and doesn't use systems biology. The entire process can be divided roughly in five major activities, with the first two steps as dry experiments (in silico), as shown in (Fig. 1.7).

DNA Microarrays. Sequence analyses, finding of genes, comparative analysis with related pathogens, predictions of thousands of proteins are to be done in real time by bioinformatic approaches performed on computer (in silico – see also Chap. 6). DNA chips (microarrays) are used to investigate the expression patterns of genes. Gene clusters can be recognized, up- and downregulated genes can be identified, and biological pathways and networks can be detected. Known and novel immunity-related genes and pathways can be described [12, 13].

1.2.2 Prediction Algorithms

A first challenge is the prediction of proteins by in silico mapping of epitopes, also called dry experiments in contrast to wet experiments on the bench. Not every protein of the huge amount of proteins of a pathogen is suitable for vaccine development. Accurate prediction algorithms are essential: e.g., cross-reactivity and autoantigens, surface expression for immune recognition, conserved regions in contrast to sequence variability, membrane proteins, and number of helices (Table 1.3).

A serious protein prediction can save time and money. The exact localization of a protein helps to determine the potential antigenic character. For example, a signal peptide (leader sequence) on the N terminus serves as an intracellular "postal code" and gives the way for exportation toward the cell surface. Such proteins are preferred because proteins of cell surface are exposed to antibodies, B cells, and T cells. The physical and chemical complexity of a protein influences the expression in a heterologous system like *E. coli*, the most commonly used organism for industrial and pharmaceutical protein production. Not every heterologous protein can be cloned, expressed, and purified.

Prediction of T Cell Epitopes. The prediction of epitopes (antigenic determinant), the binding portion of an antigen, helps to define possible vaccine targets. If the antigen is a protein, the epitope is a short peptide. MHC class I molecules present peptides 8–10 amino acids in length and are

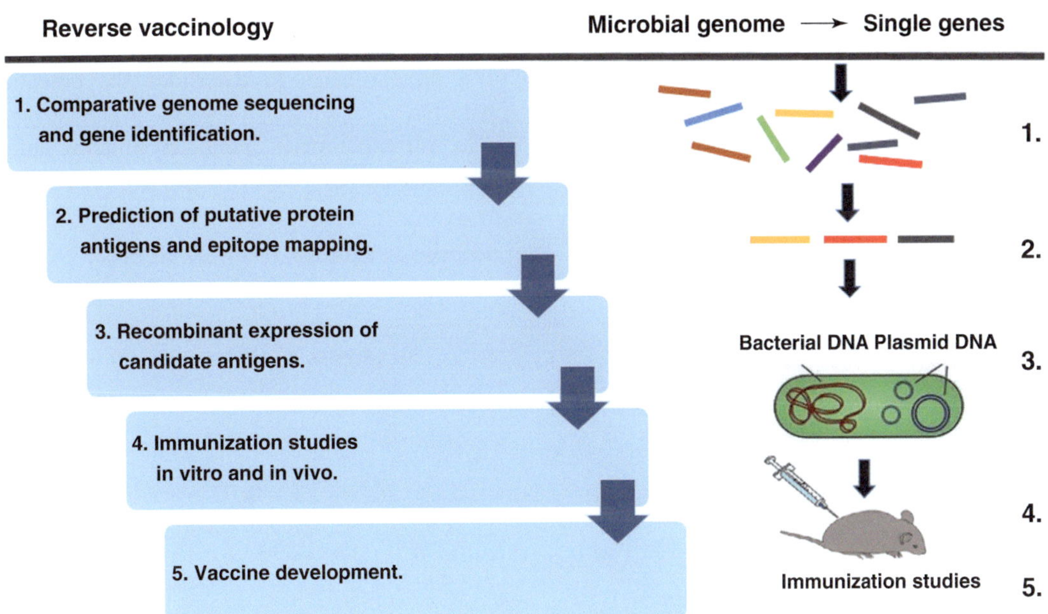

Fig. 1.7 Key strategy of reverse vaccinology. Reverse genetics starts the functional analysis of a gene by gene sequencing. The entire pathogenic genome can be screened using bioinformatic approaches to identify novel genes for vaccination. Once decoded, these genes are filtered for desirable attributes and can be well manipulated by various techniques. After recombinant expression and purification of the candidate antigens, the immunological effect on the organism will be studied in vivo

Table 1.3 In silico selection criteria for novel antigens

Antigen selection criteria	Impact	Consequence
Cross-reactivity	Specificity of an antigen as degree to which an immune response discriminates between antigenic variants	Vaccine antigens appear similar to the immune system; cross-reactivity does not necessarily mean cross-protection
Autoantigens	Humoral and/or cell-mediated immune response	Rejection of identified autoantigens
Conserved regions vs. sequence variability	Preferential targeting of conserved antigen regions	Genetic diversity is a major challenge in the design of vaccines
Localization of antigens	Intracellular trafficking of antigens and expression patterns on the membrane surface	Exportation and expression on cell surface as prerequisite for antigen–antibody recognition
Number of helices	Stable secondary α-helix structure for immunodominant T cell epitopes (helices correlate to conservation of antigen region)	Preference for immunodominant vs. subdominant epitopes

recognized by CD8+ T cells, resulting in a cellular response. In silico T cell epitope prediction ranges 90–95 % positive hits. Several bioinformatic databases are available [14–20].

Prediction of B Cell Epitopes. Prediction of B cell epitopes is much more complicated [21]. B cell epitopes consist of a continuous and discontinuous structure (Fig. 1.8). A continuous epitope is defined by the linear primary amino acid sequence of the antigen interacting with antibodies. A discontinuous epitope is defined by the conformational, characterictical 3D shape of a protein. Discontinuous epitopes generate the majority of all antibody-binding epitopes, but as yet the epitope prediction is mainly for linear epitopes with a poor hit rate [22, 23].

Already the secondary structure of a protein almost resists for prediction much less a higher protein structure. Once produced in *E. coli*, each recombinant candidate antigen undergoes a series of biochemical and immunological experiments. Protein chips were developed for high-throughput screening to study activities, functions, and interactions of proteins [24]. Known and novel immunity-related proteins and pathways can be detected.

Proof of Concept. The combination of genomics and proteomics is a powerful approach to identify novel vaccine candidates and the computer helps to select putative antigens out of thousands of proteins [25].

At the end of each in silico experiment, the proof of concept must be done in wet experiments, in cell cultures combined with immunization studies in animal models. This is the Lackmus test, not less. Figure 1.9 gives a schematic overview of reverse genetics embedded in systems vaccinology.

The approach to define new antigens starts with dry experiments (in silico), bioinformatic studies to compare genomics data on DNA level. On RNA and protein level transcriptional control, pathways and networks are analyzed. Selection criteria and accurate prediction algorithms for B and T cells and the innate immune response are essential for prediction of novel protein antigens. The exact localization of a protein helps to determine the potential antigenic character.

In wet experiments, predicted proteins are constructed, cross-checked (DNA microchips, mass spectrometry, protein

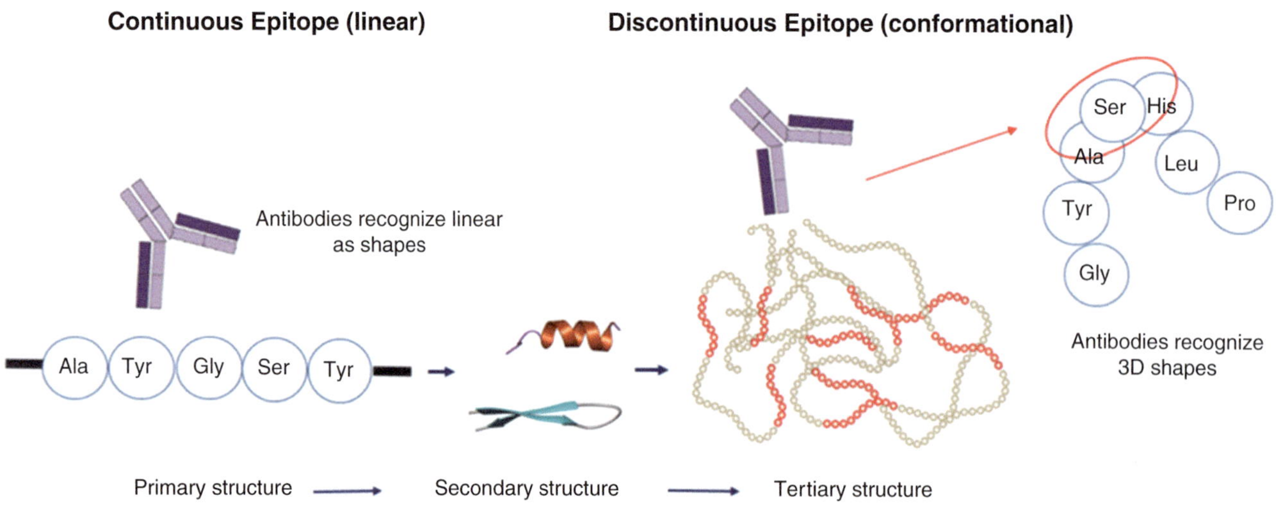

Fig. 1.8 B cell epitopes consist of a continuous and discontinuous structure. The continuous epitope is defined by the linear primary amino acid sequence of the antigen, whereas the discontinuous epitope is defined by the conformational, characterictical 3D shape of a protein. The majority of all antibodies against B cell epitopes is generated against discontinuous epitopes

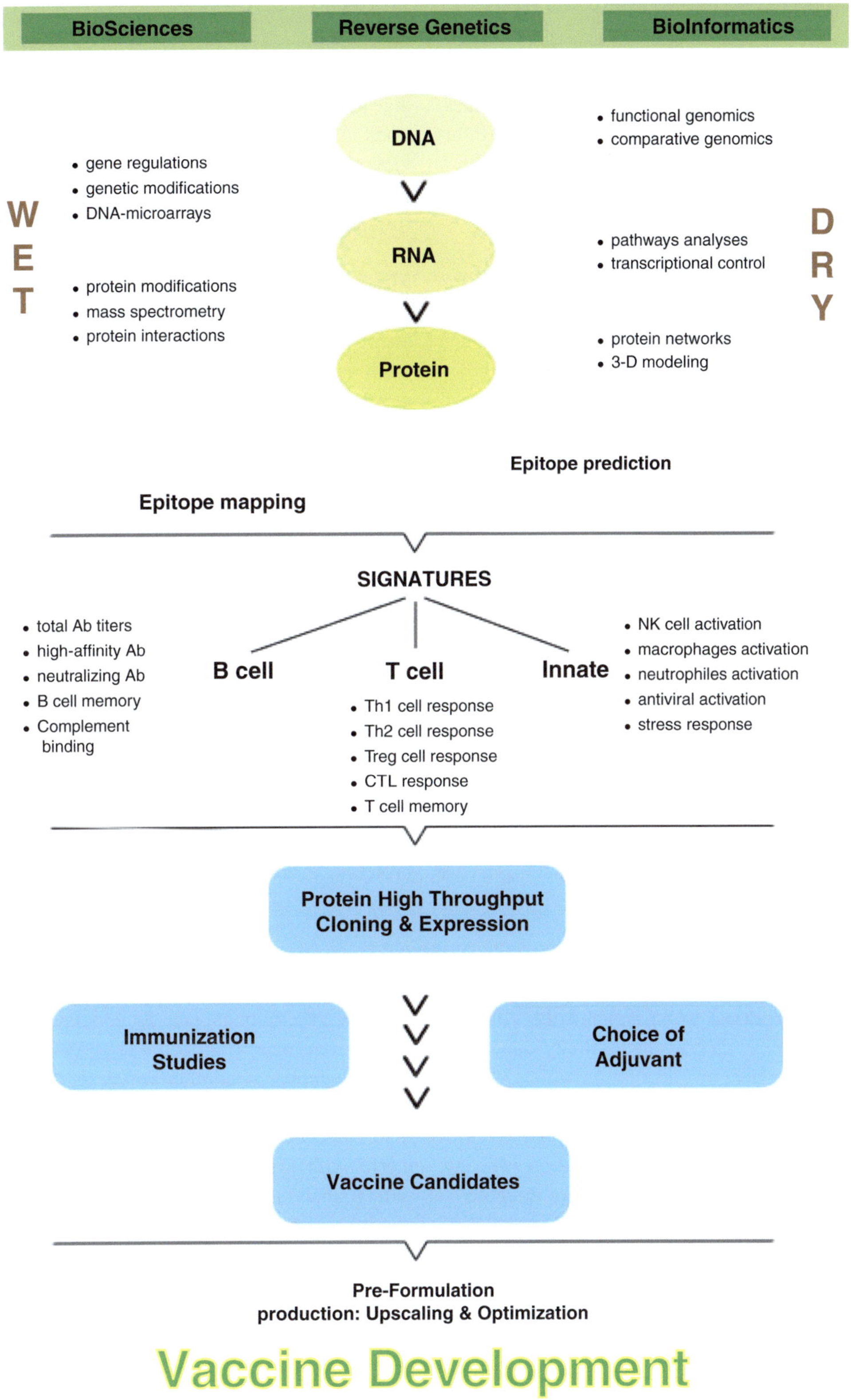

Fig. 1.9 Schematic overview of reverse genetics combined with systems vaccinology

networks), and tailored by molecular genetic tools. High-throughput cloning and expression systems deliver thousands of antigens. In vitro and in vivo immunization studies supported by bioinformatics data deliver candidate vaccines. The physical and chemical complexity of a protein influences the expression in a heterologous system like *E. coli*, the most commonly used organism for industrial and pharmaceutical protein production.

Not every heterologous protein can be cloned, expressed, and purified. Upscaling and optimization of the production process for selected pre-formulated candidate vaccines is the last step before entering the clinical development process.

Bioinformatics. Meanwhile, reverse vaccinology has been applied to a large number of bacterial pathogens. Despite the rapid progress in bioinformatics and the development of better tools to manage the huge amount of information, we are facing enormous problems. Still the most important unmet needs are HIV, tuberculosis (TB), and malaria (WHO). The only currently licensed vaccine against TB, BCG (bacille Calmette–Guérin), is in use since 90 years and is not effective enough. A better, improved modern TB vaccine is strongly needed. Moreover, there are no vaccines available for infections with West Nile virus, dengue virus, hepatitis C, etc. Even the development of a standard flu vaccine every year is a race against the time (see also Chap. 11). And what about highly variable pathogens causing persistent and latent infections, as HIV or HCV? Neither a prophylactic nor a therapeutic vaccine is available. The genes of these pathogens are identified, but the bioinformatic approach, from genome to vaccine, does not work. Why?

Limitations. The identification of novel antigens is comparatively simple in contrast to understand the complex immune reactions in vivo, such as the antibody-dependent enhancement (ADE) in dengue vaccination which leads to an increase of infectivity. Also the establishment of a local immunosuppressive milieu by anti-inflammatory cytokines (see Chap. 2) diminishes the vaccination efficacy. Our knowledge of factors triggering the tissue microenvironment influencing B and T cell functions is absolutely poor. And how to design a vaccine against TB, a frequent coinfection for HIV in the Third World, if on one hand the TB vaccine needs a strong T cell epitope [26] and on the other hand the HI virus targets T cells? Until now there is no licensed vaccine against human respiratory syncytial virus (HRSV), an important respiratory pathogen especially for newborns, although the genome is sequenced and all proteins are detected since 1997. Obstacles are the immature immune system of newborns and the Th2-dominated immune response resulting in a vaccine-enhanced disease [27].

Holistic Vaccinology. We have to go deeper and understand biological systems as series of more or less dependent subsystems like the immune system, the nerve system, or the digestive system influencing each other by dynamic functions. And based on this insight, we must develop a holistic view on vaccinology. The human genome encodes for 22,000 genes. There is a need to learn more about the regulations of (immuno) genes.

MicroRNA. To date, more than 1,500 microRNAs (miRNA) are identified as regulator of gene activity (http://mirbase.org/index.shtml). miRNAs turn a gene on or off. Such small RNA molecules are important for B and T cell development and influence the immune response [28–31]. What are the specific signals for miRNAs and in which temporal sequence? Unsolved essential problems are also that some pathogens can't be cultivated in cell cultures, or for some pathogens no animal model does exist. We are developing cheap vaccines for the Third World. But the severe poverty is the real cause of many infections. Chronic hunger may modulate the immune system through T cell repertoire and still undiscovered other immune functions. Chronic hunger in early life dramatically impacts the programming of the young thymus, a very crucial phase, having long-term effects on T cell development (see Chaps. 2 and 3).

The Crux with 'Omics. Maybe it's correct that we are living in the era of "'omics unlimited" [32]. Genomics and proteomics are well established and sufficiently describe these fields of main activities for vaccines. Meanwhile, there is an inflation of 'omics, such as allergenomics, bibliomics, cellomics, CHomics, chronomics, cross-omics, diagnomics, fragonomics, functomics, operomics, or recently vaccinomics, etc. To understand this proliferating 'omics nonsense, you need a large glossary and the collaborative support of another database, the Vaccine Ontology (VO; http://www.violinet.org/vaccineontology/) with more than 5,000 terms (in 2012) with increasing tendency. What a crux with all these 'omics and terms. The same is for statistical analysis. The more complicated statistics in a clinical trial, the more a critical mind is needed. A vaccine works or not.

We live in an era of 'omics where we no longer think, we google. Matthias Giese

Databases and statistics are not the holy grail; a traditional hypothesis-driven research of complex structures and experimental validation is still strongly needed. "*Imagination is more important than knowledge. For knowledge is limited to all we now know and understand, while imagination embraces the entire world, and all there ever will be to know and understand.*" (Albert Einstein)

1.3 Biomarkers

The preclinical research phase is essential for the success of clinical development. Genomics and proteomics offer various tools to develop biomarkers to identify immune correlates of vaccine efficacy also for already licensed and novel vaccine developments especially for therapeutic vaccines for chronic infections or cancer diseases. Meanwhile, the huge hive of literature to "correlates of protection" is so confusing that focus in this chapter is given only on laboratory parameters.

A biomarker is not per se a protein:

A biomarker is a characteristic that is objectively measured and evaluated as an indicator of normal biological processes, pathogenic processes or pharmacologic responses to a therapeutic intervention [33].... (Biomarkers Definitions Working Group, 2001). Generally, three types of novel biomarkers are of interest (Table 1.4).

With molecular tools, the traces of a vaccination can be followed up in real time and checked for molecular signatures on cell, protein, DNA, and RNA level. The type of dendritic cell (DC) carrying the antigen can be measured, the type of toll-like receptor (TLR) and NF-kB-activated genes can be detected, and the direction of immune response with all effector arms can be predicted. With cDNA microarrays, the response of host immune genes can be characterized and by comparative analysis between vaccine and non-vaccine genes associated with protection can be isolated. Lots of putative biomarkers can be detected in blood samples as a snapshot of vaccination. To control a disease by vaccination may also include the study of chromosomal region that underlies genetic variation in response to the vaccination.

One biomarker is not sufficient; a panel of various markers for innate and acquired immune factors, from genes to proteins to immune cells, is needed to be capable of characterizing the host response to vaccination. A robust panel will consist of real correlates combined with essential surrogates.

Biomarkers for YFV Vaccine. Yellow fever virus (YFV) is a small RNA virus and causes mild infection with fever, headache, or in 15 % of all cases a life-threatening acute hemorrhagic disease. The WHO estimates 30,000 deaths every year in unvaccinated populations mainly in Africa. By using cDNA microarrays to investigate gene expression patterns and additional bioinformatics, the efficacy of the yellow fever vaccine YF-17B could be evaluated [34]. Until now, over 600 million people were immunized with this live-attenuated vaccine.

Lots of various laboratory parameters were measured before and over 60 days following the vaccination, e.g., B cells, CD4+, CD8+ T cells, TLRs, gene expressions, transcription factors, cytokines, and more. Aim of this study was to find molecular signatures correlating with the high magnitude of CD8+T cells and the antibody titer. Surprisingly, the correlating biomarkers were some genes within the innate stress response system shaping the CD8+T cell response [35]. Stress is known to be a potent immune modulator.

A novel class of biomarkers are serum microRNAs (miRNA). Many studies have demonstrated that miRNA expression profiles in patient suffering on a chronic disease (cancer, infections, autoimmunity) and healthy individuals are significantly different (see personalized vaccines in this chapter).

Table 1.4 Various types of biomarkers

Prognostic biomarkers	• **these biomarkers are based on the difference in selected characteristics between normal and pathogenic processes**
Predicitive biomarkers	• **these biomarkers assess the possible therapeutical effect of a drug/vaccine in a pathogenic process**
Response biomarkers	• **these biomarkers measure the real therapeutical effect of a drug vaccine in a pathogenic process**

1.3.1 Correlate of Protection

Almost all licensed vaccines work through induction of antibodies, which neutralize or opsonize a pathogen making a bacterium or a cell susceptible for phagocytosis. For lots of classical vaccines, the serum antibody IgG titer correlates with vaccine-induced immunity [36].

Discrepancy. There is a discrepancy observed in most diseases that the measured immune response does not correlate with the vaccine-induced protection. We measure a protection, but in many cases the mechanism of immune protection is poorly known. In clinical descriptions, the terms "correlate" and "surrogate" are used for an immune response that is responsible for protection and an immune response of unknown players measured by a substitute [37]. In vaccine field trials, immune correlates or surrogates are evaluated to predict protection from infection or disease at both individual and population level, across populations, genders, and ages [38–40].

Immunological Endpoints. Correlates of protection are defined, immunological endpoints that can predict vaccine efficacy. They can be derived from animal models that recapitulate disease; randomized, controlled efficacy studies in humans; experimental challenge models in human volunteers; and, observational epidemiological field studies (including case-control studies) comparing immune status in naturally infected versus exposed individuals who remain asymptomatic. This knowledge is extremely valuable to move candidates through the regulatory pathway for clinical testing. It also allows for post-licensure vaccine evaluation and optimization, comparing formulations, immunization schedules, or other modifications to the final product. A correlate allows one to predict the performance of a vaccine in different populations and settings and to compare vaccine candidates. National regulatory agencies typically accept well-defined immunological endpoints as the basis for licensure in cases where efficacy studies cannot be conducted or are not warranted.

Historically, correlates of protection have relied on the measurement of the titer of the antibody response upon vaccination as simple linear function to viral replication. A new definition was necessary, because protective immunity may not even correlate with the humoral response.

The US Food and Drug Administration (FDA) defines a "correlate of protection" as laboratory parameter that has been shown to be associated with protection from clinical disease. (FDA Guidance for Industry, 1997, report no. 97 N-0029, IV.C. Efficacy)

1.4 Systems Biology

The central dogma of molecular biology that DNA makes RNA makes protein by Francis Crick (1956) is still the framework to understand the basic mechanisms of living organisms but not sufficient to explain all aspects of a complex life. Epigenetic changes during life have added a new dimension to our understanding of the relationship between genotype and phenotype and challenge the linear causality from gene to protein function. In this sense "*…systems biology…is about putting together rather than taking apart, integration rather than reduction. It requires that we develop ways of thinking about integration that are as rigorous as our reductionist programs, but different.…It means changing our philosophy, in the full sense of the term*" (Denis Noble, *The music of life: Biology beyond the genome*. Oxford: Oxford University Press, 2006).

Antibodies provide the first line of defense that can prevent an early infection and correlate with protection. In case of an intracellular pathogen, antibodies can't prevent the replication and don't protect. This is where T cells come into play and the measurement of T cell immunity is a more accurate correlate of efficacy.

Integrative Biology. To understand the immunological mechanisms of vaccination, the chronological steps of antigen uptake, processing, and presentation to B and T cells can now be studied in detail (see Chap. 2). Using single genomic and single proteomic data, we are more and more able to understand the complex biological network of innate and acquired immunity. We are right in the middle of systems biology (also called integrative biology), investigating the (immuno-) biology as a whole, with all immune cells, cytokines, and interactions with the environment [41]. Rightly we speak of an immune system and should never forget the holistic complex.

1.4.1 Therapeutic EAV Vaccine

We are using systems biology in our laboratory to develop a therapeutic vaccine for persistent infections with equine arteritis virus (EAV) as a model system for humans. EAV, a small ss(+)RNA virus of the family of Arteriviridae, causes respiratory diseases and abortions.

The vaccine development has started backward. First, we investigated the putative escape strategies in vitro by DNA chips (Fig. 1.10) and found that EAV upregulates 12 interferon (IFN)-related genes and downregulates 2 IFN-related genes. One of this downregulated gene was the IFN-γ-

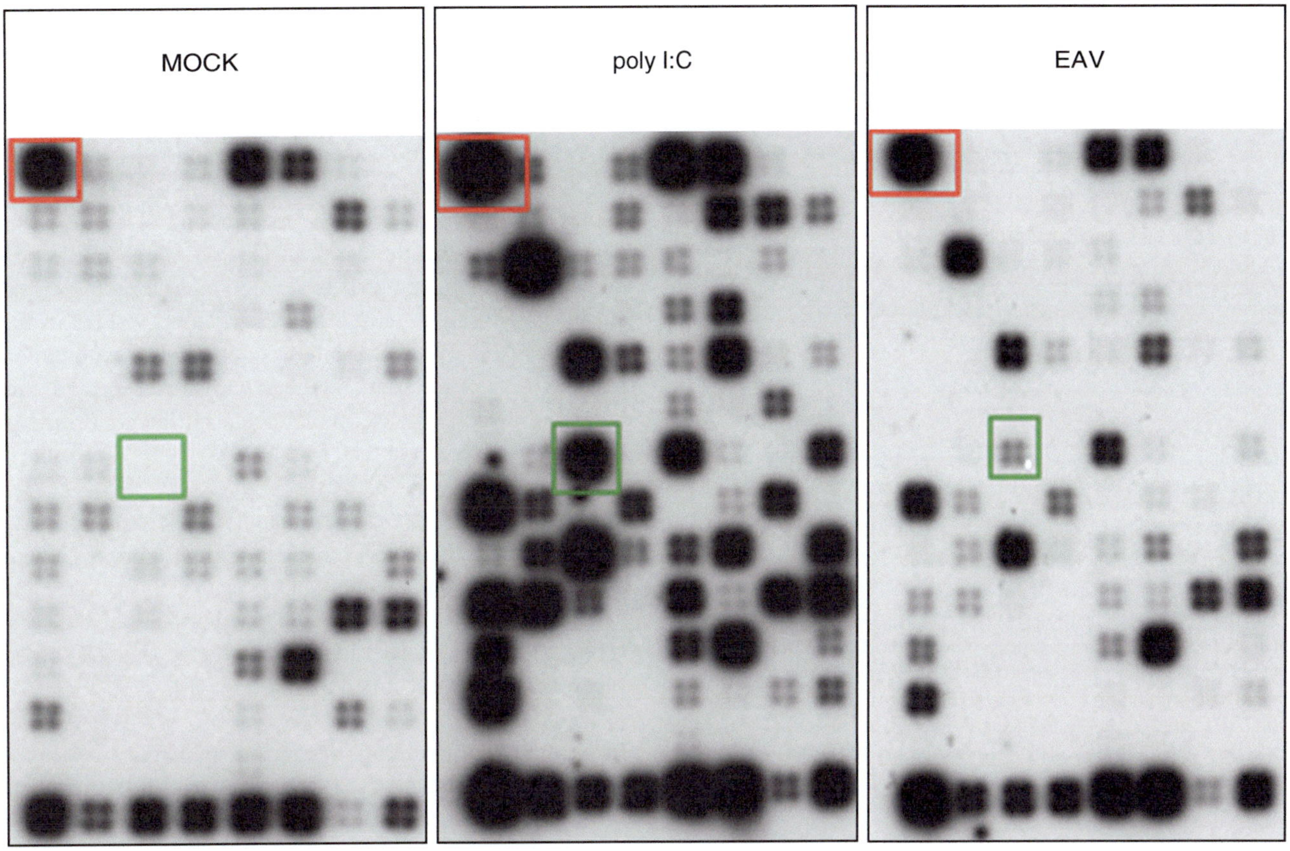

Fig. 1.10 OligoGEArrays with RNA of C2C12 cells: untreated MOCK control, polyI:C treatment, infection with EAV control genes: GAPDH (*red spot*), IFN beta (*green spot*), and EAV-upregulated and EAV downregulated genes can be detected in direct comparison with the MOCK and polyI:C control (Anett Heinrich-Schulz, PhD thesis 2010, M. Giese)

inducible protein (Ifl30, acc.no. NM-023065), an essential biomarker for the persistence of EAV in vitro.

In additional experiments, we could measure that the intracellular peptide transportation system TAP (transporter-associated peptides, also transporter associated with antigen processing) was downregulated following the infection with EAV and last but not least the MHC I molecules. With all results taken together, we assumed that EAV triggers a cascade of intracellular and antigen-processing-related events to escape the immune response (Fig. 1.11).

T Cell Vaccine. With this knowledge that EAV reduces the cellular immunity, we developed a multivalent DNA T cell epitope vaccine based on two envelope proteins together with the intracellular nucleocapsid protein [42]. In several therapeutic vaccination trials, we found that this vaccine is able to cure persistent EAV-infected horses via a strong CD8+ T cell activity (measured in an autologous cytotoxic T cell assay) dependent on the virus load. But with too much virus in the body, the vaccine treatment fails.

The measurement for the vaccine efficacy is the serum level of IFN-γ. Starting from backward, from the biology of the virus, IFN-γ accurately correlates with the virus load in vitro. The correlation to the virus load in vivo needs further studies. However, IFN-γ could be confirmed as biomarker for the grade of EAV infection in horses and vv as hallmark for the efficacy of a therapeutic vaccination. The more virus, the less IFN-γ and the less therapeutic efficacy of the vaccine. The less virus, the more IFN-γ and the more vaccine efficacy.

IFN-γ, produced by T cells, NK cells, is an immunomodulator influencing not only the expression of MHC I and II but also B and T cell differentiation.

The only licensed vaccine against tuberculosis (TB) is bacille Calmette–Guérin (BCG). The protective mechanisms of this vaccine are poorly understood. However, IFN-γ is established as one biomarker for the BCG vaccine efficacy [43, 44].

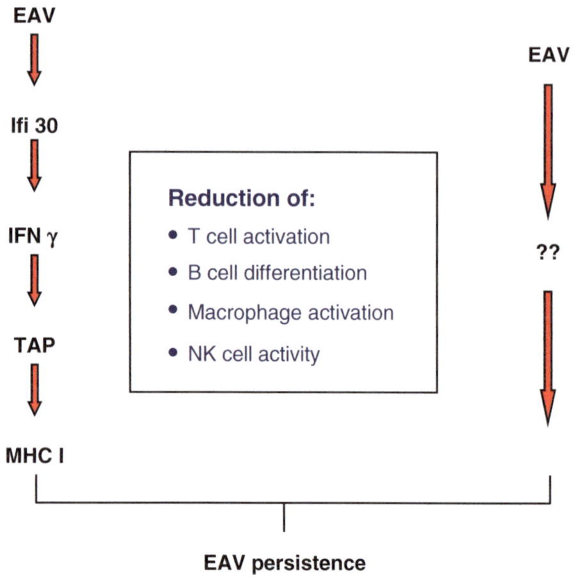

Fig. 1.11 Development of EAV persistence. After entering the target cell, EA virus suppresses among other genes the interferon-inducible gene 30, Ifi 30. The protein encoded by Ifi 30 plays an important role in the MHC presentation. The lack of IFN-γ provokes a lower expression of TAP resulting in a diminished presentation of antigen via MHC I and the persistence of EAV. This downregulation seems to be part of the EAV evasion strategy. Further research is needed to uncover additional escape mechanisms of EAV

1.5 Personalized (P) Vaccines: The 3 Bs: Bedside-Bench-Bedside

P (personalized) vaccines use patient's antigens, tissues, or cells which are manipulated ex vivo and reinjected to the same patient as autologous vaccine, a procedure mainly used in oncology (see Chap. 12).

1964. The first scientific report on an experimental autologous cancer vaccine is published [45].

1994. Thirty years later, in December 1994, the first commercial approach of an anti-melanoma vaccine has started a multicenter clinical trial in Vienna [46].

Anti-melanoma Vaccine. Melanoma cells were isolated from a patient and sent to our laboratory. In a first step, the cancer cells were largely expanded in roller bottles and inactivated by cobalt-60 radiation. For the following gene transfer of interleukin 2 (IL-2), adenovirus 5 (Ad5) was chosen as vector. IL-2 was linked to Ad5 via a complex streptavidin–biotin bridge. Readout was the expression rate of IL-2 in vitro.

The whole laboratory process took several weeks and was going along with problems such as the successful isolation of a sufficient number of cancer cells for propagation, slow or no cell growth, and fluctuating transfection rates. The gene-modified irradiated cancer cells were s.c. reinjected to the patient. The theoretical concept behind this autologous cell vaccine is to present the immune system a panel of melanoma cancer antigens in combination with IL-2 as immune enhancer. In practice, this vaccine did not work, and after phase II, the study was finished.

At least two main reasons can be identified for this failure: (1) already after the second application, anti-vector antibodies in all patients could be measured. The vaccine was neutralized. (2) But the basic mistake was done in the preclinical development, where a non-metastasizing (local encapsulated tumor) mouse model was used instead of the more realistic B-16 melanoma model. The correlation between IL-2 expression and the therapeutic efficacy in this non-metastasizing mouse model could not be confirmed in the clinical trial.

2010. Almost 50 years after the first experimental study with autologous cancer vaccines, first FDA approved a dendritic cell (DC) therapeutic cancer vaccine [47]. Since the first clinical trial in the 1990s with ex vivo-manipulated DCs, about 50 more clinical trials were initiated, but DC-based vaccines have largely failed until today [48].

Immunological Profiling. P vaccines are mainly developed for cancer patients; however, they are also useful for patients suffering on chronic infections, metabolic disorders, and autoimmune diseases. The aim of individual profiling is to understand the patient-specific interplay between disease and immune system and to tailor a vaccine fitting with measured individual biological conditions. The prerequisite for a P vaccine is the collection of individual data starting with the age, gender, family history and the analysis of results from (epi-) genomic epidemiology studies to define general genetic variants and combined with the regular monitoring of the physiological state. Because generally the patient comes first to the doctor when he has fallen ill, the healthy baseline of gene and protein data are missing and also a longitudinal profile of healthy conditions is not available which limits the use of genomics and proteomics.

Fingerprints. The medical profiling starts with disease-associated fingerprints, a gene-profiling technique using DNA microarrays. To simplify the complexity of up or downregulated genes, analysis by grouping related genes based on their pathways will be done. Identification of active pathways is more predictive as the collection of different genes [49]. Loss or gain function of genes can be investigated by differential display and subtractive hybridization [50]. The vaccine-induced immune response is also monitored by functional gene and protein analysis using DNA/RNA and protein array technologies.

PBMC. Peripheral blood mononuclear cell (PBMC) can be easily isolated and stimulated in vitro, and the gene expression profile can be routinely measured. In a clinical study with melanoma patients in which the patients got a therapy with IFN-α, it was found that the gene expression profile of in vitro IFN-α-stimulated PBMCs was similar to the gene expression of PBMCs following IFN-α treatment in vivo. This demonstrates the great benefit of gene analysis of individual PBMCs in vitro as predictor for immune response [51]. The molecular profiling of PBMCs raised to a key function in personalized medicine.

MicroRNAs. miRNAs are a class of highly conserved noncoding small RNAs that regulate gene expression at the post-transcriptional level (http://mirbase.org/index.shtml). miRNAs turn a gene on or off. Such small RNA molecules are important for B and T cell development and influence the immune response [28–31]. The first miRNA, *lin-4*, was isolated in the nematode *C. elegans* in 1993.

Blood and Plasma Samples. miRNAs are single-stranded endogenous RNAs of about 22 nucleotides (nt). Base pairing via complementary sequences within mRNA molecules results in gene silencing, either translational pausing, or most commonly, transcript degradation (Fig. 1.12). Stable endogenous miRNAs in bodily fluids (serum, plasma, urine) are used as diagnostic, prognostic, and predictive biomarkers. These circulating miRNAs escape degradation by ribonuclease activity. Moreover, targeted gene silencing via miRNAs is investigated for therapeutic treatments [52]. Numerous cancer-specific miRNAs have been identified [53]. For example, plasma concentration of miR-192 was significantly higher in patients with pancreatic cancer than in healthy individuals.

The first evidence that miRNAs are not only associated with the development of the immune system but also with

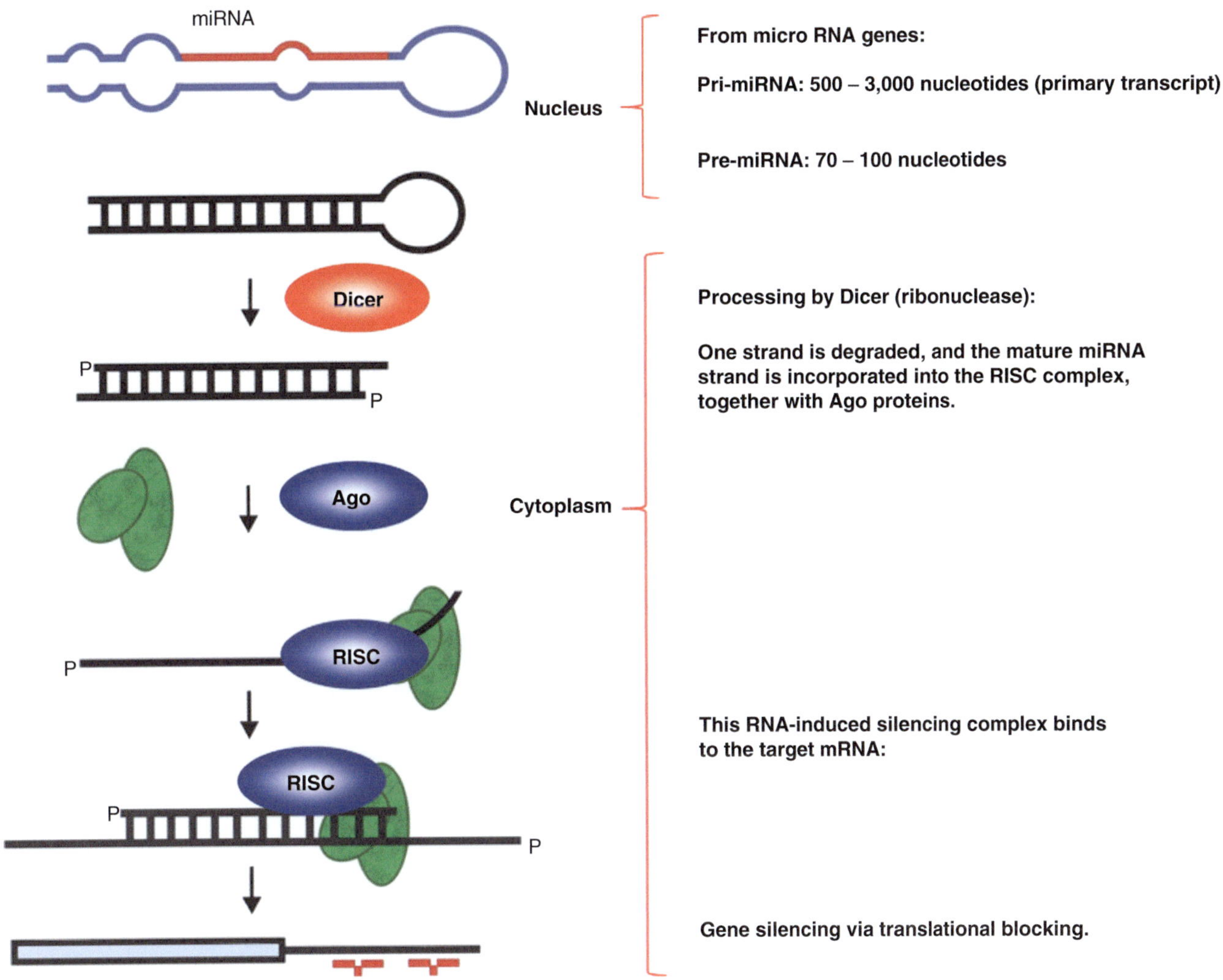

Fig. 1.12 Highly conserved microRNAs are encoded by specific genes in the nucleus. Upon gene activation, the double-stranded pri-miRNA is recognized by a nuclear protein that cuts the RNA into the precursor-miRNA (Pre-miRNA). Pre-miRNA hairpins are exported out of the nucleus and are cleaved by the enzyme dicer in the cytoplasm. The mature miRNA is part of an active RNA-induced silencing complex (RISC) containing dicer and associated Ago proteins. Gene silencing may occur either via mRNA degradation or preventing mRNA from being translated (translational blocking) (Modified scheme on the basis of Jörg Hartig, University of Konstanz/Germany)

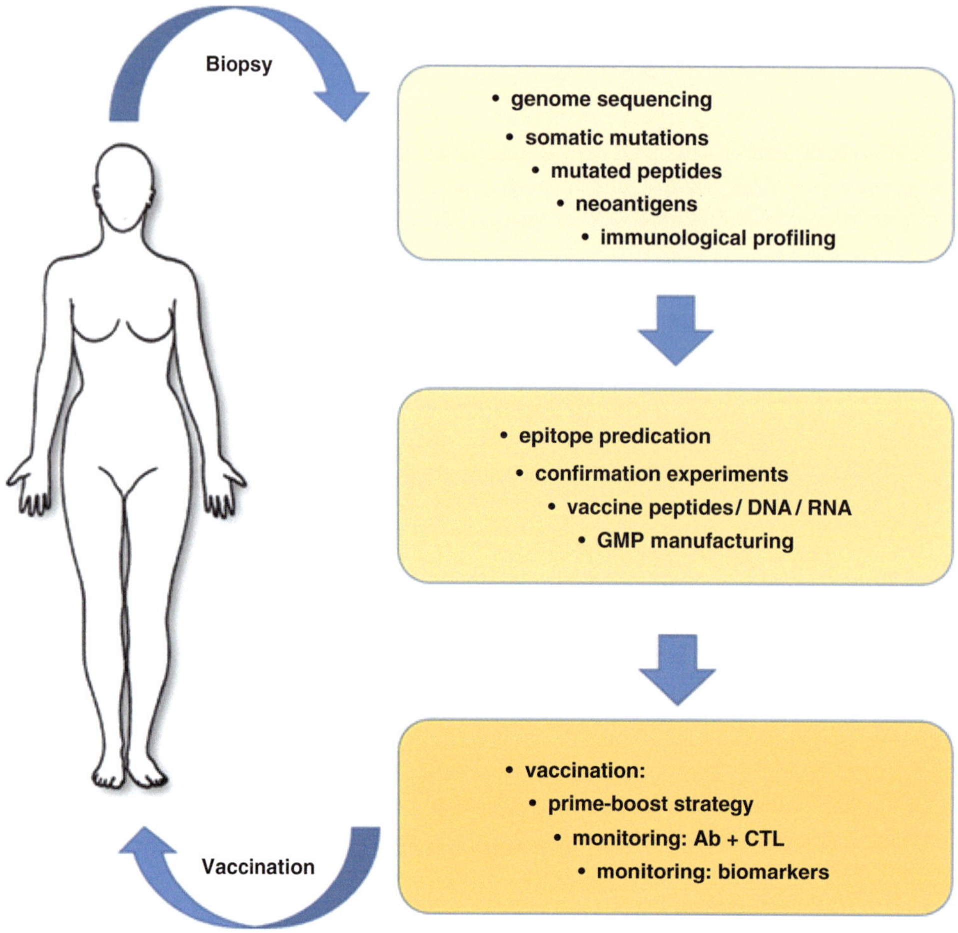

Fig. 1.13 Personalized (P) vaccine development based on a three-step approach: (1) Collection of gene and protein data. The immunological profiling uses DNA microarrays for disease-oriented fingerprints, leading to the identification of mutated peptides or neoantigens (cancer) as potential vaccine candidates. Loss or gain function of genes can be investigated by differential display and subtractive hybridization. (2) Epitope-based vaccine development either as peptide or nucleic acid vaccine or in combination (prime-boost). (3) Vaccination regime. The vaccine-induced immune response is monitored by the antibody titer and cytotoxic T cell (CTL) response and specific biomarkers

the function of both the innate and the adaptive arms came from patients affected by immunological disorders. Studies with knockout mice confirmed these observations.

Stable endogenous miRNAs in bodily fluids are used as diagnostic, prognostic, and predictive biomarkers. Moreover, targeted gene silencing via miRNAs is investigated for therapeutic treatments [52]. Numerous cancer-specific miRNAs have been identified [53]. Profiling of miRNAs in individual PBMCs, or more generally in blood and plasma samples, can be used for prediction of (immune) response of an individual anticancer treatment [54, 55]. Also in acute or chronic viral diseases, such as hepatitis A or B, a prognostic and predictive circulating miRNA biomarker can be used for the development and monitoring of therapeutic P vaccines [56–58].

Activity-Based Protein Profiling. The functional analysis of proteins instead of the mere recording of various proteins offers a platform for monitoring active proteins, referred to as activity-based protein profiling (ABPP) [59]. A chemical reagent, consisting of a reactive group (RG) and a tag, binds covalently to the active site of an enzyme. Inactive enzymes cannot bind an RG. A tag is a reporter such as a fluorophore or an affinity label such as biotin for measuring this chemoproteomic complex. ABPP can be used to study virus–host interactions by profiling serine hydrolases [60] and to develop individual P vaccines against chronic viral infection. Serine hydrolases are involved in a variety of physiological and pathological processes, also in viral infection [61].

For translation of data from active pathways, or the interpretation of protein–protein interactions and networks, bioinformatic tools are indispensable to filter the huge amount of data [62, 63].

One Gene, Different mRNAs. In summary, P vaccines use personal bioinformatic data from systems biology to design patient-specific individual vaccines for cancer diseases, chronic infections, and noncancer–noninfectious (NINC) disorders (Fig. 1.13). The personal genetic profiling for prediction of diseases, the management of a therapy, or the development of individual vaccines should belong into the hands of specialized accredited clinical genetic services and laboratories and not into the hands of private companies offering a direct-to-consumer DNA profiling. DNA fingerprints alone are not sufficient; they must be interpreted in the context with systems biology.

There is no one-to-one relationship between the analyzed DNA and the transcribed mRNA and the translated protein.

Cells can use alternative splicing resulting in various mRNAs, and proteins undergo posttranslational modifications. Therefore, one gene can result in different mRNAs, finally in different proteins with different functions and different interactions with other proteins. Moreover, a serious genetic profiling is always linked with advice from clinical geneticists. The availability of a personalized medicine is of course no guarantee for recovery from a severe illness. Lots of tests have only limited informative value and can therefore not provide accurate individual predictions. Each test result is only a fractal-like use of a complex biological system, another piece in an unlimited puzzle.

1.6 Therapeutic Window for Vaccination

The efficiency of the immune system decelerates during life alone due to the immunosenescence (see Chap. 5). Age-associated immune changes take place in the innate and acquired immune systems and affect not only lymphocytes but also myeloid cells with a change in pro-inflammatory cytokines. Also chronic infections caused by certain pathogens, such as CMV and HIV, remodel the immune system toward aged T cells. The loss of immune competence is also a major risk for many cancer diseases [64]. Immunosenescence and diseases reduce the efficacy of therapeutic vaccines.

A therapeutic window (TW) as part of the medical profiling should be based on a risk analysis of various parameters, e.g., cell samples, DNA and RNA arrays, and protein analysis. The measurement of a TW maybe the last chance to successfully reactivate most immune functions before the imbalance of the immune system will get irreversibly. The TW is not comparable to the pharmacological window, the well-defined range of a drug, between the effective dosage and the toxic amount of dosage.

Vaccine-induced long-term effects require adequate innate and acquired immune functionality, especially a diverse repertoire of T cells that can be measured by genomic and proteomic approaches during medical profiling. New antigens are recognized mainly by naive T cells. A loss of T cell repertoire diversity correlates with an impaired immune response. Therapeutic vaccines can also face functionally exhausted T cells thus do not respond properly to therapeutic vaccination. Therefore, a therapeutic vaccination should ideally combine the blocking of inhibitory pathways with stimulatory signals for the activation of CD8+ T cells, the major effector cells against cancer and chronic viral infections.

1.6.1 Balance

It seems easier to describe what an immunological disease-related imbalance does mean then to explain the immune homeostasis in healthy patients. The immune system is ambiguous, protective, and harmful – immunity on the one hand and calculated immunopathology on the other hand – and is well balanced by redundant regulatory mechanisms [65, 66]. The maintenance of the immune homeostasis with the ability to accurately regulate duration and intensity of humoral and cellular response is the basis for health, also against the early onset of many tumors (Fig. 1.14).

The Immune Surveillance Hypothesis. The healthy and young immune system is able to control at least in part growth of tumors. In 1863, Rudolf Virchow discovered active leukocytes in tumor tissues. And it was Paul Ehrlich in 1909 who postulated a "body's own protection system" against tumor cells. "The immune surveillance hypothesis" was born and elaborated in the 1950s and 1960s: T cell-mediated immunity evolved as a specific defense against cancer cells and that T cells constantly patrol the body, searching for abnormal body cells [67]. Until today, there are many clinical data demonstrating the correlation between the immune system/surveillance and the development of tumors: spontaneous remission of colon carcinoma, acute myeloid leukemia, or remission of lung and liver metastases of lung cancer (NSCLC). As long as the tumor load is controlled by the immune system, as long as this balance between diseases and innate and acquired immunity works, the life is not threatened. The same is for infectious disease.

1.6.2 Hip-Hop Balance

The correlation of immune dysfunctions and the development of tumors are also described, such as modification of T cells, T cell anergy, reduced expression of molecules of signal pathways, and reduced cytokine production. The immune-risk phenotype (IRP) is defined as CD4/CD8 ratio. In healthy conditions, the number of CD4+ T cells is higher as the number of CD8+CD28- Treg cells (formerly called T-suppressor cells), and the CD4/CD8 ratio is rarely less than 1.0. The ratio may drop as low as 0.1 during a progressive disease. In the case of HIV infection, the decline of CD4+ T cells is proportional to the virus load – the higher the virus titer the more rapid the decline. As described ear-

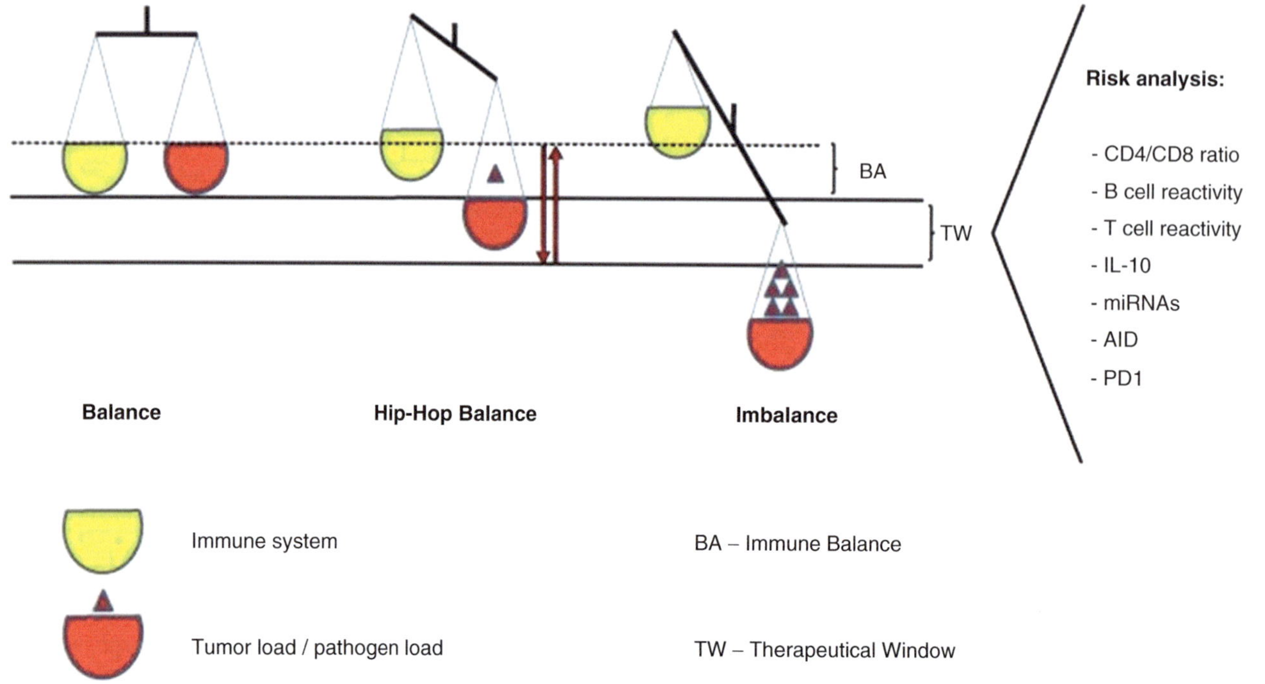

Fig. 1.14 Therapeutic window. The analysis of bodily fluids (blood, plasma, urine) *can* provide useful data on the current immune status of the patient. In healthy conditions, e.g., the number of CD4+ T cells is higher as the number of CD8+CD28- Treg cells and the CD4/CD8 ratio is rarely less than 1.0. Immunosenescent cells highly express senescence markers such as PD1, AID and CD57, and the overall activities of B and T cells are diminished. The status of Hip-Hop balance gives a chance for therapeutic vaccination before the immunological imbalance gets irreversible

lier with the therapeutic vaccine against EA virus, the efficacy strongly depends on the virus load – too much virus load and the vaccine treatment fails. Treg cells can damp the antitumor T cell response; therefore, the number of Treg cells can be used as prognostic factor [68, 69]. There are lots of host factors from cytokines to B and T cell reactivity which can be used as determinants of a therapeutic vaccine response.

The Hip-Hop balance is defined as an immunological condition in which the disease has partially destroyed some effector and regulatory functions, but the immune system can recover and respond to vaccination due to its redundancy. This is *the* therapeutic window and should be defined for each personalized vaccine.

1.6.3 Imbalance

Back to the clinical trial of 1994, and the anti-melanoma vaccine, the tumor burden in all patients was so massive that some patients died during the treatment. The balance of T cell subsets and their location within tumor tissues is a prognostic factor for the immunotherapeutic efficacy. The accumulation of Treg cells at the tumor site combined with a decrease of functional cytotoxic T cells (CTLs) is of bad prognosis. The immune system got imbalanced:

Immunosenescence. Immunosenescence is not limited only to the normal process of aging but also linked to chronic diseases or malnutrition. It's a multicell and multifactorial process in the innate and acquired system. A multiple decline of major immune functions includes also the immunodominance: one epitope is dominant and triggers the response, and all other epitopes are subdominant and don't mount for an effective response. Immunosenescent individuals have a diminished ability for immunodominance resulting in a weak and more diffuse immune response. Immunosenescent B cells show an impaired ability to undergo immunoglobulin class switch recombination (CSR) measured by a reduced antibody production. Activation-induced cytidine deaminase (AID) is essential for immunoglobulin (Ig) gene CSR and somatic hypermutation (SHM). The AID expression in immunosenescent B cells is significantly reduced compared to young individuals.

Replicative Senescence. Another drawback of immunosenescence is the telomere shortening of senescent CD8+ T cells, the replicative senescence. It does not affect only the replicative potential but also significantly antiviral effector functions, such as IFN-γ production or antigen-specific cytotoxicity. Senescent T cells lack important co-stimulatory molecules such as CD28 and CD27 but highly express senescence markers: PD-1, CD57, and KLRG-1.

This count to a lesser extends for CD4+ T cells but especially for CD8+ T cells which develop the most functional defects.

Risk Analysis. Some laboratory parameters for this imbalance can be isolated from blood and plasma such as chronic pro-inflammatory cytokines, T and B cells (reactivity), immunosenescence markers like AID or PD-1, and miRNAs which are associated, e.g., with advanced stage of cancer [70]. Stable endogenous miRNAs in bodily fluids (serum, plasma, urine) are used as diagnostic, prognostic, and predictive biomarkers.

A risk analysis of several parameters before vaccination could help to understand the current disposition of the immune system: makes a therapeutic vaccination sense or not?

References

1. Luytjes, W., Krystal, M., Enami, M., Parvin, J.D., Palese, P.: Amplification, expression, and packaging of foreign gene by influenza virus. Cell **59**, 1107–1113 (1989)
2. Enami, M., Luytjes, W., Krystal, M., Palese, P.: Introduction of site-specific mutations into the genome of influenza virus. Proc. Natl. Acad. Sci. U. S. A. **87**, 3802–3805 (1990)
3. Tan, L.K., Carlone, G.M., Borrow, R.: Advances in the development of vaccines against Neisseria meningitidis. N. Engl. J. Med. **362**, 1511–1520 (2010). doi:10.1056/NEJMra0906357
4. McAleer, W.J., et al.: Human hepatitis B vaccine from recombinant yeast. Nature **307**, 178–180 (1984)
5. Hollinger, F.B., Troisi, C.L., Pepe, P.E.: Anti-HBs responses to vaccination with a human hepatitis B vaccine made by recombinant DNA technology in yeast. J. Infect. Dis. **153**, 156–159 (1986)
6. Stephenne, J.: Production in yeast versus mammalian cells of the first recombinant DNA human vaccine and its proved safety, efficacy, and economy: hepatitis B vaccine. Adv. Biotechnol. Processes **14**, 279–299 (1990)
7. Finne, J., Leinonen, M., Makela, P.H.: Antigenic similarities between brain components and bacteria causing meningitis. Implications for vaccine development and pathogenesis. Lancet **2**, 355–357 (1983)
8. Fleischmann, R.D., et al.: Whole-genome random sequencing and assembly of Haemophilus influenzae Rd. Science **269**, 496–512 (1995)
9. Pizza, M., et al.: Identification of vaccine candidates against serogroup B meningococcus by whole-genome sequencing. Science **287**, 1816–1820 (2000)
10. Sette, A., Rappuoli, R.: Reverse vaccinology: developing vaccines in the era of genomics. Immunity **33**, 530–541 (2010). doi:10.1016/j.immuni.2010.09.017
11. Giuliani, M.M., et al.: A universal vaccine for serogroup B meningococcus. Proc. Natl. Acad. Sci. U. S. A. **103**, 10834–10839 (2006). doi:10.1073/pnas.0603940103
12. Gay, C.G., et al.: Genomics and vaccine development. Rev. Sci. Tech. **26**, 49–67 (2007)
13. Bambini, S., Rappuoli, R.: The use of genomics in microbial vaccine development. Drug Discov. Today **14**, 252–260 (2009). doi:10.1016/j.drudis.2008.12.007
14. Helmberg, W.: Bioinformatic databases and resources in the public domain to aid HLA research. Tissue Antigens **80**, 295–304 (2012). doi:10.1111/tan.12000
15. De Groot, A.S., Berzofsky, J.A.: From genome to vaccine–new immunoinformatics tools for vaccine design. Methods **34**, 425–428 (2004). doi:10.1016/j.ymeth.2004.06.004
16. Wang, P., et al.: A systematic assessment of MHC class II peptide binding predictions and evaluation of a consensus approach. PLoS Comput. Biol. **4**, e1000048 (2008). doi:10.1371/journal.pcbi.1000048
17. He, Y., Xiang, Z., Mobley, H.L.: Vaxign: the first web-based vaccine design program for reverse vaccinology and applications for vaccine development. J. Biomed. Biotechnol. **2010**, 297505 (2010). doi:10.1155/2010/297505
18. Schafer, J.R., Jesdale, B.M., George, J.A., Kouttab, N.M., De Groot, A.S.: Prediction of well-conserved HIV-1 ligands using a matrix-based algorithm, EpiMatrix. Vaccine **16**, 1880–1884 (1998)
19. Rammensee, H., Bachmann, J., Emmerich, N.P., Bachor, O.A., Stevanovic, S.: SYFPEITHI: database for MHC ligands and peptide motifs. Immunogenetics **50**, 213–219 (1999)
20. Ehrenmann, F., Kaas, Q., Lefranc, M.P.: IMGT/3Dstructure-DB and IMGT/DomainGapAlign: a database and a tool for immunoglobulins or antibodies, T cell receptors, MHC, IgSF and MhcSF. Nucleic Acids Res. **38**, D301–D307 (2010). doi:10.1093/nar/gkp946
21. Gowthaman, U., Agrewala, J.N.: In silico tools for predicting peptides binding to HLA-class II molecules: more confusion than conclusion. J. Proteome Res. **7**, 154–163 (2008). doi:10.1021/pr070527b
22. Blythe, M.J., Flower, D.R.: Benchmarking B cell epitope prediction: underperformance of existing methods. Protein Sci. **14**, 246–248 (2005). doi:10.1110/ps.041059505
23. Barlow, D.J., Edwards, M.S., Thornton, J.M.: Continuous and discontinuous protein antigenic determinants. Nature **322**, 747–748 (1986). doi:10.1038/322747a0
24. Sharma, A., et al.: Identification of potential universal vaccine candidates against group A Streptococcus by using high throughput in silico and proteomics approach. J. Proteome Res. **12**, 336–346 (2013). doi:10.1021/pr3005265
25. Flower, D.R., Macdonald, I.K., Ramakrishnan, K., Davies, M.N., Doytchinova, I.A.: Computer aided selection of candidate vaccine antigens. Immunome Res. **6**(Suppl 2), S1 (2010). doi:10.1186/1745-7580-6-S2-S1
26. Hanekom, W.A.: The immune response to BCG vaccination of newborns. Ann. N. Y. Acad. Sci. **1062**, 69–78 (2005). doi:10.1196/annals.1358.010
27. Kim, J.Y., Chang, J.: Need for a safe vaccine against respiratory syncytial virus infection. Korean J. Pediatr. **55**, 309–315 (2012). doi:10.3345/kjp.2012.55.9.309
28. Fernando, T.R., Rodriguez-Malave, N.I., Rao, D.S.: MicroRNAs in B cell development and malignancy. J. Hematol. Oncol. **5**, 7 (2012). doi:10.1186/1756-8722-5-7
29. Okada, H., Kohanbash, G., Lotze, M.T.: MicroRNAs in immune regulation–opportunities for cancer immunotherapy. Int. J. Biochem. Cell Biol. **42**, 1256–1261 (2010). doi:10.1016/j.biocel.2010.02.002
30. Malan-Muller, S., Hemmings, S.M., Seedat, S.: Big effects of small RNAs: a review of microRNAs in anxiety. Mol. Neurobiol. **47**(2), 726–739 (2012). doi:10.1007/s12035-012-8374-6
31. Asirvatham, A.J., Magner, W.J., Tomasi, T.B.: miRNA regulation of cytokine genes. Cytokine **45**, 58–69 (2009). doi:10.1016/j.cyto.2008.11.010
32. Kandpal, R., Saviola, B., Felton, J.: The era of 'omics unlimited. Biotechniques **46**(351–352), 354–355 (2009). doi:10.2144/000113137
33. Biomarkers Definitions Working Group: Biomarkers and surrogate endpoints: preferred definitions and conceptual framework. Clin. Pharmacol. Ther. **69**, 89–95 (2001). doi:10.1067/mcp.2001.113989
34. Gaucher, D., et al.: Yellow fever vaccine induces integrated multilineage and polyfunctional immune responses. J. Exp. Med. **205**, 3119–3131 (2008). doi:10.1084/jem.20082292

35. Pulendran, B., Li, S., Nakaya, H.I.: Systems vaccinology. Immunity **33**, 516–529 (2010). doi:10.1016/j.immuni.2010.10.006
36. Plotkin, S.A.: Vaccines: correlates of vaccine-induced immunity. Clin. Infect. Dis. **47**, 401–409 (2008). doi:10.1086/589862
37. Plotkin, S.A.: Correlates of protection induced by vaccination. Clin. Vaccine Immunol. **17**, 1055–1065 (2010). doi:10.1128/CVI.00131-10
38. Qin, L., Gilbert, P.B., Corey, L., McElrath, M.J., Self, S.G.: A framework for assessing immunological correlates of protection in vaccine trials. J. Infect. Dis. **196**, 1304–1312 (2007). doi:10.1086/522428
39. Le Polain de Waroux, O., Maguire, H., Moren, A.: The case-cohort design in outbreak investigations. Euro Surveill. **17**, pii: 20202 (2012)
40. Halloran, M.E., Longini Jr., I.M., Struchiner, C.J.: Design and interpretation of vaccine field studies. Epidemiol. Rev. **21**, 73–88 (1999)
41. Wang, K., Lee, I., Carlson, G., Hood, L., Galas, D.: Systems biology and the discovery of diagnostic biomarkers. Dis. Markers **28**, 199–207 (2010). doi:10.3233/DMA-2010-0697
42. Giese, M., et al.: Stable and long-lasting immune response in horses after DNA vaccination against equine arteritis virus. Virus Genes **25**, 159–167 (2002)
43. Weir, R.E., et al.: Comparison of IFN-gamma responses to mycobacterial antigens as markers of response to BCG vaccination. Tuberculosis (Edinb.) **88**, 31–38 (2008)
44. Abebe, F.: Is interferon-gamma the right marker for bacille Calmette-Guerin-induced immune protection? The missing link in our understanding of tuberculosis immunology. Clin. Exp. Immunol. **169**, 213–219 (2012). doi:10.1111/j.1365-2249.2012.04614.x
45. Aswaq, M., Richards, V., McFadden, S.: Immunologic response to autologous cancer vaccine. Arch. Surg. **89**, 485–487 (1964)
46. Stingl, G., et al.: Phase I study to the immunotherapy of metastatic malignant melanoma by a cancer vaccine consisting of autologous cancer cells transfected with the human IL-2 gene. Hum. Gene Ther. **7**, 551–563 (1996). doi:10.1089/hum.1996.7.4-551
47. Hovden, A.O., Appel, S.: The first dendritic cell-based therapeutic cancer vaccine is approved by the FDA. Scand. J. Immunol. **72**, 554 (2010). doi:10.1111/j.1365-3083.2010.02464.x
48. Lesterhuis, W.J., et al.: Dendritic cell vaccines in melanoma: from promise to proof? Crit. Rev. Oncol. Hematol. **66**, 118–134 (2008). doi:10.1016/j.critrevonc.2007.12.007
49. Khatri, P., Sirota, M., Butte, A.J.: Ten years of pathway analysis: current approaches and outstanding challenges. PLoS Comput. Biol. **8**, e1002375 (2012). doi:10.1371/journal.pcbi.1002375
50. Munir, S., Singh, S., Kaur, K., Kapur, V.: Suppression subtractive hybridization coupled with microarray analysis to examine differential expression of genes in virus infected cells. Biol. Proced. Online **6**, 94–104 (2004). doi:10.1251/bpo77
51. Zimmerer, J.M., et al.: Gene expression profiling reveals similarities between the in vitro and in vivo responses of immune effector cells to IFN-alpha. Clin. Cancer Res. **14**, 5900–5906 (2008). doi:10.1158/1078-0432.CCR-08-0846
52. Sibley, C.R., Seow, Y., Wood, M.J.: Novel RNA-based strategies for therapeutic gene silencing. Mol. Ther. **18**, 466–476 (2010). doi:10.1038/mt.2009.306
53. Chen, P.S., Su, J.L., Hung, M.C.: Dysregulation of microRNAs in cancer. J. Biomed. Sci. **19**, 90 (2012). doi:10.1186/1423-0127-19-90
54. Gamez-Pozo, A., et al.: MicroRNA expression profiling of peripheral blood samples predicts resistance to first-line sunitinib in advanced renal cell carcinoma patients. Neoplasia **14**, 1144–1152 (2012)
55. Ng, E.K., et al.: Circulating microRNAs as specific biomarkers for breast cancer detection. PLoS One **8**, e53141 (2013). doi:10.1371/journal.pone.0053141
56. Elfimova, N., et al.: Circulating microRNAs: promising candidates serving as novel biomarkers of acute hepatitis. Front Physiol. **3**, 476 (2012). doi:10.3389/fphys.2012.00476
57. Cortez, M.A., Calin, G.A.: MicroRNA identification in plasma and serum: a new tool to diagnose and monitor diseases. Expert Opin. Biol. Ther. **9**, 703–711 (2009). doi:10.1517/14712590902932889
58. Ajit, S.K.: Circulating microRNAs as biomarkers, therapeutic targets, and signaling molecules. Sensors (Basel) **12**, 3359–3369 (2012). doi:10.3390/s120303359
59. Liu, Y., Patricelli, M.P., Cravatt, B.F.: Activity-based protein profiling: the serine hydrolases. Proc. Natl. Acad. Sci. U. S. A. **96**, 14694–14699 (1999)
60. Shahiduzzaman, M., Coombs, K.M.: Activity based protein profiling to detect serine hydrolase alterations in virus infected cells. Front Microbiol. **3**, 308 (2012). doi:10.3389/fmicb.2012.00308
61. Steuber, H., Hilgenfeld, R.: Recent advances in targeting viral proteases for the discovery of novel antivirals. Curr. Top. Med. Chem. **10**, 323–345 (2010)
62. Bindea, G., Galon, J., Mlecnik, B.: CluePedia Cytoscape plugin: pathway insights using integrated experimental and in silico data. Bioinformatics **29**(5), 661–663 (2013). doi:10.1093/bioinformatics/btt019
63. Henderson-Maclennan, N.K., Papp, J.C., Talbot Jr., C.C., McCabe, E.R., Presson, A.P.: Pathway analysis software: annotation errors and solutions. Mol. Genet. Metab. **101**, 134–140 (2010). doi:10.1016/j.ymgme.2010.06.005
64. Pawelec, G., Derhovanessian, E., Larbi, A.: Immunosenescence and cancer. Crit. Rev. Oncol. Hematol. **75**, 165–172 (2010). doi:10.1016/j.critrevonc.2010.06.012
65. Barnaba, V., Paroli, M., Piconese, S.: The ambiguity in immunology. Front Immunol. **3**, 18 (2012). doi:10.3389/fimmu.2012.00018
66. Germain, R.N.: Maintaining system homeostasis: the third law of Newtonian immunology. Nat. Immunol. **13**, 902–906 (2012). doi:10.1038/ni.2404
67. Ostrand-Rosenberg, S.: Immune surveillance: a balance between protumor and antitumor immunity. Curr. Opin. Genet. Dev. **18**, 11–18 (2008). doi:10.1016/j.gde.2007.12.007
68. Wilke, C.M., Wu, K., Zhao, E., Wang, G., Zou, W.: Prognostic significance of regulatory T cells in tumor. Int. J. Cancer **127**, 748–758 (2010). doi:10.1002/ijc.25464
69. Ogino, S., Galon, J., Fuchs, C.S., Dranoff, G.: Cancer immunology–analysis of host and tumor factors for personalized medicine. Nat. Rev. Clin. Oncol. **8**, 711–719 (2011). doi:10.1038/nrclinonc.2011.122
70. Huang, L., et al.: Downregulation of six microRNAs is associated with advanced stage, lymph node metastasis and poor prognosis in small cell carcinoma of the cervix. PLoS One **7**, e33762 (2012). doi:10.1371/journal.pone.0033762

Basic Vaccine Immunology

2

Contents

The most outstanding aspects of the immune responses following a vaccination are described here. But it is beyond the scope of this chapter to describe in detail all immunological functions. We focus on a more general description on what is known of the vaccine immunity.

2.1 Chemical Nature of Antigens

Viruses, bacteria, parasites, and fungi are permanent natural threats of our life. Also different types of allergies against pollen, mold fungus, animal hairs, or house dust mites are able to provoke an antigen-induced antibody response. Also environmental allergens, natural or industrial-produced ultrafine carbon particulate matter (PM), can cause allergies and promote asthma. PM is deposited in alveoli leading to a pro-inflammation response.

Antigens are able to induce a specific immune response (Table 2.1). So manifold the world of antigens (Ag) looks like all known antigens (except of industrial PM) can be classified into five groups depending on their chemical nature (Fig. 2.1): proteins, glycoproteins, carbohydrates, lipids (lipoproteins), and nucleic acids. The nomenclature of antigens is presented in Table 2.2.

Table 2.1 Definition of antigen

Modern definition of antigen	• **An antigen is able to induce a specific immune response.**
Classical definition of antigen	• **An antigen is able to being bound by an antibody via surface epitopes.**

M. Giese, *Introduction to Molecular Vaccinology*, DOI 10.1007/978-3-319-25832-4_2

Antigen	Chemical structure	Antigenic recognition site
Pure protein	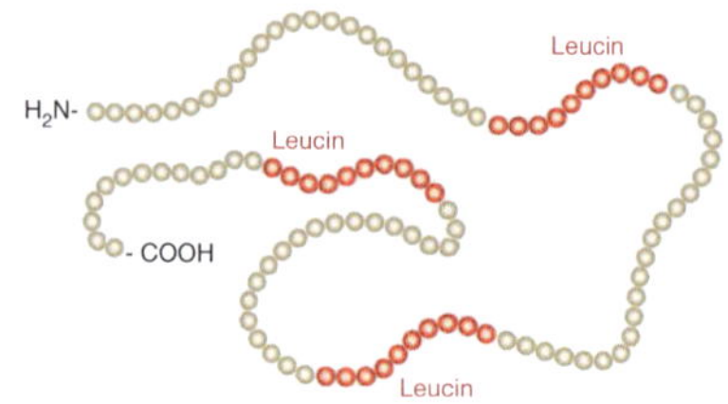	Leucine-rich repeats (LRR)-domain consisting of 2-45 LL repeats, with each repeat about 20-30 residues long.
Glyco-protein	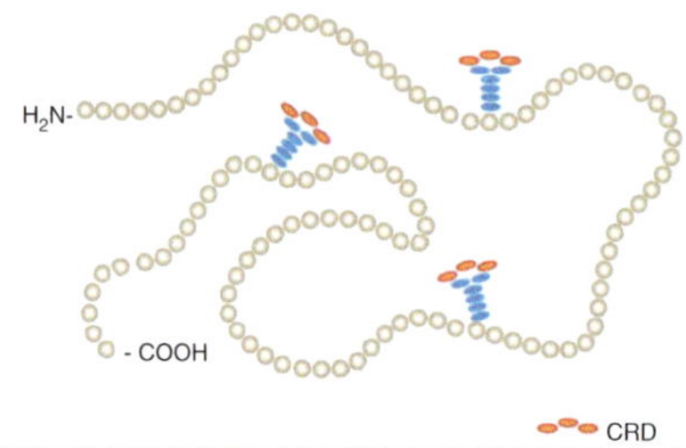	Complex sugars, such as mannose, glucose or galactose, via their carbohydrate-recognition domain (CRD).
Lipids	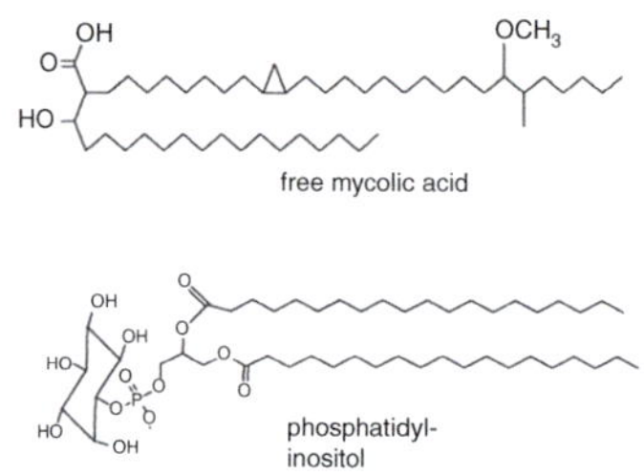	Chain lenght is recognized of diverse sets of mostly bacterial lipids, glycolipids, and lipopeptides.
Carbo-hydrates	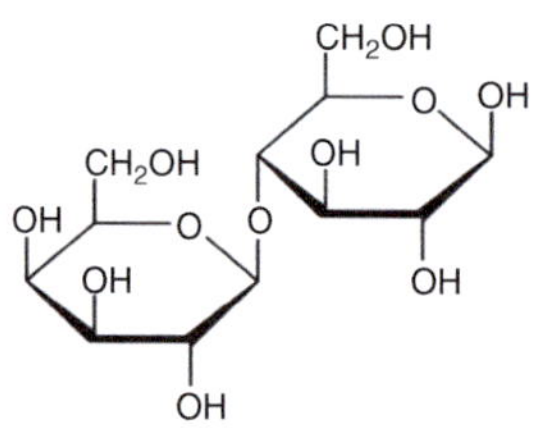	Recognition of mannose, fucose, galactose, glucan oligosaccharides via C-lectin like receptors.
Nucleic acids	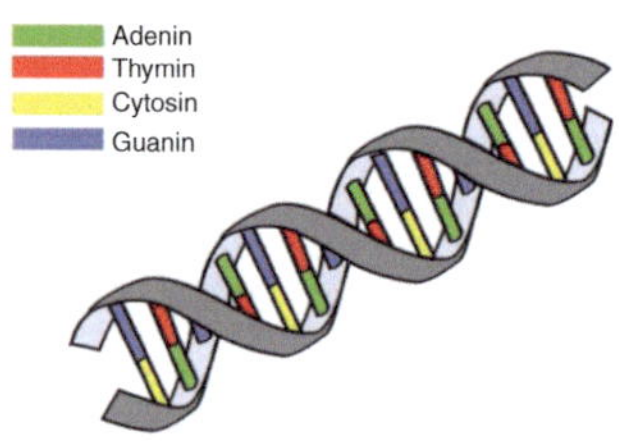	**DNA**: Recognition of bacterial DNA by the hypomethylation (CpG) compared to vertebrate DNA. **RNA**: Recognition by primary nucleotide sequence, secondary and tertiary structure, or intracellular localization.

Fig. 2.1 Chemical nature of antigens.

Each protein is encoded by genes and constructed of one or more chains of amino acids (primary sequence) linked by peptide bonds. The basic function of a protein is given by the tertiary structure, a stable three-dimensional structure. Many proteins are complexed with different sugars, like mannose, glucose, or modified by lipids (glycoproteins or lipoproteins). Glycoproteins are recognized as antigenic structure by their carbohydrate-recognition domain (CDR).

Lipids can be recognized by their different chain lengths. Lipid antigens bind to CD1 molecules where their polar lipid head group is exposed to CD1 restricted T cells. After binding to TCR, these T cells interact with macrophages, dendritic cells, NK cells, B cells, and T cells, thereby contributing to innate and acquired immune responses.

Various carbohydrates without protein binding are recognized via the C-lectin-like receptors.

Compared to vertebrate DNA, microbial DNA (bacteria, viral, fungi) is hypomethylated and can be detected by Toll-like receptor 9. In contrast to DNA the antigenic character of foreign RNA is based especially on structural differences and the intracellular localization

Table 2.2 Nomenclature for antigens

Description	Definition	Mode of action
Antigen (Ag)	Classical: a structure able to being bound by an antibody via surface epitopes Modern: any structure able to induce a specific immune response	T dependent: Ag needs assistance of T helper cells to induce antibody formation *or* T independent: Ag (polysaccharides) binds to and stimulates B cells directly
Epitope (also antigenic determinant)	Distinct molecular features on the surface of an antigen	Binding part for B cell, T cell receptor or Fab part of antibody
Decoy epitope	A molecular dummy which mimics the neutralizing epitope	First wave of antibodies directed against the decoy epitope
Antigenic molecules	Large biological polymers with *n*-epitopes	Various antibodies can bind to this antigenic molecule
Cross-reacting antigens	Several antigens with an epitope in common	Antibodies targeted to one antigen are able to react with the same epitope on all other antigens
Cognate antigen	"Déjà vu" antigen – Ag is already known	Recall of B and T cell response
Self-antigen (autoantigen)	Host-encoded proteins, cell debris	1. In healthy immunity: no T cell response but apoptosis of T cells 2. Sick immunity: lack of apoptosis leading to a T cell response against self
Non-self-antigen	Foreign structure which is not naturally found inside the body	B and T cell response
Superantigen (sAg)	A class of powerful mostly bacterial (also viral) antigens acting like toxins	Nonspecific polyclonal T activation but with massive pathological cytokine release
Particulate antigen	Particulate nature of an antigen in contrast to…	Live (inactivated) virus vaccines. Probably depot effect, strong B and T cell response
Soluble antigen	…soluble nature of an antigen – Ag remains in solution after the particles of virus/bacterium have been removed (e.g., toxins)	Subunit protein vaccines
Neoantigen	A newly acquired and individually tumor-derived antigen	B and T cell response
Hapten	Small molecule (≤1000 Da) that stimulates the production of antibody only when coupled to a larger molecule (carrier molecule)	Hapten–carrier complex as stimulant

2.1.1 Epitopes

Epitopes or antigenic determinants are distinct molecular features of an antigen. Depending on the nature and the size of antigen, several different epitopes can decorate an antigen. This epitope region of the antigen is recognized by specific antibodies, which bind to and remove the antigen from the body. In this case the epitopes are neutralizing epitopes. There are also non-neutralizing epitopes produced by some viruses as part of their escape strategy and called decoy epitopes.

A decoy is a molecular dummy and mimics the neutralizing epitope in order to bind the first wave of antibodies. Thus the body is unable to set a robust immune response up in the first beginning of the infection and the viruses can spread over the body. Antibodies against the neutralizing epitopes appear only late [1]. The decoy epitope can be located near the neutralizing epitope and separated by a short region (arterivirus) but earlier expressed as the neutralizing form. Or the decoy epitope is mimicking a viral membrane glycoprotein but expressed also as a secretory form catching the antibodies before they can bind to the membrane (filovirus) [2]. The different types of epitopes are illustrated in Fig. 2.2.

Redundant PRR System. Pathogen recognition receptors (PRRs) identify invaders by their unique, highly specific, and highly conserved pathogen-associated molecular patterns, PAMPs. All sensors use PAMPs also to discriminate "self" from "non-self." This redundant PRR system guarantees to detect a pathogen in parallel by different sensors. If one sensor fails, another PRR is active to trace this antigen. This high level of redundancy could be one reason why estimated 98 % of all infections in a healthy patient are detected and cured by the immune systems. PRRs and PAMPs are discussed later.

Pathogen recognition receptors are special cell surface, intracellular, and also secreted receptors, collectively called pathogen recognition receptors ubiquitously distributed in the body; they recognize various antigenic structures, thereby initiating an innate and acquired immune response. PRRs are discussed in detail later in this chapter.

Self-antigens (cell debris, host-encoded proteins) are presented to T cells by dendritic cells (DCs) without any co-stimulatory molecules resulting in apoptosis of these T cells. Self-antigens, usually tolerated by the immune systems, become dangerous if the immune controlling fails.

2.1.2 Different Immunogenicity

The various antigens can be different in the quantitative and qualitative immune response, also in the duration and efficacy. The immunogenicity of an antigen is determined by several factors:

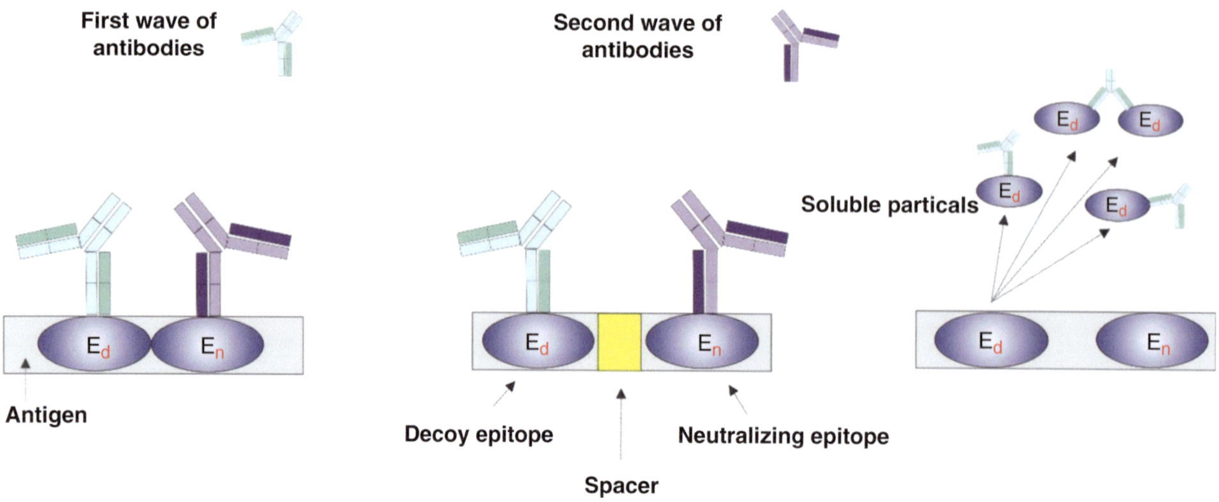

Fig. 2.2 Epitopes are distinct molecular features of an antigen. The epitope region (E_n) of the antigen is recognized by neutralizing antibodies. A decoy epitope (E_d) is a molecular dummy and mimics the neutralizing epitope in order to bind the first wave of useless antibodies. The decoy epitope can be located near the neutralizing epitope and separated by a short region (arterivirus) but earlier expressed as the neutralizing form or expressed as a secretory molecule

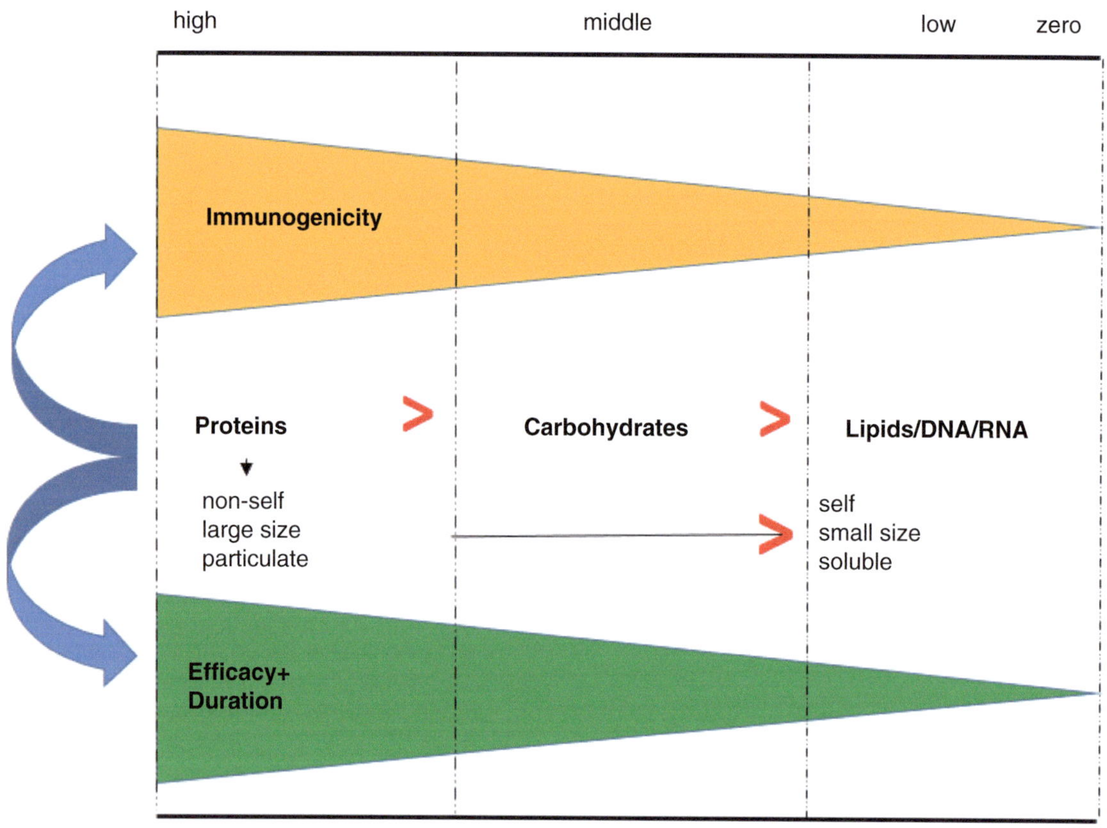

Fig. 2.3 Antigenic differences of proteins, carbohydrates, lipids, and nucleic acids in immunogenicity, efficacy, and duration of immunity

- Proteins are more immunogenic than lipids and carbohydrates.
- Chemical and structural differences of an antigen to a self-antigen.
- The size and complexity of an antigen, more epitopes for binding of antibodies.
- Particulate antigens are more immunogenic than soluble antigens (Fig. 2.3).

If the antigen shares similarity with a host protein, a poor immune response is most likely the consequence due to epitope mimicry and autoimmunity can be triggered, targeting both the antigen and host protein(s) [3]. Not only proteins can elicit the latter but also polysaccharides. This became evident from vaccines in meningococcal bacteria which could not be used for *Neisseria meningitides* because of the induction of polysaccharide-based autoimmunity [4]. A highly complex foreign protein, for which no similar structured self-antigen does exist, will be recognized as invader and induce a strong immune response.

2.2 Antigen-Presenting Cells

At best a vaccine will induce a complete immune response, comprising of components of innate and acquired immunity and humoral and cellular activities. Thereby B and T cells, monocytes, macrophages, natural killer cells (NK), granulocytes, or antigen-presenting cells (APCs) such as dendritic cells act in concert triggered by various cytokines, together with complement factors and antibodies.

APCs are in the early front for each vaccination and target cells for antigens. APCs bind different antigens and connect the innate and the acquired immunity. They use congenital, evolutionary highly conserved patterns to recognize various antigens in order to activate B and T cells. Thus, the acquired immunity is regulated by innate immunological components (Fig. 2.4).

PRRs and PAMPs. The antigen recognition is part of the innate system and controlled by two corresponding elements. The first element are the pattern recognition receptors (PRRs) [5] expressed on the cell surface or located in endosomes or in cytoplasm. The counterpart are the pathogen-associated molecular pattern (PAMP), exclusively expressed on microbes. Microbes, organized in one class, share the same PAMP [6].

The main drivers for the specific antigen (Ag) presentation are three types of professional APCs, monocytes [7]/macrophages [8], B cells [9], and dendritic cells belonging to the white blood cells (Table 2.3). All APCs are produced by hematopoietic stem cells in the bone marrow.

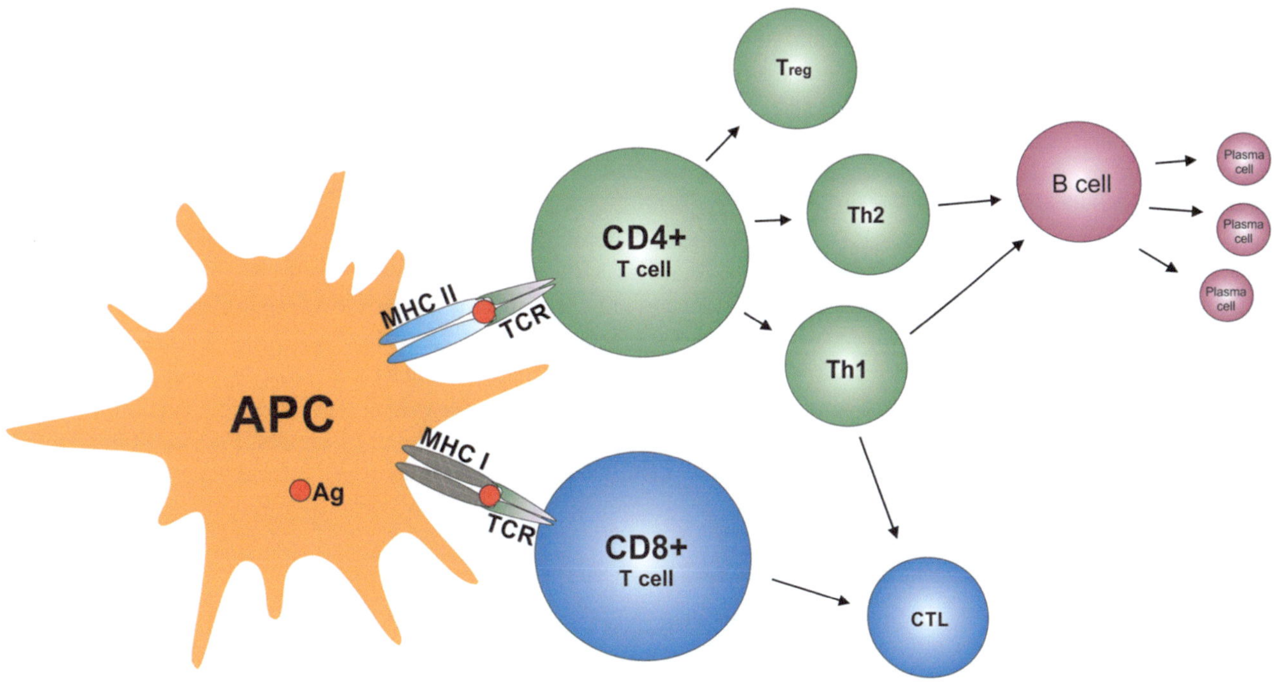

Fig. 2.4 Process of a T cell based immune reaction. Antigen-presenting cells (*APCs*) bind different antigens and connect the innate and the acquired immunity. They use highly conserved patterns to recognize antigens (*Ag*), to process them, and finally to present parts of the Ag via their major histocompatibility protein complex (*MHC*) I or II to T cells for activation (*TCR* T cell receptor, *Treg* T regulatory cell, *Th1/2* T helper cells, *CTL* cytotoxic T lymphocyte)

Table 2.3 Professional antigen-presenting cells (APCs)

Cell type	Location	Function	Marker	Reference
Monocytes: 1. Classical 2. Intermediate 3. Nonclassical	Blood	Phagocytosis, Ag presentation	CD14+, CD16– CD14+, CD16+ CD14+, CD16++	[3]
Macrophages	Tissue	Phagocytosis, Ag presentation	CD14+, CD40+, CD64+	[4]
B cells	Blood, lymphoid organs	Ag presentation, antibodies, regulation	CD19+, CD20+, CD21+	[5]
Dendritic cells	Tissue	Ag presentation	See Table 2.4	

2.2.1 Dendritic Cells

Monocytes/macrophages exhibit only a limited capacity to activate naïve T cells, and the antigen presentation by B cells mainly serves as auto-presentation for antibody production. Especially dendritic cells (DCs) are the real professional cells for Ag presentation to T cells. DCs are mobile and can move as immature cells in the blood, and once activated they migrate from blood to different tissues to secondary lymphoid organs. DCs are the main gatekeepers of the immune system. DCs possess complete molecular equipment to take-up antigens and to process and present antigens to induce an immune response. DCs acquire only soluble antigen via endocytosis.

It's not surprising that DCs are in the focus of vaccine development since two decades. DCs are present in lots of tissues, lymphoid and non-lymphoid, including brain [10], mainly abundant in tissues where external and internal environments run across: skin, lung, and gastrointestinal tract. Thereby, DCs are essential both for the immunotolerance and for induction of a protective response via MHC I and MHC II, in combination with co-stimulatory molecules such as B7 and pro-inflammatory cytokines. DCs are composed of a network of different subsets, which can be phenotypically and functionally differentiated.

Immature DCs. As immature cells DCs are always in motion to patrol through the body and to capture antigens at any time. They are sentinel cells of the immune system. At this stage the MHC molecules (HLA in humans) are only to a less extent prevalent. Also the co-stimulatory signals are absent, necessary for the complete activation of T cells.

DCs cannot be detected and differentiated by any exclusive cell marker. Rather, a combination of markers, presence and absence, are used to identify DCs. Furthermore, the differentiation is complicated by the fact that monocytes, macrophages, and DC share a common macrophage–DC progenitor and monocytes/macrophages can be developed into DCs after specific stimulation. Table 2.4 shows the functional subsets of DCs [11–15].

Depending on their ontogenetic origin, DCs are divided into a myeloid (also called conventional or classical) and a lymphoid line (nonconventional) [16]. Myeloid DCs (mDCs) are most similar to monocytes and can be divided into several subsets and are divided in migratory DCs and the lymphoid tissue-resident DCs. Surface marker for mDCs are CD11c+,CD11b+, CD1a+, and sometimes CD103+. These peripheral DCs are located in the epidermis as Langerhans cells (LC), in the skin dermis, moreover in the mucosa, and interstitial spaces. All mDCs but LCs produce large amounts of different Th2 cytokines such as IL-4 and IL-10. Following the Ag capture and processing, mDCs migrate to regional lymph nodes in order to present the peptide antigens and to activate both CD4+ and CD8+ T cells.

Lymphoid DCs are referred as plasmacytoid DCs (pDCs) and look like plasma cells. They circulate in the blood stream and are characterized by their ability to produce huge amount of type I interferon [17] and other Th1 cytokines. To this, pDCs must be activated by viruses. Embedded in lymphoid and in peripheral tissues, pDCs form the group of lymphoid

Table 2.4 Functional subsets of dendritic cells (DCs) in peripheral human blood

Subsets of DCs	Localization	Hallmark and marker	Reference
Myeloid (m)DCs: (*conventional DCs*)			
Dermal (d)DCs Langerhans Cs Brain (bDCs) Interstitial (iDCs)	Dermis Epidermis Brain Interstitium	Th2 cytokines (IL-4, IL-10) and CD1a+, CD14+ CD1a+, CD1b–, CD1c– CD11b+, CD103+ CD11c+,CD11b+, CD1a+	[7] [8] [9] [10]
Plasmacytoid (p)DCs (*nonconventional DCs*)	Blood, lymphoid organs	Th1 cytokines, interferon α, CD11c–, CD11b–, CD1a+	[11]

tissue-resident DCs. Surface markers are CD11c−, CD11b−, CD1a+. DC subsets can also be differentiated by their lifespan and especially by their anatomical localization. Thus, the specific function of a DC is adjusted to its localization [18].

2.2.2 Langerhans Cells: First Line of Defense

Langerhans cells (LCs) are a subset of skin DCs, radioresistant, and also found in the mucosa of the nose, mouth, or in the genital tract, and play a key role in the first line of defense. In particular, Langerhans cells in the basal and suprabasal layers of epidermis are in a strategic advantageous position to capture vaccine antigens, process them, and migrate to draining lymph nodes. Almost 2 % of all epidermal cells are LCs. Following the antigen capture, LCs migrate through the dermis to the lymph vessels (Fig. 2.5).

Two different surface receptors of LCs capture glycoproteins via endocytosis (pinocytosis and phagocytosis), the C-type lectin receptor DEC-205 (CD205), and the langerin receptor (CD207). During maturation LCs express MHC I and II molecules.

2.2.3 Lectin and Lectin-Like Receptors

Many cells of the immune systems, DCs, monocytes, macrophages are provided with lectin or lectin-like receptors (LLR). These LLRs are pathogen recognition receptors and perform the same functions as the family of Toll-like receptors (TLR). The lectin-like receptor DEC-205 (CD205) is part of the macrophage mannose receptors (MMR) family and recognizes terminal monosaccharide residues of microbes and fungi via the carbohydrate-recognition domain (CRD).

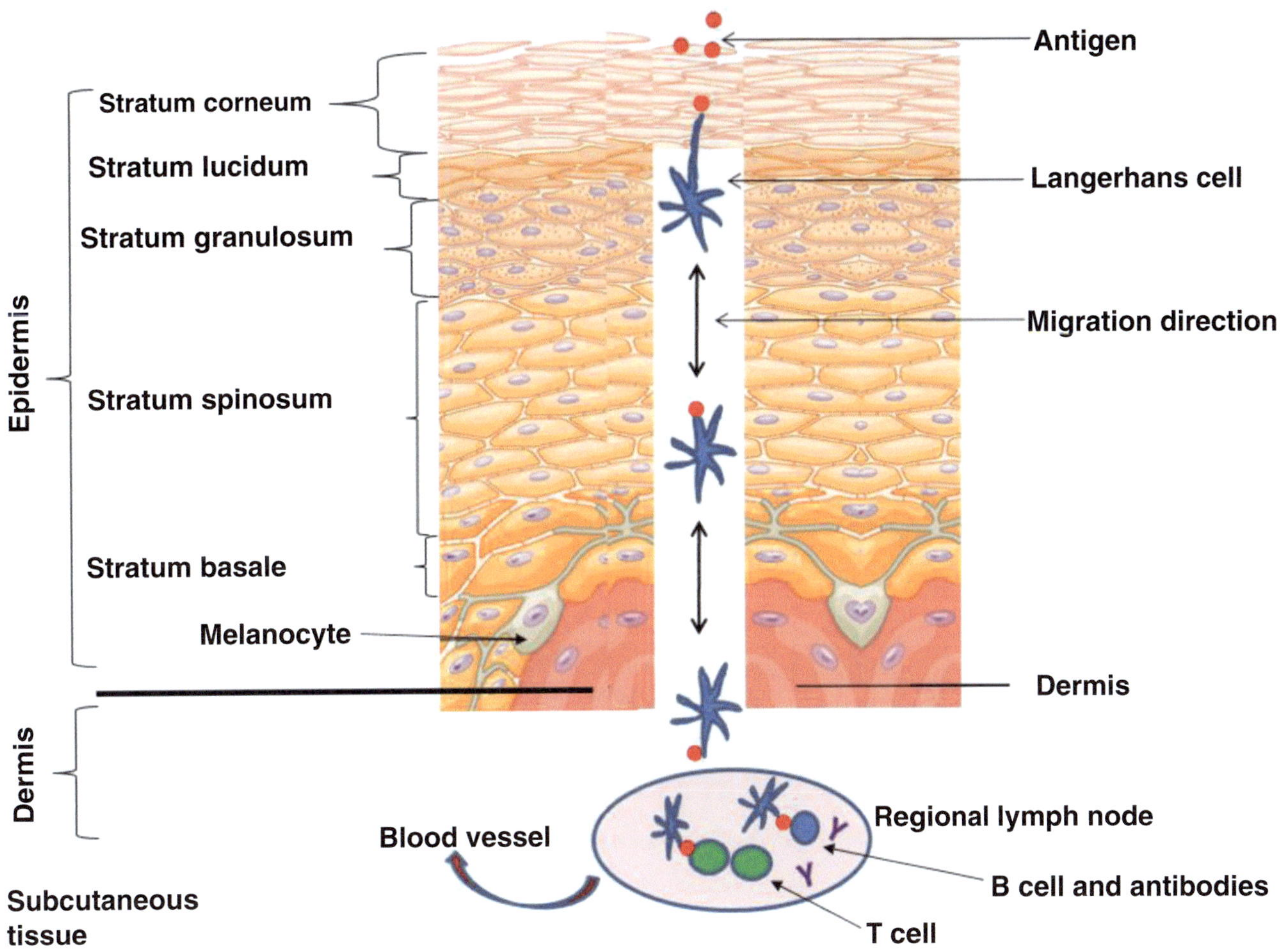

Fig. 2.5 Migration of Langerhans cells. Langerhans cells (LCs) are a subset of skin DCs and also found in the mucosa of the nose, mouth, or in the genital tract and play a key role in the first line of defense. LCs in the basal and suprabasal layers of epidermis are in a strategic advantageous position to capture vaccine antigens, process them, and migrate to draining lymph nodes. LCs control the space to the hard skin, as well as the inner space to the dermis. LCs mainly capture bacterial and fungal antigens, also allergens, but no viral antigens

Multi-merization. Also the langerin receptor (CD207), member of the type II receptor family, recognizes and processes microbial glycoproteins. The difference between CD205 and CD207 is the different recognition of end-standing sugars. The more diverse the carbohydrates look like in the body, the more diverse the carbohydrate-recognition domains of LLRs [19]. Even lowest differences in the glycosylation pattern compared to the wild type activate a suitable LLR that binds with high affinity to its specific carbohydrate antigen. This implicates a very high degree of variability of the LLR binding domain. Another possibility of LLRs against foreign carbohydrate antigens is the multi-merization of LLRs. As response to repetitive carbohydrate units of a given antigen, the LLR can form and consequently augment the binding capacity. Figure 2.6 illustrates the characteristic structure of a C-lectin-like receptor.

The C-type lectin and langerin receptors are generally used to identify Langerhans cells: LC (CD 207$^+$/CD205$^+$). Intradermally applied antigen is taken up by LCs within some minutes via these receptors. Even large molecules such as antibodies are able to cross the basal membrane which separates the epidermis from the dermis and are taken up by the dendrites of LCs [20].

At the same time these dendrites can expand to the opposite direction and, by passing the tight junctions, penetrate into the stratum corneum of epidermis without damage and take-up antigens [12]. Hence, LCs control the space to the hard skin as well as the inner space to the dermis. LCs are mobile and literally sentinel cells of the immune system.

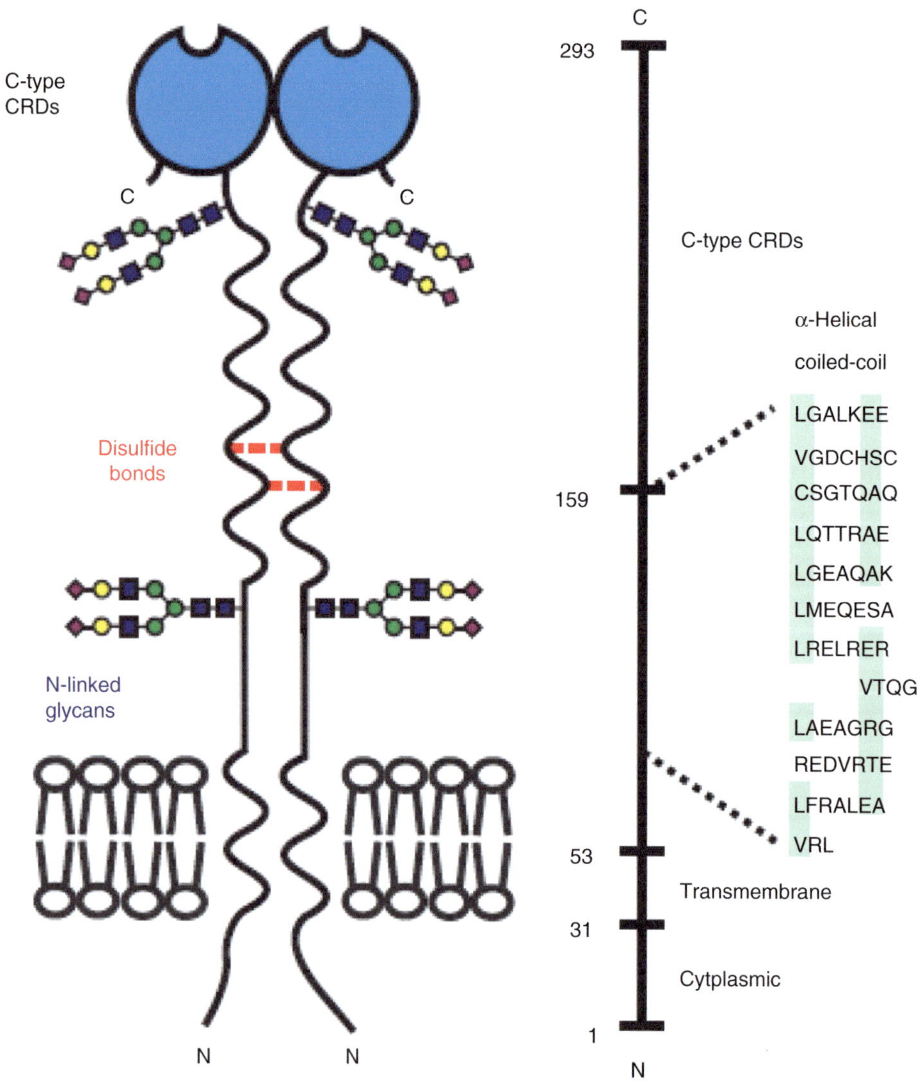

Fig. 2.6 The characteristic structure of a C-lectin-like receptor. Eukaryotic cells recognize numerous antigens by C-lectin-like receptors. One receptor is LSECtin (liver and lymph node sinusoidal endothelial cell C-type lectin). The figure describes the typical domain organization of LSECtin (*CRD* carbohydrate-recognition domain). LSECtin is a member of the type 2 receptor group of transmembrane proteins containing C-type lectin-like domains (CTLDs). The cytoplasmic tail of LSECtin contains a motif which may direct receptor internalization (Credit: Powlesland et al.; copyright © 2007 by the American Society for Biochemistry and Molecular Biology)

However, LCs mainly capture bacterial and fungal antigens, also allergens, but no viral antigens [21].

Once taken up LCs present the processed antigens via cross priming to CD8+ T cells and induce a strong cellular immune response. During this activation step, LCs produce lots of IL-15 and also IL-6 and IL-8. These essential cytokines support the maturation of cytotoxic T lymphocytes (CTLs) [22].

2.2.4 Cross Priming

Cross priming was first described in 1976 [23] and stands for the presentation of exogenously captured antigens such as debris from apoptotic or necrotic cells by APCs such as LCs to CD8+ T cells via MHC I molecules. In contrast to direct (classical) priming, it is the presentation of endogenously synthesized antigens from intracellular pathogens. Cross priming could be also another redundant mechanism of the immune system to make sure that a CTL response can be developed against such viruses which cannot infect APCs or infect APCs and deactivate the processing and presentation mechanism like MCMV [24]. The role of cross priming in natural viral infections remains controversial [25]. Cross priming is required for vaccination.

2.2.4.1 Effector Mechanisms

Once primed and activated, CD8+ cytotoxic T lymphocytes (CTLs) have a large repertoire of effector mechanisms to destroy the target cells:

- Cytotoxic proteins, e.g., perforin and granzyme A, granzyme B [26].
  In this process the direct cell-to-cell contact by the T cell receptor (TCR) and MHC I is essential.
- CTLs directly bind to the Fas-ligand (CD95L) by the Fas receptor on the target cell. This activates the caspase cascade leading to apoptosis [27].
- CTLs secrete large amount of TNF and IFN-γ. TNF binds to its receptor on the target cell, inducing apoptosis, whereas IFN-γ enhances the expression of MHC I and Fas-ligand, resulting as well in apoptosis of the target cell [28].

Figure 2.7 shows the cross priming and direct priming of CD8+ CTLs and effector mechanisms against a target cell.

2.2.5 Capture of Antigens by Dendritic Cells

The different layers of the skin are constructed like a phalanx. Could a pathogen successfully invade the epidermis, the next front line is the dermis with dermal dendritic cells (dDCs), member of the myeloid DCs family. These cells are also motile, express high levels of MCH II molecules, and can cross present viral antigens other than LCs. Two distinct populations can be described: dDCs CD1a+ and dDCs CD14+. These both populations are phenotypically and functionally quite different.

The first one exhibits a typical dendritic morphology with DC typical markers such as CD1, CD83, or CD208. Another feature is the uptake of antigens, processing, and migration to the lymph node with activation of T cells. The other subpopulation exhibits a macrophage morphology and with typical macrophage marker, such as CD14, CD68, or CD209. Those dDCs also exert a typical macrophage function, the phagocytosis of bacteria and viruses. But among these two subpopulations, there are also hybrids, phagocytotic dDCs with a dendritic morphology [11]. The common ontogenesis helps to explain this mixture of dendritic cells and macrophages. DCs can develop from macrophages following a specific stimulation. GM-CSF induces CD1, and LPS induces CD14 dendritic cells.

DC and Cytokines. In contrast to LCs, which produce little cytokines except for IL-15, especially dDCs secrete large amount of different cytokines following stimulation of CD40: IL-1α/β, IL-6, IL-7, IL-8, IL-10, IL-12, GM-CSF, TNF-α, TGF-β [29, 30]. Most of all these cytokines are produced by both dDCs subpopulations, but IL-10 is only secreted by CD14-DCs. The pattern of pro-inflammatory and anti-inflammatory cytokines indicates the direction of immune response.

2.2.6 Impact of Skin for Vaccine Development

The skin is the largest human organ. Dependent from the body size, the skin decorates 1.5–2.0 m^2 (16.1–21.5 sq. ft.). The skin is the anatomical barrier from tissue injury and pathogens and the largest immunological organ (Fig. 2.8).

A transcutaneous immunization (TCI) targets LC and other DCs. A topical application delivers the vaccine antigens to LCs of the epidermis. Needle-free and noninvasive methods are hydrogel patches containing biodegradable nanoparticles such as chitosan as carrier, liposomes, or other polymers like polyethylene glycol-based gels (PEG). Hydrophilic macromolecules as peptides/proteins cannot penetrate across the skin and need a carrier. One limitation of this application method seems that only soluble and no particulate antigens are able to induce an immune response [31]. The particle size, the hydrophilicity/hydrophobicity of the carrier, may influence the uptake by phagocytosis.

A low-invasive method are microneedle patches. Such patches are able to carry different kinds of antigens, from DNA to peptide/protein or inactivated or live virus. Lower

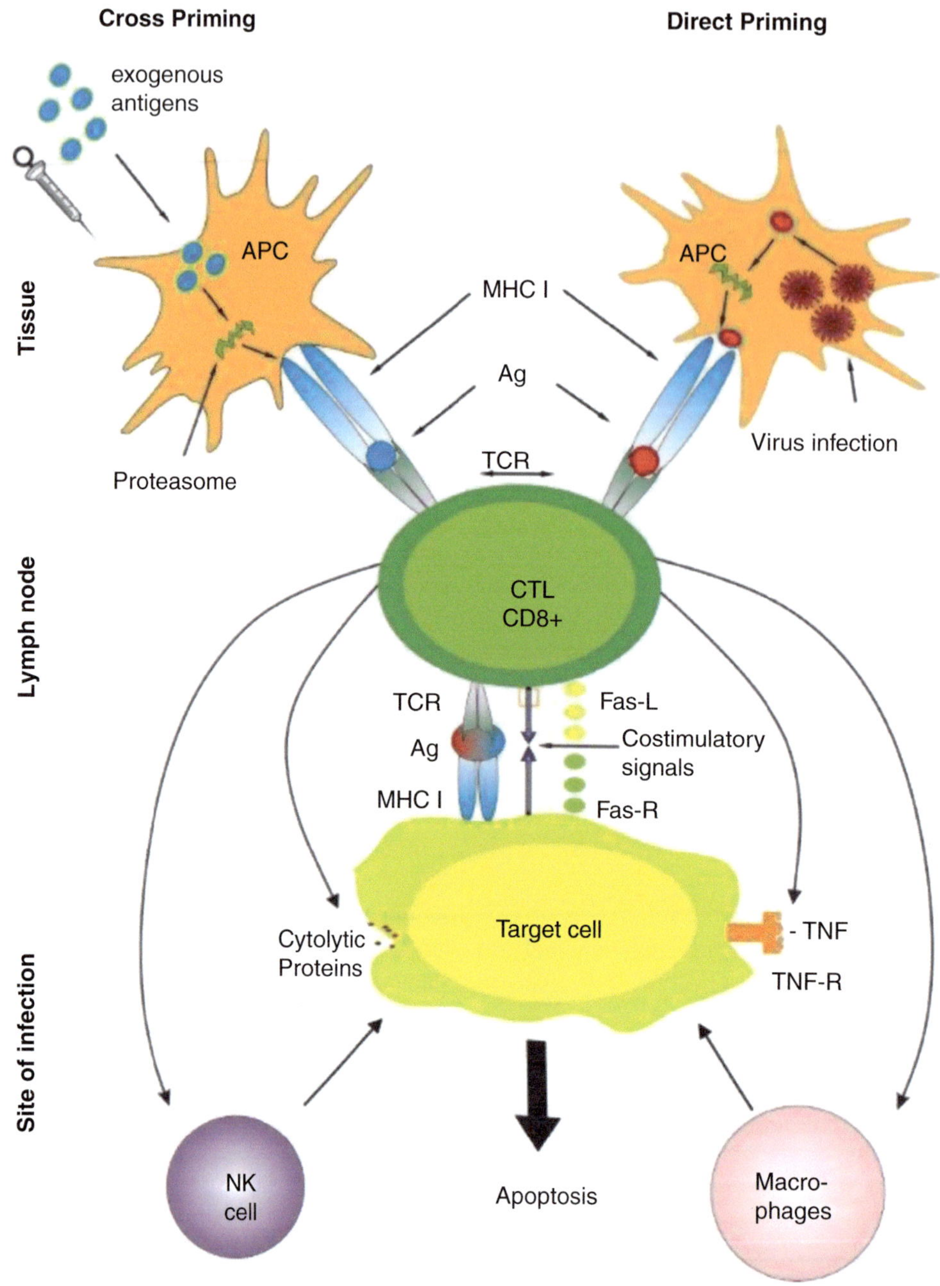

Fig. 2.7 Cross priming compared to direct priming with activated CTLs. Cross priming stands for the presentation of exogenously uptake of antigens such as debris from apoptotic or necrotic cells by APCs. Also DNA vaccination uses cross priming for activation of the cellular immune response. In contrast, direct (classical) priming stands for the presentation of endogenously synthesized antigens from intracellular pathogens. After intracellular processing, the antigens are presented via MHC I to CD8+ cytotoxic T lymphocytes. The activated CTL recognizes via its T cell receptor (*TCR*) the cognate antigen on the surface of a target cell. Several effector mechanisms can destroy the target as described before

vaccine doses are required compared to a classical intradermal injection. Needles are robust enough to penetrate the skin and to painlessly deliver the vaccine to LCs. This simple, safe, effective, and low-cost device is suitable for self-administration.

The application of antigens via electroporation targets DCs of the dermis. The electric pulses reversibly change the permeability of the cell membrane and therefore the antigen can penetrate the cell.

Besides this simple in vivo targeting of APCs by cutaneous immunization routes, a more complicated ex vivo method for direct targeting DCs was developed as whole cell vaccine. DCs were isolated from patient's blood, cultivated in vitro, and challenged with an antigen, e.g., a tumor

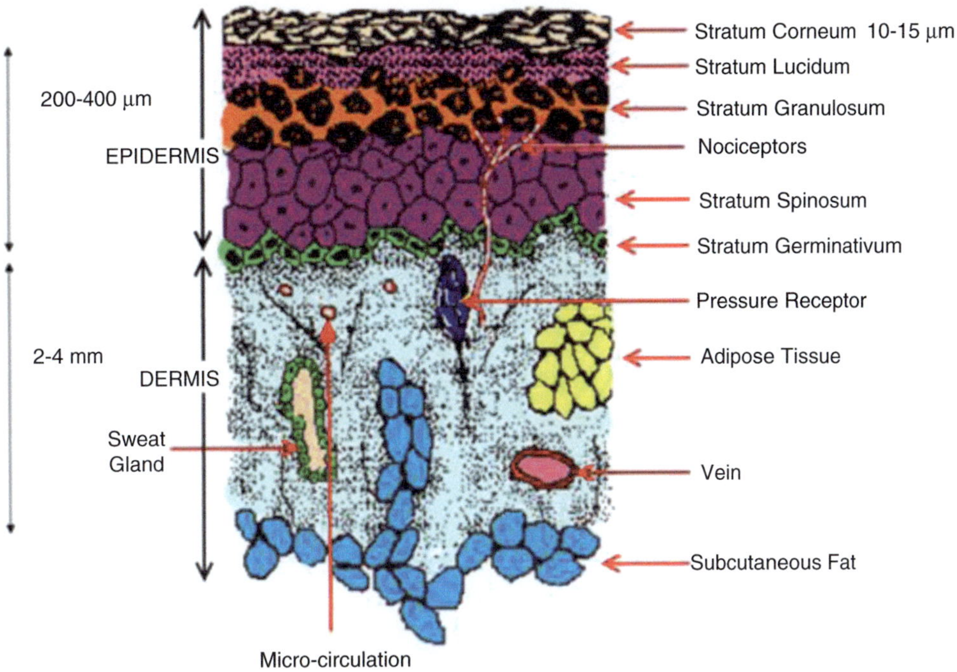

Fig. 2.8 Diagrammatic representation of the major features of the skin anatomy

antigen (TA). By the uptake of the TAs, the maturation of the DCs is activated and the TAs are processed. After a complex procedure in the laboratory of 3–5 days, the patient is injected with his autologous TA loaded DCs which in vivo alert T and B cells. In 2010 the US FDA has approved Sipuleucel-T, the first personalized cellular autologous immunotherapy for the treatment of advanced prostate cancer [32].

Various delivery technologies for vaccines are discussed in Chap. 10.

2.3 Inflammation and Cytokines

Inflammation is following a microbial infection by bacteria, viruses, fungi, or other pathogens. Further inducers for inflammation are trauma or toxins, reactive T cells, and more. The function of an inflammatory reaction is to prevent an infection at a very early start by producing pro-inflammatory cytokines such as IL-1, IL-6, IL-8, and TNF-α. Other cytokines exert a pleiotropic nature acting both pro-inflammatory and anti-inflammatory [33].

2.3.1 Pro-inflammatory Cytokines

IL-1 and TNF operate in a synergistic manner and upregulate a cascade of genes, e.g., for type II phospholipase A2 (PLA2) and cylooxygenase-2 (COX-2), or the inducible NO synthetase (iNO) resulting in the production of chemotactic enzymes. These enzymes attract new immune cells like macrophages, NK cells, or neutrophils to the site of infection. At the same time blood vessels dilate and become more permeable. Other cytokines such as IL-4, TGF-β, and especially IL-10 control and suppress the inflammation process, and hence they support the healing. These cytokines act as anti-inflammatory and account for the pivotal immune balance. Therefore, every therapeutic intervention of the immune homeostasis must be very carefully calculated.

2.3.2 Anti-inflammatory Cytokines

IL-10 plays a key role in immune suppression besides IL-4 and TGF-β. IL-10 is a master cytokine, powerfully monitoring the immunopathological milieu after infections. IL-10 is under normal conditions essential to regulate the inflammation. Different T cell subsets produce IL-10, such as Th1, Th2, and Th17, but also eosinophils and neutrophils [34], NK cells, DC, and B cells [35, 36]. This cell variability and redundancy in anti-inflammatory cytokine production gives rise to a multiple immune regulation on multiple levels with the only aim to suppress the inflammatory response triggered by IFN-γ, IL-2, or TNF and other pro-inflammatory cytokines (Table 2.5).

Table 2.5 Major pro- and anti-inflammatory cytokines

Pro-inflammatory cytokines	Major producer cells	Main functions
IL-1	Macrophages Fibroblast endothelial cells	Inducing the release of IL-2 Influencing growth/differentiation of B cells Causing fever Inducing synthesis of acute phase proteins Tissue damage
IL-2	T cells	Acts as T cell growth factor (*TCGF*)
IL-6	Macrophages Fibroblasts	Influencing B cell maturation (B cell stimulatory factor 2) Inducing synthesis of acute phase proteins
IL-8	Macrophages/monocytes Endothelial cells	Chemoattractant for neutrophils, basophils, and T cells Potent angiogenic factor
IL-12	Macrophages DCs	IL-12 promotes the development of Th1 responses; powerful inducer of IFN-γ production by T and NK cells
TNF-α (or cachectin)	Macrophages Lymphoid cells Mast cells, endothelial cells	Stimulating the acute phase response Chemoattractant for neutrophils Stimulation of inflammatory lipid prostaglandin E2 (PGE_2)
IFN-γ	Macrophages DCs NK cells Th1 cells	Activation of macrophages Induction of MHC II molecules
Anti-inflammatory cytokines	**Major producer cells**	**Main functions**
IL-13	Th2 cells	Molecular bridge between allergic inflammatory cells to the nonimmune cells: altering physiological functions by cell to cell contact
IL-10 (master cytokine)	Macrophages Th1, Th2, Th17 eosinophils Neutrophils NK cells DC B cells	Downregulation of Th1 cytokine expression Downregulation the expression of MHC II Co-stimulatory molecules on macrophages IL-10 can block NF-kappa B activity
IL-4	Th2 cells	Stimulation of activated B and T cells IL-4 decreases the production of Th1 cells, and of IL-12, IFN-γ of DCs and macrophages
IL-1Ra	Macrophages/monocytes Neutrophils	Antagonist of IL-1receptor and inhibits IL-1 activities
TGF-β	Secreted by many cell types including macrophage	TGF-β induces apoptosis in numerous cell types TGF-β appears to block the activation of lymphocytes and monocyte-derived phagocytes Immunosuppressive effects on several immune cells

Because IFN-γ and IL-2 are important for the establishment of a cellular response, the impact of IL-10 leads to a shift from a mainly Th1 response toward a mainly Th2 response. Not only the T cell-mediated immunity but also the maturation and function of DCs are influenced by this cytokine, and the overall cytokine pattern has changed following IL-10 secretion. IL-10 acts directly on APC cells to decrease accessory molecules such as B7, necessary for MHC I and II. Otherwise, IL-10 stimulates the proliferation of CD4+ T cells, thereby enhancing a humoral response.

IL-10 is a key cytokine bridging the innate and acquired immune reactivity, on the one hand constitutively produced by macrophages and on the other hand produced by T cells after specific stimulation.

2.3.3 IL-10 as Biomarker

IL-10 takes a special role in some intracellular infections by diverse pathogens. Some bacteria, fungi, viruses, or parasites induce IL-10 by binding to their specific pattern recognition receptor (PRR) and activating gene expression. For this reason, IL-10 can be also used as biomarker, as surrogate marker of some infections. The level of IL-10 production seems to be dependent on the intensity of the PRR stimulation. TNF will be immediately downregulated; consequently, the complete inflammatory response falls down. Because of the lack of TNF, probably the main inducer, the apoptosis gets down.

The significant contribution of IL-10 to chronic infections must be considered critically. In these special conditions, IL-10 acts as *devil molecule* because it prevents a strong inflammation response and so avoiding the clearance of the pathogen [37]. Obviously, various microorganisms enact escape strategies of targeted induction of IL-10 for their persistence.

Leishmaniasis is caused by an obligate intracellular and zoonotic parasite of the genus *Leishmania*, causative agent for a group of related diseases such as viscerale (VL), cutaneous, or mucosal/mucocutaneous leishmaniasis as far as fatal systemic infection.

The estimated worldwide prevalence is 12 million cases, annual mortality of 60,000, occurring in 4 continents, endemic in 88 countries, 72 of which are developing countries. According to WHO, two million people will be newly infected annually.

IL-10 and Vaccination. A special situation is given to VL as an important opportunistic coinfection associated with HIV, an underestimated combination. Both pathogens reinforce each other. There is as yet no effective vaccine. One reason is given to the escape strategy of *Leishmania* spp., evasion by IL-10. BALB/c mice were primed by a DNA vaccine, coding either for LACK (*Leishmania* homolog of receptors for activated C-kinase) or for TRYP (tryparedoxin peroxidase) and boosted by the corresponding antigen in modified vaccinia virus Ankara (MVA) and challenged by L. major. LACK-vaccinated mice developed a high level of IL-10 due to Treg cells. The Th1 response was at the same time downregulated, resulting in a lack of IFN-γ and TNF production. But the blocking of IL-10 receptors enhanced the IFN-γ production up to 3.5-fold. Conclusion: The DNA/MVA-LACK vaccine did not work. Other than the vaccination with TRYP, the level of IL-10 was low, but the level of IFN-γ high. TRYP-vaccinated mice were fully protected after the challenge with L. major [38].

Low IFN-γ and High IL-10. These studies demonstrate that *Leishmania* spp. are able to survive and persist by using the host cytokine IL-10. Furthermore, the level of IL-10 titer in correlation to the level of IFN-γ could be a predictive biomarker of the success of a vaccination. The choice of an appropriate antigen will influence the direction of response, toward a Th1 or Th2, toward a cellular or humoral reactivity.

In order to monitor the clinical process of vicerale leishmaniasis infection, the level of IL-10 titer is measured among others. The correlation to the parasite load is significant. Also the corresponding titer of IFN-γ is significant: A low IFN-γ titer goes along with a high titer of IL-10. So, the titer of IL-10 is an indirect biomarker for the severeness of this parasitic infection [39]. Other pathogens, like *Trypanosoma cruzi*, *Klebsiella pneumoniae*, or *Candida albicans*, also highjack IL-10 to prevent an immune attack.

IL-10 as Virokine. The impact of IL-10 as an immune modulator is also expressed in the context with some viruses. Such viruses code for their own IL-10 homolog (vIL-10) and can directly influence the immune response against them. The first vIL-10 was described for Epstein–Barr virus (EBV) in 1990 [40]. The homology on protein level to the huIL-10 is 70 %.

There are also viruses not possessing their own gene encoding such as virokines. These viruses circumvent the lack of vIL-10 by expressing a special viral protein which upregulates the host production of IL-10 [41].

Meanwhile IL-10 is also used as prognostic factor for some cancer diseases. A high IL-10 expression is significantly associated with aggressive clinical manifestations in melanoma and squamous cell carcinoma [42, 43].

2.4 Therapeutic Vaccines and the Immunosuppressive Environment

Pro-inflammatory cytokines such as interleukin-1β (IL-1β), interleukin-6 (IL-6), and tumor necrosis factor-α (TNF-α) are responsible for the initiation of inflammation in response to infections, tissue damage, or cancer development [44]. This activates a cell-mediated immune response. Anti-inflammatory cytokines are also released to fine-tune and to balance this immune reaction and to limit the sustained inflammatory reactions.

2.4.1 Immunosuppression

The central role of IL-10 is to supervise the inflammation reaction, whether in microbial infections or in cancer diseases. IL-10 suppresses effector functions of macrophages, T cells, B cells, NK cells, and mast cells. Other cytokines are also involved in controlling the inflammation, such as TGF-β, by blocking IL-1α/β of monocytes/macrophages by IL-1 receptor analogist (IL-1Ra); IL-4, by blocking the binding of pro-inflammatory cytokines to their specific receptors; IL-6, by inhibition of TNF or other cytokines such as IL-1; or IL-11, by promoting a Th2 response (Fig. 2.9).

Dichotomous Nature. It must be noted that with the exception of IL-1Ra and further soluble cytokine receptors, all anti-inflammatory cytokines have a dichotomous nature and can also perform pro-inflammatory activities [45].

In all immunosuppressive events, the aim of anti-inflammatory cytokines is to downregulate T effector functions resulting in a local immunosuppressive milieu. Only with this prior condition, pathogens can persist and tumor cells can proliferate. The immune regulatory network has changed from protection against pathogens to a severe protection of the nested pathogens.

As some microbial pathogens encode for own IL-10 as part of their escape strategy as some tumors secrete IL-10 or TGF-β also as part of their escape strategy enhancing the local dominance of anti-inflammatory molecules and the establishment of an immunosuppressive environment to evade the protective immune response. Also tumor-associated macrophages secrete many cytokines which promote immunosuppression [46].

Any therapeutic vaccination has to overcome this strong bastion of anti-vaccine activities where the antigen presenta-

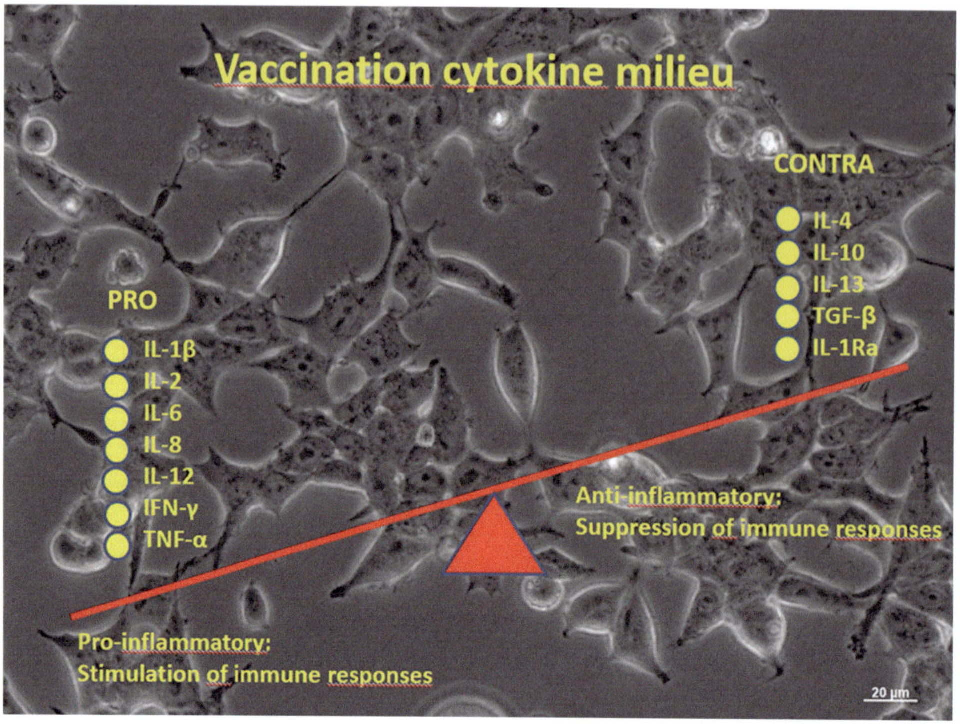

Fig. 2.9 A therapeutic vaccine is confronted with a strong bastion of anti-vaccine activities. CONTRA: Anti-inflammatory cytokines downregulate T effector functions resulting in a local immunosuppressive milieu. The immune regulatory network has changed from protection against pathogens to a severe protection of the nested pathogens. CTL activities are reduced; antigen presentation by DCs is abolished. PRO: For vaccination pro-inflammatory cytokines have to prepare the necessary immune milieu. Without this prerequisite, a therapeutic vaccination does not work (Photo: 293-TK cells by S. Giese, University of Freiburg/Germany)

tion by DCs or the MHC I and II is reduced or abolished, the CTL activities reduced or stopped. The failure of such vaccines is to restore not effectively the T cell immunity against the persisting pathogens and then maintain this status of restored inflammatory response against the status of immunosuppression. The fact alone that bacteria, viruses, and parasites use pathogen-encoded or host-encoded proteins to survive within the host demonstrates the high priority of pro-inflammatory cytokines and the related essential cellular activities as defense strategy against invading microorganisms and cancer diseases.

Based on this knowledge, a therapeutic vaccine must fulfill at least three fundamental functions as shown in Table 2.6.

Table 2.6 Therapeutic vaccine functions

Anti-inflammatory:
Dam up the anti-inflammatory process

↓

Pro-inflammatory:
Reconstitution of the pro-inflammatory environment

↓

T cell immunity:
Repeated exposure of multiple antigens to reconstitute the T cell immunity

2.5 Pathogen Recognition

The long cascade of an antigen-specific immune reaction is started upon the recognition of an antigen by APCs via their pathogen recognition receptors (PRR) to generate a B and T lymphocyte immune response.

These germline-encoded PRRs are part of the innate immune system and cross link the innate with the acquired immunity which depends on clonal expansion of B and T cells. There is a permanent cross talk between innate and acquired immunity with a clear hierarchy. The PRRs form the base of a highly efficient and redundant receptor network for permanent monitoring of pathogens and dangerous self-antigens. PRRs are expressed on the cell surface or are located in endosomes or in cytoplasm. This redundant system guarantees that a pathogen can be detected in parallel by different sensors. If one sensor fails another, PRR is active to trace this antigen. This high level of redundancy could be one reason why estimated 98 % of all infections in a healthy patient are detected and cured by the immune systems.

Pattern Recognition Receptors (PRR). The theoretical basis of the mechanisms of pathogen recognition was developed by Charles Janeway. In 1989, he postulated that each APCs would express pattern recognition receptors (PRR), recognizing pathogens on a specific conserved pattern of molecular structures called "pathogen-associated molecular patterns" (PAMPs) [47].

2.5.1 Non-Toll-Like Receptors

In addition to Toll-like receptors (TLRs), meanwhile other classes of innate PRRs, chemically and structurally different from TLRs were described. As against TLRs little is known about the precise molecular mechanisms of most of all non-TLRs:

1. *NLRs* – nucleotide binding and oligomerization domain (NOD) – like receptors (NLRs). From the human NLR family are to date 22 members known, the most prominent are NOD1 and NOD2 which control bacterial infections and inflammation [48].
2. *RLRs* – the retinoid acid-inducible gene I (RIG-I)-like receptors (RLRs). This family comprises three members, the retinoic acid-inducible gene I (RIG-I), the melanoma differentiation-associated gene 5 (MDA5), and laboratory of genetics and physiology 2 (LGP2), and plays a key role in sensing viral RNA [49].
3. *CLRs* – C-type lectin receptors. Members of this diverse family of 17 subfamilies act as soluble PRR or also membrane bound. Dectin-1 and dectin-2 receptors mainly detect mannose and glucan structures and, besides these dominant carbohydrates, also proteins and lipids. CLRs have been implicated especially in anti-fungus immunity [50, 51].
4. *DNA sensors*, i.e., DAI, the DNA-dependent activator of IFN-regulatory factors, or AIM2 (absent in melanoma 2), or the indirect sensing of dsDNA by the RNA Polymerase III, a polymerase which transcribes AT-rich dsDNA into dsRNA, which in turn is now able to activate (RIG-I)-like receptors [52]. These DNA sensors recognize cytosolic DNA [53].

Toll Gene of *Drosophila*. In 1996, the first Toll PRR was characterized in *Drosophila* [54], and only one year later the first "Toll-like" receptor (TLR) was described in humans [55]. The Toll gene of *Drosophila* was isolated in 1988, and the Toll protein is characterized as an integral membrane protein with a cytoplasmic and a large extra cytoplasmic domain [56].

In contrast to most of TLRs which are mainly sensors for extracellular pathogens, non-TLRs are located within the cell [57]. Table 2.7 gives and overviews the different classes of PRRs.

The immense significance of the germline-encoded PRRs for the immune defense against pathogens is highlighted by their high quantity and distribution within the animal kingdom, from arthropods to vertebrates, from insects to mammals, the whole evolution preserved in this receptor family.

Table 2.7 Classes of different PRRs, ligands, and cellular distribution

Toll-like receptors	Ligand	Cellular distribution
TLR2/1	Triacyl lipopeptides,soluble lipoproteins	B-cells, NK-cells, DCs, macrophages, fibroblast cells, epithelial cells and endothelial cells
TLR2	Peptidoglycan, Lipoteichoic acid, Lipoarabinomannan, Zymosan	B-cells, NK-cells, DCs, macrophages, fibroblast cells, epithelial cells and endothelial cells
TLR4	LPS, flavolipin	B-cells, NK-cells, DCs, macrophages, fibroblast cells, epithelial cells and endothelial cells
TLR5	Flagellin	B-cells, NK-cells, DCs, macrophages, fibroblast cells, epithelial cells and endothelial cells
TLR6/2	Diacyl lipopeptides	B-cells, NK-cells, DCs, macrophages, fibroblast cells, epithelial cells and endothelial cells
TLR3	dsRNA	B-cells, NK-cells, DCs, macrophages, fibroblast cells, epithelial cells and endothelial cells
TLR7	ssRNAs rich in guanosine or uridine	B-cells, NK-cells, DCs, macrophages, fibroblast cells, epithelial cells and endothelial cells
TLR8	ssRNAs rich in guanosine or uridine	B-cells, NK-cells, DCs, macrophages, fibroblast cells, epithelial cells and endothelial cells
TLR9	unmethy. CpGs, Hemozoin in parasites	B-cells, NK-cells, DCs, macrophages, fibroblast cells, epithelial cells and endothelial cells
TLR10	the most probable ligand seems to be a bacterial peptide	lymphoid tissues such as spleen, lymph node, thymus, and tonsil

NOD-like receptors	Ligand	Cellular distribution
NOD1	γ-D-glutamyl-*m*-diaminopimelic acid	e.g. DCs
NOD2	muramyl-dipeptide (MDP)	e.g. DCs
NLRP1	activated by lethal toxin	e.g. DCs
NLRP3	Pathogen derieved toxins e.g. M2 of influenza	e.g. DCs
NLRP7	acylated lipopeptides	e.g. DCs

RIG-like receptors	Ligand	Cellular distribution
RIG-1	dsRNA with blunt ends, ssRNA with 5' triphosphate, RNA panhandle structure	all cells except for pDCs
MDA5	long synthetic dsRNA RNaseL-cleaved self-RNAs with monophosphate ends	all cells except for pDCs
LGP2	neg./pos. regulator for RIG-1/MDA5	all cells except for pDCs

C-type lectin receptors	Ligand	Cellular distribution
Dectin-1	β-1,3-glucan (fungal pathogens)	Phagocytic immune cells
Dectin-2	high-mannose structures	predominantly expressed on tissue macrophages, DCs and inflammatory monocytes
Macrophage-inducible C-type lectin	variety of endogenous and exogenous ligands e.g. SAP130, α-mannan, trehalose dimycolate, mycobacterial cord factor	predominantly expressed by activated macrophages

DNA sensors	Ligand	Cellular distribution
AIM2	cytosolic DNA	macrophages
p202		
IFI16	cytosolic DNA	
IFIX		
DDX41		

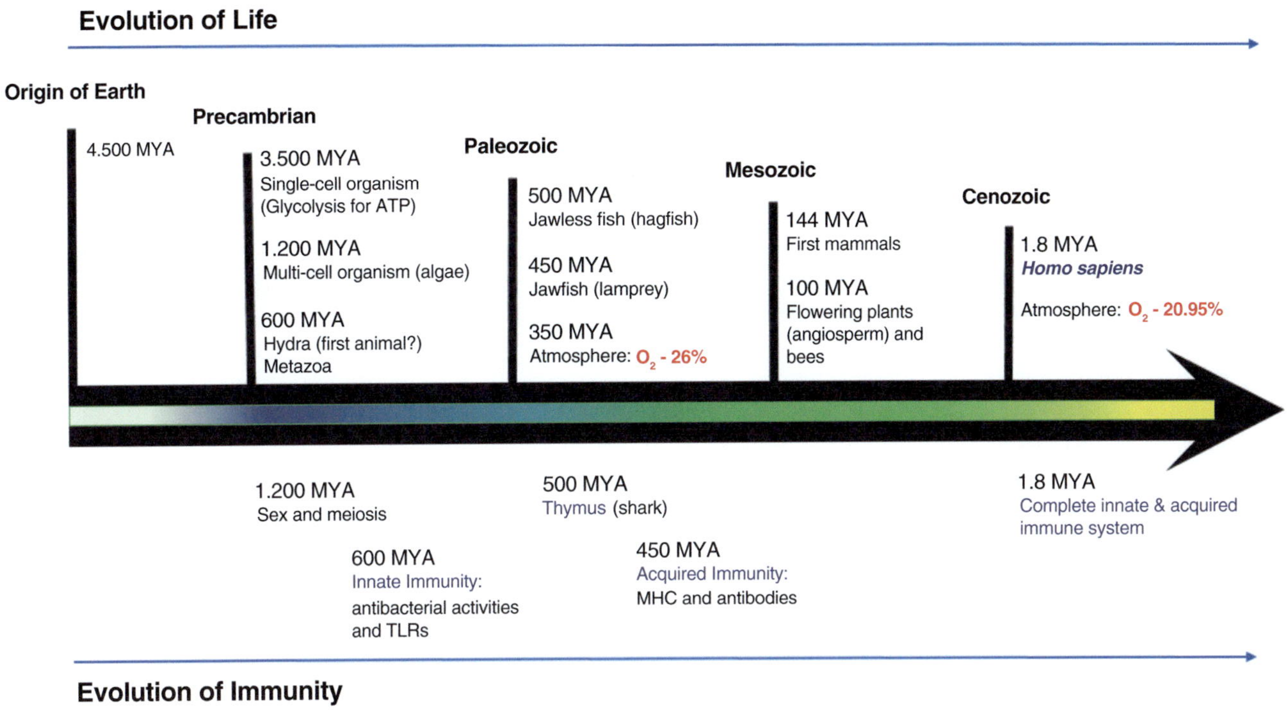

Fig. 2.10 Short timeline of evolutionary major events in the development from innate to acquired immunity, measured in millions of years ago (MYA) (Figure prepared for this book by S. Giese, Institute of Virology, University of Freiburg/Germany)

500 PRRs. A study from 2007 counts for around 500 PRRs, among them 177 TLRs, detected in 77 distinct organisms [58]. Insects don't have a specific acquired immunity, but only an innate, like plants. In addition, the discovery of the evolutionarily ancient PRRs emphasizes the dominant role of the innate immunity against the mammalian-acquired immunity.

The pacemaker of the immune response cascade is the innate system, even though innate and acquired immunity work hand in hand. A short view on the evolution of key steps toward the development of a complete immune system is shown in Fig. 2.10 and illustrates the ancient role of the innate immunity.

Different PRRs work together to sense an individual pathogen and to adjust immune defenses to its evolving virulence structures displayed during infection.

Dependent on their functions, PRRs can be divided into two functional groups as shown in Table 2.8.

Table 2.8 Types of PRRs dependent on their functions

Scanvenger receptors	• **Responsible for phagocytosis of microorganisms without relaying intracellular signals, e.g., mannose receptors.**
Signaling receptors	• **With relaying intracellular signals for triggering the innate and acquired immunity, e.g., TLRs.**

2.5.2 Toll-Like Receptor

TLRs are the best-characterized sensors among the heterogeneous group of PRRs and recognize both exogenous and endogenous pathogen-associated molecular patterns (PAMPs), but also endogenous damage-associated molecular patterns (DAMPs). DAMPs arise from cancer cells, necrotic cells, tissue injury, or degradation processes.

Currently there are 10 TLRs discovered in humans, 13 in mouse. The TLR10 is restricted to humans only.

Distribution. TLRs can be found in DCs, macrophages, and monocytes, T cells, B cells, and NK cells. Moreover, TLRs are also expressed on normal tissue cells, such as endothelial cells and fibroblasts; on muscle cells; and on cartilage and osteochondral tissues, namely, on chondrocytes, osteoblasts, and osteoclasts. Recently, TLR expression was also detected in fat tissue, on adipocytes [59], in the liver, on hepatocytes [60], and in the spleen [61]. This broad ubiquitous distribution of TLRs on various cells, in different tissues, and in different organs underlines the systemic significance for the innate immunity with its inflammation responses and the development of an acquired immunity [62] (Fig. 2.11).

TLRs and Cell Surface. The TLR1, TLR2, TLR4, TLR5, TLR6, and TLR10 are located on the cell surface. They are type 1 α-helical transmembrane glycoproteins: The leucine-rich ectodomain comprises the ligand-binding site, a single membrane-standing α-helix, and a cytoplasmic Toll/interleukin-1 receptor (TIR) domain, responsible for the downstream signal transduction. These cell surface TLRs are specialized to recognize and bind structures of gram-negative and gram-positive bacteria.

TLR1 recognizes soluble lipoproteins, e.g., *Neisseria meningitides*. TLR2 recognizes lipoproteins and also glycolipids of, e.g., *Mycoplasma* and *Treponema maltophilum*. TLR2 acts as heterodimer together with TLR1, TLR6, or TLR10. TLR2 is also specialized on fungal ligands like zymosan.

Lipopolysaccharide. One of the best investigated pathogenic structures is lipopolysaccharide, LPS. TLR4 binds LPS via interacting with the myeloid differentiation protein, MD-2, forming a tandem TLR4/MD-2. This tandem is the molecular basis for binding of lipid A, the biologically active component of LPS (for a schematic figure of LPS, see Chap. 7). In this process, the coreceptor MD-2 is responsible for binding of the fatty acids by binding the acyl groups [63].

Additional nonbacterial ligands for TLR4 other than lipid A are, e.g., gp52 envelope protein of MMT-virus, or fusion protein of RS virus, or endogenous ligands, such as the heat shock proteins HSP60, HSP70.

TLR5 is the only TL receptor for binding pure proteins. TLR5 recognizes a highly conserved region of bacterial flagellins, and thus this receptor is able to recognize and bind a broad spectrum of microbes.

Little is known of TLR10 with the exception that TLR10 and TLR1 form a heterodimer. It is speculated that TLR10 recognizes bacterial peptides.

In summary, TLR1, TLR2, TLR4, TLR5, TLR6, and TLR10 are specialized to bind bacterial and other pathogenic lipoproteins, glycolipids and lipopolysaccharides, beyond that viral envelop proteins or endogenous structures described from tissue damage or other degradation processes, such as heat shock proteins.

TLRs and Nucleic Acids. TLR3, TLR7, TLR8, and TLR9 are located in the endosome and recognize exclusively nucleic acids in terms of bacterial, viral, or host-derived DNA and RNA. TLR3 binds dsRNA and can also be activated by the synthetic dsRNA polyI:C. Furthermore, this receptor binds host-derived mRNA and tRNA.

The special character of TLR3 as antivirus receptor is demonstrated by the induction of type I interferons (IFNs) and the subsequent innate antiviral activities after binding to TLR3. Natural dsRNA normally arises during viral replication. However, natural-derived dsRNA is only a weak activator of TLR3 in vitro. TLR7 preferentially expressed on pDCs, like TLR8, and TLR9 bind ssRNA and are activated especially by viruses causing chronic infections. The activation of these receptors also induces IFNs. TLR9 recognizes unmethylated bacterial ssDNA, CpGs, but also viral DNA, e.g., HSV1,2 [64, 65] in contrast to other nucleic acid binding receptors.

TLR7 and Virus. Inactivated viral vaccines use TLR7. This could be very clearly demonstrated with inactivated whole influenza A virus. The viral RNA was bound by TLR7 on pDCs leading to a massive production of IFN-α. It is important to note that the process of virus inactivation does not influence the binding properties and hence does not also influence the endosomal receptor capacities, in contrast to a recombinant flu vaccine which is only composed of proteins, or a split vaccine, where the viruses are destroyed by detergents, and the viral RNA is eliminated by purification procedures. An activation of TLR7 by recombinant or split vaccines does not happen [66, 67].

TLR9 and CpG. The natural bacterial backbone of a DNA vaccine itself is able to activate the TLR9. But this natural adjuvant effect is very weak probably due the fact that the vaccine pDNA is mainly a dsDNA and not ssDNA. To improve this weak adjuvant effect, several synthetic species-specific CpGs can be incorporated into the DNA vector on the same plasmid or on an extra plasmid [64].

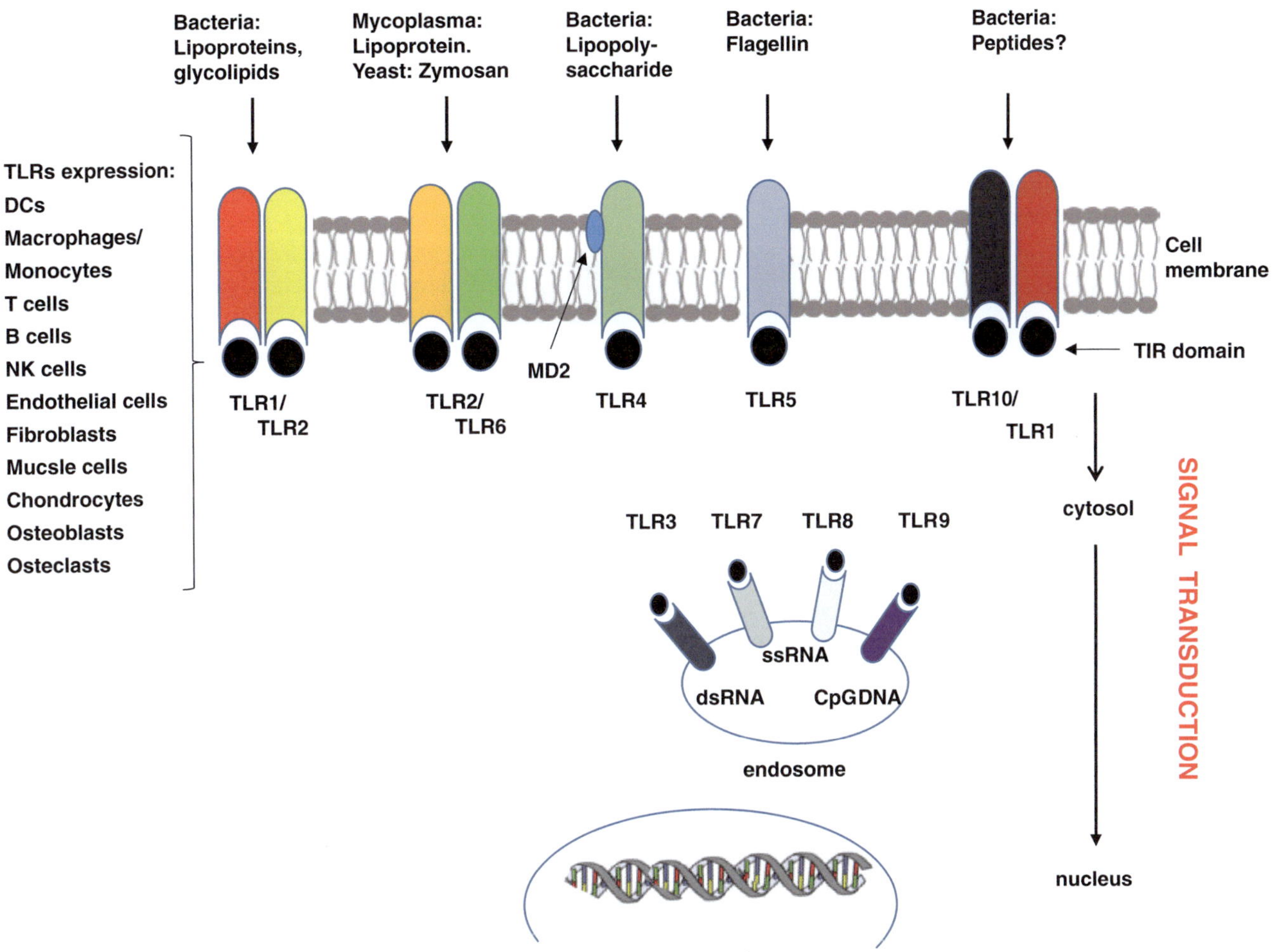

Fig. 2.11 Toll-like receptors and known ligands. TLRs recognize pathogen-derived ligands by their ectodomains and trigger innate immune responses via signal transduction leading to activation of target genes. Currently there are 10 TLRs discovered in humans, 13 in mouse. TLR10 is restricted to humans only. TLR1, TLR2, TLR4, TLR5, TLR6, and TLR10 are located on the cell surface and are type 1 α-helical transmembrane glycoproteins: The leucine-rich ectodomain comprises the ligand-binding site, a single membrane-standing α-helix, and a cytoplasmic TIR domain, responsible for the downstream signal transduction. TLR3, TLR7, TLR8, and TLR9 are located in the endosome and recognize exclusively nucleic acids in terms of bacterial, viral, or host-derived DNA and RNA. This broad ubiquitous distribution of TLRs on various cells, in different tissues, and in different organs underlines the systemic significance for the innate immunity with its inflammation responses

2.6 PAMPs: Pathogen-Associated Molecular Patterns

TLRs and also other PRRs identify bacteria, viruses, fungi, protozoa, and parasites by their unique, highly specific, and highly conserved pathogen-associated molecular patterns, PAMPs. All sensors use PAMPs also to discriminate "self" from "non-self." Not all ligand-recognition mechanisms are fully understood. Major PAMP ligands (shown in Fig. 2.1) and known structural features are:

1. *Lipids*: Chain lengths are recognized, e.g., triacyl (TLR1), diacyl (TLR2), and hexa-acyl of LPS (TLR4). The conserved pattern of LPS is the lipid A. The immunostimulant monophosphoryl lipid A (MLP) used as adjuvant contains only five lipid chains. And, in contrast to the natural LPS, the inflammatory activity is about 100 less and a weak activator of the innate immune response [68].
2. *Proteins*: The leucine-rich repeat (LRR) domain consisting of 2–45 LL repeats, with each repeat about 20–30 residues long is the target PAMP for PRRs. These PRRs contain themselves a LL domain and the resulting receptor-ligand complex consists of a protein–protein interaction [69].
3. *Carbohydrates*: Complex sugars form with protein glycoproteins or with lipid glycolipids. Some TLRs and CLRs recognize complex sugars, such as mannose, glucose, or galactose, via their carbohydrate-recognition domain (CRD), a domain within the lectin multidomain protein [70].
4. *RNA*: Many PRR sensing RNA are known for recognizing not only non-self but also self RNA under pathological

conditions. Therefore, several RNA recognition features are essential for the identification of "non-self" RNA, e.g., primary nucleotide sequence, secondary and tertiary structure, or intracellular localization [71].

5. *DNA*: The molecular pattern for PRR recognition of bacterial DNA is the stringent hypomethylation compared to vertebrate DNA. Microbial DNA contains a high frequency of unmethylated cytosine–phosphate–guanine (CpG) dinucleotides [72].

2.7 DAMPs: Damage-Associated Molecular Patterns

It is a commonplace to talk about immune system's ability to react against foreign pathogens. But perhaps the immune system does not react explicitly not a bit against non-self, but react only against any "danger," irrespectively of the source. This danger hypothesis was presented first by Matzinger in 1994 [73]: "For many years immunologists have been well served by the viewpoint that the immune system's primary goal is to discriminate between self and non-self. I believe… that its primary driving force is the need to detect and protect against danger…."

DAMPs or Alarmins. Today danger signals are defined analogous to PAMPs as endogenous host-encoded proteins which are released after cellular stress, tissue injury, and necrotic cell destruction, in the complete absence of any pathogen. Those molecules are collectively called damage-associated molecular patterns, DAMPs, sometimes also called alarmins. Many DAMPs are nuclear or cytosolic proteins, and also extracellular matrix proteins (ECM), which are either upregulated or released following tissue injury. These normally hidden proteins send a signal "danger" resulting in a sterile inflammation. Substances in this process released from damaged cells change now from the intracellular reducing to the extracellular oxidizing milieu, leading to a dramatical change of the extracellular redox milieu.

Oxidative Stress. One consequence of this disordered redox milieu could be a chronic inflammation. Examples of such substances are different so-called leaderless secretory proteins (LSPs), like high mobility group B 1 molecule, HMGB 1, or IL-18. These proteins are strong mediators of inflammation and be involved in the oxidative stress [74, 75]. DAMPs like PAMPs are bound by the same set of PRRs. DAMP ligands are described for TLR1, TLR2, TLR3, TLR4, TLR7, TLR8, and TLR9 [76]. There is also a synergy described between endogenously derived DAMPs and exogenously derived microbial PAMPs leading to a common innate immune response [77].

Besides intra- and extracellular proteins, lipoproteins, glycoproteins, or nonproteins like genomic DNA and RNA molecules, some major DAMP ligands which can activate the immune system are:

1. *Mitochondrial DAMPs, MTDs.* Peptides and DNA from mitochondria, the intracellular organelles responsible for providing the energy of a cell, and released after cell disruption after trauma [78].
2. *High mobility group B 1 molecule, HMGB 1.* An ubiquitous nuclear chromatin-associated protein which acts as a transcription factor and is released, e.g., from necrotic but not apoptotic cancer cells or actively secreted by macrophages during the early pro-inflammation phase [79].
3. *Heat shock proteins, HSPs.* A family of highly conserved ubiquitous proteins acting as chaperons and responsible for the correct folding and transport of proteins. Hsp90, e.g., plays an important role in antigen presentation and maturation of DCs and is released by necrotic cells [80].
4. *S-100 proteins.* A family of at least 21 members of calcium-binding proteins, and beside other functions in cell grow, differentiation also involved in inflammation. Some S-100 proteins are useful as tumor markers, and the release of the intracellular S100A8 or S100A9 into the extracellular medium is a strong danger signal [81].
5. *Hyaluron acid fragments, HA.* A carbohydrate polymer, non-sulfated glycoglycans, and part of the extracellular matrix (ECM). Degradation products of HA can be found rapidly after tissue injury at the site of inflammation [82].

2.8 TLR Intracellular Signal Cascade and Immune Response

The only function of antigen binding to TLR or another PRR, regardless of the origin, PAMP, or DAMP, is to induce an immune response against this captured antigen. This response must be reasonable, a balance between Th1and Th2 actions, a more Th2 or a more Th1 response, or a switch between Th1 and Th2. This response should also be effective and not directed against phantoms such as decoy epitopes. Based on these assumptions, the immune reaction must be time limited, coordinated, controlled, well appropriate, and leading to a memory effect.

To meet all these assumptions, a precisely adjusted signal cascade to the individual situation within the APC usually happens. The final outcome is the specific activation of selected immune-relevant genes. Thereby, about 150 genes can be activated and expressed. The cross talk within the signal cascade is essential in order that a protective and not pathological immune response will be induced. A set of mitogen-activated protein (MAP) kinases governs the activation of the signal cascade. A MAP feature is the three-tiered classical pathway; three kinases are connected in series. In contrast to classical MAPKs, a two-tiered system is described for atypical MAPKs (Fig. 2.12).

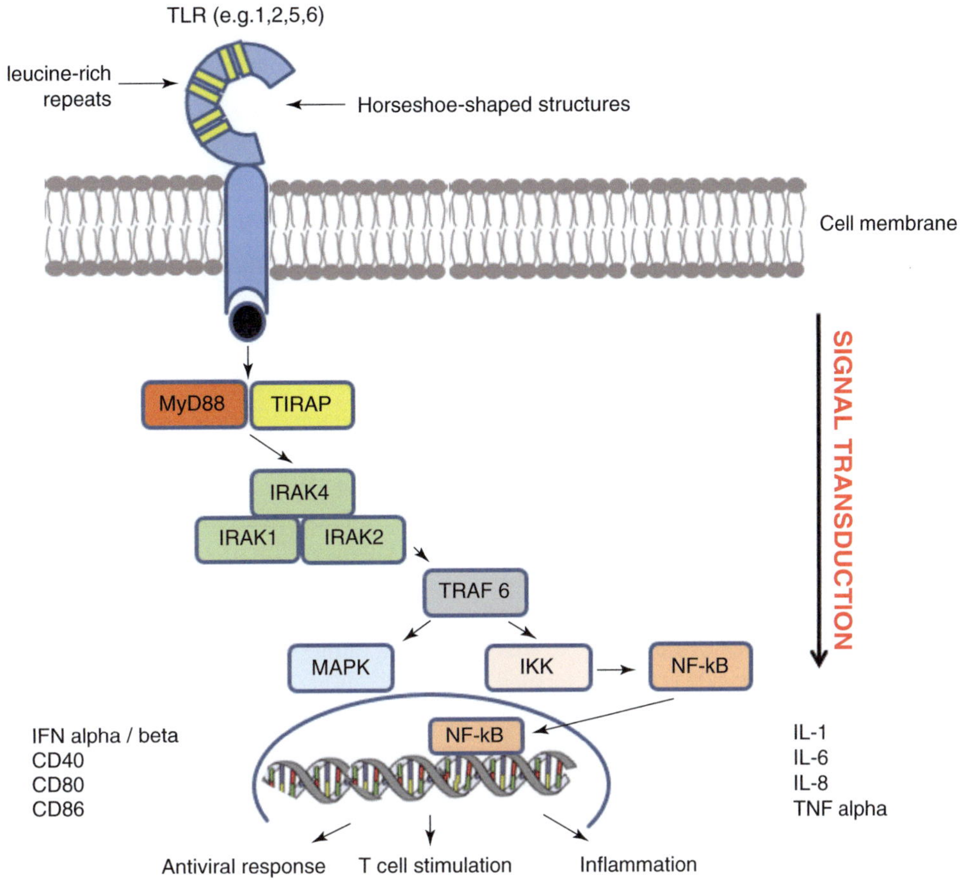

Fig. 2.12 Signal transduction via TLR. All TLRs share a common structural framework in their extracellular, ligand-binding domains. These domains all adopt horseshoe-shaped structures built from leucine-rich repeats. Ligand binding leads to downstream signaling whose structural basis consists of a set of mitogen-activated protein (*MAP*) kinases which governs the activation of the signal cascade. The TIR domain is the essential molecular key which connects the immune stimulus with a proper immune response. TIR recruits subsequently an adaptor molecule out of cytoplasm. The main adaptor molecules are Myd88 and TRIF. About 150 genes can be activated via NF-kB or AP-1, another transcription factor, and expressed

2.8.1 Toward Gene Activation

There are five main steps of TLR-dependent signal cascade:

1. *Binding of adaptor molecules*
The ligand binds to the N-terminal leucine-rich extracellular domain of TLRs and dimerizes the ectodomains, forming now a horseshoe structure. This results in a conformation change of the cytoplasmic TIR intracellular domains, forming now a TIR–TIR homodimer. The TIR domain (Toll/interleukin 1 receptor) is the essential molecular key which connects the immune stimulus with a proper immune response and highly conserved among all other TLRs. The TIR dimer recruits subsequently an adaptor molecule out of cytoplasm. Five different cytoplasmic adaptor molecules are available, each able to bind to TIR [83, 84]. (Table 2.9).

Together with different cell types, these different adaptor molecules account for a large variability in gene expression and hence for the different immune activities.

Table 2.9 Adaptor molecules for the TLR-mediated pathways

MyD88	• Myeolid differentiation primary response gene 88
TRIF	• TIR- domain containing adaptor inducing IFN β
TIRAP	• TNF receptor associated protein
TRAM	• Sterile alpha and Armadillo motif containing protein

The main adaptor molecules are Myd88 and TRIF. Two pathways are distinguished, a MyD88-dependent and a MyD88-independent pathway.

Most of all TLRs use MyD88. TLR3 uses TRIF, and TLR4 uses MyD88 and TRIF. TLR2, TLR4, and TLR6 are located within the cell membrane and use the adaptors TIRAP instead of MyD88 and TRAM for TRIF.

2. *Activation of IKK complex*
The N-terminus of MyD88, so-called death domain (DD, a bundle of characteristic six alpha-helices, found in all apoptotic proteins) is involved in the binding of IRAK (IL-1 receptor-associated kinase, a serine/threonine kinase family). IRAK is self-activated by autophosphorylation and binds to TRAF-6 after dissociation (TRAF-6, TNF-receptor-associated factor 6). The activated TRAF-6 activates the IKK complex, composed of IKK-γ also known as NEMO (inhibitor of kappa-B kinase), and the two catalytic subunits IKK-α (or IKK1) and IKK-β (or IKK2). The activation of IKK is the crucial step toward the release of transcription factors and a hallmark of the NF-kB (nuclear factor kappa-light-chain-enhancer of activated B cells) pathway.

3. *Release of transcription factors*
TRAF-6 interacts with enzymes catalyzing the formation of polyubiquitin chains. These ubiquitins are required for IKK activation and end in two distinct pathways Ubiquitin is attached to IkB protein, part of the cytoplasmic NF-kB-IkB complex and inhibitor of NF-kB. IkB is thereby labeled for proteolytic degradation. This inactivation of IkB starts the pathway for NF-kB which is now on the path into the nucleus. NF-kB is the most prominent transcription factor among a large group. The other pathway starts also with the ubiquitinated IkB protein and involves the c-Jun N-terminal kinase (JNK) for activation of AP-1 (activator protein1). AP-1 translocates also into the nucleus, just as IFR3, another transcription factor.

4. *Activation of genes via NF-kB*
NF-kB is often called "central mediator of the immune response." More than 150 genes are controlled by this transcription factor [85]. Almost all of these genes are directly involved in the immune response. Based on the inducible gene regulation, the organism is able to react very quickly and very targeted on negative influences, such as infections (oxidative) stress or tissue injury. A dysregulation of NF-kB contributes to a pathoimmunity and is also discussed to play a major role in cancer diseases, because NF-kB also controls genes responsible for cell proliferation [86, 87] (Table 2.11).

NF-kB is no single protein, rather a complex of some proteins with a unique feature, the Rel homology domain (RHD) composed of 300 aa.

The RHD is also part of other transcription factors and responsible for the protein–DNA linkage. The NF-kB complex forms homo- and heterodimers, and by association with IkB, NF-kB quiets in cytoplasm. The dissociation of IkB activates NF-kB following translocating into the nucleus and binding to a specific 10 bp DNA site, called kB. The best-known complex in mammalian cells is composed of the proteins p50 and RelA, also known as NF-kB.

Table 2.10 Activation steps after ligand binding to TLRs

1. Binding of adaptor molecules
↓
2. Activation of IKK complex
↓
3. Release of transcription factors
↓
4. Activation of genes via NF-kB
↓
5. Release of activated immune molecules

NF-kB dimer has no intrinsic enzymatic activity and only mediates the transcriptional control of target genes, because the structure of the dimer does not allow a direct binding to nucleosomal DNA. The dimer binds to a co-regulator, such as histone acetyltransferases (HATs) and histone deacetylases (HDACs). These co-regulators are enzymatic active and shift acetyl groups. DNA expression is regulated by acetylation and deacetylation. After opening the chromatin structure through histone acetylation, the preinitiation complex (PIC) is assembled and helps the RNA polymerase II to activate the transcription via binding to the TATA box of the promoter, the transcription start site of any gene [88]. Table 2.10 summarizes the different steps necessary for activation of immune-related genes.

5. *Release of activated immune molecules*
The transient change in the gene expression by NF-kB or another transcription factor is quick and enables the immune system to a prompt and robust response against danger, PAMP, or DAMP, arranged by any PRRs, such as TLRs.

TLRs are expressed on DCs, monocytes and macrophages, T cells, B cells, and NK cells, furthermore on endothelial cells and fibroblasts; on muscle cells; on chondrocytes, osteoblasts, and osteoclasts; on adipocytes; on hepatocytes; and on splenocytes. This ubiquitous distribution assists a ubiquitous immune reaction.

Besides the differential activation of TLRs by PAMPS and DAMPs, the cell type has great impact on the selection of immune genes and ultimately on the production and secretion of cytokines, receptors, acute phase proteins (APPs), regulator proteins (Reg P), or growth factors (GF).

Therefore, the diversity of the immune activities strongly depends on various stimuli, different PRRs/TLRs, and respectively the cell-type-specific transcriptional profiles within the stimulated cell.

If viruses activate NF-kB as part of their escape strategy to regulate their replication, an immunopathological reaction will succeed [89, 90]. In this case a viral encoded motif binds to the kB site by bypassing the normal signaling pathway. A directed cytokine gene activation follows in support of an intact, not disturbed, viral replication. And as discussed before, IL-10 again acts as immunosuppressive provirus cytokine.

Table 2.11 TLR signaling to target immune and nonimmune genes via NF-kB

Cytokines	Receptors	APPs	Reg P	GF	Others
IFN-β	MHC I	Tissue F1	TAP1	GM-CSF	p53
IFN-γ	B7.1	CRP	ICAM-1	G-CSF	IRF-1
IL-1 α/β	CD48	CF C4	ELAM-1	M-CSF	IRF-2
IL-2	IgG heavy c.	CF B	FAS-ligand	PDGF Bc	IkBα
IL-6	IgE heavy c.		IAPs		c-myc
IL-8	Ig light c.				c-myb
IL-9	TNFr				junB
IL-12	CD23				
IL-15	CD69				
TNF-α/β					

Abbreviations: *APPs* acute phase proteins, *Reg P* regulatory proteins, *GF* growth factors, *IFN* interferon, *IL* interleukin, *TNF* tumor necrosis factor, *MHC* major histocompatibility complex, *B7.1* co-stimulator of T cells, *CD48* lymphocytes antigen, *Ig* immunoglobulin heavy/light chain, *TNF* tumor necrosis factor receptor, *CD23* cell surface molecule, *CD69* C-type lectin protein, *Tissue F1* tissue factor 1, *CRP* C-reactive protein, *CF C4* complement factor C4, *CF B* complement factor B, *TAP1* transport protein for ER, *ICAM* 1 intracellular adhesion molecule, *ELAM* 1 endothelial cell leukocyte adhesion molecule, *FAS* ligand inducer of apoptosis, *IAPs* inhibitors of apoptosis, *CSF* colony stimulating factors/granulocyte/monocyte/macrophage, *PDGF Bc* platelet derived growth factor B chain, *p53* tumor suppressor, *IRF* interferon regulatory factor, *IkB* inhibitor of Rel/NF-kB, c-myc/c-myb/junB-proto-oncogene

HBsAg and NF-kB. The hepatitis B virus surface Ag (HBsAg), covering 90 % of the surface of hepatitis B virus (HBV), is part of a prophylactic vaccine and binds to NF-kB [91]. The findings from this binding studies and the observed viral manipulation of targeted immune genes could contribute to the development of therapeutic antivirus vaccines.

To this day there is no licensed drug which can directly block the activity of NF-kB, interesting not only for oncology. NF-kB can be easily experimentally manipulated and be blocked under controlled laboratory conditions. However, also after 25 years of intensive NF-kB research, the fears are massive that a therapeutic inhibition could induce non-predictable and uncontrollable gene suppression with fatal outcomes.

2.8.2 Impact of TLRs on Vaccine Development

TLRs identify pathogens and intracellular danger signals on distinct structures, PAMPS and DAMPs. In addition, lots of TLRs are involved in diseases, such as TLR2, TLR7, and TLR9 in systemic lupus erythematosus (SLE), and in the production of autoantibodies; TLR2 in bacterial and viral infections; TLR4 in allergy or rheumatoid arthritis, various infection diseases, asthma, cardiac, and liver disease; and TLR3, TLR4, TLR7, and TLR9 in malignant melanoma.

TLRs bridge the innate and acquired immunity. Also the type of immune response, Th1 or Th2, is triggered by them. What an opportunity to develop ligands for some TLRs which dependent on the disease would promote a cellular activity, e.g., for viral infections, cancer, or more dam the humoral response up, e.g., in allergic asthma. TLRs are therapeutic targets and can be manipulated by agonists and antagonists [92].

Agonists binding to some TLRs are developed as vaccine adjuvants. Already licensed is Fendrix® as adjuvant for hepatitis B vaccine: HBsAg is adjuvanted by AS04C, containing monophosphoryl lipid A (MPL). MPL is structurally related to LPS (see also Chap. 7) and a ligand for TLR4. It is reported that a full protection could be achieved after two immunizations in contrast to three immunization steps with a traditional alum-adjuvanted HBsAG vaccine.

In November 2012, the US Food and Drug Administration (FDA) Vaccines and Related Biological Products Advisory Committee (VRBPAC) granted Heplisav®, again a HBsAg-based vaccine but in this case combined with a synthetic CpG oligodeoxynucleotides (CpG ODN), an immunostimulatory sequence (ISS) and ligand for TLR9. The VRBPAC also reviewed and evaluated data concerning a theoretical risk that vaccines with these CpG adjuvants might cause autoimmune diseases.

CpG ODN. The immunostimulating capacity of CpG ODN was first described by Krieg in 1995 [93]. He discovered that unmethylated CpG motifs, repeated cytosines followed by guanines and with a phosphodiester backbone, are widely distributed in microorganisms but absolutely rare in vertebrates. So unmethylated ssCpG ODNs are considered PAMPs and are used to trigger the immune response. TLR9 is constitutively expressed only in B cells and plasmacytoid dendritic cells. It is not fully understood whether a specific sequence of CpGs, internal palindromes, or modifications of the phosphates are responsible for the immunostimulation or specific structures such as loops at both ends of the molecule. Accordingly the synthesized CpGs, 18–28 nucleotides in length, are very heterogeneous.

Besides CpGs adjuvants which synergistically act, CpGs are meanwhile clinically tested as adjunctive immunotherapy after chemo treatment in some cancer diseases [94]. The efficacy of CpGs as mono immunostimulant without a tumor-associated antigen is indeed disappointing. A significant prolongation of the survival time could not be achieved so far, so that an approved immunotherapy for cancer patients based on CpGs does not exist as yet.

Antagonists of TLRs are in preclinical and clinical development. LPS binds to TLR4 and is involved in sepsis. Lipid A derivates and other compounds block the LPS binding site of TLR4 and consequently inhibit the signal cascade. TLR2 and TLR4 are involved in cardiovascular diseases, in the progression of arteriosclerosis. A reduced expression of both receptors by an antagonist shows an anti-arteriogenic effect.

2.9 T Cells

While the innate immunity is based among others on highly conserved receptor structures, fixed in the germ line, the acquired immunity is characterized by clonal expansion of B and T cells. These cells carry antigen-specific receptors, whose diversity is dependent on gene rearrangements.

Following the capture of antigens by immature DCs via TLRs/PRRs, DCs migrate from non-lymphatic tissue via blood or lymph vessels to a lymph node, where they mature, process, and present the captured antigens via MHC to the T cell receptors (TCR) of naïve T cells.

2.9.1 Priming

A T cell needs three distinct signals for a complete activation, called priming (Fig. 2.13). In addition to the presentation of antigen (signal 1), co-stimulatory molecules (signal 2) are essential for a complete T cell priming and furthermore pro-inflammatory molecules (signal 3). If the T cell fails to receive signal 2, it dies on apoptosis.

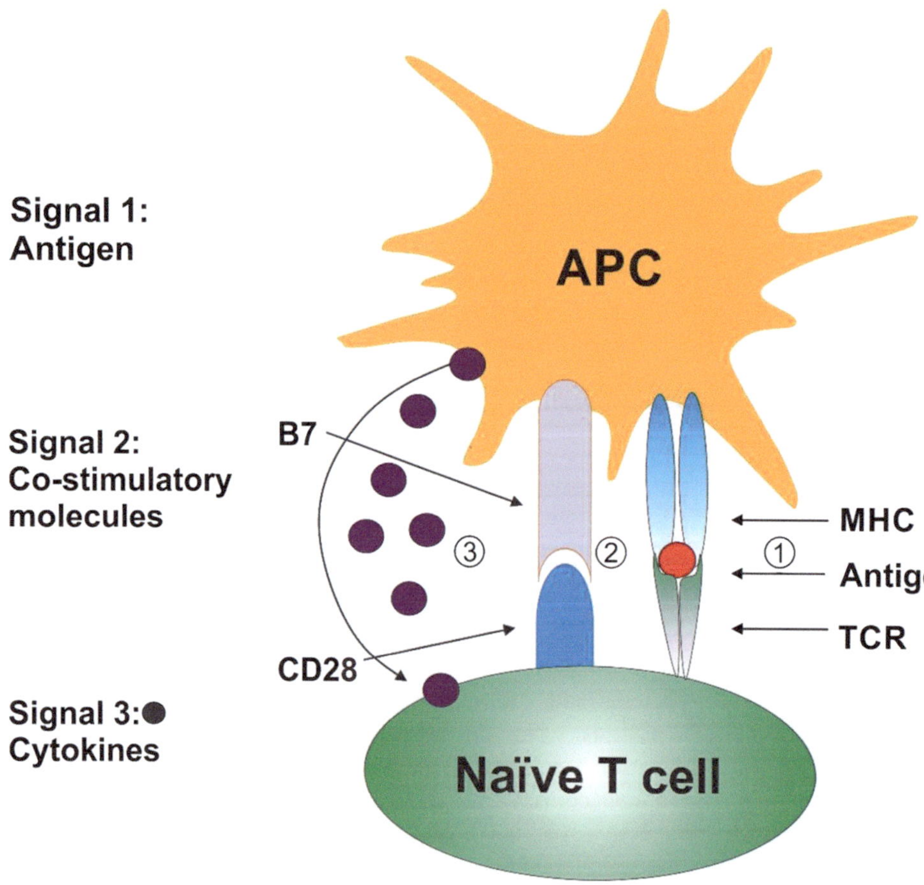

Fig. 2.13 T cell priming. In addition to the presentation of antigen (signal 1), co-stimulatory molecules B7 and CD28 (signal 2) are essential for a complete T cell priming and furthermore pro-inflammatory molecules (signal 3). If the T cell fails to receive signal 2, it dies on apoptosis (*APC* antigen-presenting cell, *MHC* major histocompatibility complex, *TCR* T cell receptor)

Cross Talk T Cells and DCs. An incomplete priming results in anergy, a functionally inactivation, but still alive, a status of tolerance. The major co-stimulatory signal of T cells is CD28 enabling T cell expansion and differentiation probably via enhancement of intracellular TCR signals [95]. CD28 binds to B7 molecules (B7.1 = CD80 and B7.2 = CD86) of DCs. At the same time, additional signal molecules are upregulated both within T cells and in DCs (written in parentheses), such as 4-1BB (4-1BBL), CD27 (CD70), and CD40 (CD40L). A very intensive cross talk takes place between T cells and DCs during this process. DCs secrete specific pro-inflammatory cytokines (signal 3) which additionally support T cells in maturation, priming, and survival, such as IL-1α, IL-6, IL-7, IL-12, IL-15, IL-18, IL-27, IL-33, IFNs, IFN γ, and TNF-α [29]. This is a quick immune response, a type 1 response.

2.9.2 T Cell Family

T lymphocytes make up 70–85 % of the lymphocytes in our bodies. There are two main groups, *helper T cells and cytotoxic T cells*, which have been given numerical names, CD4+ and CD8+ T cells. After complete priming, T cells differentiate to various effector cells, CD4+ T helper cells (Th), with the traditional subsets Th1, Th2, a recently identified IL-17-producing subset Th17 [96], T follicular helper cells (T_{Fh} cells are specialized to regulate B cell response) [97] regulatory T cells [98] (Treg, formerly known as suppressor T cells), and CD8+ T cytotoxic T cells (CTLs). Subsets of T cells and their functions are summarized in Table 2.12.

The importance of regulatory T cells is becoming increasingly apparent in all aspects of immunity. They have not only a central function in early life (see Chap. 4) but seem also to control vaccine immunogenicity in adults [99]. Depletion of Treg cells in murine models prior to vaccination has been shown to enhance immune responses to some vaccines. Treg-mediated suppression of T cells, B cells, monocytes, macrophages, and eosinophils is performed by the production of soluble factors such as IL-10, TGF-β, and IL-35. In addition, Treg cells also produce high levels of the immunosuppressive adenosine which is discussed in Chap. 4.

All these T cells mainly subsequently migrate into the blood and to the site of infection or danger. Thereby T cells express migration receptors, enabling to infiltrate into peripheral tissues. The common feature of the large T cell family is the unique T cell receptor (TCR).

Table 2.12 T cell family

Subsets of T cells	Function
1. T helper cells	Support of other immune cells by releasing cytokines
Th1	Cellular immune response: IL-2, IL-12, IFN-γ, TNF-α
Th2	Humoral immune response: IL-4, IL-5, IL-6, IL-10, TGF-β
Th17	Family of related pro-inflammatory cytokines (IL-17A, IL-17F, and IL-22 against bacterial and fungal infections)
T follicular helper cell (T_{Fh})	Regulation of B cell response within B cell follicles of secondary lymph organs
T regulatory cell (Treg)	Suppression or downregulation of induction and proliferation of effector T cells; responsible for creating the balance between the pro- and anti-inflammatory immune response
2. Cytotoxic T lymphocyte (CTL)	Killer effect on cancer/infected cells by release of cytotoxins perforin, granzymes, and *granulysin*

CD4+ Th1 cells produce cytokines, such as IL-2, IL-12, and IFN-γ, and support a cellular immunity arranged, e.g., by macrophages and CD8+ cytotoxic T lymphocytes (CTLs). Those immune cells kill infected cells by granzyme B and perforin and secrete IFN-γ and TNF-α. CD4+ Th2 cells produce IL-4, IL-5, IL-6, IL-10, and IL-13 to support B cell activation resulting in a humoral immunity. The development from an immature to a mature and primed T effector cell takes 3–5 days.

T Cell–B Cell Connection. B cells, another type of APCs, bind, internalize, and process antigens in complex with MHC II molecules and present to CD4+ T follicular helper cells (T_{Fh} cells), primed with the cognate antigen. T_{Fh} cells migrate into the B cell follicles of secondary lymph organs where they recognize via the TCRs this MHC II–antigen complex and activate the B cell to the production of antibodies.

The Cycle Is Closed. Antigen-presenting cells broadly distributed through the body bind danger signals, whether pathogen or host derived, via ubiquitous TLRs/PRRs. Following the processing and presentation, up to 150 genes are expressed within the APC, ready to induce an immune response. The vaccine antigen mimics danger signals and occupies the same immune activation process like a pathogen. For a general overview, see Fig. 2.14.

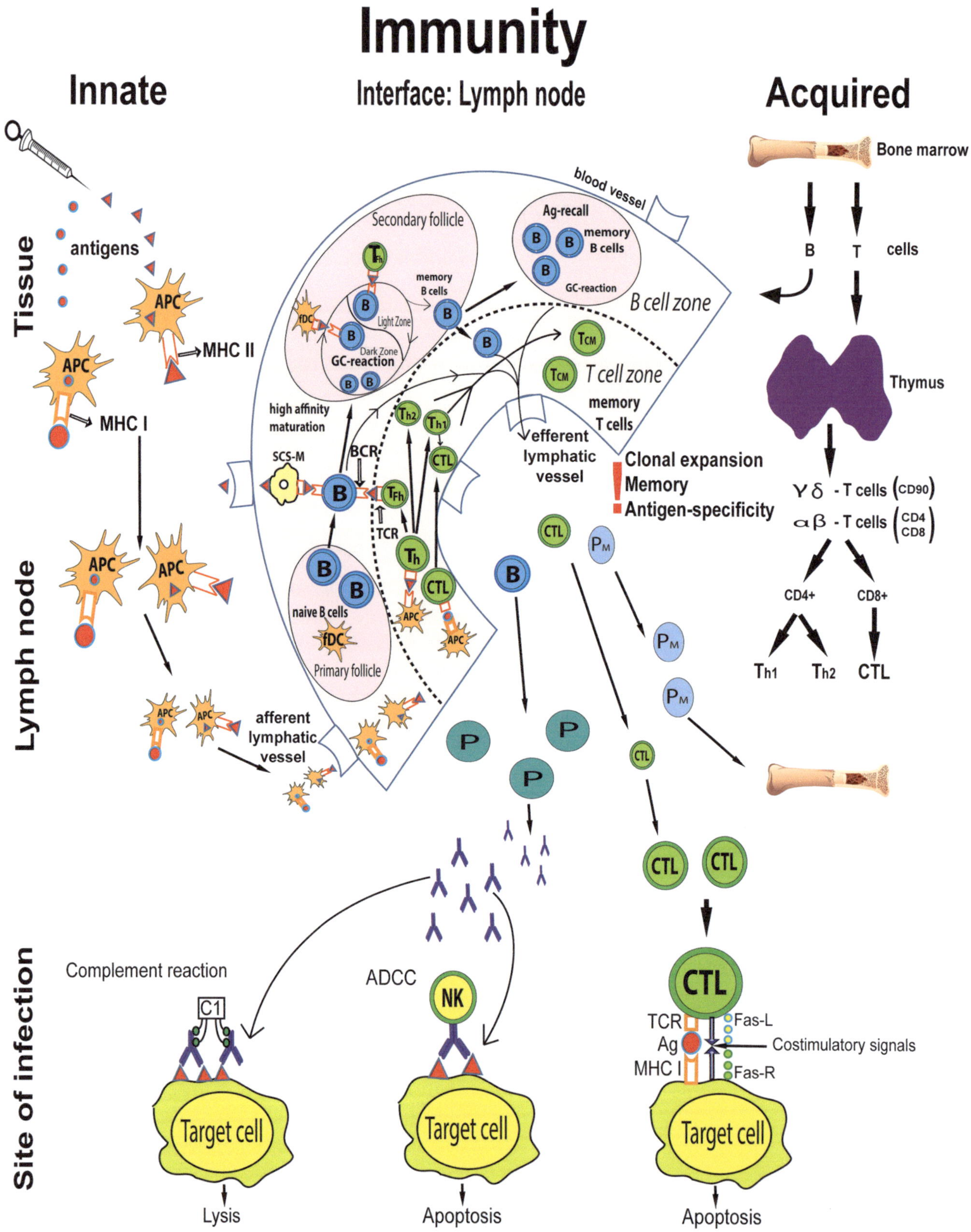
Immunity
Innate
Interface: Lymph node
Acquired
Tissue
antigens
APC
MHC II
MHC I
Lymph node
afferent lymphatic vessel
Site of infection
Secondary follicle
memory B cells
Light Zone
Dark Zone
GC-reaction
fDC
high affinity maturation
SCS-M
BCR
TCR
Th2
Th1
CTL
Tfh
Th
naive B cells
Primary follicle
Ag-recall
memory B cells
GC-reaction
blood vessel
B cell zone
TCM
T cell zone
memory T cells
efferent lymphatic vessel
Clonal expansion
Memory
Antigen-specificity
Bone marrow
B T cells
Thymus
γδ - T cells (CD90)
αβ - T cells (CD4 CD8)
CD4+
CD8+
Th1
Th2
CTL
PM
P
Complement reaction
C1
ADCC
NK
TCR
Ag
MHC I
Fas-L
Costimulatory signals
Fas-R
Target cell
Lysis
Apoptosis
Apoptosis

Fig. 2.14 The interaction of innate and acquired immunity upon vaccination
All lymphocytes (B cells, plasma cells, T cells, or natural killer cells) originate from a common progenitor cell which develops from a hematopoietic stem cell within the bone marrow
T cells migrate to the cortex of the thymus to undergo maturation in an antigen-free environment. Upon maturity, there are several forms of T cells (MHC-restricted αβ T cells, Treg cells, etc., and non-MHC-restricted γδ T cells) – all are ready to migrate to peripheral lymphoid tissue.
Lymph nodes (LN) are the interface between the innate and the acquired immunity. Upon intramuscular injection of a vaccine, antigens (Ag) are captured by antigen-presenting cells (APC such as DCs) and transported to the local LN where they are presented to T and B cells via MHC molecules. Ag can also enter the LN without APC and will be captured by residual subcapsular sinus (SCS) macrophages for presentation.
B cell development in LN is regulated by T follicular helper cells (T_{Fh}): (1) APC primed T_{Fh} cells encounter in the primary B cell follicle of LN naïve B cells that process cognate antigens relayed by SCS macrophages. This T and B cell interaction provokes a rapid clonal expansion and differentiation of B cells into short-lived plasma cells and the production of IgM antibodies, the earliest antibody. (2) Following expansion and immunoglobulin class switching to IgG, IgA, and IgE, the germinal center (GC) reaction in the secondary follicle of LN begins which is the crucial basis for the generation of memory B cells, whereas in the extracellular follicle LN short-lived plasma cells secrete antibodies. (3) The GC reaction is carried out in a cycle of different steps. B cells scan follicular DCs for antigens in the dark zone of secondary follicle with the commitment to B cell memory. T_{Fh} cells support these B cells in the light zone and drive high-affinity maturation of antigen-specific B cells into nonsecreting memory B cells and long-lived secreting plasma cells to distally function at infectious tissues.
One part of these B cells, however, doesn't leave the secondary follicle but reenters the GC cycle and undergoes another round of affinity maturation. The GC cycle reactions can continuously produce stable long-lived memory B cells.
Following cognate antigen recall memory, B cells are reactivated by memory T_{Fh} cells with a rapid proliferation of antibody-secreting memory plasma cells and induction of another GC reaction. Memory plasma cells (P_M) survive in the bone marrow and provide continuously serum antibodies to the body.
T cells develop to effector cells and central memory cells (T_{CM}). T_{CMs} are able to migrate and circulate in blood and therefore are believed to be the circulating interconversion pool for other memory T cells.
The unique hallmark of the acquired immunity is the clonal expansion, the memory effect, and the antigen specificity.
Target Killing After education B and T cells leave the LN and migrate to the site of infection. Cytotoxic T lymphocytes (CTLs) kill target cells following direct cell-to-cell contact and release cytotoxic or other proteins. Antibodies bind to cell surface antigens leading to an antibody-dependent cell-mediated cytotoxicity (ADCC), mediated by NK cells. The classical complement pathway is activated to lyse a target cell by binding of the C1 complex to antigen-bound antibody molecules

2.10 Immune Memory

The anamnestic immune memory relies on cells of the acquired immune system, such as B and T cells. At this the duration of the immune memory differs dependent from the disease, the immune status and the age of the patient, and of the type of vaccine.

Basically, a natural infection can lead to a life-long immunity, and a live vaccine results in a longer immunity than a recombinant vaccine. Responsible for the maintenance of specific memory immunity are special memory B and T cells. This is the conceptual basis of a vaccination. T cell memory in humans can be detected for up to 75 years [100].

2.10.1 Memory CD4+ T Cells

At the end of the immune response, most CD4+ T cells undergo apoptosis. Only a small pool of effector memory CD4+ T_{EM} cells survives and continues to produce cytokines as a support of ongoing immune activities. There are roughly two groups of T_{EM} cells: memory CD4+ T cells which are less differentiated and highly differentiated multifunctional T cells. These highly differentiated cells can be distinguished by a diverse pattern of cytokines, like IL-2, IFN-γ, and TNF-α, resulting in a different level of protection [101]. Memory CD4+ T cells keep their ability to migrate through peripheral tissue, and they are predominant in peripheral tissue, such as localized dermal layer of the skin among all memory T cells. CD4+ T cells produce IL-2 and help B cell differentiation into antibody-producing plasma cells and account to secondary expansion of memory CD8+ T cells [102, 103].

2.10.2 Memory CD8+ T Cells

Also the majority of T effector cells undergoes apoptotic cell death and immediately disappears from the circulation after clearance of the pathogen. Only a small population (up to 10 %) of memory T cells remains which can very quickly respond to a reinfection with a cognate antigen or cognate vaccine antigen. The maintenance of these long-living memory T cells is antigen independent but dependent on cytokines mainly through IL-7, also known as T cell survival cytokine and IL-15.

Another difference to effector T cells is the increased proliferation capability and longevity of memory T cells. This includes the increased expression of inhibitory molecules such as programmed cell death protein (PD1) and the loss of effector functions, like the loss of production of granzymes, IFN-γ, or IL-12. Additio*n*ally, the transcription of NF-kB-dependent (cytokine) genes will be reduced in memory T cells by an inhibitor of NF-kB.

2.10.3 Subsets of Memory T Cells

Three major subsets (in contrast to some literature speaking of only two) of memory T cells (CD4+ and CD8+) are identified based on their anatomical localization and functional status [104–107]: central memory T cells (T_{CM}), effector memory T cells (T_{EM}), and tissue-resident memory T cells (T_{RM}).

T_{CM} cells express homing receptors for lymph nodes, CD62L, and CCR7, residing in secondary lymphatic organs with a high proliferative but low effector potential [108]. T_{CM} cells are able to migrate and circulate in blood and therefore are believed to be the circulating and interconversion pool for other memory T cells.

T_{EM} cells produce cytotoxic proteins, reside in non-lymphoid tissues, are only low proliferative, circulate also in blood vessels, and provide efficient and rapid protection against systemic infections and only a limited efficiency against local infections. The pool of T_{EM} cells declines over time resulting in a progressive conversion to T_{CM} cells.

T_{RM} cells don't migrate and circulate. They prefer to reside in tissues that are either confronted with pathogens in the first line of defense, like the skin, intestinal (lung and gut), and vaginal mucosa tissue, or in such tissues which are highly sensitive to pathogens, like brain tissue. These cells exert effector functions and produce different cytotoxic molecules like granzyme B. Table 2.13 gives an overview on memory T cells.

Persisting antigen is not required for maintenance of memory T cells [109] but the tissue-specific microenvironment influences the expression of migration receptors such as CD103+. Nonspecific local inflammatory cytokines are sufficient to arm T_{RM} cells [110]. This protection by embedded T_{RM} cells in peripheral sites can last over years.

2.10.4 Pasta Cells

The rapid change from resting naïve T cells to highly differentiated, active, and migrating T effector cells, afterward the rapid reduction of these effector cells and the generation of memory T cells, again provided with the ability to a rapid proliferation and rapid reduction on demand, postulates a precise regulation of lymphocyte homeostasis.

Any kind of dysregulation leads a severe, sometimes life-threatening, immune disease.

One key mechanism to control this homeostasis is the regulation of metabolism. In this process the production of energy in resting T cells switches from fatty acid oxidation and decarboxylation of glucose in citrate cycle and respiratory chain to an aerobic glycolysis (oxygen is present within the cell) in activated T cells [111]. Rapidly growing tumor cells produce energy as well from glycolysis in the presence of oxygen.

Warburg Effect. This discovery was described very early by Warburg and he was awarded the Nobel Prize in Physiology in 1931 [112]. Activated T cells and cancer cells have a high demand on energy which can only be covered via glycolysis.

Table 2.13 Subsets of human memory CD4+/8+ T cells

Cell type	Localization	Marker	Function
T_{CM}	Blood, spleen, lymph nodes	CD62L+++ CCR7+ CD45RA−	Peripheral protection, circulating T cell pool, IL-2 production
T_{EM}	Blood, spleen, liver, peripheral organs	CD62L± CCR7− CD45RA+	Fast and robust peripheral protection, cytotoxic proteins, IFN-γ
T_{RM}	Skin, mucosa (lung, gut, vagina), salivary glands, brain	CD62L− CCR7− CD103+ CD69+	Fast and robust local protection, cytotoxic proteins

The fatty acid metabolism to generate energy in the form of ATP, called β-oxidation, yields the most ATP on energy per gram. In this process long carbon chain of the fatty acid is split into acetyl CoA, which enters the citric acid cycle (also known as tricarboxylic acid (TCA) cycle). One gram of fatty acids is approximately 9 kcal (37 kJ), compared to 4 kcal (17 kJ) for 1 g of carbohydrates (Fig. 2.15).

While the oxidative decarboxylation of fatty acids is located in mitochondria, the glycolysis takes place in cytoplasm of the cell and can be activated very quickly in the presence of glucose. The benefit of this cytoplasmic location for activated T cell is the rapid offer of energy as ATP. This tremendous adjustment of metabolism enables T cells to effective activities against pathogens, against danger. T cells can rapidly grow and proliferate, differentiate, migrate, and secrete cytokines.

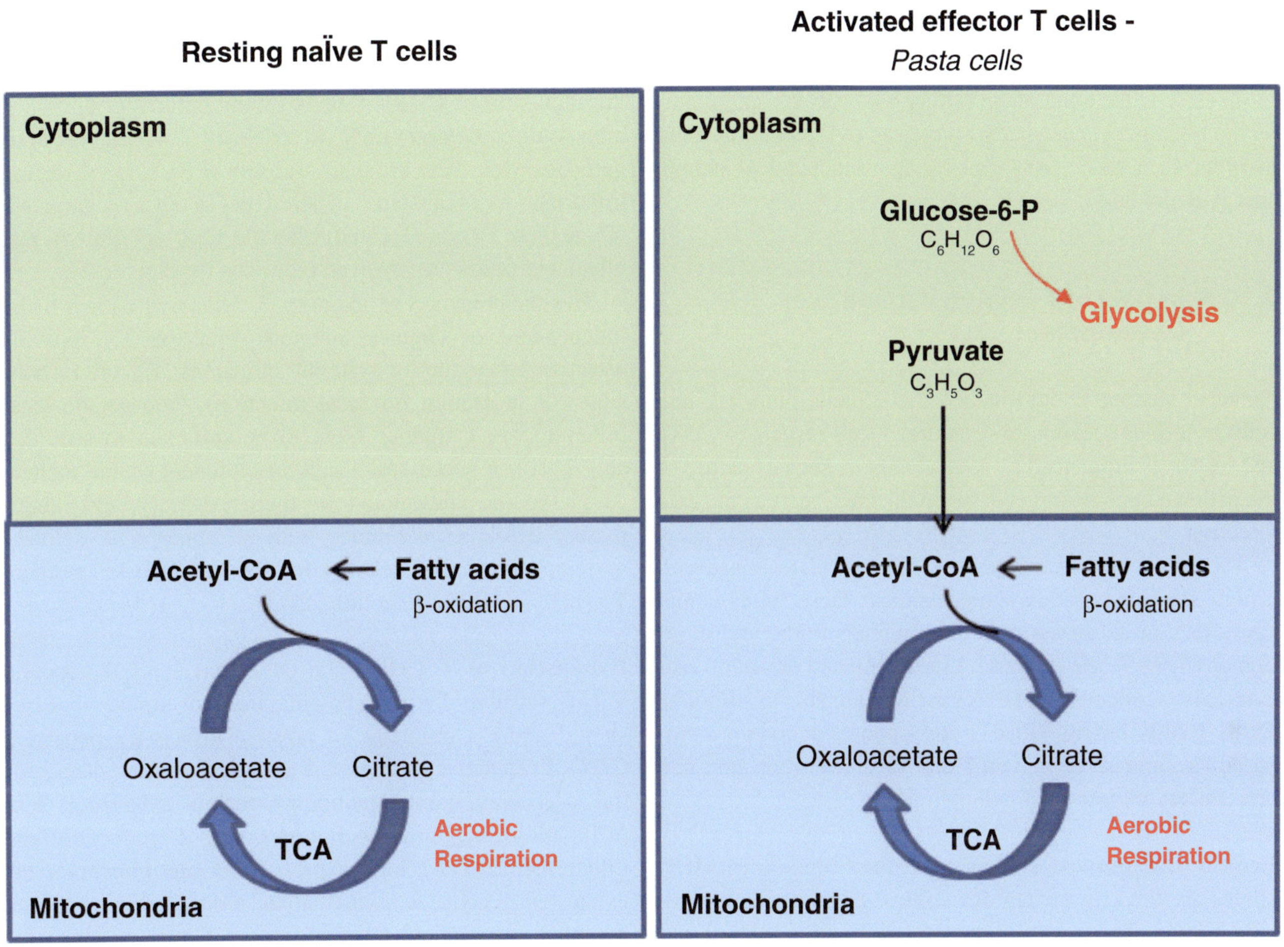

Cytoplasm (Glycolysis)

$$C_6H_{12}O_6 + \text{Enzymes} + 2(\text{NAD}) \longrightarrow C_3H_5O_3 + 2(\text{NADH})$$

Mitochondria (Aerobic Respiration)

$$2(C_3H_5O_3) + 6(O_2) + \text{Enzymes} \longrightarrow 6(CO_2) + 6(H_2O) + 38\ \text{ATP}$$

Fig. 2.15 Resting T cells generate energy in the form of ATP, from fatty acid metabolism, called β-oxidation. In this process long carbon chain of the fatty acid are split into acetyl CoA, which enter the citric acid cycle, also known as tricarboxylic acid (*TCA*) cycle. Activated T cells have a high demand on energy which can only be covered via glycolysis. While the oxidative decarboxylation is located in the mitochondria, the glycolysis takes place in the cytoplasm of the cell

Extrinsic factors control the increased metabolism. The T cell receptor (TCR) plays a key function. TCR regulates the expression of the glucose transporter, Glut1. Without TCR signals, the expression of Glut1 is decreased, resulting in a reduced absorption of glucose, subsequently leading to nutrient stress and apoptosis [113, 114]. IL-7 plays an additional key function in the metabolic switch. IL-7 promotes glucose uptake through activation of Akt kinases [115]. If this metabolic switch is absent, e.g., due to defect of enzymes, or lack of glucose, T cells will develop anergy.

Pasta Cells. After completing the mission, effector T cells turn into resting T cells and the metabolism changes back to mitochondrial fatty oxidation and oxidative decarboxylation: *Pasta cells* – like a marathon runner who eats carbohydrates on the obligatory pasta party on the eve of the marathon run in order to activate very quickly this biochemical simple energy depot later.

2.10.5 Impact of T Cells on Vaccine Development

An ideal vaccine should induce a complete, humoral, and cellular immune response. A natural T cell response, CD4+ and CD8+, is influenced by several factors, such as nature of the pathogen and its target tissue in the host, acute or chronic infection.

Vaccines for generating a robust CD8+ T cell response with a high effector capacity should address these fundamental key issues in an appropriate quality, magnitude, and duration of CD8+ T cell response. Live attenuated or vector vaccines, also replicons and DNA vaccines, are able to stimulate CD8+ T cells, but not killed or conventional peptide/protein-based vaccines. Research on T cell vaccines is concentrated on accurate, conserved T cell epitopes.

Length of Epitopes. Epitopes and their binding to MHC alleles are the requirement for epitope presentation to specific T cells. The length of peptides differs for MHC I and MHC II, depending on the allele between 8 and 11 for MHC I, respectively, between 13 and 25 residues for MHC II. By comprehensive series of epitope mapping using a panel of synthesized overlapping peptide sequences (peptide library), TCR binding sites can be identified and characterized. The prediction of novel T cell epitopes and thus the screening of vaccine candidates is also done by in silico methods [116] (see Chap. 6). However, wet experiments must follow and confirm or drop the identified epitopes.

Since 2007 the Immune Epitope Database and Analysis Resource (IEDB) provides a catalogue of T and B cell epitopes and tools to predict novel epitopes [117, 118]. Currently, data from 197,005 T cell, 221,898 MHC binding, and 7621 MHC ligand elution assays are listed in this catalogue. The access to IEDB's website is free: http://www.iedb.org.

The most gallant and definitely most difficult approach to activate CD8+ T cell is the isolation of antigens which directly bind to MHC I molecules [119]. Despite lots of efforts, there is no successful clinical trial with a protein-based T cell vaccine. A recent study, peptide pulsing of fresh blood cells ex vivo, could help to control an HIV infection via induction of CD8+ T cells [120]. A broader approach aims to directly target DCs via a defined TLR selected antigen. However, there are many subsets of DCs. It's therefore important to understand which type of DCs is targeted, where these DCs are located, what the TLR repertoire is, and which cytokines are involved (adjuvant development).

The maintenance of memory T cells was shown to be independent of cognate antigens. Whereas T_{EM} provide effective protection for systemic infections, T_{RM} are responsible for protection for local infections. Nonspecific local inflammatory cytokines seem to be sufficient to arm T_{RM} cells [110]. A successful T cell development should include a high specific adjuvant to force these necessary local inflammatory cytokines combined with an appropriate delivery system, such as skin delivery for activation of skin resident T_{RM} cells in HSV-1 infection [121].

Exhaustion of T Cells. The development of therapeutic T cell vaccines for chronic infections or cancer diseases should address problems of adverse effects by persistent CD8+ T cell activation. These T cell vaccines have the potential to generate immunopathology, such as exhaustion (loss of functions, beginning with a loss of IL-2 production) and inflammation. PD-1 high expression is one biomarker for exhausted T cells. A mathematical model helps to predict potential immune adverse effects of T cell vaccines for chronic viral infections [122].

2.10.6 Memory B Cells

The measurement of antibodies in response to a vaccine is presumed to be level of protection and duration. This vaccine immunogenicity is only an indication for a possible protection but definitely not equal to the real factual protection. There are also some reports of patients who developed antibodies after vaccination but indeed are not protected. Last but not the least, some pathogens induce a primary immune response but after their clearance a memory response is missing and the body is not protected against a reinfection with the same pathogen. This is the case, e.g., for respiratory syncytial virus (RSV), causative agent of respiratory disease in infants, morbidity in children and adults [123, 124].

Like T cells also B cells generate long-lived memory cells following the primary antigen contact. And also like memory T cells, memory B cells are able to persist without a new antigen contact [125, 126].

2.10.6.1 Memory Subtypes

Two B cell subtypes are described [127]: memory B cells and memory plasma cells. Memory B cells reside in secondary lymphoid organs and memory plasma cells survive in the bone marrow and provide continuously serum antibodies to the body (Table 2.14).

The ever measured longest survival of memory plasma cells in man, about ten decades, was found in people born on or before 1915. Survivors to the 1918 H1N1 influenza virus pandemic were enrolled in a study and tested for antibody response to the recombinant 1918 hemagglutinin (HA) protein. All survivors possess neutralizing antibodies to this H1N1 pandemic virus which also cross react with a genetically similar HA of 1930 influenza infection [128].

2.10.6.2 Affinity Maturation

Immature B cells develop into mature B cells in secondary lymphoid organs. After protein vaccination B cell development in lymph nodes (LN) is regulated by T_{Fh} cells and following in three phases [129]:

Phase 1
DC-primed T_{Fh} cells encounter in the primary B cell follicle of LN naïve B cells that process cognate antigens relayed by subcapsular sinus (SCS) macrophages [130]. This T and B cell interaction via CD27/CD70 provokes a rapid clonal expansion and differentiation of B cells into short-lived plasma cells and the production of IgM, the earliest immunoglobulin.

Phase 2
Following expansion and immunoglobulin class switch to IgA, IgE, and IgG, the germinal center (GC) reaction in the secondary follicle of LN begins which is the crucial basis for the generation of memory B cells, whereas in the extracellular follicle, LN short-lived plasma cells secrete antibodies.

Phase 3
The GC reaction is carried out in a cycle of different steps. B cells scan follicular DCs for antigens in the dark zone of secondary follicle. T_{Fh} cells support these B cells in the light zone and drive affinity maturation of antigen-specific B cells into nonsecreting memory B cells and long-lived secreting plasma cells to distally function at infectious tissues. One part of these antigen-specific memory B cells, however, doesn't leave the secondary follicle but reenters the GC cycle and undergoes another round of affinity maturation. The GC cycle reactions can last up to 8 months after protein vaccination [131] and continuously produce stable long-lived memory B cells. Following cognate antigen recall memory B cells are reactivated by memory T_{Fh} with a rapid proliferation of antibodies secreting memory plasma cells and induction of another GC reaction. But a survival cytokine, like IL-7 described for T cells, does not exist for B cells. Figure 2.16 summarizes subsets of memory T and B cells.

Table 2.14 Subsets of human memory B cells

Cell type	Localization	Marker	Function
Memory B cell	Secondary lymphoid organs (spleen, lymph nodes, tonsils, Peyer's patches)	CD19+ CD20+ CD27+ CD38–	Cell pool for rapid production of memory plasma cells; secondary GC reactions
Memory plasma cell	Bone marrow	CD19+ CD20– CD27+ CD38+++	High-affinity antibodies after recall

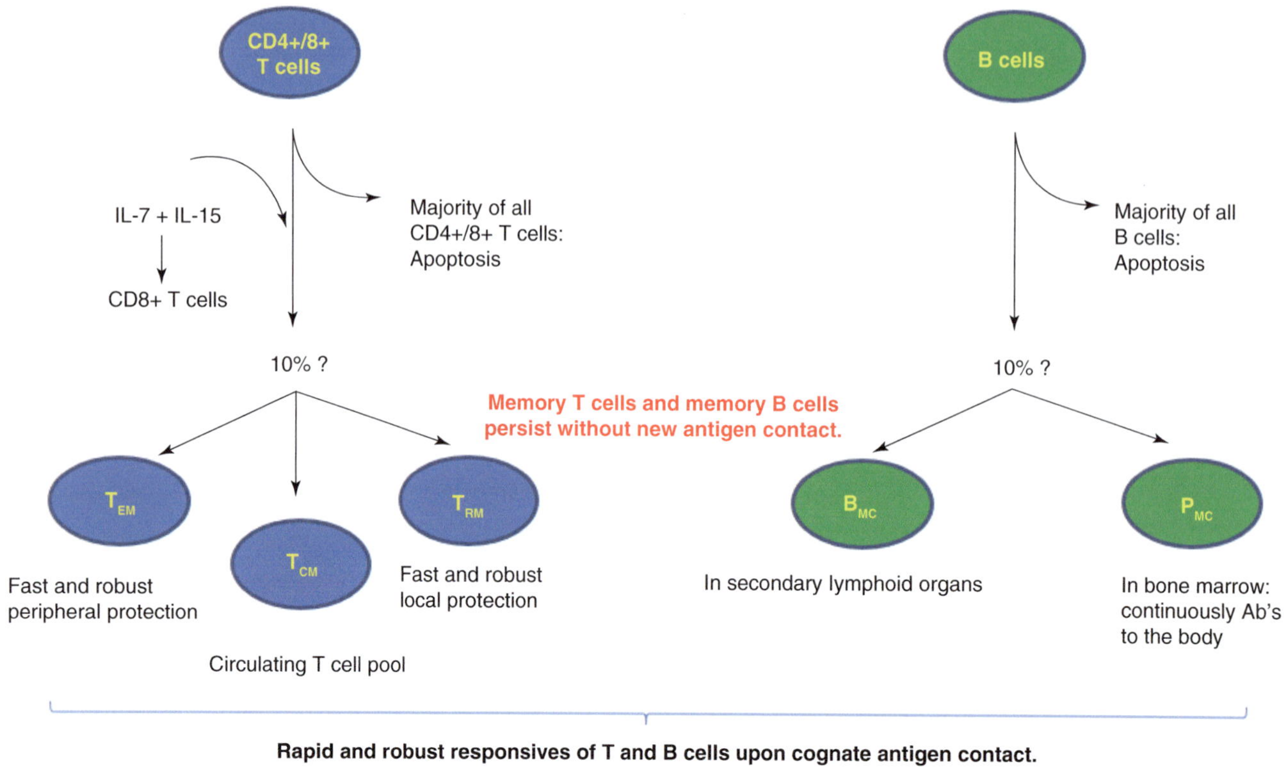

Fig. 2.16 Subsets of memory T and B cells. Responsible for the maintenance of specific memory immunity are special memory B and T cells. This is the conceptual basis of a vaccination. Only a small population (up to 10 %) of memory T and B cells remains which can very quickly respond to a reinfection with a cognate antigen or cognate vaccine antigen. The maintenance of these long-living memory T cells is antigen-independent but dependent on cytokines mainly through IL-7, also known as T cell survival cytokine, and IL-15. No survival cytokines for memory B cells do exist. $T_{EM/CM/RM}$ effector memory T cells/central memory T cells/tissue-resident memory T cells, $B_{MC/PMC}$ B memory cell/Plasma memory cell

2.11 Booster and Vaccination Strategies

Antigens. At the beginning of this chapter, we introduced the palette of different antigens: glycoproteins, lipoproteins, carbohydrates, glycolipids, and nucleic acids.

As the chemical nature of antigens are different, so are the induced immune responses. The different vaccine types correspond to the pathogen's nature, like attenuated live virus/bacterial vaccines, inactivated virus/bacterial vaccines, conjugate and polysaccharide vaccines, recombinant protein, and DNA/RNA vaccines.

The nature of an antigen, like the chemical structure (the more complex, the more immunogenic), the size (the larger the molecule the more immunogenic), and the physical form (particulate antigens than more immunogenic than soluble ones), determines the kind of immune response.

The exposure of proteins and nucleic acids to their corresponding PPRs/TLRs on T cells leads to an acquired, T cell-dependent immune response. A key specificity of this is the development of a memory response. The establishment of a long-lived immunological memory is critical for a revaccination, a booster. Once primed by a vaccination (or natural infection), the second response upon a booster mounts generally the antibody and CTL response to the cognate antigen.

Lipid Antigens. Bacterial polysaccharides (*S. pneumoniae*, *S. typhi*, *H. influenzae*) and lipids activate the innate immune system without involvement of CD4+ T cells. Lipid antigens are recognized by CD1 molecules on, e.g., Langerhans cells, following presenting the lipid–CD1 complex in a MHC-independent way to invariant NKT (iNKT) cells [132, 133]. iNKT cells are a subset of natural killer (NK) cells which are a subset of T cells.

Polysaccharide Antigens. Two classes of polysaccharide antigens have been described: thymic-independent type 1 antigens (TI-1) activate directly B cells by binding to the B cell receptor (BCR), first signal, and binding to a TLR on B cells, the second signal. TI-2 antigens bind to BCRs, first signal resulting in clustering, the second signal (see Chap. 6). This CD4+ T cell-independent activation leads antibody production. Lipopolysaccharides provoke a TI-1 response via binding to TLR4.

However, B cell response is short-lived, memory B cells are not produced (only generated upon T cell-dependent activation), and therefore a booster cannot enhance the antibody response. Moreover, as shown recently, a booster with a pure polysaccharide vaccine can lead to a state of immune tolerance or hyporesponsiveness caused by apoptosis of memory B cells [134, 135].

Conjugate vaccines, the carbohydrate is coupled to a protein carrier, first developed for infants (newborns are unable to make antibodies to repeating polysaccharide antigens due the immaturity of their B cell receptors (see also Chap. 4)) induced by a complete T and B cell response are now also used in adults and elderly with significant better results than immunization with pure polysaccharide [136].

Prime Boost. Traditionally revaccinations are given by homologous booster. Heterogeneous prime-boost strategies involve two different vector platforms for the same antigen and are in (pre)clinical studies especially for chronic infections, such as HIV, malaria, and TB. The combination of recombinant (rec) vectors used for prime boost can be very different. But the basic principle in all these prime-boost regimes is the application of different vaccine constructs targeting the same antigen.

But prime boost can be also the administration of vaccine antigens in the same or different formulations by different routes, e.g., mucosal and parenteral [137]. This mucosal–parenteral prime boost is discussed in more detail in Chap. 3.

A cancer-specific variation of prime boost is the passive immunization with therapeutic antibodies as priming and the active immunization against the same epitope as boosting (Table 2.15).

Mechanisms. 20 years after the first prime-boost vaccination, the mechanisms behind this remain unclear. More clear are the results, mostly increase of CD8+ T cell numbers with increased lytic capacity and broader antibody specificities with improved antibody quality. These results reflect that antigens presented by different platforms could bind to different TLRs so broadening the B and T cell response. Also the use of plasmid DNA as prime offers naïve and correct folded proteins to the immune system. These DNA-encoded proteins share dominant and subdominant epitopes leading to a broader response. In contrast, recombinant proteins share mostly immunodominant epitopes resulting in a narrow response only.

Drawbacks DNA. However, the bottleneck of a DNA vaccine is the low immunogenicity. Pure naked DNA does not work and must be supplemented with a strong adjuvant (M. Giese, unpublished results).

Drawback Vector. The drawback of any viral vector as prime or boost is the antibody response against the vector. Repeated administrations of a viral vector vaccine automatically induce neutralizing antibodies that dramatically reduce the efficacy of this vaccine. One of the most used viral vectors is adenovirus serotype 5 (Ad5). The seroprevalence is very high, and preexisting immunity also reduces the efficacy of this vector [138]. To circumvent this handicap, other human but also simian adenovirus serotypes [139] , such as Ad26 and Ad35, are under investigation. They differ inter alia in their innate profile and immunological potential. Not every tested adenovirus is able to strongly prime CD4+ and CD8+ T cells. The same is for pox viral vectors; they are limited to prime CD8+ T cells but are a potent boost for CD8+ T cells. The lessons learned from these experiments are the right temporal order.

Summary. To summarize this vaccine strategy, prime boost is superior in eliciting a robust complete immune response compared to DNA, protein, or vector vaccines alone. Some single vaccines fail on their own but work in combination. Nevertheless, we are far from a miracle linked to prime boost. The clinical phase III HIV vaccine RV-144 trial in Thailand, a prime-boost strategy, resulted in 30 % protection only [140]. Further research is needed.

Table 2.15 Prime-boost strategies

Prime-boost strategies		
Priming	**Boosting**	**Reference**
Priming with recombinant (rec) virus A	Boosting with rec virus B	[134]
Priming with DNA vaccine	Boosting with rec virus	[135]
Priming with DNA vaccine	Boosting with rec protein	[136]
Priming with virus-like particle (VLP)	Boosting with DNA	[137]
Priming with rec protein	Boosting with rec virus	[138]
Priming with mucosal vaccine	Boosting with parenteral vaccine (and vv)	(Experimental approaches)
Cancer: Priming: passive via monoclonal antibodies	Boosting: active immunization against the same epitope (Chap. 12)	(Experimental approaches)

References

1. Thaa, B., Sinhadri, B.C., Tielesch, C., Krause, E., Veit, M.: Signal peptide cleavage from GP5 of PRRSV: a minor fraction of molecules retains the decoy epitope, a presumed molecular cause for viral persistence. PLoS One **8**, e65548 (2013). doi:10.1371/journal.pone.0065548
2. Ito, H., Watanabe, S., Takada, A., Kawaoka, Y.: Ebola virus glycoprotein: proteolytic processing, acylation, cell tropism, and detection of neutralizing antibodies. J. Virol. **75**, 1576–1580 (2001). doi:10.1128/JVI.75.3.1576-1580.2001
3. Oldstone, M.B.: Molecular mimicry and immune-mediated diseases. FASEB J. **12**, 1255–1265 (1998)
4. Jones, D.: Reverse vaccinology on the cusp. Nat. Rev. Drug Discov. **11**, 175–176 (2012). doi:10.1038/nrd3679
5. Kratky, W., Reis e Sousa, C., Oxenius, A., Sporri, R.: Direct activation of antigen-presenting cells is required for CD8+ T cell priming and tumor vaccination. Proc. Natl. Acad. Sci. U. S. A. **108**, 17414–17419 (2011). doi:10.1073/pnas.1108945108
6. Takeda, K., Akira, S.: Toll-like receptors in innate immunity. Int. Immunol. **17**, 1–14 (2005). doi:10.1093/intimm/dxh186
7. Ziegler-Heitbrock, L., et al.: Nomenclature of monocytes and dendritic cells in blood. Blood **116**, e74–e80 (2010). doi:10.1182/blood-2010-02-258558
8. Khazen, W., et al.: Expression of macrophage-selective markers in human and rodent adipocytes. FEBS Lett. **579**, 5631–5634 (2005). doi:10.1016/j.febslet.2005.09.032
9. Ding, Q., et al.: Regulatory B cells are identified by expression of TIM-1 and can be induced through TIM-1 ligation to promote tolerance in mice. J. Clin. Invest. **121**, 3645–3656 (2011). doi:10.1172/JCI46274
10. Gottfried-Blackmore, A., et al.: Acute in vivo exposure to interferon-gamma enables resident brain dendritic cells to become effective antigen presenting cells. Proc. Natl. Acad. Sci. U. S. A. **106**, 20918–20923 (2009). doi:10.1073/pnas.0911509106
11. Ochoa, M.T., Loncaric, A., Krutzik, S.R., Becker, T.C., Modlin, R.L.: "Dermal dendritic cells" comprise two distinct populations: CD1+ dendritic cells and CD209+ macrophages. J. Invest. Dermatol. **128**, 2225–2231 (2008). doi:10.1038/jid.2008.56
12. Ouchi, T., et al.: Langerhans cell antigen capture through tight junctions confers preemptive immunity in experimental staphylococcal scalded skin syndrome. J. Exp. Med. **208**, 2607–2613 (2011). doi:10.1084/jem.20111718
13. Zozulya, A.L., et al.: Intracerebral dendritic cells critically modulate encephalitogenic versus regulatory immune responses in the CNS. J. Neurosci. **29**, 140–152 (2009). doi:10.1523/JNEUROSCI.2199-08.2009
14. Barchet, W., Cella, M., Colonna, M.: Plasmacytoid dendritic cells – virus experts of innate immunity. Semin. Immunol. **17**, 253–261 (2005). doi:10.1016/j.smim.2005.05.008
15. Hart, D.N., McKenzie, J.L.: Interstitial dendritic cells. Int. Rev. Immunol. **6**, 127–138 (1990)
16. Kushwah, R., Hu, J.: Complexity of dendritic cell subsets and their function in the host immune system. Immunology **133**, 409–419 (2011). doi:10.1111/j.1365-2567.2011.03457.x
17. Vremec, D., et al.: Production of interferons by dendritic cells, plasmacytoid cells, natural killer cells, and interferon-producing killer dendritic cells. Blood **109**, 1165–1173 (2007). doi:10.1182/blood-2006-05-015354
18. Chopin, M., Allan, R.S., Belz, G.T.: Transcriptional regulation of dendritic cell diversity. Front Immunol. **3**, 26 (2012). doi:10.3389/fimmu.2012.00026
19. Cambi, A., Figdor, C.G.: Dual function of C-type lectin-like receptors in the immune system. Curr. Opin. Cell Biol. **15**, 539–546 (2003)
20. Flacher, V., et al.: Epidermal Langerhans cells rapidly capture and present antigens from C-type lectin-targeting antibodies deposited in the dermis. J. Invest. Dermatol. **130**, 755–762 (2010). doi:10.1038/jid.2009.343
21. Allan, R.S., et al.: Epidermal viral immunity induced by CD8alpha+dendritic cells but not by Langerhans cells. Science **301**, 1925–1928 (2003). doi:10.1126/science.1087576
22. Oh, S., Perera, L.P., Burke, D.S., Waldmann, T.A., Berzofsky, J.A.: IL-15/IL-15Ralpha-mediated avidity maturation of memory CD8+ T cells. Proc. Natl. Acad. Sci. U. S. A. **101**, 15154–15159 (2004). doi:10.1073/pnas.0406649101
23. Bevan, M.J.: Cross-priming for a secondary cytotoxic response to minor H antigens with H-2 congenic cells which do not cross-react in the cytotoxic assay. J. Exp. Med. **143**, 1283–1288 (1976)
24. Snyder, C.M., Allan, J.E., Bonnett, E.L., Doom, C.M., Hill, A.B.: Cross-presentation of a spread-defective MCMV is sufficient to prime the majority of virus-specific CD8+ T cells. PLoS One **5**, e9681 (2010). doi:10.1371/journal.pone.0009681
25. Freigang, S., Egger, D., Bienz, K., Hengartner, H., Zinkernagel, R.M.: Endogenous neosynthesis vs. cross-presentation of viral antigens for cytotoxic T cell priming. Proc. Natl. Acad. Sci. U. S. A. **100**, 13477–13482 (2003). doi:10.1073/pnas.1835685100
26. Henkart, P.A.: CTL effector functions. Semin. Immunol. **9**, 85–86 (1997)
27. Nagata, S.: Fas-mediated apoptosis. Adv. Exp. Med. Biol. **406**, 119–124 (1996)
28. Andersen, M.H., Schrama, D., Thor Straten, P., Becker, J.C.: Cytotoxic T cells. J. Invest. Dermatol. **126**, 32–41 (2006). doi:10.1038/sj.jid.5700001
29. de Saint-Vis, B., et al.: The cytokine profile expressed by human dendritic cells is dependent on cell subtype and mode of activation. J. Immunol. **160**, 1666–1676 (1998)
30. Ueno, H., et al.: Harnessing human dendritic cell subsets for medicine. Immunol. Rev. **234**, 199–212 (2010). doi:10.1111/j.0105-2896.2009.00884.x
31. Matsuo, K., et al.: A low-invasive and effective transcutaneous immunization system using a novel dissolving microneedle array for soluble and particulate antigens. J. Control. Release **161**, 10–17 (2012). doi:10.1016/j.jconrel.2012.01.033
32. Sheikh, N.A., et al.: Sipuleucel-T immune parameters correlate with survival: an analysis of the randomized phase 3 clinical trials in men with castration-resistant prostate cancer. Cancer Immunol. Immunother. (2012). doi:10.1007/s00262-012-1317-2
33. Dinarello, C.A.: Proinflammatory cytokines. Chest **118**, 503–508 (2000)
34. Cyktor, J.C., Turner, J.: Interleukin-10 and immunity against prokaryotic and eukaryotic intracellular pathogens. Infect. Immun. **79**, 2964–2973 (2011). doi:10.1128/IAI.00047-11
35. Maynard, C.L., Weaver, C.T.: Diversity in the contribution of interleukin-10 to T-cell-mediated immune regulation. Immunol. Rev. **226**, 219–233 (2008). doi:10.1111/j.1600-065X.2008.00711.x
36. Brooks, D.G., McGavern, D.B., Oldstone, M.B.: Reprogramming of antiviral T cells prevents inactivation and restores T cell activity during persistent viral infection. J. Clin. Invest. **116**, 1675–1685 (2006). doi:10.1172/JCI26856
37. Netea, M.G., et al.: Toll-like receptor 2 suppresses immunity against Candida albicans through induction of IL-10 and regulatory T cells. J. Immunol. **172**, 3712–3718 (2004)
38. Stober, C.B., Lange, U.G., Roberts, M.T., Alcami, A., Blackwell, J.M.: IL-10 from regulatory T cells determines vaccine efficacy in murine Leishmania major infection. J. Immunol. **175**, 2517–2524 (2005)
39. Verma, S., et al.: Quantification of parasite load in clinical samples of leishmaniasis patients: IL-10 level correlates with parasite load in visceral leishmaniasis. PLoS One **5**, e10107 (2010). doi:10.1371/journal.pone.0010107

40. Moore, K.W., et al.: Homology of cytokine synthesis inhibitory factor (IL-10) to the Epstein-Barr virus gene BCRFI. Science **248**, 1230–1234 (1990)
41. Dolganiuc, A., et al.: Hepatitis C virus core and nonstructural protein 3 proteins induce pro- and anti-inflammatory cytokines and inhibit dendritic cell differentiation. J. Immunol. **170**, 5615–5624 (2003)
42. Mahipal, A., et al.: Tumor-derived interleukin-10 as a prognostic factor in stage III patients undergoing adjuvant treatment with an autologous melanoma cell vaccine. Cancer Immunol. Immunother. **60**, 1039–1045 (2011). doi:10.1007/s00262-011-1019-1
43. Chen, C.J., et al.: High expression of interleukin 10 might predict poor prognosis in early stage oral squamous cell carcinoma patients. Clin. Chim. Acta **415**, 25–30 (2013). doi:10.1016/j.cca.2012.09.009
44. Lee, S.J., et al.: Identification of pro-inflammatory cytokines associated with muscle invasive bladder cancer; the roles of IL-5, IL-20, and IL-28A. PLoS One **7**, e40267 (2012). doi:10.1371/journal.pone.0040267
45. Opal, S.M., DePalo, V.A.: Anti-inflammatory cytokines. Chest **117**, 1162–1172 (2000)
46. Hao, N.B., et al.: Macrophages in tumor microenvironments and the progression of tumors. Clin. Dev. Immunol. **948098**, 2012 (2012). doi:10.1155/2012/948098
47. Janeway Jr., C.A.: Approaching the asymptote? Evolution and revolution in immunology. Cold Spring Harb. Symp. Quant. Biol. **54**(Pt 1), 1–13 (1989)
48. Krishnaswamy, J.K., Chu, T., Eisenbarth, S.C.: Beyond pattern recognition: NOD-like receptors in dendritic cells. Trends Immunol. (2013). doi:10.1016/j.it.2012.12.003
49. Ng, C.S., Kato, H., Fujita, T.: Recognition of viruses in the cytoplasm by RLRs and other helicases – how conformational changes, mitochondrial dynamics and ubiquitination control innate immune responses. Int. Immunol. **24**, 739–749 (2012). doi:10.1093/intimm/dxs099
50. Palm, N.W., Medzhitov, R.: Pattern recognition receptors and control of adaptive immunity. Immunol. Rev. **227**, 221–233 (2009). doi:10.1111/j.1600-065X.2008.00731.x
51. Akira, S.: Innate immunity and adjuvants. Philos. Trans. R. Soc. Lond. B Biol. Sci. **366**, 2748–2755 (2011). doi:10.1098/rstb.2011.0106
52. Ablasser, A., et al.: RIG-I-dependent sensing of poly(dA:dT) through the induction of an RNA polymerase III-transcribed RNA intermediate. Nat. Immunol. **10**, 1065–1072 (2009). doi:10.1038/ni.1779
53. Cridland, J.A., et al.: The mammalian PYHIN gene family: phylogeny, evolution and expression. BMC Evol. Biol. **12**, 140 (2012). doi:10.1186/1471-2148-12-140
54. Lemaitre, B., Nicolas, E., Michaut, L., Reichhart, J.M., Hoffmann, J.A.: The dorsoventral regulatory gene cassette spatzle/Toll/cactus controls the potent antifungal response in Drosophila adults. Cell **86**, 973–983 (1996)
55. Medzhitov, R., Preston-Hurlburt, P., Janeway Jr., C.A.: A human homologue of the Drosophila Toll protein signals activation of adaptive immunity. Nature **388**, 394–397 (1997). doi:10.1038/41131
56. Hashimoto, C., Hudson, K.L., Anderson, K.V.: The Toll gene of Drosophila, required for dorsal-ventral embryonic polarity, appears to encode a transmembrane protein. Cell **52**, 269–279 (1988)
57. Meylan, E., Tschopp, J., Karin, M.: Intracellular pattern recognition receptors in the host response. Nature **442**, 39–44 (2006). doi:10.1038/nature04946
58. Lata, S., Raghava, G.P.: PRRDB: a comprehensive database of pattern-recognition receptors and their ligands. BMC Genomics **9**, 180 (2008). doi:10.1186/1471-2164-9-180
59. Fortis, A., Garcia-Macedo, R., Maldonado-Bernal, C., Alarcon-Aguilar, F., Cruz, M.: The role of innate immunity in obesity. Salud Publica Mex. **54**, 171–177 (2012)
60. Benias, P.C., Gopal, K., Bodenheimer Jr., H., Theise, N.D.: Hepatic expression of toll-like receptors 3, 4, and 9 in primary biliary cirrhosis and chronic hepatitis C. Clin. Res. Hepatol. Gastroenterol. (2012). doi:10.1016/j.clinre.2012.07.001
61. Zhu, W., et al.: Overexpression of toll-like receptor 3 in spleen is associated with experimental arthritis in rats. Scand. J. Immunol. **76**, 263–270 (2012). doi:10.1111/j.1365-3083.2012.02724.x
62. Medzhitov, R.: Toll-like receptors and innate immunity. Nat. Rev. Immunol. **1**, 135–145 (2001). doi:10.1038/35100529
63. Ohto, U., Fukase, K., Miyake, K., Satow, Y.: Crystal structures of human MD-2 and its complex with antiendotoxic lipid IVa. Science **316**, 1632–1634 (2007). doi:10.1126/science.1139111
64. Bauer, S., et al.: Human TLR9 confers responsiveness to bacterial DNA via species-specific CpG motif recognition. Proc. Natl. Acad. Sci. U. S. A. **98**, 9237–9242 (2001). doi:10.1073/pnas.161293498
65. Boivin, N., Menasria, R., Piret, J., Boivin, G.: Modulation of TLR9 response in a mouse model of herpes simplex virus encephalitis. Antiviral Res. **96**, 414–421 (2012). doi:10.1016/j.antiviral.2012.09.022
66. Geeraedts, F., et al.: Superior immunogenicity of inactivated whole virus H5N1 influenza vaccine is primarily controlled by Toll-like receptor signalling. PLoS Pathog. **4**, e1000138 (2008). doi:10.1371/journal.ppat.1000138
67. Koyama, S., et al.: Plasmacytoid dendritic cells delineate immunogenicity of influenza vaccine subtypes. Sci. Transl. Med. **2**, 25ra24 (2010). doi:10.1126/scitranslmed.3000759
68. Park, B.S., et al.: The structural basis of lipopolysaccharide recognition by the TLR4-MD-2 complex. Nature **458**, 1191–1195 (2009). doi:10.1038/nature07830
69. Ng, A., Xavier, R.J.: Leucine-rich repeat (LRR) proteins: integrators of pattern recognition and signaling in immunity. Autophagy **7**, 1082–1084 (2011)
70. Lloyd, D.H., Viac, J., Werling, D., Reme, C.A., Gatto, H.: Role of sugars in surface microbe-host interactions and immune reaction modulation. Vet. Dermatol. **18**, 197–204 (2007). doi:10.1111/j.1365-3164.2007.00594.x
71. Dalpke, A., Helm, M.: RNA mediated Toll-like receptor stimulation in health and disease. RNA Biol. **9**, 828–842 (2012). doi:10.4161/rna.20206
72. Heeg, K., Dalpke, A., Peter, M., Zimmermann, S.: Structural requirements for uptake and recognition of CpG oligonucleotides. Int. J. Med. Microbiol. **298**, 33–38 (2008). doi:10.1016/j.ijmm.2007.07.007
73. Matzinger, P.: Tolerance, danger, and the extended family. Annu. Rev. Immunol. **12**, 991–1045 (1994). doi:10.1146/annurev.iy.12.040194.005015
74. Rubartelli, A., Lotze, M.T.: Inside, outside, upside down: damage-associated molecular-pattern molecules (DAMPs) and redox. Trends Immunol. **28**, 429–436 (2007). doi:10.1016/j.it.2007.08.004
75. Khanna, A.: Interleukin-18, a potential mediator of inflammation, oxidative stress, and allograft dysfunction. Transplantation **91**, 590–591 (2011). doi:10.1097/TP.0b013e31820d3b82
76. Piccinini, A.M., Midwood, K.S.: DAMPening inflammation by modulating TLR signalling. Mediators Inflamm. (2010). doi:10.1155/2010/672395 (2010)
77. Yanai, H., et al.: HMGB proteins function as universal sentinels for nucleic-acid-mediated innate immune responses. Nature **462**, 99–103 (2009). doi:10.1038/nature08512
78. Zhang, Q., et al.: Circulating mitochondrial DAMPs cause inflammatory responses to injury. Nature **464**, 104–107 (2010). doi:10.1038/nature08780
79. Hirsiger, S., Simmen, H.P., Werner, C.M., Wanner, G.A., Rittirsch, D.: Danger signals activating the immune response after trauma. Mediators Inflamm. **2012**, 315941 (2012). doi:10.1155/2012/315941

80. Basu, S., Binder, R.J., Suto, R., Anderson, K.M., Srivastava, P.K.: Necrotic but not apoptotic cell death releases heat shock proteins, which deliver a partial maturation signal to dendritic cells and activate the NF-kappa B pathway. Int. Immunol. **12**, 1539–1546 (2000)
81. Ichikawa, M., Williams, R., Wang, L., Vogl, T., Srikrishna, G.: S100A8/A9 activate key genes and pathways in colon tumor progression. Mol. Cancer Res. **9**, 133–148 (2011). doi:10.1158/1541-7786.MCR-10-0394
82. Termeer, C., et al.: Oligosaccharides of Hyaluronan activate dendritic cells via toll-like receptor 4. J. Exp. Med. **195**, 99–111 (2002)
83. O'Neill, L.A., Fitzgerald, K.A., Bowie, A.G.: The Toll-IL-1 receptor adaptor family grows to five members. Trends Immunol. **24**, 286–290 (2003)
84. Zhang, Q., Zmasek, C.M., Cai, X., Godzik, A.: TIR domain-containing adaptor SARM is a late addition to the ongoing microbe-host dialog. Dev. Comp. Immunol. **35**, 461–468 (2011). doi:10.1016/j.dci.2010.11.013
85. Pahl, H.L.: Activators and target genes of Rel/NF-kappaB transcription factors. Oncogene **18**, 6853–6866 (1999). doi:10.1038/sj.onc.1203239
86. Baker, R.G., Hayden, M.S., Ghosh, S.: NF-kappaB, inflammation, and metabolic disease. Cell Metab. **13**, 11–22 (2011). doi:10.1016/j.cmet.2010.12.008
87. Ben-Neriah, Y., Karin, M.: Inflammation meets cancer, with NF-kappaB as the matchmaker. Nat. Immunol. **12**, 715–723 (2011). doi:10.1038/ni.2060
88. Hayden, M.S., Ghosh, S.: NF-kappaB, the first quarter-century: remarkable progress and outstanding questions. Genes Dev. **26**, 203–234 (2012). doi:10.1101/gad.183434.111
89. Griffin, G.E., Leung, K., Folks, T.M., Kunkel, S., Nabel, G.J.: Activation of HIV gene expression during monocyte differentiation by induction of NF-kappa B. Nature **339**, 70–73 (1989). doi:10.1038/339070a0
90. Rong, B.L., et al.: HSV-1-inducible proteins bind to NF-kappa B-like sites in the HSV-1 genome. Virology **189**, 750–756 (1992)
91. Jan, R.H., et al.: Hepatitis B virus surface antigen can activate human monocyte-derived dendritic cells by nuclear factor kappa B and p38 mitogen-activated protein kinase mediated signaling. Microbiol. Immunol. **56**, 719–727 (2012). doi:10.1111/j.1348-0421.2012.00496.x
92. O'Neill, L.A., Bryant, C.E., Doyle, S.L.: Therapeutic targeting of Toll-like receptors for infectious and inflammatory diseases and cancer. Pharmacol. Rev. **61**, 177–197 (2009). doi:10.1124/pr.109.001073
93. Krieg, A.M., et al.: CpG motifs in bacterial DNA trigger direct B-cell activation. Nature **374**, 546–549 (1995). doi:10.1038/374546a0
94. Jahrsdorfer, B., Weiner, G.J.: CpG oligodeoxynucleotides as immunotherapy in cancer. Update Cancer Ther. **3**, 27–32 (2008). doi:10.1016/j.uct.2007.11.003
95. Butte, M.J., et al.: CD28 costimulation regulates genome-wide effects on alternative splicing. PLoS One **7**, e40032 (2012). doi:10.1371/journal.pone.0040032
96. Ouyang, W., Kolls, J.K., Zheng, Y.: The biological functions of T helper 17 cell effector cytokines in inflammation. Immunity **28**, 454–467 (2008). doi:10.1016/j.immuni.2008.03.004
97. Deenick, E.K., Ma, C.S.: The regulation and role of T follicular helper cells in immunity. Immunology **134**, 361–367 (2011). doi:10.1111/j.1365-2567.2011.03487.x
98. Sakaguchi, S.: Regulatory T cells: key controllers of immunologic self-tolerance. Cell **101**, 455–458 (2000)
99. Macatangay, B.J., Szajnik, M.E., Whiteside, T.L., Riddler, S.A., Rinaldo, C.R.: Regulatory T cell suppression of Gag-specific CD8 T cell polyfunctional response after therapeutic vaccination of HIV-1-infected patients on ART. PLoS One **5**, e9852 (2010). doi:10.1371/journal.pone.0009852
100. Hammarlund, E., et al.: Duration of antiviral immunity after smallpox vaccination. Nat. Med. **9**, 1131–1137 (2003). doi:10.1038/nm917
101. Rudolph, M., Hebel, K., Miyamura, Y., Maverakis, E., Brunner-Weinzierl, M.C.: Blockade of CTLA-4 decreases the generation of multifunctional memory CD4+ T cells in vivo. J. Immunol. **186**, 5580–5589 (2011). doi:10.4049/jimmunol.1003381
102. Litjens, N.H., et al.: IL-2 producing memory CD4+ T lymphocytes are closely associated with the generation of IgG-secreting plasma cells. J. Immunol. **181**, 3665–3673 (2008)
103. Williams, M.A., Tyznik, A.J., Bevan, M.J.: Interleukin-2 signals during priming are required for secondary expansion of CD8+ memory T cells. Nature **441**, 890–893 (2006). doi:10.1038/nature04790
104. Kaech, S.M., Cui, W.: Transcriptional control of effector and memory CD8(+) T cell differentiation. Nat. Rev. Immunol. **12**, 749–761 (2012). doi:10.1038/nri3307
105. Sallusto, F., Langenkamp, A., Geginat, J., Lanzavecchia, A.: Functional subsets of memory T cells identified by CCR7 expression. Curr. Top. Microbiol. Immunol. **251**, 167–171 (2000)
106. Okada, R., Kondo, T., Matsuki, F., Takata, H., Takiguchi, M.: Phenotypic classification of human CD4+ T cell subsets and their differentiation. Int. Immunol. **20**, 1189–1199 (2008). doi:10.1093/intimm/dxn075
107. Keshavarz Valian, H., et al.: CCR7(+) central and CCR7(-) effector memory CD4 (+) T cells in human cutaneous leishmaniasis. J. Clin. Immunol. **33**, 220–234 (2013). doi:10.1007/s10875-012-9788-7
108. Vazquez-Cintron, E.J., et al.: Protocadherin-18 is a novel differentiation marker and an inhibitory signaling receptor for CD8+ effector memory T cells. PLoS One **7**, e36101 (2012). doi:10.1371/journal.pone.0036101
109. Lau, L.L., Jamieson, B.D., Somasundaram, T., Ahmed, R.: Cytotoxic T-cell memory without antigen. Nature **369**, 648–652 (1994). doi:10.1038/369648a0
110. Mackay, L.K., et al.: Long-lived epithelial immunity by tissue-resident memory T (TRM) cells in the absence of persisting local antigen presentation. Proc. Natl. Acad. Sci. U. S. A. **109**, 7037–7042 (2012). doi:10.1073/pnas.1202288109
111. Michalek, R.D., Rathmell, J.C.: The metabolic life and times of a T cell. Immunol. Rev. **236**, 190–202 (2010). doi:10.1111/j.1600-065X.2010.00911.x
112. Bensinger, S.J., Christofk, H.R.: New aspects of the Warburg effect in cancer cell biology. Semin. Cell Dev. Biol. **23**, 352–361 (2012). doi:10.1016/j.semcdb.2012.02.003
113. Maciver, N.J., et al.: Glucose metabolism in lymphocytes is a regulated process with significant effects on immune cell function and survival. J. Leukoc. Biol. **84**, 949–957 (2008). doi:10.1189/jlb.0108024
114. Jacobs, S.R., et al.: Glucose uptake is limiting in T cell activation and requires CD28-mediated Akt-dependent and independent pathways. J. Immunol. **180**, 4476–4486 (2008)
115. Finlay, D.K.: Regulation of glucose metabolism in T cells: new insight into the role of Phosphoinositide 3-kinases. Front. Immunol. **3**, 247 (2012). doi:10.3389/fimmu.2012.00247
116. Khan, J.M., Kumar, G., Ranganathan, S.: In silico prediction of immunogenic T cell epitopes for HLA-DQ8. Immunome Res. **8**, 14 (2012)
117. Beaver, J.E., Bourne, P.E., Ponomarenko, J.V.: EpitopeViewer: a Java application for the visualization and analysis of immune epitopes in the Immune Epitope Database and Analysis Resource (IEDB). Immunome Res. **3**, 3 (2007). doi:10.1186/1745-7580-3-3
118. Kim, Y., Sette, A., Peters, B.: Applications for T-cell epitope queries and tools in the Immune Epitope Database and Analysis

Resource. J. Immunol. Methods **374**, 62–69 (2011). doi:10.1016/j.jim.2010.10.010
119. Herd, K.A., et al.: Cytotoxic T-lymphocyte epitope vaccination protects against human metapneumovirus infection and disease in mice. J. Virol. **80**, 2034–2044 (2006). doi:10.1128/JVI.80.4.2034-2044.2006
120. De Rose, R., et al.: Control of viremia and prevention of AIDS following immunotherapy of SIV-infected macaques with peptide-pulsed blood. PLoS Pathog. **4**, e1000055 (2008). doi:10.1371/journal.ppat.1000055
121. Torti, N., Oxenius, A.: T cell memory in the context of persistent herpes viral infections. Viruses **4**, 1116–1143 (2012). doi:10.3390/v4071116
122. Johnson, P.L., et al.: Vaccination alters the balance between protective immunity, exhaustion, escape, and death in chronic infections. J. Virol. **85**, 5565–5570 (2011). doi:10.1128/JVI.00166-11
123. Walsh, E.E.: Respiratory syncytial virus infection in adults. Semin. Respir. Crit. Care Med. **32**, 423–432 (2011). doi:10.1055/s-0031-1283282
124. Graham, B.S.: Biological challenges and technological opportunities for respiratory syncytial virus vaccine development. Immunol. Rev. **239**, 149–166 (2011). doi:10.1111/j.1600-065X.2010.00972.x
125. Zinkernagel, R.M.: On natural and artificial vaccinations. Annu. Rev. Immunol. **21**, 515–546 (2003). doi:10.1146/annurev.immunol.21.120601.141045
126. Maruyama, M., Lam, K.P., Rajewsky, K.: Memory B-cell persistence is independent of persisting immunizing antigen. Nature **407**, 636–642 (2000). doi:10.1038/35036600
127. Caraux, A., et al.: Circulating human B and plasma cells. Age-associated changes in counts and detailed characterization of circulating normal CD138- and CD138+ plasma cells. Haematologica **95**, 1016–1020 (2010). doi:10.3324/haematol.2009.018689
128. Yu, X., et al.: Neutralizing antibodies derived from the B cells of 1918 influenza pandemic survivors. Nature **455**, 532–536 (2008). doi:10.1038/nature07231
129. McHeyzer-Williams, M., Okitsu, S., Wang, N., McHeyzer-Williams, L.: Molecular programming of B cell memory. Nat. Rev. Immunol. **12**, 24–34 (2012). doi:10.1038/nri3128
130. Phan, T.G., Gray, E.E., Cyster, J.G.: The microanatomy of B cell activation. Curr. Opin. Immunol. **21**, 258–265 (2009). doi:10.1016/j.coi.2009.05.006
131. Dogan, I., et al.: Multiple layers of B cell memory with different effector functions. Nat. Immunol. **10**, 1292–1299 (2009). doi:10.1038/ni.1814
132. Juno, J.A., Keynan, Y., Fowke, K.R.: Invariant NKT cells: regulation and function during viral infection. PLoS Pathog. **8**, e1002838 (2012). doi:10.1371/journal.ppat.1002838
133. Pena-Cruz, V., Ito, S., Dascher, C.C., Brenner, M.B., Sugita, M.: Epidermal Langerhans cells efficiently mediate CD1a-dependent presentation of microbial lipid antigens to T cells. J. Invest. Dermatol. **121**, 517–521 (2003). doi:10.1046/j.1523-1747.2003.12429.x
134. O'Brien, K.L., Hochman, M., Goldblatt, D.: Combined schedules of pneumococcal conjugate and polysaccharide vaccines: is hyporesponsiveness an issue? Lancet Infect. Dis. **7**, 597–606 (2007). doi:10.1016/S1473-3099(07)70210-4
135. Brynjolfsson, S.F., et al.: Hyporesponsiveness following booster immunization with bacterial polysaccharides is caused by apoptosis of memory B cells. J. Infect. Dis. **205**, 422–430 (2012). doi:10.1093/infdis/jir750
136. Paradiso, P.R.: Pneumococcal conjugate vaccine for adults: a new paradigm. Clin. Infect. Dis. **55**, 259–264 (2012). doi:10.1093/cid/cis359
137. Woodland, D.L.: Jump-starting the immune system: prime-boosting comes of age. Trends Immunol. **25**, 98–104 (2004). doi:10.1016/j.it.2003.11.009
138. Mast, T.C., et al.: International epidemiology of human pre-existing adenovirus (Ad) type-5, type-6, type-26 and type-36 neutralizing antibodies: correlates of high Ad5 titers and implications for potential HIV vaccine trials. Vaccine **28**, 950–957 (2010). doi:10.1016/j.vaccine.2009.10.145
139. O'Hara, G.A., et al.: Clinical assessment of a recombinant simian adenovirus ChAd63: a potent new vaccine vector. J. Infect. Dis. **205**, 772–781 (2012). doi:10.1093/infdis/jir850
140. Rerks-Ngarm, S., et al.: Vaccination with ALVAC and AIDSVAX to prevent HIV-1 infection in Thailand. N. Engl. J. Med. **361**, 2209–2220 (2009). doi:10.1056/NEJMoa0908492

Mucosal Immunity

3

Contents

3.1 Mucosal Barrier

The immune system can be divided into four main compartments:

- The systemic immune system, which monitors the blood for infectious agents.
- The cutaneous immune system, which patrols the skin for pathogens breaking in the skin via breaches or bites.
- The mucosal immune system, monitoring various mucosal surfaces for pathogens, such as the gastrointestinal tract (GI). Other mucosal surfaces coat the respiratory tract, the urinary tract, and the urogenital tract.
- The CNS with the blood–brain barrier and immune-reduced properties.

The mucosal surfaces exceed 300 m^2 in humans. Most harmful pathogens enter the body through these mucosal surfaces by ingestion, inhalation, or sexual contact. The first contact of all these pathogens is a single-layer epithelium covered by mucus and antimicrobial molecules. But also vaccines have to cross this massive barrier from mucus and cells.

The gut, nasal, upper respiratory and salivary, mammary, lacrimal, and other glands consist of a single layered epithelium (Fig. 3.1).

Mucins. Mucous secretion is a viscous colloid, produced by globlet cells, and this gel is a natural chemical barrier. Mucus is rich in glycoproteins and water. The glycoproteins are known as mucins (MUCs). Most mucins are secreted onto mucosal surfaces, and only some mucins are membrane bound. Mucins bind to pathogens in order to protect the epithelium for invasion. Besides MUCs also antiseptic enzymes (produced by Paneth cells), such as lysozyme or lactoferrin, and immunoglobulins, especially secretory IgA are active. (Paneth cells are named after Joseph Paneth (1857–1890), an Austrian physiologist.)

Secretory IgA. The secretory component of sIgA protects the immunoglobulin from being degraded by proteolytic

M. Giese, *Introduction to Molecular Vaccinology*, DOI 10.1007/978-3-319-25832-4_3

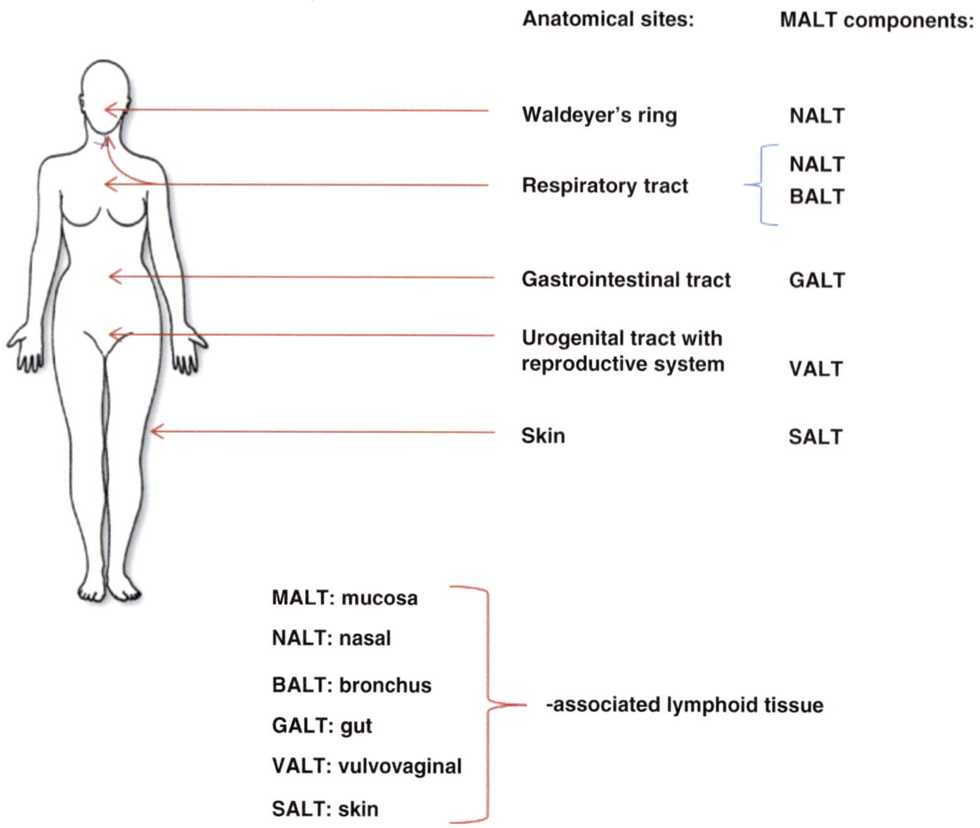

Fig. 3.1 Sites of mucosal immune systems

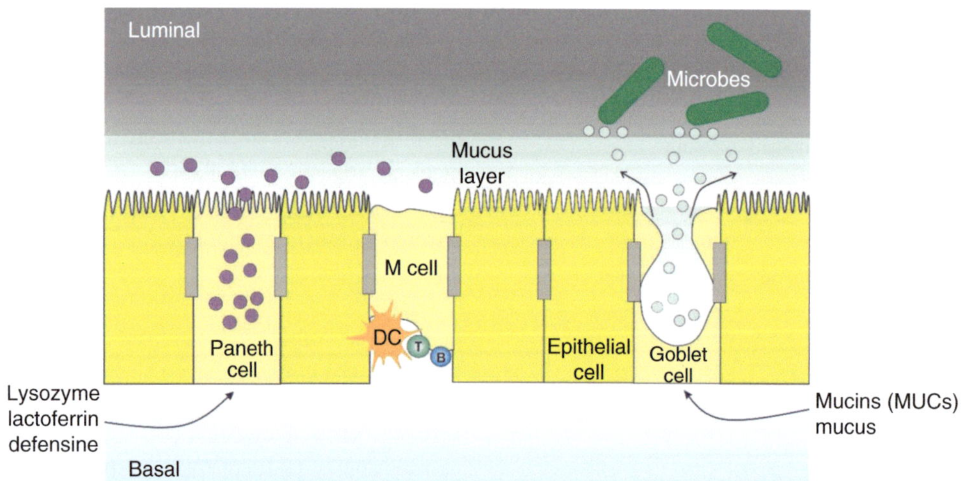

Fig. 3.2 Mucosa structure. Pathogens enter the body through mucosal surfaces by ingestion, inhalation, or sexual contact. The first contact of all these pathogens is a single-layer epithelium covered by mucus and antimicrobial molecules. But also vaccines have to cross this massive barrier from mucus and cells. Mucous secretion is produced by globlet cells and this gel is a natural chemical barrier. Mucus is rich in glycoproteins (mucins) and water. Paneth cells produce antiseptic enzymes such as lysozyme or lactoferrin and defensin. M cells (microfold) transport microorganisms and particles from the lumen to immune cells (DCs, T and B cells) across the epithelial barrier and thus are important in stimulating mucosal immunity

enzymes; thus, sIgA can survive in the harsh gastrointestinal tract environment and provide protection against microbes that multiply in body secretions.

Microorganisms that have successfully passed this first barrier find excellent living conditions in parts of the alimentary canal, in particular the ileum and the colon. Therefore, mucosa, the thin layer which lines body cavities and passages, has frontline status in immunity, making these tissue ideal sites for vaccine application (Fig. 3.2).

Mucosa vaccines are required because parenteral vaccines, although effective in eliciting systemic immune response, are ineffective in stimulating mucosal immunity against various mucosal pathogens [1].

3.2 MALT System

3.2.1 MALT Components

The mucosa-associated lymphoid tissue (MALT) is a diffuse lymphoid tissue along all mucosal surfaces populated by lymphocytes such as T cells and B cells, as well as plasma cells and macrophages. It is secondary immune tissues where antigen sampling occurs and immune responses are initiated. The MALT system is mostly subdivided into four main components, the nasal-associated lymphoid tissue (*NALT*), the bronchus-associated lymphoid tissue (*BALT*), the gut-associated lymphoid tissue (*GALT*), the skin-associated lymphoid tissue (*SALT*), and additional mucosa-associated lymphoid tissues as described in Table 3.1.

Main Components. The cellular basis of all MALT tissues is two main components, an inductive site and an effector site. The upper inductive site is the site where antigens are captured, processed and specific immune responses are initiated, and the lower effector site, glandular tissues and the Lamina propria (LP) region, where antibodies are produced and cell-mediated immune response takes place. There is a constant migration from the upper site to the lower (Fig. 3.3).

One main effector function is the production of IgA in antigen-specific reactions and the IgA secretion across mucosal surfaces. Th1 and cytotoxic T cell-mediated reactions can also occur, the later resulting in immunotolerance.

3.2.2 Immunotolerance

Two adaptive homeostatic mechanisms normally preserve mucosal integrity:

1. Immune exclusion mediated by secretory antibodies to inhibit penetration of potentially dangerous microorganisms and proteins
2. Immunosuppression in the gut to counteract hypersensitivity against innocuous organisms or antigens – known as "oral tolerance"

The oral immunotolerance is important for normal physiology, not less than important for our survival. An immune response against pathogens is highly requested, but it would be self-destructive to mount an immune response against components of the food. Immune cell activation therefore differs between the MALT and other lymphoid tissues. MALT cells do not mix with other immune cells outside of MALT, and MALT cells express specific homing receptors allowing their homing during circulation. Finally, MALT plasma cells produce a secretable form of immunoglobulin A

Table 3.1 Components of the MALT system

Anatomical system of the body	Inductive sites	Effector sites	Lymphoid structures
Respiratory tract	Nasopharynx-associated lymphoid tissue (NALT)	Nasopharyngeal mucosa	Waldeyer's pharyngeal ring: Adenoids (pharyngeal tonsils) Palatine tonsils Lingual tonsils Tubal tonsils
	Bronchus-associated lymphoid tissue (BALT)	Bronchial mucosa – lower respiratory tract	Peyer's patches Isolated lymphoid follicles
	Larynx-associated lymphoid tissue (LALT)	Larynx	Laryngeal tonsils Lymphoid follicles Lymphoid follicles with germinal centers
Digestive system	Salivary duct-associated lymphoid tissue (DALT)	Salivary glands	Lymphoid follicles
	Gut-associated lymphoid tissue (GALT)	Gastrointestinal mucosa	Peyer's patches Lymphoglandular complexes Isolated lymphoid follicles cryptopatches Appendix
Skin	Skin-associated lymphoid tissue (SALT)	Keratinocytes, Langerhans cells	Skin trophic T cells Lymphatic endothelial cells
Ocular system	Conjunctiva-associated lymphoid tissue (CALT)	Conjunctiva	Lymphoepithelium Lymphoid follicles with B and T cell zones Adjacent blood vessels that have thickened endothelia Lymphoid vessels
	Lacrimal duct-associated lymphoid tissue (LDALT)	Ocular tissues	Lymphoid follicles
Reproductive system	Vulvovaginal-associated lymphoid tissue (VALT)	Urogenital tract	Lymphoid follicles
Excretory system	Rectal lymphoepithelial tissue	Gastrointestinal mucosa	Lymphoid follicles

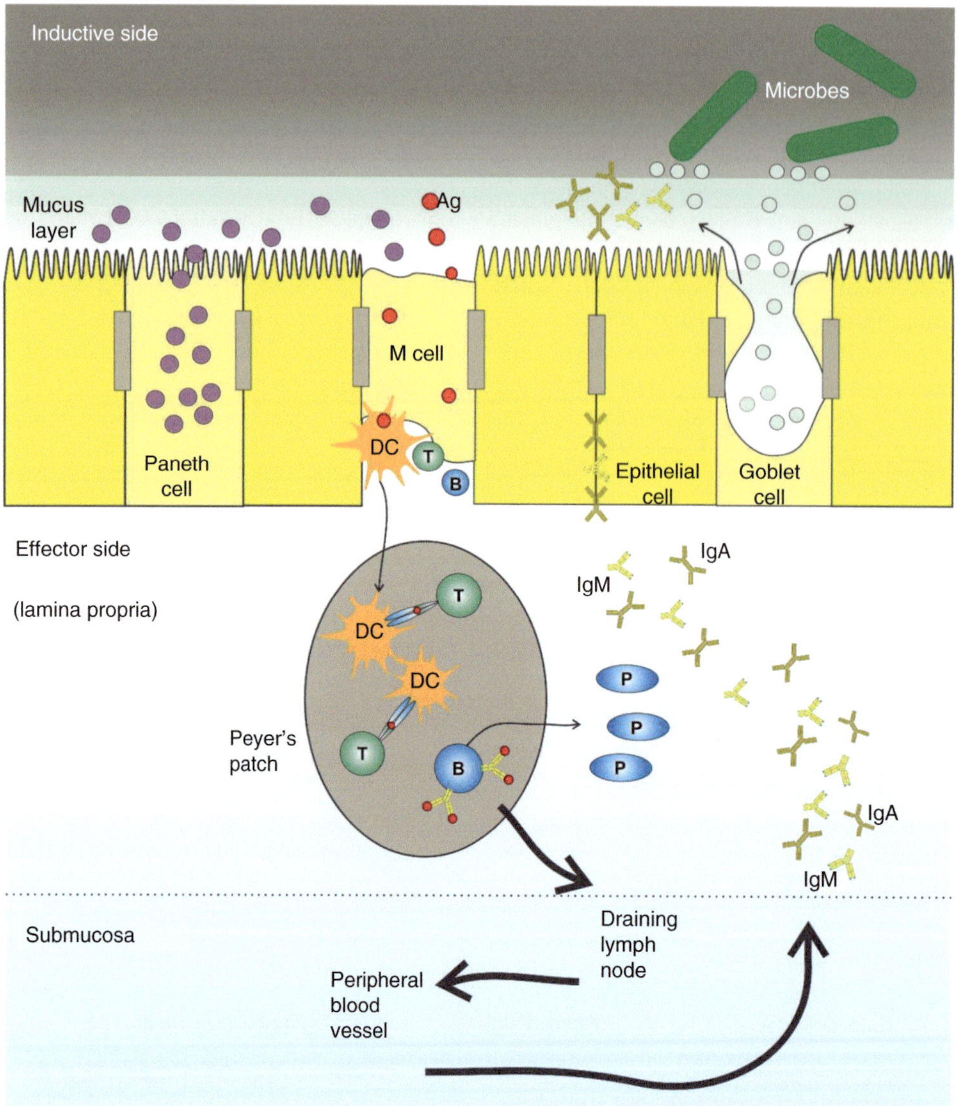

Fig. 3.3 Cross talk between upper and lower MALT region. The cellular basis of all MALT tissues is two main components, an inductive site and an effector site. The upper inductive site is the site where antigens are captured, e.g., by M cells and DCs, processed and specific immune responses are initiated, and the lower effector site, where antibodies are produced and cell-mediated immune response takes place. MALT plasma cells produce a secretable form of immunoglobulin A (sIgA) dimers which can be taken up by epithelial cells and then released onto the epithelial surface. T cells, B cells, and memory cells are stimulated upon encountering antigen in Peyer's patches, organized lymphoid nodules. There is a constant migration from the upper site to the lower. Lymph nodes within the submucosa transport the immune response to peripheral blood vessels

(sIgA) dimers which can be taken up by epithelial cells and then released onto the epithelial surface.

In summary the mucosal immune response differs from systemic immune responses:

- Secretory IgA as dimer is the major immunoglobulin isotype.
- The MALT system produces the most antibodies.
- In the MALT system, there exist the most effector T cells (the majority of all T and B cells, ≥75 %, exist within MALT).
- Lymphoid cells have two functional sites, an inductive and an effector site.
- The enteric bacterial flora is a major stimulus for the development of mucosa immune system.

3.3 Nasal Vaccination[1]

Nasal delivery of vaccines occurred over a millennium ago in China, where ground scabs from small pox lesions, presumably containing live virus, were sniffed. Figure 3.4 illustrates this ancient vaccination method.

3.3.1 NALT

The nasal mucosa is complex and includes important elements of the immune system. Therefore, it is an ideal route of delivery for a noninvasive vaccine delivery. The anatomy of the nasal cavity is shown in Fig. 3.5. The ciliated surfaces of the nasal turbinates deliver mucus to the floor of the nasal cavity and from there to the throat, site of the Waldeyer's ring, consisting notably of adenoids and tonsils [3]. Mucociliary clearance disposes of ambient particulates that deposit on the nasal epithelium. Normal mucociliary clearance rates are approximately 45–90 min from the proximal to distal points in the nasopharynx [4]. The intent of any nasal vaccine delivery system is to achieve a residence time at the nasal mucosa sufficient to elicit the desired immunological and hopefully protective response.

Nasal vaccine delivery proposes to target the nasal-associated lymphoid tissue (NALT). The principle on which this approach depends is to present the selected antigen to the NALT and Waldeyer's ring and ultimately to the immunologically important M cells and dendritic cells. These cells are responsible for producing an immune response through antigen presentation to circulating lymphocytes.

The Waldeyer's ring is de facto no ring but an aggregation of lymphoid tissues located at the openings of the respiratory and digestive tract (Fig. 3.6).

The two most common (and effective) nasal delivery devices are either multiple- or single-dose pumps, examples of which deliver calcitonin, to treat osteoporosis, and corticosteroids, to treat allergic rhinitis, respectively [5]. However, these FDA-approved products require solution or suspension formulations which are not the most desirable preparations for vaccines. Recently, the use of powder aerosols for vaccination has been proposed with attendant advantages of increased residence time and greater opportunity for antigen presentation [5, 6].

[1]Nasal dry powder vaccine delivery technology by *Anthony J. Hickey, Herman Staats, Chad J. Roy, Kenneth G. Powell, Vince Sullivan, Ginger Rothrock and Christie M. Sayes* in Molecular Vaccines – From Prophylaxis to Therapy, Volume 2, Springer-Verlag Wien, 2013, Ed. Matthias Giese.

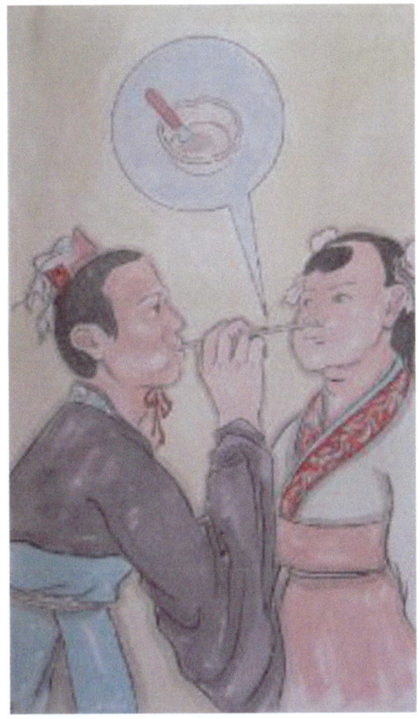

Fig. 3.4 Smallpox nasal vaccination via dry powder. Voltaire, 1694–1778, observed "… the Chinese go about it (inoculation) in a different fashion they make no incision but give smallpox through the nose, like snuff. This way is pleasanter (than cutaneous delivery), but it comes to the same thing…" [2]

3.3.2 Anthrax Vaccine and Nasal Application

The mortality associated with inhalation or pulmonary anthrax, along with recent concerns regarding the possibility of the causative microorganism being used as a weapon, necessitates the development of a vaccine that is easily administered and requires minimal storage and distribution controls that can be rapidly deployed. Inhalation anthrax is considered to be the most deadly form of anthrax.

Bacillus Anthracis. The causative organism of anthrax is *Bacillus anthracis* (*B. anthracis*). This organism is associated with infections of animals and results in skin and pulmonary disease in humans following contact with infected animals or animal products [7]. Pulmonary anthrax is a particularly insidious, and if untreated, fatal form of the disease.

A unique component of the life cycle of *B. anthracis* is the formation of spores as a method of withstanding stressful environmental conditions. Anthrax spores, in common with those of other organisms, are exquisitely suited to dispersion in air. Spores then deposit throughout the respiratory tract. The ability of these spores to retain their viability through extremes of environmental stress for decades or centuries

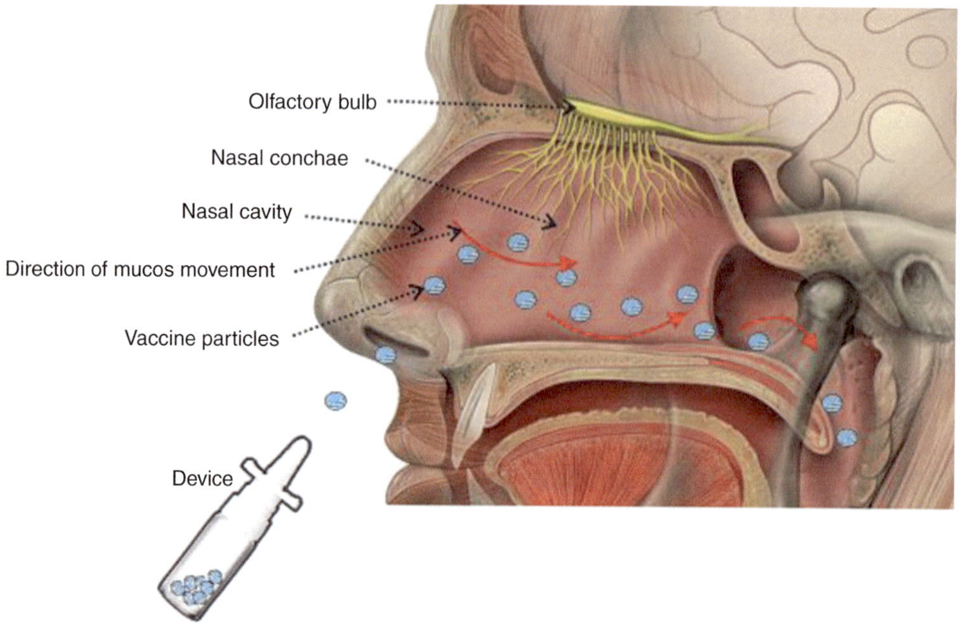

Fig. 3.5 Schematic anatomy of the nasal cavity (Figure by M. Giese Heidelberg, Germany)

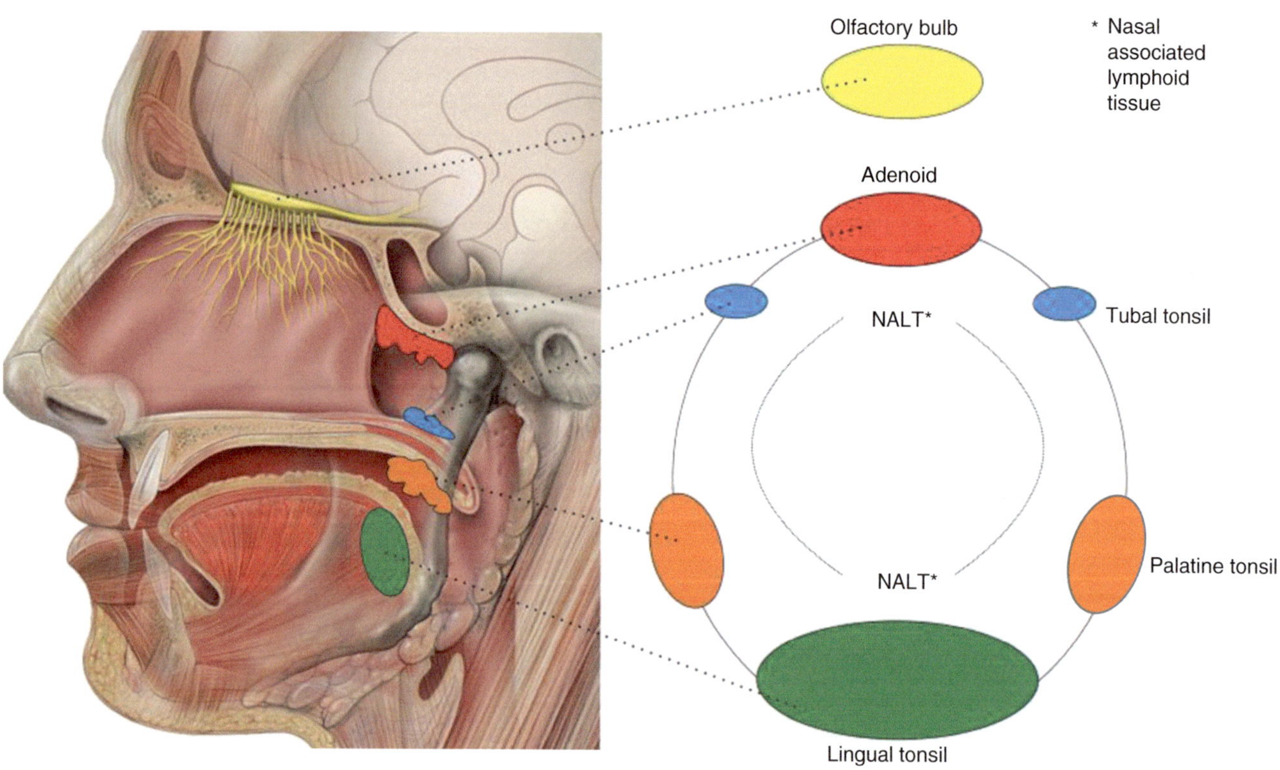

Fig. 3.6 Schematic anatomy of the Waldeyer's ring (Figure by M. Giese Heidelberg, Germany)

poses a public health risk. The virulence, ease of delivery, and long-term stability of *B. anthracis* spores rendered them a source of great concern throughout the middle of the twentieth century at the height of state-sponsored biological weapons development and, more recently, regarding bioterrorism.

After the terrorist action in the United States of September 11, 2001, the demand for biodefense measures increased following the incident in which letters contained "weaponized" anthrax powders [8, 9]. The immediate demand was for drugs (e.g., ciprofloxacin) to treat infected individuals. The need for vaccines that could be stockpiled and quickly distributed with the minimum storage considerations (special packaging or temperature) in quantities sufficient to contain an outbreak, particularly for health-care providers and military personnel, also became a research and development focus [10]. In this context, vaccines for protection and drugs for treatment have been developed for this specific application over the past decade.

Current Vaccine. In general, the practice of presenting live organisms as a vaccine system, albeit in an attenuated state, is an elevated health risk. The previously mentioned example for smallpox treatment in China and Europe was undoubtedly a risky procedure because the prospects of contracting disease were significant. Similarly, for anthrax, the use of a virulent organism would be a questionable strategy. The current vaccine, BioThrax (Emergent Solutions), uses culture filtrate, which presents all of the important antigens (lethal factor [LF], protective antigen [PA], and edema factor [EF]) [10] (Fig. 3.7).

Recombinant Vaccines. The emphasis for novel immunization strategies for protection against anthrax has been the use of recombinant protective antigen, which has demonstrated protection in animal models of disease [11]. Indeed, it has just been announced that an rPA vaccine, SparVaxTM (PharmAthene), is entering further phase II trials. However, it has been suggested that adjuvancy is required to ensure a sufficiently robust response. This may be achieved through coadministration of an adjuvant molecule of which there are many but most notably monophosphoryl lipid A (MPL) – an FDA-approved drug, referred to as Ceravix, and safely used in human studies with a nasal *Norovirus* vaccine.

Alternatively, a physical approach may be taken using small targeting particles (nanoparticles) that would deliver the antigen effectively to the NALT. Nanoparticles have a particular propensity for this purpose and have been shown for many years to be effective as carriers and adjuvants [12–14]. It is important to note that despite the mucosal route of administration, an IgA response is not thought to be significant in protection from anthrax [11].

Currently, we might add not only is it "pleasanter" (needle-free) and that it "amounts to the same thing" (a protective immune response), but with current technology, it is stable on storage, easy to use, and inexpensive. The delivery of particles in a stable dispersible form lends itself to the use of dry particles. The ability to spray dry particle suspensions has been demonstrated for a number of vaccine applications [15]. Specific to this discussion, Fig. 3.8 outlines the

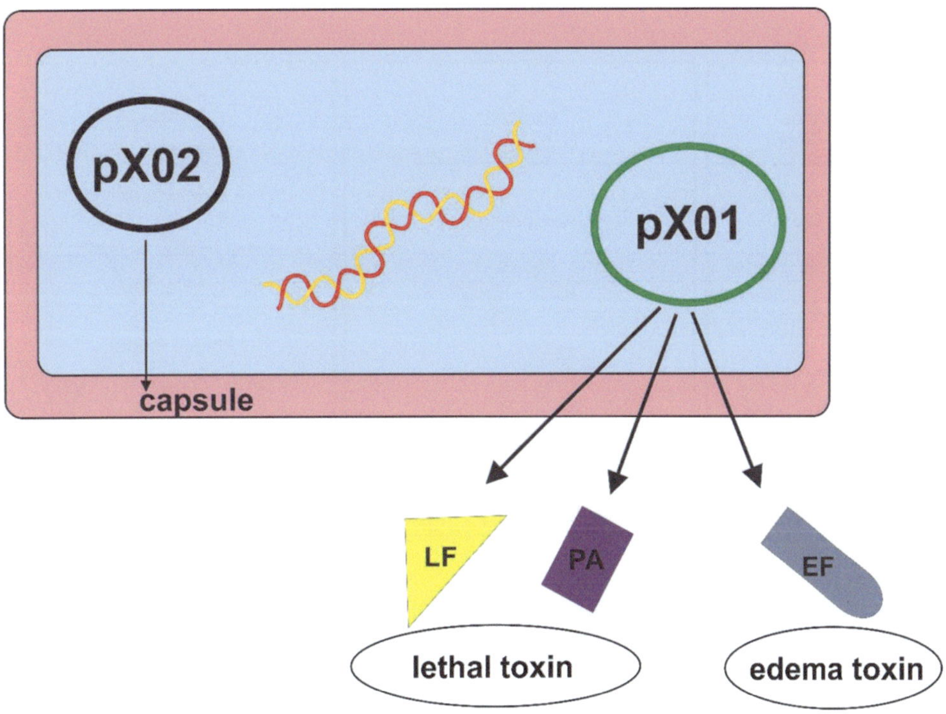

Fig. 3.7 Bacillus anthracis antigens. The main virulent factors are encoded on two extrachromosomal double-stranded plasmids, pXO1 (189 kb, anthrax toxin complex) and pXO2 (96 kb, capsule). The toxin is a complex of three plasmid-encoded proteins: lethal factor (*LF*), edema factor (*EF*) on the plasmid one, and the protective antigen (*PA*) which ushers the two toxic proteins LF and ED in host cells (Figure by M. Giese Heidelberg, Germany)

components needed for the development of a safe and effective technologically advanced nasal vaccine system.

3.3.3 Components of Nasal Vaccines

3.3.3.1 Formulation

In order to develop vaccine formulations that would have potential for worldwide distribution, dry powders must be able to be stored long-term without refrigeration and be administered without the use of needles. Spray-dried, freeze-dried, and spray-freeze-dried powders have demonstrated equivalent immunogenicity to conventional liquid formulations with the potential advantage that dry powders can circumvent the problem of the cold chain which is often associated with liquid vaccine formulations. These techniques can be paired with conventional and novel nanoparticle fabrication methodologies such as precipitation, homogenization, and top-down manufacturing to generate dry powders of loose nanoparticle aggregates having aerodynamic diameters suitable for mucosal delivery as has previously been demonstrated for inhaled formulations.

3.3.3.2 Devices

There are only a few nasal powder delivery devices available commercially or in clinical development [16]. One such device is shown in Fig. 3.9. While formulation and powder morphology play key roles in targeting deposition to the nasal tissues, it is essential that the powder be deaggregated and efficiently delivered from the device.

Key device attributes fall into two categories: those affecting clinical efficacy and those human factors reflective of the human–device interaction.

Firstly, the emitted dose fraction from the device needs to be as large as possible. Secondly, the emitted dose must be in a form that reaches the targeted tissue.

Particles smaller than 10 μm can be carried deeper into the lung tissue which may not be desirable, while particles larger than 50 μm may have difficulty reaching immunoresponsive tissues.

The challenge is in obtaining the proper deaggregation of the particles without excessive energy input. Moving air is generally used to deaggregate and propel the particles into the airway. However, excess airflow can force the particles to pass the targeted region so that they "pass through" without settling and eliciting an immune response.

From the human factor perspective, the device should be intuitive and easy to handle. Devices are currently targeted for administration by clinicians, but possible applications include biodefense vaccines where delivery by untrained personnel may be desired. Finally, the device should be unit dose; there is no need for a multidose format, and it would be

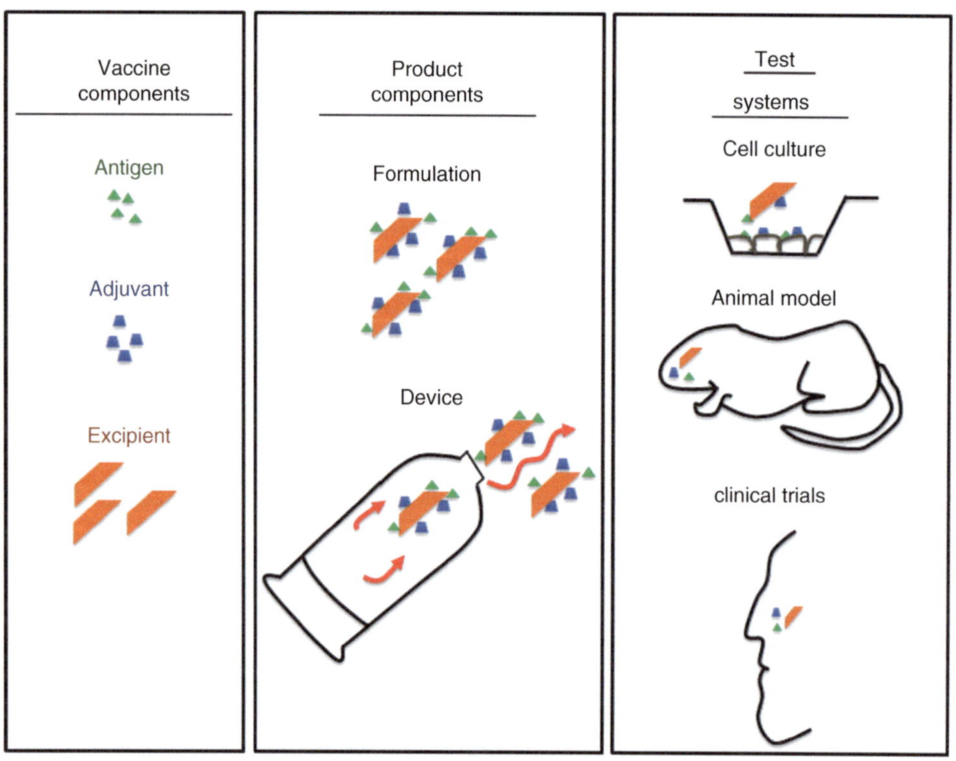

Fig. 3.8 Schematic of the key elements of the vaccine product and the methods of evaluation as presented in this chapter

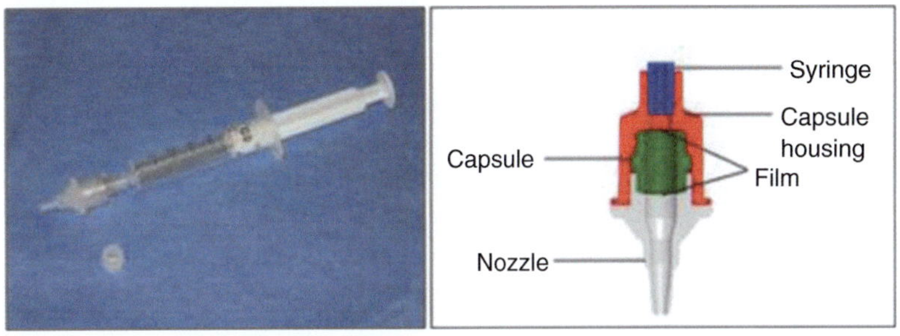

Fig. 3.9 The BD Solovent® device for nasal vaccine administration [17]. This device depends on "burstable membranes" that rupture under syringe air pressure during use. This results in a gentle pop and the expulsion of the dose

unnecessarily risky to use the same device on multiple people. Furthermore, the device should not be "reloadable" for unintended use.

3.3.3.3 Adjuvants for Nasal Immunization

Alum. Aluminum salts (alum) have been used as adjuvants with great success for almost a century and have been particularly effective at promoting protective humoral immunity. However, alum is not optimally effective for diseases where cell-mediated immunity is required for protection. Furthermore, classical biological adjuvants, such as Freund's adjuvant, have shown improved efficacy for protection in animal models, yet the toxicity profiles prevent widespread adoption for human use. In particular, there is demand for safe and nontoxic adjuvants able to stimulate cellular immunity without undue toxicity and adjuvants suitable for use with mucosally delivered recombinant and subunit vaccines. Novel particle and biological adjuvants offer a means to overcome the deficiencies of classical adjuvant technologies.

Modern Mucosal Adjuvants. A human study was recently performed using a nasally delivered dry powder vaccine containing a Norwalk virus-like particle (VLP) immunogen (i.e., monophosphoryl lipid A [MPL]) as the adjuvant and chitosan as a mucoadhesive [18]. The Norwalk VLP was well tolerated and immunogenic in humans, suggesting that a dry powder vaccine formulation for use in humans is feasible. Polymeric nanoparticles have also demonstrated dual functionality as antigen delivery systems with added adjuvant effect [19]. We postulate that dry powder polymeric nanoparticle aerosols containing recombinant protective antigen (rPA) delivered from a commercial device and targeted to the nasal mucosa will protect nonhuman primates from challenge with airborne anthrax.

Adjuvants, in the context of vaccines, may be functionally defined as any substance able to augment the immunogenicity of the vaccine antigen. Adjuvants are beneficial since they are able to enhance the percentage of vaccines that achieve protective immunity at the completion of the vaccination regimen [20], and they are able to increase the magnitude of immune responses induced [20], reduce the antigen dose required to induce protective immunity [21], and/or reduce the number of immunizations needed to induce protective immunity [22]. In general terms, adjuvants either enhance antigen delivery to or enhance the activation state of dendritic cells, the primary antigen-presenting cell that initiates the development of adaptive immunity after vaccination [23].

Nanogels. Adjuvants can increase the immunogenicity of nasally delivered vaccines by enhancing antigen delivery to the host. A recent study by Kiyono et al. [24] described the use of cationic nanogels as adjuvants for nasally delivered protein antigens. Although the cationic nanogels did not enhance the activation state of nasal dendritic cells, the cationic nanogels significantly enhanced the immunogenicity of the nasal vaccine due to improved antigen retention in the nasal cavity that was associated with better antigen delivery to nasal dendritic cells [24]. A nanoemulsion adjuvant system is also being developed as a nasal vaccine adjuvant [25–27] and has been described as "… does not contain a proinflammatory component but penetrates mucosal surfaces to load antigens into dendritic cells." [27]

Dry Powders. Dry powders produced by spray-freeze-drying (SFD) liquid vaccine formulations also provide a vaccine adjuvant strategy to enhance the immunogenicity of nasally delivered vaccines [28] when compared to nasal immunization with liquid vaccine formulations. Since other studies have demonstrated that increased nasal retention of vaccine formulations correlates with increased immunogenicity of the vaccine [24, 29, 30], it is possible that dry powder vaccine formulations augment the immunogenicity of nasally delivered vaccines by increasing antigen retention in the nasal cavity to ultimately improve antigen delivery to the nasal dendritic cells for better induction of antigen-specific adaptive immunity.

TLR Ligand Adjuvants. Adjuvants may also activate the host innate immune system to enhance the induction of antigen-specific adaptive immunity after nasal immunization [31, 32]. Adjuvants that activate the innate immune system are typically thought to activate dendritic cells [33] to increase their ability to induce antigen-specific adaptive immune responses. A wide range of mucosal adjuvants able to activate the innate immune system include pro-inflammatory cytokines [34, 35] and Toll-like receptor ligands (TLR ligands; monophosphoryl lipid A, CpG oligodeoxynucleotides, imiquimod) [33, 34, 36]. Although cholera toxin and related toxins are known to provide effective mucosal adjuvant activity, adverse events associated with the use of toxin-based adjuvants [37, 38] will likely limit their use in human vaccines. Cytokines and TLR ligand adjuvants have been used as nasal vaccine adjuvants in human clinical studies with acceptable safety profiles suggesting that adjuvanted nasally administered vaccines may be feasible with additional optimization and safety evaluations [35, 39].

A general overview on adjuvants and their mode of action is presented in Chap. 7.

3.3.4 Mechanisms of Particle Uptake

Many of the markers of toxicity are also pro-inflammatory mediators. This type of induced response is desirable to achieve a protective immunity from vaccines. Individual parameters may be associated with specific phenomena (e.g., caspase and oxygenase or extracellular cytoplasm leakage caused by peroxy radical formation on cellular membranes). However, these acellular markers may not be indicative of the entire tissue system – it is important to consider the combined response in terms of magnitude and duration of each cellular response as a signature of transition from reversible "transient" to irreversible "toxic" response. For example, the oxidative stress as indicated by the REDOX (i.e., reduction or oxidation) state of glutathione has been used to indicate this transition from normal transient phenomenon to toxic cell response [40–42].

Conclusions from the literature have led to the premise that there are two primary physicochemical properties of small particles, including nanoparticles, which influence their stability, mobility, and toxicity. These two primary physicochemical properties are as follows: (1) surface modification or conjugation to other molecules and (2) physical contact with cells. The former influences particle aggregation state, determines individual particle suspendability, and affects susceptibility to degradation. The latter affects cellular uptake mechanism substantially.

Particle Size. Particles that are less than 20 nm can transport across the cytoplasmic membrane and accumulate in a variety of subcellular components. Particles (or aggregates of particles) between 20 and 200 nm have the potential to be taken up into cells via active transport mechanism of *clathrin* or caveolin pit formation. Particles (or aggregates of particles) larger than 200 nm are readily endocytosed via macropinocytosis (Fig. 3.10).

Ultimately, most particles sequester in membrane-bound vesicles where the acidification process begins. The acidification process usually breaks the particle down into their ions or molecules, releasing then a concentrated dose to specific tissues most vulnerable to particle deposition. While not all mechanisms are known within this general field of study, most agree that cellular uptake plays a large role in a cell's and a tissue's response to particles.

Studies have shown that exposure to particles in both in vitro and in vivo systems may cause production of inflammatory biomarkers [41, 43–46]. After engineered particles are internalized by cell, such as phagocytes, the inflammatory cascade may be triggered. Inflammation is the complex biological response of cells and tissues to harmful pathogens and other toxicants. It is both a proactive mechanism to remove these harmful pathogens and to initiate production of repair enzymes. Unchecked inflammation can lead to a host of diseases, such as asthma, atherosclerosis, and rheumatoid arthritis; therefore, it is normally tightly regulated by the body. Figure 3.11 graphically depicts the four distinct steps in a particle-induced inflammatory cascade.

Critical Parameters. The critical performance parameters for nanoparticle-based vaccines would include:

- Particles that are less than 100 nm in diameters (a.k.a. nanoparticles*) that contain antigen that is released over a one-week time period.
- A spray-freeze-dried aggregate of approximately 20 μm in aerodynamic diameter.
- The spray-freeze-dried aggregates should deaggregate into primary particles in less than 15 min. This short time period is due to the fact that mucociliary clearance rates of 45–90 min require rapid deaggregation to allow individual particles to access the mucosa.
- Ideally, the product should be room temperature stable for a few years.

(* a.k.a. nanoparticles: nanometer-sized cluster nanoparticles)

3.3.5 Animal Models for Anthrax

Aerosol Delivery. The in vivo testing and evaluation of a new vaccine formulated for aerosol delivery requires careful consideration of factors relating to the appropriateness of the species and delivery modality as it relates to the immunogen and the corresponding infectious disease agent.

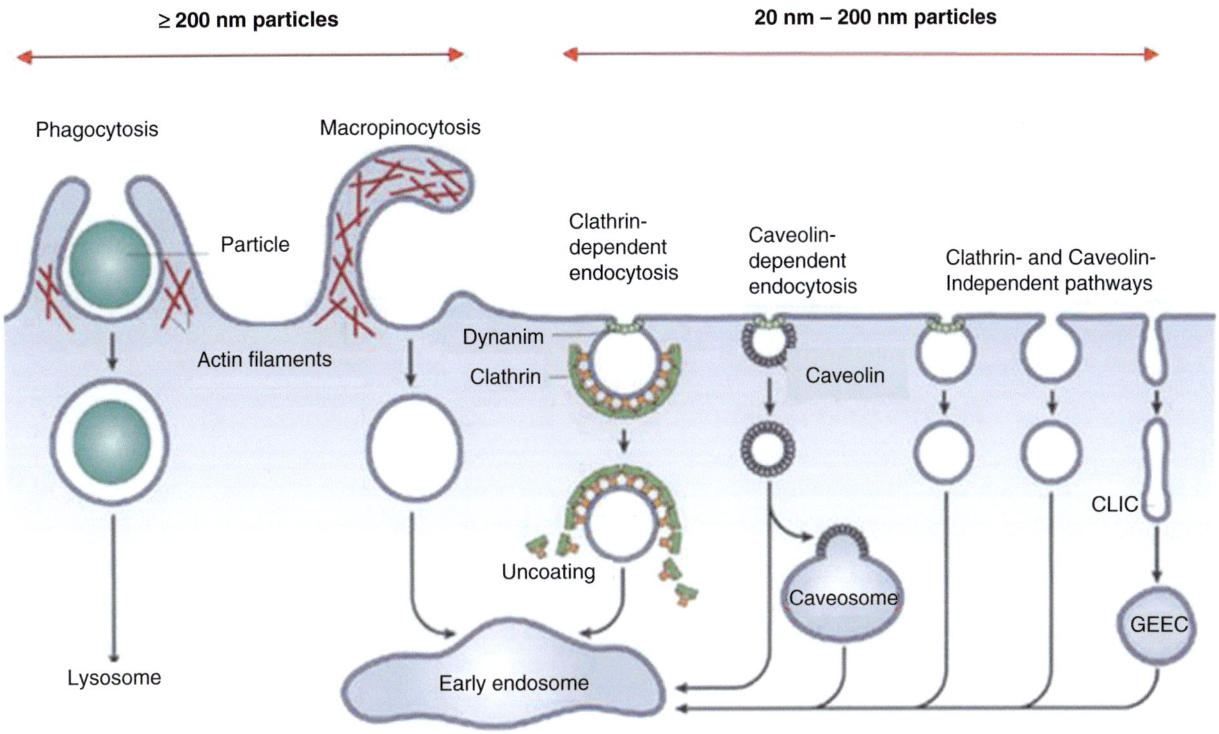

Fig. 3.10 Large particles, 200 nm in size or larger, can be taken up by phagocytosis, and smaller particles between 20 and 200 nm are taken up by clathrin- or caveolin-dependent active mechanisms. Most internalized cargos are delivered to the early endosome, also clathrin- or caveolin-independent particles, transported via tubular carriers (*CLIC*). Some transport routes may first traffic to intermediate compartments, such as the caveosome or glycosylphosphatidylinositol-anchored protein-enriched endosomal compartments (*GEEC*) (Credit: Mayo and Pagano [127])

The rationale underpinning evaluation in a particular species is determined at least in part upon the predicted serological and/or mucosal immune response in that particular species. There is a narrow range of species available for use in these types of studies because the availability of well-characterized and documented infectious disease models is generally lacking.

In addition, matching the selected modality of vaccination in the animal model with the ultimate clinical administration route can further limit choices. Many delivery platforms do not cater to a seamless adaptation in a preclinical setting; this is especially the case where an inhalation device requires any sort of respiratory compliance maneuver to assure dosing. Thus, one is faced with the logistical challenge of providing a surrogate delivery platform for vaccination delivery for the animal experiments.

Rabbit Model. Specific to vaccination and the immune response, selection of the species that will produce the desired immune response is many times predicated upon past studies using similar immunogens with familiar targets. Selection of the rabbit in the establishment of a clinical correlate of immunity against anthrax, for example, uses a previous characterized animal model with robust serological antibody production from a culture filtrate vaccine product (anthrax vaccine adsorbed, AVA) [47].

Inhalation anthrax in the rabbit has been well documented and provided a well-characterized model of infection that can be used to test efficacy of a particular vaccine formulation [48]. In this particular example, the model and corresponding immune response was used to establish an in vitro correlate of immunity (α-PA IgG) predictive of clinical efficacy of the vaccine formulation. The establishing of a correlate of immunity would have not been possible if the basis of the model (inhalation anthrax in the rabbit) and the corresponding marker of immunity (α-PA IgG) had not been first characterized.

Superantigen-Associated Shock. Choice of species in the use of animal models also requires critical assessment of the interspecies-specific biological responses prior to selection. The available animal models for investigation of superantigen-associated shock (Sag), for example, is heavily dependent upon the richness of MHC-II receptors in the

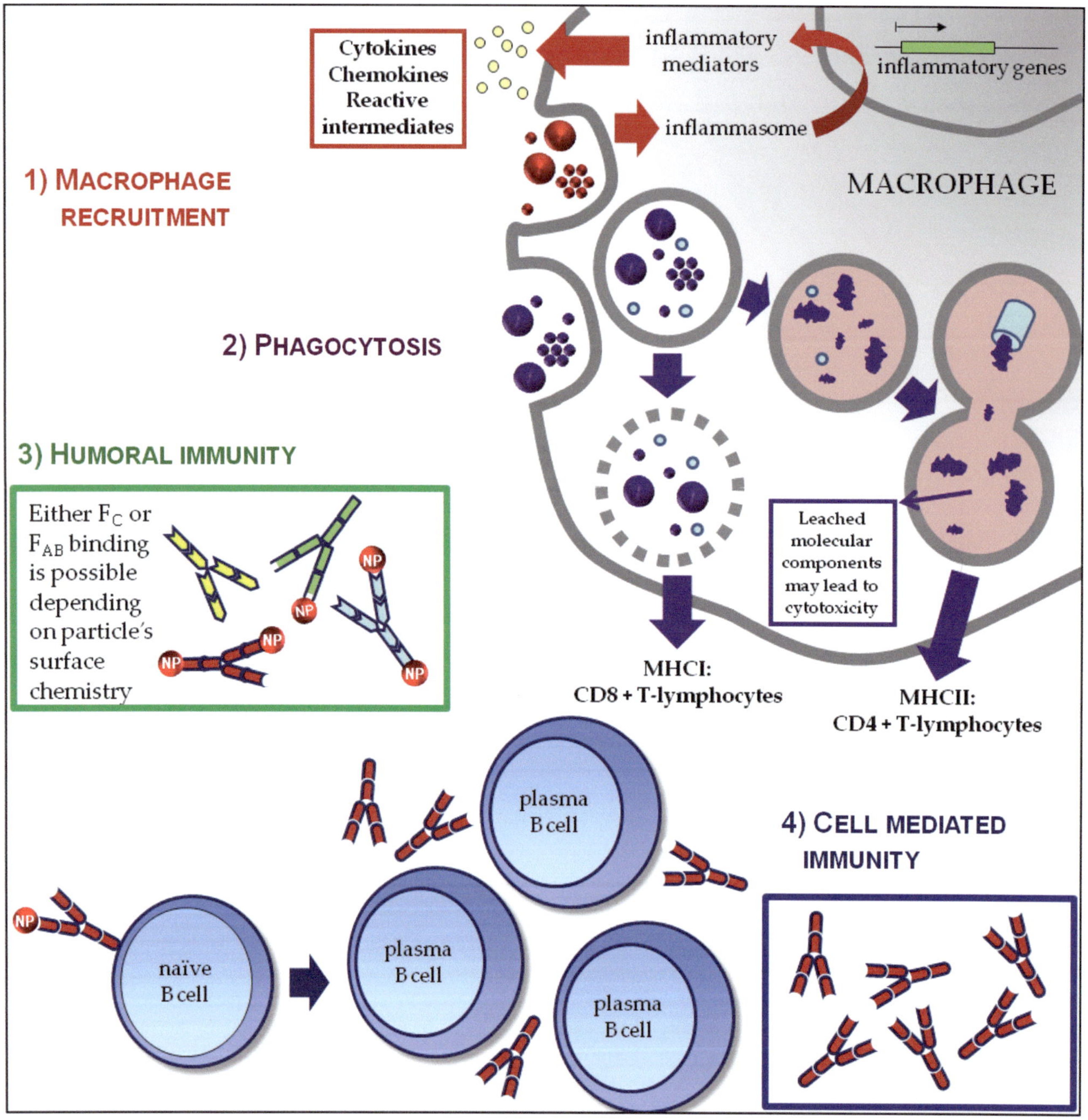

Fig. 3.11 General mechanisms of cellular toxicity after inhalation of particles. Presumed steps in triggering either cell-mediated or humoral immunities include: (*1*) inhaled particles induce macrophage recruitment to mediate inflammation with cytokines and nitric oxide, causing local tissue damage; (*2*) individual particles are phagocytosed and acidified in macrophage endocytic pathway, causing cytotoxic release molecular components; (*3*) specific to nanometer-sized particles, binding to nonspecific subsets of naive humoral repertoire is possible; and (*4*) particles are recognized by a specific B cell paratope, which clonally expands plasma cells, secreting particle-specific antibodies, clearing the particles

animal species. Direct binding of Sag toxins to circulating T cells is mediated through the MHC-II receptor and therefore represents a critical pathway in the subsequent inflammatory response. Rodents and rodent-like species are generally nonresponsive to challenge with purified staphylococcal and streptococcal enterotoxemic shock due to the lack of circulating MHC-II receptors.

Although these receptors are found in great abundance in phylogenetically higher life forms such as the primate, larger animals are generally used as disease models much more sparingly and only at selected intervals compared to rodent species. Rodent models are still used as a disease model of Sag-induced toxicity through the use of co-stimulatory mediators such as lipopolysaccharide (LPS) or through the use of

Table 3.2 Licensed nasal vaccines

Target pathogen (region)	Licensed vaccine	Details of vaccine	Ref.
Influenza (USA)	FluMist® (quadrivalent nasal influenza vaccine)[a]	Live attenuated influenza virus A/H1N1, A/H3N2, and two influenza B strains	[51]
Influenza (Europe)	Fluenz® (quadrivalent nasal influenza vaccine)[a]	Live attenuated influenza virus A/H1N1, A/H3N2, and two influenza B strains	[51]
Influenza (India)	Nasovac-S® (trivalent)	Live attenuated influenza virus A/H1N1, A/H3N2, and one influenza B strain	[52]

[a]Same manufacturer

transgenics that express for MHC-II [49, 50]. The particular example of animal models of Sag-induced toxicity punctuates the requirement for critical assessment of predictive response prior to design of a study that may incorporate challenge for determination of efficacy of a vaccine product.

3.3.6 Licensed Nasal Vaccines

Only three of the nasal vaccines have been licensed until today and are commercially available for prevention of influenza (Table 3.2). They consist of live attenuated organisms obtained by egg-based manufacturing and reassortant technology (FluMist®, Fluenz®, Nasovac-S®). These vaccines have been successful in preventing disease in specific target populations: FluMist® and Fluenz® are approved for use in persons 2 through 49 years of age living in industrialized countries, infants, and school-age children in developing countries (Nasovac-S®).

3.3.7 Limitations of Nasal Vaccines

The large mucosal surface and the high vascularization of the tissue make the nasal delivery of vaccines an attractive route for immunization. However, there are serious hurdles limiting the potential of nasal vaccination:

1. Short residence time of the antigen and adjuvant in the nasal cavity due to the rapid muco-nasal clearance rate (15–30 min).
2. From this follows only a short time for a successful uptake through the mucosal barrier.
3. Dose volume is restricted from 25 to 200 μl due to the anatomy of the nasal cavity.
4. The pH of the nasal mucosa (pH 5.5–6.5) influences the activity and stability of the antigen.
5. Nasal enzymes, proteases and nucleases, attack the antigen.
6. A lack of safe and powerful adjuvants resulting in an insufficient immune response.
7. Finally, pathological conditions in the upper and lower respiratory tract like tonsillitis, pharyngitis, and allergies. In addition, also cold and a running nose are bottlenecks for nasal immunization.

The consequences of these hurdles mean to develop delivery systems to overcome the physicochemical barriers. For that matter, nanotechnology could offer tools to increase the residence time and to stabilize the formulation (micro- and nanotechnology in Chap. 8). But using nanoparticles can be also of some limitations, see Table 3.3. Several particulate delivery systems have been developed for nasal delivery in the recent years: liposomes, ISCOMs, polymeric micro- and nanoparticle, and virus-like particles (VLPs) to mention only some innovative systems. The major problem with suitable mucosal adjuvants still remains to be solved.

3.3.8 Olfactory System and Enterotoxin Adjuvant

In mammals, the sense of smell is performed by the olfactory system which is divided in two distinct parts: a *main olfactory system* and an *accessory olfactory system*. The main olfactory system detects airborne substances, while the

Table 3.3 Limitation and implications for nasal vaccination

Physicochemical barriers	Implications
Short residence time (15–30 min)	Poor uptake of antigen
Restricted dose volume	Low content of antigen and adjuvant
Acid pH of nasal mucosa	Influences antigen activity and stability
Nasal enzymes	Degradation of antigen
Lack of safe and powerful adjuvants	Weak immunity
Pathological respiratory tract conditions	Vaccine is nonapplicable

accessory olfactory system senses fluid-phase stimuli. Inhaled substances, also particular vaccines, contact the main olfactory epithelium (OE) which contains various olfactory receptors. Olfactory neurons (ON) transduce receptor activation signals axonal to the olfactory bulbs (OBs), which belongs to the central nervous system.

Viral upper respiratory infections can damage the olfactory epithelium and cross the brain–blood barrier to invade the brain [53].

Some enterotoxins, given intranasally as adjuvants for protein antigens, could also target the olfactory nerves/epithelium (ON/E) and olfactory bulbs and cause neuroinflammation.

Bell's Palsy. Nasaflu Berna®, an intranasal influenza subunit vaccine and applied as a spray, was introduced in Switzerland in 2000 and already withdrawn from the market in 2001 because of a possible association with Bell's palsy, a transient facial paralysis. The results of several studies in animals raised concerns that the used adjuvant heat-labile toxin (LT) from *Escherichia coli* may be an inflammatory mediator and responsible for the adverse neurologic events [54]. In a mouse model, intranasally applied LT from *E. coli* induced inflammatory responses in meninges, the olfactory nerve, and glomerular layers of the OB.

Blood–Brain Barrier. The development of neurological side effects is specifically promoted by the neuron-binding compounds, such as A-B moiety of heat-labile enterotoxins. The process of antigen trafficking into the ON/E and subsequently the endocytosis into the nerve cell requires ADP-ribosyltransferase activity of the A subunit of the enterotoxin-based adjuvant, as well as binding to GM1 gangliosides on neuroepithelial cells (monosialoganglioside) by the B subunit. These binding activities are prerequisites for the damage and increased permeability of ON/E. The blood–brain barrier is leaky for vaccine proteins. Cytokine release with neuroinflammation and apoptosis of neurons is the consequence [55] (Fig. 3.12 and Chap. 7, LPS).

Nanoparticles and CNS. Some nasal adjuvants can destroy the blood–brain barrier (BBB) as discussed, and unwanted substances will enter the central nervous system via the olfactory system. Also pathological incidents can temporary break the BBB down.

The rapidly evolving area of nanoparticles and the wide range of applications have major impact on our lives. Metallic nanoparticle, e.g., are used for their antimicrobial properties in everyday products ranging from deodorants to personalized computer devices. Other nanoparticles are included in toothpastes, beauty products, sunscreens, batteries, solar cells, coatings, drug delivery systems, etc. Nanotechnologies

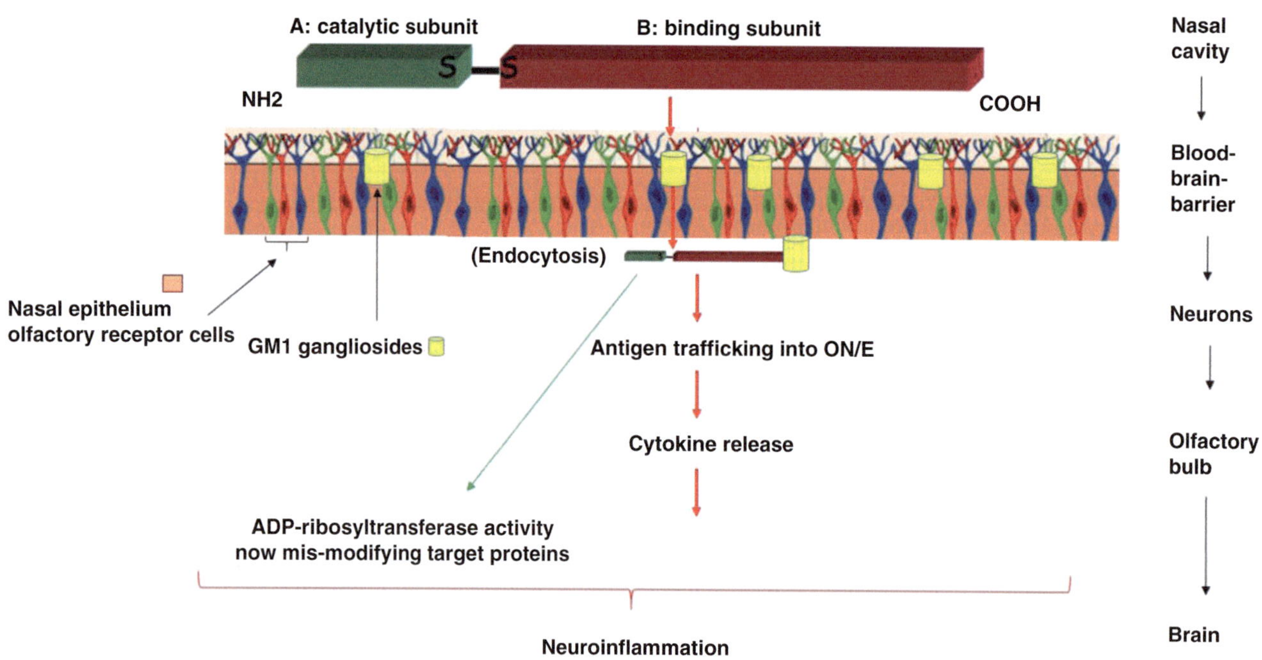

Fig. 3.12 A-B moiety of heat-labile enterotoxins crossing the blood–brain barrier. Inhaled substances, also particular vaccines, contact the main olfactory epithelium (OE) which contains various olfactory receptors. Olfactory neurons (ON) transduce receptor activation signals axonal to the olfactory bulbs (OBs). The process of antigen trafficking into the olfactory nerves/epithelium (*ON/E*) and subsequently the endocytosis into the nerve cell requires ADP-ribosyltransferase activity of the A subunit of the enterotoxin-based adjuvant, as well as binding to GM1 gangliosides on neuroepithelial cells (monosialoganglioside) by the B subunit. A damaged blood–brain barrier leads to the release of cytokines resulting in neuroinflammation (Figure by M. Giese Heidelberg, Germany)

seem to have an endless future and have progressively increased in many industrial and medical applications.

Despite the great progress in nanotechnologies, we should realize that the current knowledge on engineered nanoparticles and their interactions with the CNS cells is extremely poor! Extremely poor! [56]

Intranasal delivery of a detoxified single deletion mutant of *E. coli* LT was associated with Bell's palsy (transient facial nerve paralysis), emphasizing the need for a careful assessment of safety of novel candidates [37]. Nanoparticles in nasal vaccine compositions could influence our brain, and we should very carefully study these influences before we decide to use them.

3.4 Oral Vaccination[2]

Oral vaccination is sought as a practical and effective way to prevent diseases caused by enteric pathogens. It has the potential to induce local immune responses providing a front line of defense at mucosal surfaces as well as systemic immunity. Compliance is also higher for oral vaccination in all ages compared with parenteral vaccination and can be easily implemented to benefit large populations. One of the goals of modern vaccinology is the development of vaccines as tools that can reduce the devastating morbidity and mortality caused by enteric diseases in children under the age of five living in developing countries.

Licensed oral vaccines against polio, rotavirus, cholera, and typhoid fever have had a major impact on reducing global disease burden and mortality. A quandary that remains to be solved is the diminished immunogenicity and efficacy of these vaccines when given to subjects living in underdeveloped areas of the world as compared to people living in industrialized nations.

Low socioeconomic status, poor living conditions, malnutrition, and natural barriers that affect people living in less privileged countries are now recognized as major determinants of vaccine performance. Novel protective antigens, adjuvants, and immunization approaches to overcome these barriers are being explored. Understanding the processes involved in the induction of immune responses by orally delivered antigens, the delicate balance between immune activation and tolerance in the gut and the association between mucosal and systemic immunity is essential to assist the development and evaluation of vaccine candidates.

[2]Gut immunology and oral vaccination by *Sharon M. Tennant, Khitam Muhsen and Marcela F. Pasetti* in Molecular Vaccines – From Prophylaxis to Therapy, Volume 1, Springer-Verlag Wien, 2013, Ed. Matthias Giese.

3.4.1 Harsh Conditions for Oral Vaccines

The passage through the gastrointestinal tract (GI) represents the primary barrier to oral vaccines owing to the many hurdles: harsh acidic environment with variable pH, degradative enzymes which can result in the destruction of the vaccine, the mucosal gel layer on the epithelium surface, the tight monolayer of endothelial cells itself present throughout the GI, and the transit time in the GI.

The pH of the stomach ranges from 1.0 to 2.0 and rises 4–6 from the proximal end to the ileum and to pH 7 in the colon. The pH variation in the GI tract attacks the vaccine formulation and also the integrity of nanoparticles. Hydrochloride acid, pepsin, trypsin, amylase, etc. degrade protein- and nucleic acid-based vaccines and, e.g., starch capsules (as carriers).

The mucosal layer lining the surface of the GI tract represents another major barrier. The average thickness varies from 170 μm (stomach) to 10 μm (ileum) to 100 μm (colon). Vaccine antigens first must surpass the mucosal gel and then be transported across the intestinal epithelium on the way to GALT. Vaccines must also circumvent the oral tolerance.

The GALT/MALT is exposed to heavy and continuous exposure of pathogens and the main entry for microorganisms. Therefore, the digestive tract is an important of the immune system with the largest mass of lymphoid tissue in the human body. The network of DCs and B and T cells is responsible for the simultaneous induction and regulation of sIgA responses and the oral tolerance.

The transit time in the GI tract can be an additional limitation for the uptake of vaccine antigens. The GI motility is characterized by two distinct states: fed and fasted with distinct motilities. The fasted state is characterized by a cycle of regular contractions (2–3 h in the stomach and small intestine) and quiescent periods (40–60 min). Feeding disrupts this pattern resulting in a period of irregular contractile activities with no pattern. This background must be taken into account when specific sites in the GI shall be targeted. Figure 3.13 summarizes the major limitations for oral vaccination.

3.4.2 Vaccine Uptake and Immunological Priming in the Intestinal Mucosa

Understanding the molecular and cellular mechanisms by which orally delivered antigens and adjuvants are sampled, processed and stimulate immune cells to develop protective immunity is critical to assist in the design of more effective oral vaccines and immunization strategies. Dissecting the host factors that influence these processes is also important when targeting specific groups (e.g., infants and young children).

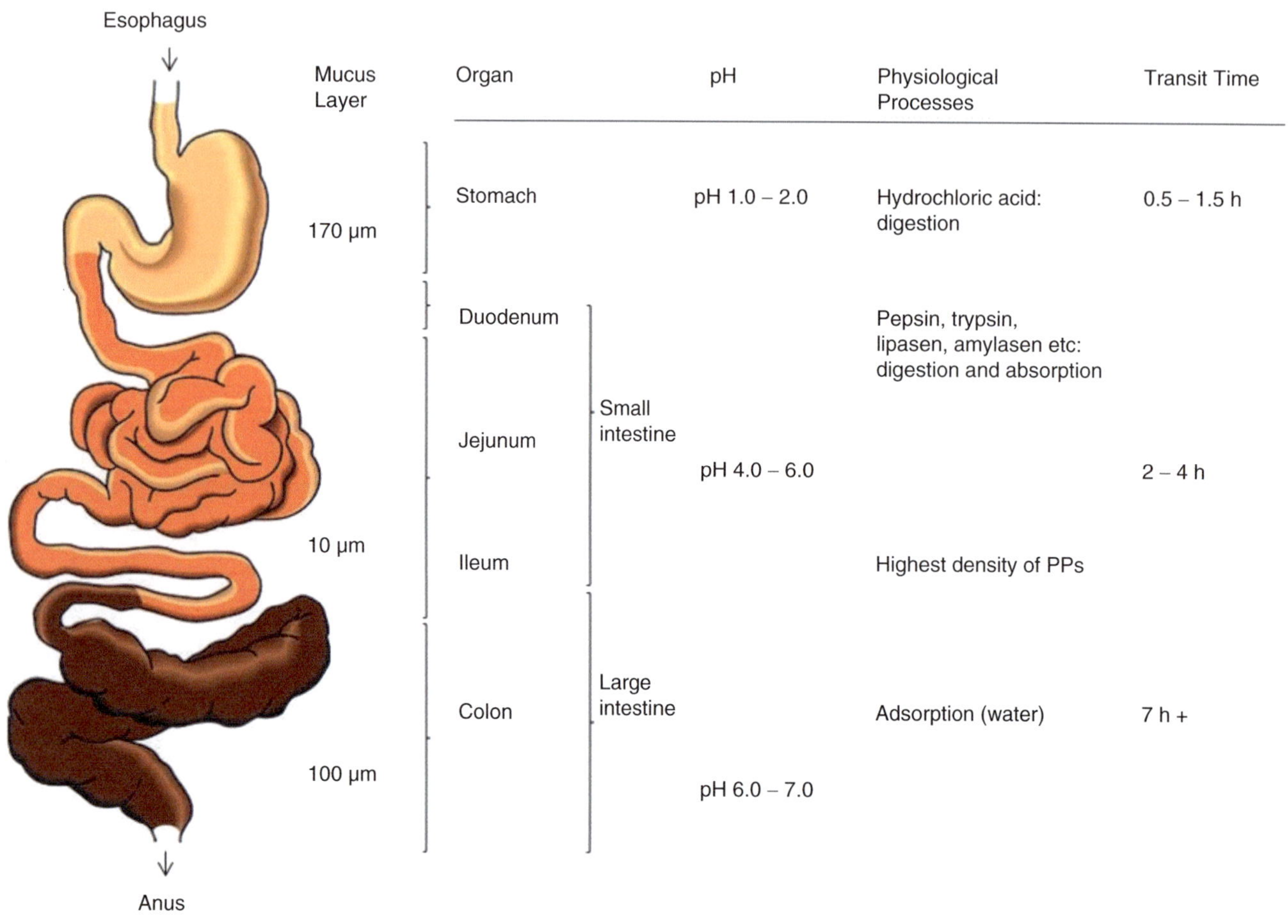

Fig. 3.13 Transit time and pH conditions in the gastrointestinal tract. The most optimal site for antigen uptake within the GI tract is the ileum of the small intestine. The transit time in the ileum lies between 2 and 4 h, and the highest density of Peyer's patches is concentrated here (Figure by M. Giese Heidelberg, Germany)

Antigens that reach inductive sites of the intestinal mucosa are captured by the microfold (M) cells within the follicle-associated epithelium (FAE) and actively transported to reach dendritic cells (DCs) and other antigen-presenting cells (APC, e.g., macrophages) underlying the FAE. Chemokines produced by the epithelial cells recruit and activate DC and B and T cells in mucosal inductive sites. Alternatively, antigens can be taken up directly by DC in the lamina propria that extends their dendrites throughout the intestinal epithelium.

Lamina propria DC has been associated with the induction of systemic IgG to orally delivered antigens, whereas DC in the Peyer's patches (PP) has been associated (mainly) with the production of intestinal T cell-dependent IgA. Antigen-loaded DC migrates to interfollicular T cell areas of the lymphoid follicles or to local/regional lymph nodes where they present antigens and stimulate naive T cells. These cells will expand and differentiate into $CD4^+$ and $CD8^+$ effector and memory T cells, Th17 or regulatory T (Treg) cells, and will migrate to the lamina propria of mucosal effector sites via efferent lymphatics and blood [56].

Peyer's Patches. Gut mucosal DC (i.e., conventional $CD11c^{hi}$, plasmacytoid DC, and CD103 DC) plays a key role in the outcome of mucosal responses by determining the nature of the T cell (i.e., effector, memory, regulatory) and B cell (i.e., IgA, IgG) responses induced and imprinting specific homing receptors (i.e., α_4/β_7, CCR9, and CCR10) on antigen-committed lymphocytes. B cells activated by vaccine antigens will cluster in the Peyer's patches or mesenteric lymph nodes (MLN) to form germinal centers (GC), a special microenvironment that promotes B cell growth and differentiation. In the GC, B cells will undergo IgA class switch and affinity maturation, becoming IgA^+ plasmablasts.

The *GC reaction* depends on cognate B cell–T cell CD40–CD40L interaction and IgA-inducing signals including TGF-β, IL-4, IL-10, and retinoic acid (RA). In the GC, B cells also interact with stromal cells called follicular dendritic cells (FDC) and receive signals and co-stimulation from follicular helper T (T_{FH}) cells, which further promote GC formation and IgA class switching (e.g., TGF-β1). The IgA^+ plasmablasts generated in the GC will migrate to the lamina propria where they will terminally differentiate into polymeric IgA-secreting plasma cells in a process that involves cytokines produced by CD4⁺ T helper cells (e.g., IL-2, IL-5, TGF-β, and IL-10), DC (e.g., RA, IL-10, TGF-β, IL-6, B cell activating factor [BAFF], and proliferation-inducing ligand [APRIL]), and intestinal epithelial cells (e.g., TGF-β, IL-6). Activation of B cells and the production of IgA through T cell-independent mechanisms have been described in mice and humans [57, 58].

Antigen Uptake. This process appears to occur in the Peyer's patches but also in isolated lymphoid follicles and in the lamina propria, which unlike the PP lack segregated T cell zones. It involves recruitment and activation of B cells that respond to antigens (or microbial products) recognized by their own receptors (including "innate receptors") or antigens presented by DC, as well as molecules such as TGF-β, BAFF, APRIL, IL-6, IL-10, and RA produced by various subsets of DC, local stromal cells, and epithelial cells. T-independent, low-affinity, "natural" IgA responses are produced against commensal organisms, whereas "classical" high-avidity T cell-dependent IgA appears to be produced by pathogenic bacteria, toxins, and viruses [59]. It should be noted, however, that while a wealth of mechanistic information on gut immunology has been derived from mouse studies, their relevance and applicability to humans remains to be determined. The processes involved in vaccine uptake and immunological priming in the gut are depicted in Fig. 3.14.

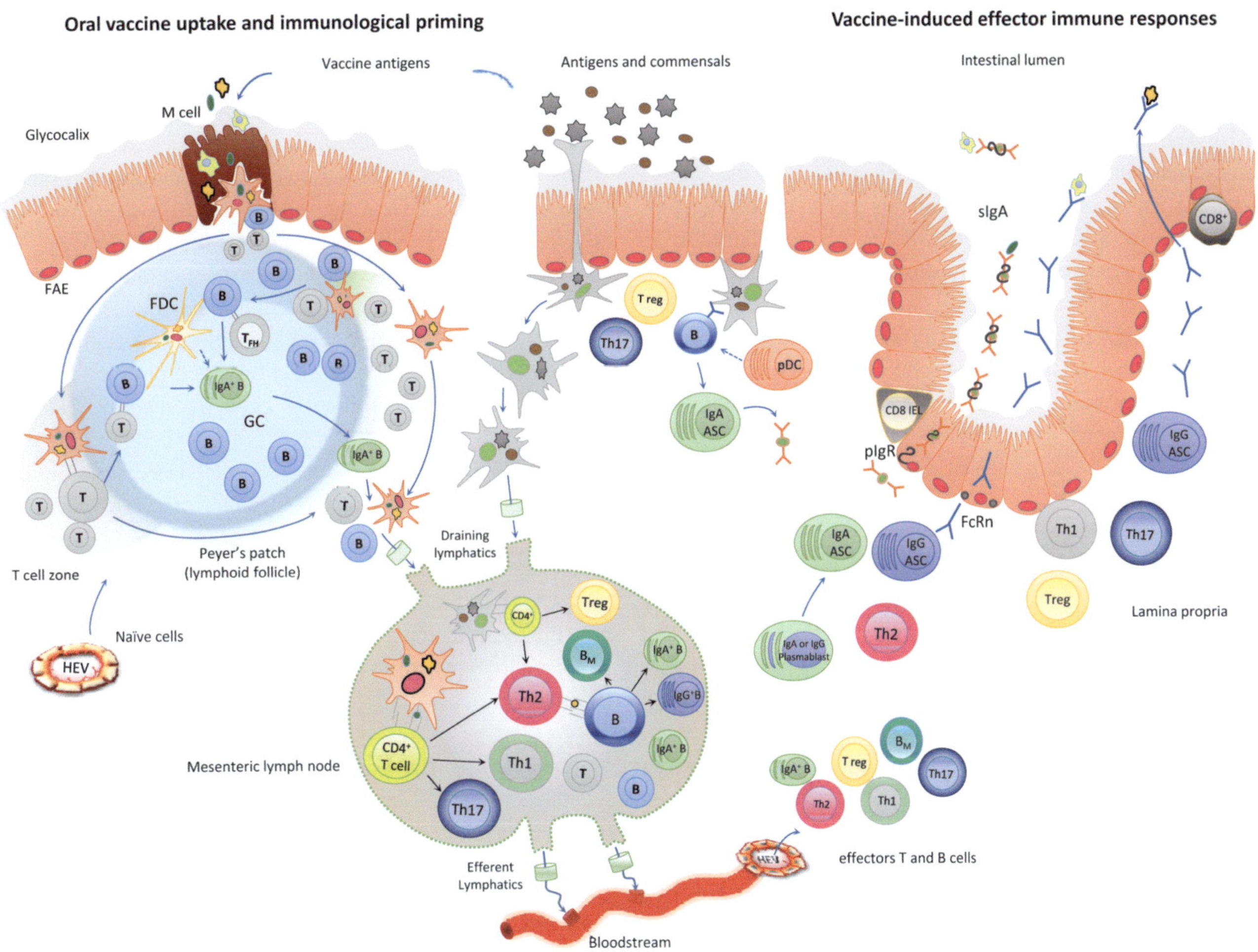

Fig. 3.14 The follicle-associated epithelium (*FAE*) contains M cells that specialize in endocytosis and rapid transport of intact antigens. Vaccine antigens are transported by the M cells across the epithelial barrier and taken up by subepithelial immature dendritic cells (*DCs*). DC within the epithelial layer of the intestinal lamina propria may also capture antigens from the lumen through their extended dendrites; some of these DCs (CD103⁺, CD11b⁺) are involved in the induction of tolerance to commensals. Immature DC as well as naive and memory lymphocytes enter the mucosa through high endothelial venules (*HEV*); these cells are attracted by chemokines (CCL20, CCL23, and CXCL16) produced by the FAE enterocytes and other mediators. DC carrying vaccine antigens migrate to the interfollicular T cell areas or to the draining lymph nodes to present antigens to naive CD4⁺T cells

3.4.3 Immunological Effectors Induced by Oral Vaccination

The main effector sites of adaptive immunity in the gut are the epithelium and the lamina propria. A large number of antigen-specific antibody-secreting cells (ASCs) and activated T cells reside in these tissues and provide a first line of defense against intestinal pathogens. A hallmark of oral vaccination is the induction of long-lived antigen-specific mucosal IgA-secreting plasma cells; this process occurs mainly in the PP and isolated lymphoid follicles.

Immune Exclusion. In a seemingly robust and self-sufficient manner, these cells produce dimeric IgA, which is transported through the epithelial barrier into the intestinal lumen via the polymeric Ig receptor (pIgR). In the lumen, secretory IgA (sIgA) binds to microbial surface antigens and prevents their attachment to the mucosal interface. Through this mechanism of "immune exclusion," IgA blocks invasion of potential pathogens [60, 61].

Mucosal sIgA can also neutralize toxins, viruses, and microbial antigens within epithelial cells or in the lamina propria and escort them out to the lumen. In addition to stopping pathogens from entry, IgA helps maintain harmony in the interplay between commensals and the host immune system. Two IgA subclasses are present in human mucosal secretions: IgA1, found primarily in saliva and the proximal small intestine (this is also the subclass found in serum), and IgA2, present mainly in the distal small intestine and colon [62]. IgA1 appears to recognize mainly proteins, whereas IgA2 recognizes polysaccharides and lipopolysaccharides (LPS) [58].

IgG is also produced by mucosal plasma cells and transported across the epithelial barrier through the neonatal Fc receptor (FcRn) [63]. It is also believed that serum IgG diffuses across the epithelial barrier by paracellular leakage and this could explain the protection induced by parenteral vaccines to some enteric pathogens (e.g., *Shigella* spp.). Both IgA and IgG can transport antigens through the epithelial cells from the intestinal lumen to the lamina propria or from the basolateral cell surface back to the lumen [64].

In mice, antibody-mediated transport of microbes through M cells has been associated with reduced inflammation and mucosal destruction. Conceivably, similar approaches that could shuttle vaccine antigens across the intestinal epithelium might provide a means to B cells are antigenically primed outside of the lymphoid follicle by interaction with DC and T cells; these activated B lymphocytes reenter the follicle, and after interaction with follicular dendritic cells (FDC), which capture migrating antigens and Treg-derived T follicular B helper (TFH) cells, they become germinal center (GC) cells. In the GC, B cells undergo IgA class switch and somatic hypermutation differentiating into IgA^+ plasmablasts (or plasma cells) and potentially memory B (B_M) cells. Effector $CD4^+$Th cells primed in the interfollicular T cell areas may also enter the B cell follicle where they activate B cells (through CD40-CD40L interaction) and release cytokines (i.e., IL-4, IL-5, IL-10, TGF-β) that induce GC reaction, leading to initial maturation of B cells and IgA isotype switching.

IgA plasma cells can also be induced through a T cell-independent mechanism that involves B cell activation by direct contact with DC and the production of B cell activation and growth factors (e.g., BAFF, APRIL, TGF-β, and nitric oxide) by distinct DC subsets (e.g., FDC and plasmacytoid DC) and epithelial cells. T-independent (low-affinity, "natural") IgA responses are induced in the PP but could also be generated in isolated lymphoid follicles and the lamina propria. Simultaneous with the activation of T and B cells, retinoic acid (RA) produced by mucosal DC imprints gut-homing receptors (i.e., $\alpha_4\beta_7$, CCR9, CCR10) on antigen-specific Th cells and IgA-committed B cells.

B and T cells activated in the gut mucosa by vaccine antigens migrate to the regional (mesenteric) lymph nodes, where they further differentiate into distinct effector populations (e.g., Th1, Th2, Treg, Th17, and B_M cells). Vaccine-specific T and B cells exit the lymph nodes through the thoracic duct and access the bloodstream, and they disseminate through circulation and reenter the mucosal effector sites. In the lamina propria, mucosal B cells terminally differentiate into plasma cells, most of which produce IgA that is exported through epithelial cells as secretory (sIgA). Mucosal IgG is produced by local plasma cells or may exudate from blood. The processes depicted are simplified; it should also be noted that the mechanisms involved in the induction of adaptive (activating or regulatory) immune responses following oral immunization are only partially understood to improve oral vaccine take. Alternatively, vaccine uptake could be enhanced by targeting antigens to the M cells, enterocytes, and DC using vectors and specific ligands [65].

Enterocytes. Like M cells, enterocytes express transcytotic receptors such as TLR2, TLR4, or α5β1 integrin, in which the integrin receptor is not located on the apical surface as on M cells but redistributed from the basolateral to the apical surface. The age-related variation in expression levels of these receptors should be assessed to ensure that the targeting vaccine strategy is applicable in both children and elderly (see also Chaps. 4 and 5). Figure 3.15 illustrates various possibilities for uptake of antigens within the intestine.

The enterocytes of the small intestine are the major intestinal cells and involved in the digestion and absorption of nutrients. Enterocytes augment the M cells which are in the focus as receptor cell for antigen uptake. M cells are very

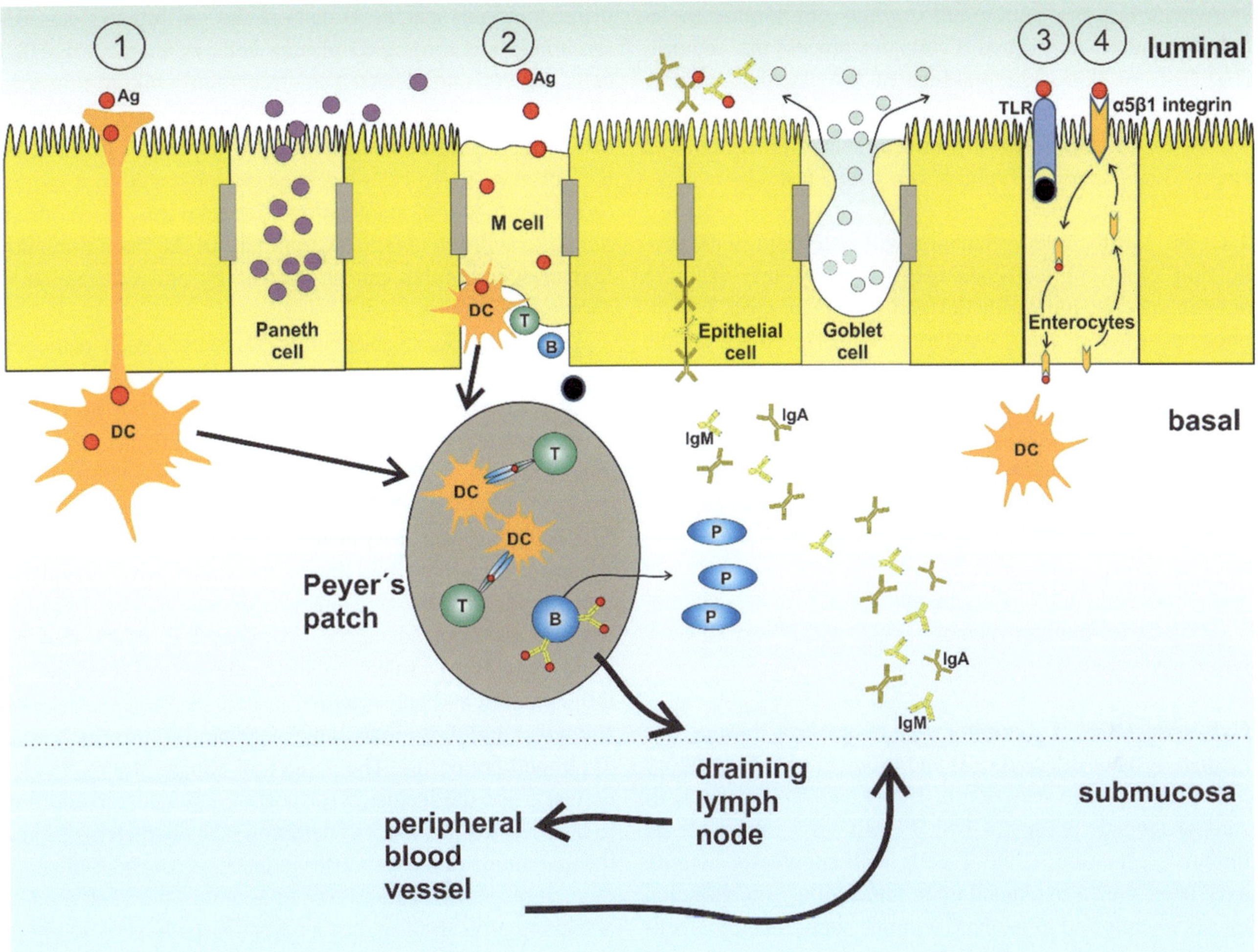

Fig. 3.15 Routes for antigen sampling. (*1*) Dendritic cells are able to capture antigens on the luminal site by their branched dendrites. (*2*) Antigens that reach inductive sites of the intestinal mucosa are captured by M cells and actively transported to reach dendritic cells (*DCs*) and other antigen-presenting cells (e.g., macrophages) underlying the FAE. (*3*, *4*) Enterocytes are most abundant in the small intestine and also suitable to uptake antigens. Like M cells, enterocytes express transcytotic receptors such as TLR2, TLR4, or α5β1 integrin. T cells, B cells, and memory cells are stimulated upon encountering antigen in Peyer's patches, organized lymphoid nodules. There is a constant migration from the upper site to the lower. Lymph nodes within the submucosa transport the immune response to peripheral blood vessels

rare (approximately 1 in 10,000,000) and for that reason alone rather suboptimal for vaccination. Most oral vaccines rely on delivery of large amounts of antigen in the hope there will be sufficient random uptake to induce an effective immune response.

In contrast, enterocytes are most abundant in the small intestine and also suitable to uptake antigens.

B and T lymphocytes primed by vaccine antigens in the intestinal mucosa migrate to the mesenteric lymph nodes, where they further differentiate. They exit the lymph nodes through the thoracic duct, access the bloodstream, and disseminate systemically to reach mucosal effector sites. The presence of circulating IgA ASC is a typical indicator of intestinal immunological priming following enteric infection or oral vaccination. These cells are detected transiently in circulation (7–10 days after antigen exposure) while migrating to effector sites or other lymphoid tissues. Virtually all IgA and some IgG ASCs induced by oral immunization express integrin $\alpha_4\beta_7$, which binds the mucosal vascular addressin cell adhesion molecule-1 (MAdCAM-1) expressed by lamina propria high endothelial venules. Many of the intestinal and all colon IgA ASCs also express CCR10 which enables them to respond to the mucosal epithelial chemokine CCL28.

Gut Homing. A smaller proportion of these orally primed ASCs express peripheral lymph node homing receptor CD62L (L-selectin), which is mainly induced after systemic immunization [66]. It is now well accepted that the local lymphoid environment, rather than the nature of the antigen, determines the homing properties of the activated lymphocytes. DC from the gut and the MLN (such as $CD103^+$ DC) stimulates IgA production and imprints gut-homing molecules on mucosally primed B cells in a process that requires RA, IL-6, or IL-5. The presence of IgA and IgG-specific ASC expressing gut-homing receptors has been demonstrated in humans following infection or oral vaccination against *V. cholerae*, *S.* Typhi, *Shigella*, and *Rotavirus*.

T Cells. Ideally, oral vaccination will also result in the production of strong cell-mediated immunity that includes antigen-specific intraepithelial and lamina propria T lymphocytes. Most of the T lymphocytes present in the lamina propria (in both mice and humans) are effector memory $CD4^+$ T cells ready for rapid defense and include the classical subsets (Th1, Th2, and Th17), Treg cells and natural killer T (NKT) cells [56]. Through interaction with $CD103^+$ DC in the lamina propria and MLN, T cells are induced to express CCR9 and $\alpha4\beta7$ acquiring the capacity to migrate to mucosal effector sites. CCL25, which is expressed by crypt epithelium cells in the jejunum and ileum, mediates chemotaxis of CCR9-bearing memory $\alpha4\beta7^{hi}$ $CD4^+$ and $CD8^+$ T lymphocytes into the lamina propria.

Cytotoxic $CD8^+$ T lymphocytes in mucosal tissues can mediate lysis of infected cells and promote an inflammatory milieu through the secretion of IFN-γ and TNF-α that activate phagocytic killing. $CD8^+$ T cells also participate in immune regulation; $CD8^+$ T cells with suppressor activity have been shown to expand upon interaction with epithelial intestinal cells and to mediate immune suppression via cell-to-cell contact. $Foxp3^+$ $CD4^+$ Treg cells also play a key role in preserving immune homeostasis and tolerance against commensal organisms and food antigens in the gut [67].

$CD4^+$Th17 Cells a subset defined by the production of Th17, are present in the lamina propria in the small and large intestine. They have been found to increase upon signals from intestinal commensals and have also been implicated in protection against *H. pylori* and other bacterial infections [32]. Th17-related cytokines such as IL-22, IL-17A, IL-17F, and granulocyte–macrophage colony-stimulating factor (GM-CSF) are important for protection against extracellular pathogens. These cytokines, however, have also been associated with the development of pathologic disorders such as inflammatory bowel diseases (IBD), which can be counteracted by $FoxP3^+$ Treg cells [68]. It is also believed that many of the functions in gut inflammation typically attributed to IL-12 and Th1 cells might be due instead to Th17 cells and IL-23. Adult volunteers who received the oral typhoid vaccine Ty21a developed $CD8^+$ T cells secreting IL17A and other cytokines, in response to vaccination [69].

B_M Cells. Another desirable attribute of oral vaccination is the capacity to induce immunologic memory. Mucosally primed antigen-specific B cells in the gut mucosa can differentiate into long-lived plasma cells or memory B (B_M) cells. B_M cells are detected in circulation while in transit to niche organs; these cells do not secrete antibody but rapidly differentiate into ASC upon antigen exposure. In humans, the presence of B_M cells has been demonstrated in response to infection or oral vaccination with rotavirus, *V. cholerae*, *Shigella*, and *Salmonella.* A summary of the main immunological effectors that can be induced by oral vaccination is shown in Fig. 3.14.

Depending on the mechanism by which each pathogen causes disease, different vaccine approaches would be needed to generate specific immunological effectors that could target distinct virulence factors and interrupt pathogenesis.

Mucosal-Parenteral Approach. A mucosal vaccine might be sufficient to prevent illness by noninvasive organisms such as *V. cholerae* and enterotoxigenic *E. coli* (ETEC), whereas a combined mucosal-parenteral approach may be more suitable to protect against pathogens that cause gut inflammation and cell destruction such as *Shigella* spp. and *Rotavirus* and those inducing a systemic disease, such as *S.* Typhi and poliovirus. The antigen of choice, the method of delivery, and the inclusion (or not) of adjuvants, in addition to host-related factors, will determine the characteristics and the magnitude of the responses induced. A careful evaluation of such responses is important to ascertain the likelihood of achieving protection against a particular pathogen in light of known immune correlates (or surrogates) of protection [70].

3.4.4 Intestinal Tolerance and Immune Regulation Related to Vaccination

There is a delicate balance between promoting the activation of the gut mucosal immune system to mount an adaptive immune response to a potential pathogen while maintaining tolerance to prevent immune disorders such as food allergy, inflammatory bowel disease (IBD), and celiac disease. It could be argued that considering the prevalent tolerogenic environment of the gut, it is counterintuitive to expect orally delivered antigens to engender a strong immune response without disturbing immune balance and physiological homeostasis. The nature of the antigen and the mode of delivery (e.g., dose) can determine the end result (immune activation or tolerance). Oral vaccines that have been the most successful involve active replication (e.g., *Rotavirus*) or strong immunogenic stimuli (e.g., live attenuated strains, immunomodulatory molecules).

Oral Tolerance. Oral tolerance refers to a specific type of peripheral tolerance and may depend on the same mechanisms. Oral tolerance originates in the intestinal immune system and may involve either anergy or deletion of T cells, or the induction of regulatory T cells, depending of the antigen dose presented by DCs: antigen expressed at high levels tends to favor deletion and anergy, whereas low doses seem to generate predominantly regulatory T cells. Together with Treg cells, other T cell subsets including TR1, Th3, and nTreg cells that make IL-10 and TGF-β help establish a local tolerogenic environment.

Large particles are typically captured by M cells and likely to undergo the normal process of antigen presentation and immunological priming, whereas soluble antigens (administered orally in a single high dose or in multiple small doses) are likely to be taken up and presented preferentially by APC in the gut to induce tolerance by clonal anergy/deletion or suppression of effector cells [71].

Several T cell subsets involved in maintaining oral tolerance and homeostasis in the gut have been described: $Foxp3^+$ $CD25^+$ $CD4^+$ nTreg cells, $CD25^-$ $Foxp3^-$ IL-10-secreting $CD4^+$Tr1 cells, and TGF-β-secreting Th3 T cells. nTreg cells develop in the thymus and are believed to mediate systemic homeostasis and prevent autoimmune disease. Both antigen-specific and antigen-nonspecific regulatory mechanisms of intestinal immunity have been described, the first involving regulatory cytokines that maintain an immunosuppressive environment and the second the generation of antigen-specific anergy or Treg cells that can maintain systemic immunologic quiescence [72].

Soluble antigens that have diffused into the lamina propria through tight junctions or translocated through transcellular transport may be taken up by special lamina propria $CD103^+$ DC, which have a unique tolerogenic phenotype [49]. These cells migrate to the MLN where they promote the differentiation of $CD4^+$ T cells into $FoxP3^+$ $CD25^+$ $CD4^+$ Treg cells through the production of RA, which acts as a cofactor for TGF-β-mediated conversion of T cells into Treg cells.

Interleukin 10. An essential component that drives and maintains mucosal tolerance is IL-10, which is produced mainly by Tr1 and nTreg cells but also by myeloid cells in the gut. Both IL-10 and TGF-β (produced by Tr1, Th3, and nTreg) have suppressive functions inhibiting production of cytokines by activated T cells, the expression of co-stimulatory molecules on APC, and the production of antibodies. The microbiota is also known to influence the induction of $Foxp3^+$ Treg cells and, as a consequence, the state of tolerance. Some of the $Foxp3^+$ Treg cells in the PP differentiate into T_{FH} cells which are involved in GC formation and support IgA responses; this agrees with IgA supporting (unperturbed) housekeeping functions at the mucosal interface.

3.4.5 Licensed Oral Vaccines and Clinical Trails

A handful of oral vaccines have been licensed and are commercially available for prevention of polio, *Rotavirus*, *S.* Typhi, and *V. cholerae* O1 (Table 3.4). They consist of live attenuated organisms obtained by tissue culture passage (Rotarix® and poliovirus) [73] or reassortant technology (RotaTeq®) [74], deletion of virulence factors (cholera) [75] or chemical mutagenesis (typhoid) [76], as well as inactivated organisms combined with immunomodulatory recombinant toxin subunits (cholera) [77].

These vaccines have been successful in preventing disease in specific target populations: infants living in industrialized countries (rotavirus vaccines), infants in developing countries (polio vaccine), and school-age children in developing countries (typhoid and cholera vaccines). Despite their success in industrialized nations, however, there is mounting evidence of their reduced immunogenic capacity and efficacy in certain subpopulations in less developed areas of the world [78].

3.4.5.1 Oral Polio Vaccine

There are three serotypes of poliovirus: 1, 2, and 3. This single-stranded RNA virus replicates in the lymphoid tissue underlying the gastrointestinal epithelium and generally produces either mild (fever and sore throat) or no symptoms. In

Table 3.4 Licensed oral vaccines

Target pathogen	Licensed vaccine	Details of vaccine	Ref.
Poliovirus	Sabin's tOPV (trivalent oral poliovirus vaccine)	Live attenuated poliovirus strains of serotypes 1, 2, and 3	[79]
Rotavirus	RotaTeq®	Pentavalent attenuated reassortant rotavirus vaccine	[80]
	Rotarix®	Live attenuated monovalent rotavirus vaccine	[81]
Salmonella Typhi	Vivotif®	Live attenuated *S.* Typhi Ty21a	[76]
Vibrio cholerae	Dukoral®	Whole killed *V. cholerae* O1 Inaba and Ogawa (El Tor and classical biotypes) admixed with recombinant cholera toxin B subunit (CTB)	[82]
	Shanchol®, MORCVAX®	Whole killed *V. cholerae* O1 strains and a O139 strain (without CTB)	[82]

<1 % of cases however, the virus disseminates to motor neurons and causes flaccid paralysis. Albert Sabin developed a trivalent oral poliovirus vaccine (tOPV) containing live strains from serotypes 1, 2, and 3 attenuated by repeated passage through nonhuman cells [79]. As part of the Global Polio Eradication Initiative, this vaccine has eliminated the transmission of wild-type polioviruses throughout the Americas, the Western Pacific, and Europe.

Type 2 poliovirus has been globally eradicated as of 1999. However, poliovirus still remains endemic in Pakistan, Afghanistan, and Nigeria.

Sabin's tOPV has been the vaccine of choice for use in poliovirus-endemic countries due to the ease of delivery, its capacity to induce lifelong immunity in the intestine (the primary site of virus entry), and the fact it can be shed in the stool and indirectly immunize other individuals in the community. Despite its overall success, however, tOPV has proven less effective in the remaining reservoirs [83]. In the states of Uttar Pradesh and Bihar in India, some children under 5 years of age have received ~15 doses of tOPV compared to 10 doses given to children elsewhere in India. Despite this high coverage, the former group developed lower immune responses to the vaccine, which has been attributed to diarrhea and other enteric infections caused by poor sanitation and high population density [84].

The composition of the vaccine may also be responsible for the reduced immunogenicity. The type 2 strain efficiently colonizes the intestine and elicits stronger immune responses than the type 1 and 3 strains. Since it is possible that the type 2 virus can outcompete the other virus strains, tOPV contains $\geq 10^{6.0}$ infectious units of type 1 virus, $10^{5.0}$ infectious units of type 2 virus, and $10^{5.8}$ infectious units of type 3 virus per dose [62]. In the states of Uttar Pradesh and Bihar in India and in other developing countries, monovalent type 1 (mOPV1) and type 3 (mOPV3) vaccines and the bivalent type 1+3 (bOPV) vaccine have been used to interrupt transmission of the type 1 and 3 polioviruses. Due to these efforts, India has been wild-type poliovirus-free since 13 January 2011.

One of the disadvantages of tOPV is the occasional reversion to virulence that causes vaccine-associated paralytic poliomyelitis (VAPP) in 1 out of 2.5 million doses. As such, in some countries where transmission of wild-type poliovirus has been successfully interrupted, tOPV has been replaced with inactivated poliovirus vaccine (IPV).

3.4.5.2 Rotavirus Vaccines

Rotavirus is a double-stranded RNA virus and the leading cause of severe gastroenteritis in children less than 5 years of age. It affects both developing and industrialized countries, and it is estimated to cause 527,000 deaths annually, the majority of which occur among children in the developing world. Effective vaccines are considered the best prophylactic intervention to reduce the burden of disease, and the WHO Strategic Advisory Group recommends their inclusion in national immunization programs.

Serotyping is based on the VP7 glycoprotein (G serotypes) and the VP4 protease-sensitive protein (P serotypes). Five strains (P[8], G1; P[4], G2; P[8], G3; P[8], G4; and P[8], G9) are commonly detected and constitute the main vaccine targets [85].

Intussusception. Two oral vaccines, RotaTeq® and Rotarix®, are currently licensed in most countries. An oral vaccine previously licensed in the United States, RotaShield®, was withdrawn from the market due to its association with intussusception, an unexpected complication that appeared shortly after the first dose in which a part of the intestine invaginates into another part of the intestine; the vaccine is no longer available. The induction of serum IgA has been associated with protection against rotavirus infection children. The levels of serum IgA but in particular the frequency of circulating rotavirus-specific IgA ASC were found to correlate with intestinal ASC measured in biopsies.

3.4.5.3 Rotarix®

Rotarix® (also known as RV1) is a live attenuated monovalent rotavirus vaccine. It is administered orally at 6–14 weeks of age and again ~4 weeks later. This vaccine contains the RIX4414 strain which is a G1P[8] serotype and is derived from the parent vaccine strain 89–12 [86]. The vaccine was attenuated by passaging 43 times.

A large multinational, double-blind phase 3 trial performed in 11 Latin American countries and Finland showed that Rotarix® is highly effective in protecting infants against severe gastroenteritis (vaccine efficacy of 85 %, $P<0.001$ vs. placebo), significantly reduces the rate of severe gastroenteritis from any cause (rate reduction of 40 %, $P<0.001$), and is not associated with an increased risk of intussusception. A post-licensure study performed in Mexico and Brazil showed that Rotarix® was associated with a short-term risk of intussusception in approximately 1 of every 51,000–68,000 vaccinated infants. However, the benefits of the vaccine far outweighs the risks as it prevented approximately 80,000 hospitalizations and 1300 deaths from diarrhea each year in these two countries.

In contrast to the excellent efficacy seen in high- and middle-income countries of Europe and Latin America, a randomized, placebo-controlled, multicenter trial in Africa (South Africa and Malawi) showed a vaccine efficacy of 61.2 %. Efficacy against severe gastroenteritis from any cause was only 30.2 %. Possible reasons for the reduced efficacy in African infants include malnutrition, coinfection with other enteric pathogens, anti-rotavirus antibodies in breast milk, and interference by the oral poliovirus vaccine.

3.4.5.4 RotaTeq®

RotaTeq® (also known as RV5) is a pentavalent attenuated rotavirus vaccine developed through reassortment of ten genes from the bovine rotavirus strain WC3 and an individual capsid gene from five of the most common human serotypes (G1, G2, G3, G4, and PIA) [80].

Three doses of the vaccine are given orally, starting at 6 to 12 weeks of age with the subsequent doses given at 4–10-week intervals. A final formulation of 12×10^7 infectious units per dose was evaluated in a large field trial performed in 70,000 infants predominantly from the United States and Finland but also from Central and South America, Europe, and Asia. The vaccine had a 98 % efficacy in protection against severe gastroenteritis, and there was no difference in the risk of intussusception between vaccine and placebo recipients. In a post-licensure study in the United States, 786,725 total doses were administered to 4- to 34-week-old infants and showed no increased risk of intussusception due to vaccination.

A combined efficacy of 33.9 % against severe rotavirus gastroenteritis and 51.2 % against very severe gastroenteritis was reported in two recent multicenter, double-blind, placebo-controlled vaccine trials performed in 4- to 12-week-old infants in Africa and Asia through the entire follow-up period [87]. These studies also showed cross-protection against non-vaccine serotypes. Although the vaccine efficacy in these trials was substantial, the values obtained were lower than in trials performed in developed countries or in developing countries in Latin America [88].

The African trial involved 5468 infants in rural sites in Ghana and Kenya and an urban area in Mali. The vaccine efficacy against severe rotavirus gastroenteritis declined from 64.2 % in the first year of life to only 19.6 % in the second year of life (resulting in an overall efficacy of 39.3 %). This reduction in efficacy was most likely due to waning immunogenicity. Serum IgA geometric mean titers (GMT) measured 14 days after the 3rd dose were 5–10 times lower than for subjects in trials performed in developed countries. Similarly, postimmunization serum neutralization antibody responses were fourfold lower for G1 and threefold lower for P1A[8] in the African subjects. The Asian trial involved 2036 infants in Matlab, Bangladesh, and urban and peri-urban Nha Trang, Vietnam [89]. Three doses of RotaTeq® resulted in a vaccine efficacy of 48.3 % against severe rotavirus disease. However, unlike the African study, the vaccine efficacy was similar in the first and second years of life (51 and 45.5 %, respectively).

Possible explanations for the lower efficacy of rotavirus vaccine in African and Asian infants are the same as for Rotarix® as well as the younger age of the infants enrolled in this study compared to other studies. Additionally, many of the infants in these trials received the oral poliovirus vaccine and RotaTeq® at the same time. It has previously been shown that coadministration of the oral poliovirus vaccine results in reduced immunogenicity of oral rotavirus vaccines.

3.4.5.5 Cholera Vaccines

Cholera is still a major global public health problem, occurring mainly in developing countries. In 2010, 317,534 cases of cholera and 7543 deaths were reported to the World Health Organization (WHO) worldwide although the true global burden is estimated at 3–5 million cases and 100,000–130,000 deaths annually. Vaccination is recommended in endemic areas in high-risk groups and during outbreaks, using available oral killed vaccines. *Vibrio cholerae* serogroups O1 and O139 are responsible for most of the cholera epidemics seen worldwide [90]. Serogroup O1 is further divided into biotypes, El Tor and classical, and serotypes, Inaba and Ogawa. An effective cholera vaccine needs to protect against both biotypes and serotypes.

V. cholerae has a high infectious dose and is acquired through fecal-oral contamination, usually via food and waterborne transmission. The disease is caused by the cholera toxin (CT) which consists of five B (binding) subunits and one A (active) subunit. The B subunits bind to GM1 ganglioside receptors and serve as a conduit for the A subunit to access the epithelial cells causing profuse secretion of water and electrolytes. Unlike other enteric infections, prior exposure to wild-type *V. cholerae* infection induces a serogroup-specific protection against clinical disease that is robust and durable [91]. The precise immunological effectors responsible for this protection are not fully known. Individuals from endemic areas infected with *V. cholerae* develop LPS-specific IgA ASC, which peaks 7 days after the onset of disease and express the gut-homing integrin receptor $\alpha4\beta7$.

Serum vibriocidal antibodies have been inversely correlated with susceptibility to infection but are unlikely the protective effector mechanism. Intestinal IgA, on the other hand, is believed to play a critical role blocking the pathogen at mucosal surfaces.

Mucosal LPS-specific IgA ASC was detected in duodenal biopsies of cholera-infected patients, even in the absence of detectable anti-LPS IgA in secretions. These cells might resume antibody production when appropriately stimulated. IgG and IgA B_M cells specific for *V. cholerae* LPS, CTB, and TcpA were found in cholera-infected patients for up to 1 year following disease, and the frequency of LPS-specific IgG B_M cells has been associated with protection against infection in household contacts of cholera patients [92]. A mucosal anamnestic response mediated by B_M cells (directed primarily to the LPS) appears to be necessary for long-term protection against cholera.

Two types of oral cholera vaccines are commercially available, both consisting of whole killed organisms. Dukoral™ contains heat- or formalin-inactivated *V. cholerae* O1 Inaba and Ogawa strains of both El Tor and classical biotypes admixed with recombinant cholera toxin B subunit (CTB). Although it is internationally licensed, it is mainly used in travelers because of its high cost [82]. Two doses are recommended, 10–14 days apart. In a randomized double-blind trial, protective efficacy was ascertained in children aged 2–15 years and women older than 15 years in rural Bangladesh. Among 62,285 subjects, vaccine efficacy after 3 years was 50 % (26 % for 2- to 5-year-olds and 63 % for older subjects). After 5 years of follow-up, protective efficacy was still 49 %.

Shanchol™ or MORCVAX contains several *V. cholerae* O1 strains and an O139 strain, without CTB, and represents a less expensive alternative. Shanchol™ was tested in 101 adults and 100 children (1–17 years old) in a cholera-endemic region: Kolkata, India. Following two doses of vaccine, 53 % of adults and 80 % of children showed seroconversion (defined as a fourfold rise in serum vibriocidal antibody titers following vaccination as compared with baseline) against *V. cholerae* O1 and only 10 % of adults and 27 % of children seroconverted for *V. cholerae* O139.

In another study performed in a cholera-endemic region, 2- to 5-year-old toddlers and 12- to 23-month-old infants living in the Mirpur area in Dhaka, Bangladesh, were given two doses of the vaccine which was safe and immunogenic in all age groups. However, in both of these studies performed in cholera-endemic regions, the geometric mean fold rise in vibriocidal antibodies in adults was lower than that seen in a non-cholera-endemic area (SonLa, Vietnam). This is most likely due to the high baseline titers observed in Kolkata and Dhaka, suggesting that pre-existing immunity due to natural infection may negatively affect the immune response of live oral attenuated vaccines. Toddlers and infants had lower baseline levels presumably due to lack of exposure to *V. cholerae* O1. In a large double-blind trial in Kolkata, India, Shanchol® showed 67 % efficacy ($P<0.0001$) against *V. cholerae* O1 diarrhea in recipients aged one year and older. Recent studies suggest that a single dose of Dukoral® or Shanchol® may be sufficient to elicit protection [93].

Compared with wild-type *V. cholerae* infection, the inactivated whole-cell cholera vaccines induce a more limited and short-lived protection in adults and particularly in children [94]. Hence, live vaccine strains that can mimic natural infection are sought to harness the immunological effectors of naturally derived immunity, ideally after a single immunization.

CVD 103-HgR is a live attenuated vaccine derived from a *V. cholerae* O1 classical biotype, Inaba serotype that contains a deletion in the gene that encodes the A subunit of cholera toxin, and also carries a gene that encodes mercury resistance (inserted into the hemolysin A [hlyA] locus). Clinical trials performed in the United States and Europe showed that a single oral dose of 5×10^8 colony-forming units (CFU) of CVD 103-HgR resulted in seroconversion (fourfold or greater rise in serum vibriocidal antibodies) in >90 and 88 % of vaccines, respectively. The vaccine was also able to protect volunteers against cholera due to both biotypes (El Tor and classical) and serotypes (Inaba and Ogawa) of *V. cholerae* O1 in challenge studies.

However, clinical trials performed in several developing countries showed diminished immunogenicity. In Indonesia, 5×10^8 CFU of CVD 103-HgR elicited seroconversion in only 16 % of 5- to 9-year-old children. Similar results were observed in 2- to 4-year-old children. Clinical trials performed in Peru and Thailand showed similar results. Nonetheless, 5×10^9 CFU of CVD 103-HgR was able to elicit high seroconversion rates in Indonesian children and Peruvian and Thai adults. CVD 103-HgR was also tested in a randomized large-scale controlled field trial in a highly endemic area of North Jakarta. Contrary to the results in US volunteers, the efficacy was low due to a decrease in the incidence of disease at the end of the study. One possible explanation is that the extensive vaccination led to indirect protection, and when the disease disappeared, the estimates of efficacy became insignificant.

In a randomized, placebo-controlled, double-blind, crossover clinical trial in Mali, lower vibriocidal seroconversion rates following immunization with CVD 103-HgR were observed among HIV seropositive versus HIV seronegative subjects. CVD 103-HgR was previously manufactured by the Swiss Serum and Vaccine Institute (Berne, Switzerland) under the trade names Orochol® and Mutacol® and licensed as a single-dose cholera vaccine. Production is being resumed by PaxVax; clinical trials are currently being performed to make it available in the United States (NCT01585181; ClinicalTrials.gov). Other live vaccines in the front line include Peru 15 (Haikou VTI Biological Institute, China); also a genetically engineered toxin-deficient strain found to be safe and immunogenic in adults and children in Bangladesh, although not yet tested in phase 3 studies; and live attenuated *V. cholerae* 638 and CTB-expressing strain VA 1.3, both attenuated El Tor derivatives.

3.4.5.6 Oral Typhoid Vaccine

Salmonella enterica serovar Typhi (*S.* Typhi) causes an acute systemic infection characterized by persistent high fever. It is a food and waterborne infection uncommon in modern industrialized countries but endemic in underdeveloped areas lacking adequate sanitary conditions. The peak incidence of typhoid fever is seen among school-age children [95]. In urban slum environments in South Asia, systematic household and health center-based active surveillance demonstrated a high incidence of bacteremic typhoid infection among febrile toddlers and preschool children. Travelers from industrialized countries to developing countries are also at increased risk of developing typhoid fever.

Natural *S.* Typhi infection induces serum antibody responses to bacterial LPS, flagella, outer membrane proteins, and other bacterial antigens, gut-derived ASC and sIgA [96]. High titers of serum IgG against the capsular Vi antigen are found in ~80–90 % of chronic biliary *S.* Typhi carriers, in 12–38 % of acute typhoid fever patients who do not become chronic carriers, but only rarely in healthy individuals from endemic areas. Proliferative responses to *S.* Typhi antigens were observed in healthy adults living in typhoid-endemic areas who have no known history of clinically overt typhoid fever. Elevated serum levels Th1-type cytokines (e.g., IFN-γ, TNF-α, IL-1, and IL-6) were seen in patients with culture-confirmed typhoid fever.

Strain Ty21a. A live attenuated oral typhoid vaccine, strain Ty21a, developed in the early 1970s by chemical mutagenesis, is licensed for use in the United States for travelers to endemic areas, and in other countries worldwide, Ty21a provides significant protection without causing adverse reactions. In large-scale efficacy field trials with Ty21a, involving approximately 514,000 schoolchildren in Chile, 32,388 in Egypt, and 20,543 subjects from 3 years of age to adults in Indonesia, no vaccine-attributable adverse reactions were found through passive surveillance.

Two formulations are licensed: enteric-coated capsules and a lyophilized vaccine to be reconstituted with buffer. In recent years, however, only the enteric-coated capsules have been commercially available. A field trial in Santiago, Chile, showed that three doses of Ty21a in enteric-coated capsules given every other day conferred 67 % protection over 3 years of follow-up. Based on these results, this formulation and dose regimen are used throughout the world, except for the United States and Canada where a four-dose regimen is used. The four-dose North American regimen is based on results of another large-scale, randomized comparative trial carried out in Chile where four doses of Ty21a in enteric-coated capsules were significantly more protective than two or three doses.

Ty21a confers a long-lived protection. Individuals who received Ty21a in two Chilean field trials were followed up for a total of 2 years, and over this period, the enteric-coated capsule formulation of Ty21a conferred 62 % vaccine efficacy, while the liquid formulation had a point estimate of vaccine efficacy of 78 % over 5 years of follow-up. Immune responses in Ty21a recipients include serum IgG against the O polysaccharide and mucosally primed O-specific ASC that are detected 7–10 days after vaccination. Most of these ASCs carry the intestinal homing integrin $\alpha_4\beta_7$. O-specific serum IgG and gut-derived ASC were found to correlate with the protection conferred by different formulations and immunization regimens of Ty21a in field trials. Intestinal sIgA antibody responses and antibody-dependent cellular cytotoxicity have also been described following oral Ty21a immunization [97]. Additionally, Ty21a stimulates strong T cell proliferative responses, Th1-type cytokine secretion (e.g., IFN-γ, TNF-α), and multifunctional $CD8^+$ cytotoxic T lymphocytes. T cell clones with T_{EM} phenotype (i.e., $CCR7^-$, $CD27^-$ $CD45RO^+$ $CD62L^-$) co-expressing gut-homing molecules (i.e., $\alpha_4\beta_7$ and CCR9) were derived from peripheral mononuclear cells of Ty21a vaccinees.

3.4.6 Environmental Barriers Associated with Oral Vaccination

There is growing recognition that oral vaccines meet a very different host in underdeveloped populations compared to industrialized nations. At a global level, one of the greatest challenges of modern vaccinology is to identify and overcome the barriers that lead to the diminished immunogenicity and reduced protection of oral vaccines in impoverished populations [98]. Some of the factors that may explain this phenomenon include small bowel bacterial overgrowth, which is indicative of environmental enteropathy in individuals living in poverty, heavy intestinal helminth infestation, malnutrition, maternal antibodies, interaction with the microbiota, and interaction with other vaccines. These factors are summarized in Table 3.5 and are herein described separately but they are interrelated [99].

3.4.6.1 Small Bowel Bacterial Overgrowth (SBBO) and Environmental Enteropathy

Many children living in poverty have small bowel bacterial overgrowth, which manifests itself as excessive colonization of the proximal intestine, and environmental (or tropical) enteropathy characterized by histopathological changes in the small intestine, including inflammation and blunting of villi. It is believed that children (and adults) living in poverty in developing countries are continually exposed to fecal contaminants, which leads to SBBO and environmental enteropathy. Interestingly, environmental enteropathy can be reversed and eventually disappears, and then the individual is transferred to a clean environment.

SBBO may be one reason why CVD 103-HgR showed reduced efficacy in clinical trials performed in developing countries. In a clinical study performed in Chile, SBBO (measured by lactulose breath H_2 test) was detected in 10 out of 178 five- to nine-year-old children. These children had lower vibriocidal geometric mean titers than other children though this was not significant (160 vs. 368, $P=0.25$). Logistic regression showed that peak H_2 (cleaved by bacterial enzymes following ingestion of lactulose) was associated with diminished vibriocidal seroconversion ($P=0.04$).

Environmental Enteropathy. SBBO and environmental enteropathy may have a direct inhibitory effect on live oral vaccines through the production of short-chain fatty acids or other small molecules, or an indirect effect, through the activation of innate immune cells (as shown by increased lymphocytes in the mucosa) and a pro-inflammatory milieu that destroys the vaccine. Alternatively, fecal contaminants may compete with the live oral vaccines for colonization sites in the gut and prevent the vaccine from accessing key receptors or cells [106].

Evidence to suggest that coinfections of the intestine affect the immune response generated by live vaccines is shown in a clinical trial performed with CVD 103-HgR in a high helminth prevalence region in Ecuador. One hundred

Table 3.5 Environmental barriers to oral vaccination

Barrier	Example of reduced immunogenicity due to the barrier or increased immunogenicity when the barrier was overcome	Ref.
Small bowel bacterial overgrowth (SBBO) and environmental enteropathy	In Chile, children with SBBO showed reduced vibriocidal seroconversion following immunization with the live oral cholera vaccine CVD 103-HgR	[100]
Malnutrition	In Bangladesh, supplementation with zinc improved vibriocidal seroconversion induced by Dukoral®	[101]
Maternal antibodies and immune components of maternal milk	In Bangladesh, temporary withholding of breast-feeding for 3 h before immunization with Dukoral® resulted in increased magnitude of vibriocidal antibodies	[102]
Microbiota	In Finland, IgA seroconversion to the live oral rotavirus vaccine RotaShield® was improved when coadministered with the probiotic *Lactobacillus casei* GG	[103]
Oral immunization of newborns	Increased seroconversion has been observed in infants given a monovalent oral poliovirus vaccine in contrast to trivalent oral poliovirus vaccines	[104]
Coadministration of vaccines	tOPV can affect the immunogenicity of oral rotavirus vaccines when coadministered	[105]

and thirty-nine children were given two doses of albendazole (a broad-spectrum anti-helminth) or placebo followed by CVD 103-HgR after the second dose. Seroconversion (serum vibriocidal responses) was higher in the albendazole group compared to the placebo group (29.3 % vs. 15.5 %) though this difference was not significant ($P=0.06$).

3.4.6.2 Malnutrition

Maternal and child malnutrition is highly prevalent in low- and middle-income countries. For example, 33 % of children in South Central Asia and 28 % of children in Eastern Africa are underweight. Many of these children have vitamin A and zinc deficiencies. Zinc is required for many cellular functions and for effective innate and acquired immunity [106]. Deficiency of vitamin A is well known for causing immune defects in the gut, affecting distinct populations of intestinal DC. In mice, the vitamin A metabolite retinoic acid is critical for trafficking of vaccine-induced T cells to the gastrointestinal mucosa and for protective vaccine efficacy [107]. Indeed, children with vitamin A deficiency have depressed immune responses compared to children who have been supplemented to normal vitamin A levels.

Zinc. Some studies have shown that supplementation of zinc or vitamin A improved immunogenicity induced by oral vaccines. In a study performed in Bangladesh, 2- to 5-year-old children were given zinc, vitamin A, or both, 1 week before the oral cholera vaccine Cholerix/Dukoral and vibriocidal titers were measured 2 weeks after vaccination [101]. The study showed that supplementation with zinc but not vitamin A improved the rates of vibriocidal seroconversion. Conversely, when sera from these children were tested for antibody to cholera toxin (CT), children who received zinc had significantly lower levels of CT antibodies than children who did not receive micronutrient supplementation. Therefore, zinc enhanced vibriocidal but suppressed CT–antibody responses to cholera vaccination. A second study in Bangladesh confirmed that zinc supplementation could increase the magnitude of vibriocidal responses induced by Dukoral [102].

Vitamin A. The effect of vitamin A supplementation on the immune response to oral polio vaccine was ascertained in a study performed in 1085 infants in Ghana. Vitamin A or placebo was given at 6, 10, and 14 weeks of age at the time the infants received their diphtheria/pertussis/tetanus (DPT) vaccine. Neutralization titers against poliovirus types 1, 2, and 3 were determined, and no significant differences were observed between the groups that received vitamin A supplementation and the placebo group. In a similar study performed in New Delhi, India, infants that were given vitamin A at 6, 10, and 14 weeks with OPV showed increased neutralizing antibody titers against poliovirus type 1 (but not type 2 or 3) compared to the placebo group (who did not receive vitamin A supplementation) [108]. These results are consistent with a previous study performed in Indonesia that found that vitamin A did not affect immune responses to any of the polioviruses.

Overall, the data suggests that zinc and to a lesser extent vitamin A supplementation may improve immune responses to oral vaccines but more studies need to be performed to determine the effect on specific vaccines.

3.4.6.3 Maternal Antibodies and Immune Components of Maternal Milk

Some live oral vaccines may be inhibited by elevated levels of antibodies in breast milk. In addition, human breast milk contains immunomodulatory molecules and cytokines that promote the development of the gut immune system, some of which have tolerogenic functions such as TGFβ, IL-10, and vitamin A [109].

The most well-known example of maternal milk interfering with vaccine take is that of rotavirus vaccines. Breast milk contains IgA antibodies that neutralize rotavirus and also lactadherin (a receptor analog) that can bind to the virus and prevent its attachment. Various studies have been performed to examine the effect of breast milk on the immunogenicity of rotavirus vaccine with mixed results. Goveia et al. [110] examined the effect of breast-feeding frequency (never breast-fed vs. sometimes breast-fed vs. exclusively breast-fed) on the ability of RotaTeq® to protect against rotavirus gastroenteritis in 5098 infants from 11 countries from three regions: Europe, the United States, and Latin America/the Caribbean.

Breast-feeding did not affect the efficacy of the vaccine. On the other hand, analysis of breast milk from Indian women has shown that it possesses high titers of IgA and neutralizing activity which could theoretically reduce vaccine potency [111]. Breast milk from Korean and Vietnamese women had slightly lower IgA and neutralizing titers, and American women had the lowest titers. A clinical trial performed in Bangladesh has shown that temporary withholding of breast-feeding for 3 h before immunization with Dukoral® resulted in an increased magnitude of vibriocidal antibodies and frequency of responders compared to subjects who just received the vaccine [102]. This difference was seen in 10- to 18-month-old infants but not in 6- to 9-month-old infants.

3.4.6.4 Microbiota

It is unclear how the gut microbiome interacts with orally delivered vaccines and affects immunization. It is known, however, that socioeconomic, geographic, and cultural settings imprint differences in gut microbiome profiles [112]. Turnbaugh et al. [113] studying the gut microbiome in obese and lean twins in the United States found that there is no single abundant bacterial phylotype in the human gut. Instead, it appears that a core gut microbiome exists at the level of metabolic functions.

This suggests that not only is the gut microbiome different between different populations but that it is also different within a population (in terms of the bacterial phylotypes). Evidence to suggest that the microbiota can alter immunogenicity induced by oral vaccines is shown in a study from Finland [103]. Investigators orally administered *Lactobacillus casei* GG in conjunction with RotaShield® vaccine to 2- to 5-month-old infants and observed rotavirus IgA seroconversion in 93 % cases versus 74 % of the placebo controls who did not receive *L. casei* ($P=0.05$). The potential to improve vaccine responses by modifying the gut microbiota in infants and the possibility of using probiotics as adjuvants and/or delivery vehicles are currently being explored [114].

3.4.7 Oral Immunization of Newborns and Coadministration of Vaccines

The immune system of newborns and older infants differs in their composition and functional capacity. It is generally accepted, however, that the neonatal immune system is not underdeveloped but rather "inexperienced" and conventional vaccines fail to activate key cells involved in antigen presentation and immune stimulation. Newborns have been shown to respond to oral polio vaccine, and protective immunity can be achieved after a single immunization at birth. Interestingly seroconversion rates are higher when newborns are given the monovalent, as opposed to the tOPV vaccine [104]. A recent study reports a reduction in Th1 and Th2 immune responses to intradermal BCG vaccination in newborns who were simultaneously given OPV but cautions about potential confounding factors.

As mentioned above, the efficacy of live oral vaccine efficacy can be affected by coadministered vaccines. The tOPV vaccine is known to affect immunogenicity to oral rotavirus vaccines when both are given to infants [105]. As more oral vaccines are licensed and added to the Expanded Program on Immunization (EPI), well-designed clinical trials will be needed to measure the effect of different vaccine combinations.

3.4.8 New Oral Vaccine Approaches for Enteric Pathogens

Live vaccines with the capacity to induce both antibodies and cell-mediated immunity embody one of the most efficient approaches to prevent disease caused by typhoid, non-typhoidal, and paratyphoid *Salmonella*. The challenge remains to generate strains that are safe and yet sufficiently immunogenic. A live attenuated, single-dose, *S.* Typhi vaccine, Typhella™ (also known as M01ZH09) proved to be safe and immunogenic in US adults and Vietnamese children [115]. This vaccine has mutations in *aroC* (aromatic biosynthesis pathway) and *ssaV* (SPI-2 type III secretion system). Larger field trials would be needed to determine its protective efficacy. A series of attenuated *S.* Typhi vaccines, CVD 908-*htrA* (with deletions in *aroC*, *aroD*, and *htrA*), and CVD 909 (CVD 908-*htrA* that constitutively expresses Vi) have been shown to be safe and immunogenic after a single dose.

While enteric fever due to *S.* Typhi has been substantially reduced, paratyphoid fever still remains. A live attenuated *S.* Paratyphi A vaccine, CVD 1902, harboring deletions in the *guaBA* and *clpX* loci and developed at the Center for Vaccine Development, University of Maryland Baltimore, is currently being tested in a phase 1 clinical trial (ClinicalTrials.gov NCT01129452). The data obtained to date suggest that the vaccine was well tolerated and immunogenic.

3.4.8.1 *Shigella* and Enterotoxigenic *E. coli* (ETEC) Vaccines

Diarrhea caused by *Shigella* spp. and ETEC remains a notable disease burden associated with substantial mortality globally but particularly in children in much of the developing world. The genus *Shigella* contains four species (or groups), *S. dysenteriae*, *S. flexneri*, *S. boydii*, and *S. sonnei*, which in turn includes one or multiple serotypes [116]. These invasive pathogens often cause profuse dysentery which is often refractory to oral rehydration. A vaccine against these pathogens is greatly needed, and such a vaccine should induce broad protection against *S. dysenteriae* I (causes epidemics of severe dysentery), all 14 serotypes of *S. flexneri* (cause endemic pediatric shigellosis), and *S. sonnei*.

A number of *Shigella* vaccine candidates based on killed or live attenuated organisms have been developed and evaluated in human studies. An inactivated *S. sonnei* whole-cell vaccine was shown to be safe and immunogenic in volunteers ingesting three to five doses of 10^{10} killed organisms. A series of live attenuated vaccines developed at Walter Reed Army Institute have been shown to protect vaccinated adult volunteers in experimental challenge studies and adult and children living in endemic areas in controlled field trials [117]. The live attenuated *S. flexneri* 2a SC602 strain harbors mutations in the plasmid-encoded gene *icsA* and the chromosomal gene *iuc*. Five clinical trials performed in the United States showed that SC602 is well tolerated and elicits mucosal immune responses. However, when the vaccine was tested in Bangladeshi adults and children, although it showed minimal vaccine shedding and reactogenicity, it also produced very minimal immune responses. A pentavalent *Shigella* vaccine consisting of multiple attenuated strains (*S. sonnei*, *S. dysenteriae* 1, *S. flexneri* 2a, 3a, and 6) is being pursued by investigators at the CVD to provide broad-spectrum protection [116], and several candidate strains containing mutations in *guaBA* and *sen/set* loci (e.g., CVD 1204, CVD 1208) have been evaluated in phase 2 studies in adult human volunteers. This approach has not yet been tested in endemic populations.

A live oral vaccine, ACE527, comprising three attenuated strains of ETEC was safe and well tolerated in humans at doses up to 10^{11} CFU in adult volunteers. In a phase 2b efficacy study whereby vaccinated and unvaccinated volunteers were challenged with ETEC 10407, this vaccine reduced the incidence and severity of diarrhea but did not meet the primary endpoints of the study in reduction of moderate to severe diarrhea. The dietary deficiency of iron in Bangladeshi volunteers has been suggested as one reason for the lower immunogenicity of this vaccine which has a mutation in iron uptake.

The development process of a recombinant vaccine against *Shigella* spp. is described in detail in Chap. 9.

3.4.8.2 Norovirus Virus-Like Particles

Noroviruses (NoV) are single-stranded, positive-sense RNA viruses that cause gastroenteritis in humans. The NoV capsid can be expressed in insect or plant cells, and it has been shown that the VP1 capsid protein can self-assemble virus-like particles (VLPs) that resemble the NoV capsid. Phase 1 clinical trials using VLPs of the prototype NoV, Norwalk virus, showed that Norwalk virus-like particles are safe and immunogenic in humans following oral and intranasal administration and protective against NoV experimental challenge [39]. Appealing features of this system include the possibility of expressing VLPs in plants, which can be ingested [118] (see also Chap. 9), and the potential to display vaccine epitopes on their surface for heterologous vaccination.

3.4.8.3 Novel Adjuvants for Mucosal Immunization

The choice of adjuvants to accompany a mucosally delivered antigen is critical as it may have a dramatic impact in the magnitude, quality, and duration of the immune responses induced. Toll-like receptor (TLR) agonists, detoxified bacterial enterotoxins, mucoadhesives, saponins, and particles are among the most extensively tested. A genetically detoxified double mutant of the *Escherichia coli* heat-labile enterotoxin (LT) harboring deletions on 192G and L211A, also known as dmLT, is presently one of the most promising oral adjuvant candidates. In mice, oral administration of dmLT was able to enhance responses to coadministered tetanus toxoid [119]. Clinical trials are ongoing to evaluate the safety and immunogenicity of dmLT fed to adult volunteers (NCT01147445; ClinicalTrials.gov). While oral adjuvants could be powerful tools to improve the immunogenicity of orally delivered antigens, they could also disturb the delicate balance between immune stimulation and tolerance, particularly during the first year of life when the gut immune system is not yet fully developed [120].

3.4.8.4 Prime–Boost Immunization

The administration of vaccine antigens in the same or different formulations by different routes (e.g., mucosal and parenteral), also known as the "prime–boost" strategy (see also Chap. 2), might provide a means to overcome the limited efficacy associated with oral vaccination and to improve responses to antigens that are poorly immunogenic. This approach could be useful to enhance the breadth and magnitude of immune responses to pathogens that breach the mucosal barrier and become systemic. Mucosal prime–parenteral boost regimens have been successful at inducing protective immunity in various animal models [121].

In humans, oral priming with *S.* Typhi vaccine strain CVD 909 followed by parenteral boost with *S.* Typhi Vi capsular antigen induced Vi serum IgG responses and classical ($CD19^+IgD^- CD27^+$) IgA and IgG B_M cells specific for bacterial antigens. The combination of OPV followed by parenteral IPV (or in reverse order) has been implemented in several countries to elicit both gut and systemic immunity, minimizing the risk of VAPP. [122] In fact, IPV was found to induce mucosal IgA only if preceded by OPV vaccination.

Israeli soldiers who received a parenteral O polysaccharide-based *Shigella* vaccine were protected against infection, and this may have been facilitated by prior natural (oral) exposure to the organism. Interest for the prime–boost strategy is growing and more studies in humans are expected in the near future.

3.5 Common Mucosal Immunity

It would be a tremendous advantage to develop a vaccine which stimulates a common mucosal immunity (CMI) response from the application site to distant mucosal sites. Mucosal tissues possess both antigen-presenting and processing cells with the potential to induce a complete, humoral, and cellular immune response including immunological memory.

The favorite prime inductive site for mucosal immunity is lymphatic tissues (MALT), in the upper respiratory tract (NALT), in the lower respiratory bronchus tract (BALT), and in the gastrointestinal tract (GALT). Other mucosal sites as the urinogenital tract are also suitable but not everywhere accepted due to cultural or religious reasons.

The antigen-specific immune response is generally initiated in the MALT, whereas the diffuse lamina propria (LT) below this lymphatic tissue is the effector site for IgA production and T cell response. Following T cell priming, lymphocytes move to distant mucosal effector compartments. Once in the circulation, the majority of activated lymphocytes home back to site where the antigen was initially took up by the DCs.

Cell Trafficking. Responsible for this homing effect (cell trafficking) are adhesion molecules expressed on the activated lymphocytes. This expression is regulated by DCs via their production of retinoic acids. The most important homing receptors in humans on activated lymphocytes are α4β7 integrin and chemokine (C-C motif) receptor 9 (CCR9) [123].

The importance of exposure of T cells to microbial elements in the gut is demonstrated by findings that a high proportion of $\alpha_4\beta_7$ neonatal T cells is found in cord blood [124].

Homing Receptors. The ligand for α4β7 integrin is the mucosal addressin cell adhesion molecule-1 (MAdCAM-1), expressed by highly endothelial venules (HEV) in the gastrointestinal tract. Lymphocytes bearing the α4β7 integrin receptor undergo extravasation in these capillaries. The chemokine receptor CCR9 on lymphocytes recognizes its chemokine ligand CCL25 which is dominantly produced by the intestinal epithelium. However, nasal immunization induces the expression of alternative adhesion molecules, α4β1 integrin, and CCR10. Their ligands are the vascular cell adhesion molecule 1 (VCAM-1) and CCL28 [125] (Fig. 3.16).

Oral immunization induces a more restricted mucosal response, as reflected by a more restricted homing receptor repertoire than nasal immunization. Nasal immunization induces antibodies in a broader range of mucosal tissues, such as saliva and the urogenital tract, but it is rather poor in

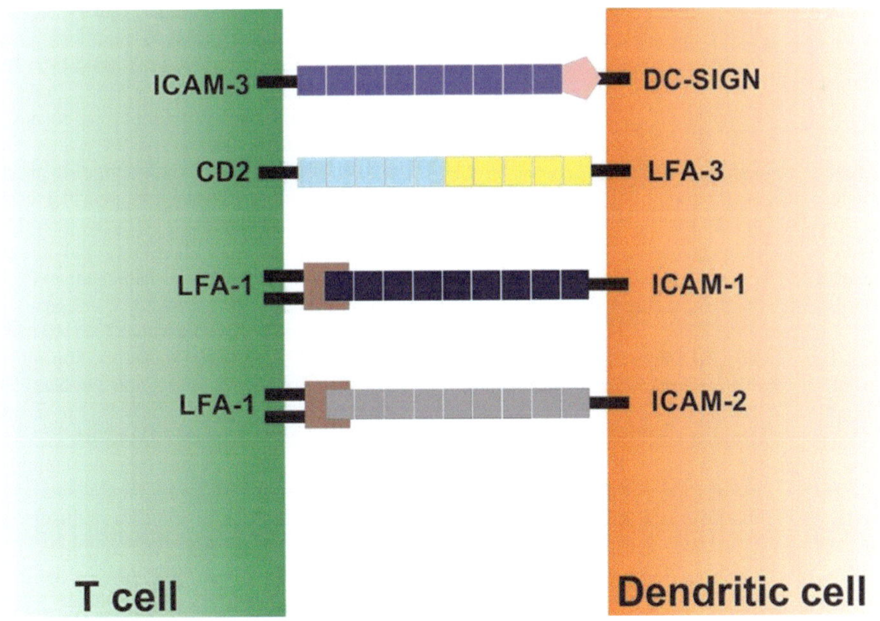

Fig. 3.16 Adhesion molecules. Once in the circulation, the majority of activated lymphocytes home back to site where the antigen was initially taken up by the DCs. Responsible for this homing effect are adhesion molecules expressed on the activated lymphocytes and corresponding receptors on dendritic cells. DC surface receptors not only facilitate antigen uptake but also mediate physical contact between dendritic cells and T cells. *ICAM-3* intercellular adhesion molecule 3, *DC-SIGN* dendritic cell-specific intercellular adhesion molecule-3-grabbing non-integrin, *CD2* cluster of differentiation 2, *LFA-3* lymphocyte function-associated antigen 3, *LFA-1* lymphocyte function-associated antigen 1, *ICAM-1* intercellular adhesion molecule 1, *ICAM-2* intercellular adhesion molecule 2 (Scheme by M. Giese Heidelberg, Germany)

stimulating intestinal immune response due to the lack of specific homing receptors.

Adhesion Molecules and Addressins. Adhesion molecules are sticky cell surface molecules involved in binding with other cells or with the extracellular matrix (ECM). They govern cell-to-cell interactions and play critical roles in a variety of biological processes, for example, in the immune system where they support, e.g., lymphocyte migration, and pairing between many less avid receptors and their ligand. Being lymphocyte homing receptors, they are also known as addressins. Adhesion molecules have also been discovered to play a critical role in the process of metastatic tumor dissemination.

This immune cell trafficking is also supported by sphingosine-1-phosphate (S1P), a bioactive lipid which recognizes its receptor, S1P1, on activated lymphocytes. S1P1 belongs to a sphingosine-1-phosphate receptor subfamily and has an important role in regulating the cell migration. This migration-associated molecule is common to both respiratory and intestinal mucosa [126].

The majority of activated lymphocytes home back to the site where the antigen was initially taken up by the DCs by using this system of homing receptors and their specific ligands. But a portion of these activated lymphocytes seed distal mucosal sites where the pathogens may also encounter. The above-described imprinting system for tissue tropism allows also some mobility to other mucosa-associated tissues and is the basis for the common mucosal immunity.

References

1. Brandtzaeg, P.: Mucosal immunity: induction, dissemination, and effector functions. Scand. J. Immunol. **70**, 505–515 (2009). doi:10.1111/j.1365-3083.2009.02319.x
2. Voltaire, F.M.A.: Philosophical Letters. Dover, New York (2003)
3. Hickey, A.J., Garmise, R.J.: Dry powder nasal vaccines as an alternative to needle-based delivery. Crit. Rev. Ther. Drug Carrier Syst. **26**, 1–27 (2009)
4. Garmise, R.J., Staats, H.F., Hickey, A.J.: Novel dry powder preparations of whole inactivated influenza virus for nasal vaccination. AAPS PharmSciTech **8**(4), 2–10, E81 (2007)
5. Hickey, A.J., Swift, D.: Aerosol Measurement, Principles, Techniques and Applications, 3rd edn, pp. 805–820. Wiley, New York (2011)
6. Garmise, R.J., et al.: Formulation of a dry powder influenza vaccine for nasal delivery. AAPS PharmSciTech **7**, E19 (2006)
7. Alcomo, I.E.: Fundamentals of Microbiology, pp. 263–266. Jones and Bartlett Publishers, Sudbury, Mass (2001)
8. Krasner, R.I.: Biological Weapons, the Microbial Challenge, pp. 335–360. ASM Press, Washington, D.C. (2002)
9. Investigation, F. B. o. Famous cases & criminals: amerithrax or anthrax investigation. www.fbi.gov/about-us/history/famous-cases/anthrax-amerithrax (2011)
10. Pharmacists, A. S. o. H.-S.: American Society of Health-System Pharmacists, pp. 360–377. Bethesda (2002)
11. Mantis, N.J., Morici, L.A., Roy, C.J.: Mucosal Vaccines for Biodefense: Critical Factors in Manufacture and Delivery, pp. 181–195. Springer, New York (2012)
12. Csaba, N., Garcia-Fuentes, M., Alonso, M.J.: Nanoparticles for nasal vaccination. Adv. Drug Deliv. Rev. **61**, 140–157 (2008)
13. Koping-Hoggard, M., Sanchez, A., Alonso, M.J.: Nanoparticles as carriers for nasal vaccine delivery. Expert Rev. Vaccines **4**, 185–196 (2005)
14. Espueles, S., Gamazo, C., Blanco-Prieto, M.J., Irache, J.M.: Nanoparticles as Adjuvant-Vectors for Vaccination, pp. 317–325. Informa Healthcare, New York (2007)
15. El-Kamary, S.S., et al.: Adjuvanted intranasal Norwalk virus-like particle vaccine elicits antibodies and antibody-secreting cells that express homing receptors for mucosal and peripheral lymphoid tissues. J. Infect. Dis. **202**, 1649–1658 (2010)
16. Administration, U. S. F. a. D.: Efficacy Testing and Surrogate Markers of Immunity Workshop Vol. http://www.fda.gov/downloads/BiologicsBloodVaccines/NewsEvents/Workshops MeetingsConferences/TranscriptsMinutes/UCM054606.pdf. Center for Biologics Research and Evaluation (2002)
17. Sewall, H.: The role of epithelium in experimental immunization. Science **62**, 293–299 (1925)
18. Wang, S.H., Kirwan, S.M., Abraham, S.N., Staats, H.F., Hickey, A.J.: Stable dry powder formulation for nasal delivery of anthrax vaccine. J. Pharm. Sci. (2011). doi:10.1002/jps.22742
19. Jain, S., O'Hagan, D.T., Singh, M.: The long-term potential of biodegradable poly(lactide-co-glycolide) microparticles as the next-generation vaccine adjuvant. Expert Rev. Vaccines **10**, 1731–1742 (2011)
20. Jacques, P., et al.: The immunogenicity and reactogenicity profile of a candidate hepatitis B vaccine in an adult vaccine non-responder population. Vaccine **20**, 3644–3649 (2002)
21. Keitel, W., et al.: Dose ranging of adjuvant and antigen in a cell culture H5N1 influenza vaccine: safety and immunogenicity of a phase 1/2 clinical trial. Vaccine **28**, 840–848 (2010). doi:10.1016/j.vaccine.2009.10.019
22. Nevens, F., et al.: Immunogenicity and safety of an experimental adjuvanted hepatitis B candidate vaccine in liver transplant patients. Liver Transpl. **12**, 1489–1495 (2006)
23. Soloff, A.C., Barratt-Boyes, S.M.: Enemy at the gates: dendritic cells and immunity to mucosal pathogens. Cell Res. **20**, 872–885 (2010). doi:10.1038/cr.2010.94
24. Nochi, T., et al.: Nanogel antigenic protein-delivery system for adjuvant-free intranasal vaccines. Nat. Mater. **9**, 572–578 (2010). doi:10.1038/nmat2784
25. Stanberry, L.R., et al.: Safety and immunogenicity of a novel nanoemulsion mucosal adjuvant W805EC combined with approved seasonal influenza antigens. Vaccine **30**, 307–316 (2012). doi:10.1016/j.vaccine.2011.10.094
26. Makidon, P.E., et al.: Nanoemulsion mucosal adjuvant uniquely activates cytokine production by nasal ciliated epithelium and induces dendritic cell trafficking. Eur. J. Immunol. **42**, 2073–2086 (2012). doi:10.1002/eji.201142346
27. Bielinska, A.U., et al.: Mucosal immunization with a novel nanoemulsion-based recombinant anthrax protective antigen vaccine protects against Bacillus anthracis spore challenge. Infect. Immun. **75**, 4020–4029 (2007). doi:10.1128/iai.00070-07
28. Amorij, J.P., et al.: Pulmonary delivery of an inulin-stabilized influenza subunit vaccine prepared by spray-freeze drying induces systemic, mucosal humoral as well as cell-mediated immune responses in BALB/c mice. Vaccine **25**, 8707–8717 (2007)
29. Gwinn, W.M., et al.: Effective induction of protective systemic immunity with nasally administered vaccines adjuvanted with IL-1. Vaccine **28**, 6901–6914 (2010). doi:10.1016/j.vaccine.2010.08.006

30. Jaganathan, K.S., Vyas, S.P.: Strong systemic and mucosal immune responses to surface-modified PLGA microspheres containing recombinant hepatitis B antigen administered intranasally. Vaccine **24**, 4201–4211 (2006)
31. Levitz, S.M., Golenbock, D.T.: Beyond empiricism: informing vaccine development through innate immunity research. Cell **148**, 1284–1292 (2012). doi:10.1016/j.cell.2012.02.012
32. Lycke, N.: Recent progress in mucosal vaccine development: potential and limitations. Nat. Rev. Immunol. **12**, 592–605 (2012). doi:10.1038/nri3251
33. Thompson, A.L., et al.: Maximal adjuvant activity of nasally delivered IL-1alpha requires adjuvant-responsive CD11c(+) cells and does not correlate with adjuvant-induced in vivo cytokine production. J. Immunol. **188**, 2834–2846 (2012). doi:10.4049/jimmunol.1100254
34. Thompson, A.L., Staats, H.F.: Cytokines: the future of intranasal vaccine adjuvants. Clin. Dev. Immunol. **2011**, 289597 (2011). doi:10.1155/2011/289597
35. Couch, R.B., et al.: Contrasting effects of type I interferon as a mucosal adjuvant for influenza vaccine in mice and humans. Vaccine **27**, 5344–5348 (2009). doi:10.1016/j.vaccine.2009.06.084, S0264-410X(09)00962-1 [pii]
36. Duthie, M.S., Windish, H.P., Fox, C.B., Reed, S.G.: Use of defined TLR ligands as adjuvants within human vaccines. Immunol. Rev. **239**, 178–196 (2011). doi:10.1111/j.1600-065X.2010.00978.x
37. Lewis, D.J., et al.: Transient facial nerve paralysis (Bell's palsy) following intranasal delivery of a genetically detoxified mutant of Escherichia coli heat labile toxin. PLoS One **4**, e6999 (2009). doi:10.1371/journal.pone.0006999
38. Mutsch, M., et al.: Use of the inactivated intranasal influenza vaccine and the risk of Bell's palsy in Switzerland.[see comment]. N. Engl. J. Med. **350**, 896–903 (2004)
39. Atmar, R.L., et al.: Norovirus vaccine against experimental human Norwalk Virus illness. N. Engl. J. Med. **365**, 2178–2187 (2011). doi:10.1056/NEJMoa1101245
40. Hayes, J.D., Pulford, D.J.: The glutathione S-Transferase supergene family: regulation of GST and the contribution of the isoenzymes to cancer chemoprotection and drug resistance. Crit. Rev. Biochem. Mol. Biol. **30**, 445–600 (1995). doi:10.3109/10409239509083491
41. Sayes, C.M., Reed, K.L., Warheit, D.B.: Assessing toxicity of fine and nanoparticles: comparing in vitro measurements to in vivo pulmonary toxicity profiles. Toxicol. Sci. **97**, 163–180 (2007). doi:10.1093/toxsci/kfm018
42. Mittler, R.: Oxidative stress, antioxidants and stress tolerance. Trends Plant Sci. **7**, 405–410 (2002). doi:10.1016/s1360-1385(02)02312-9, Pii s1360-1385(02)02312-9
43. Warheit, D., et al.: Comparative pulmonary toxicity assessment of single-wall carbon nanotubes in rats. Toxicol. Sci. **77**, 117–125 (2004)
44. Gurr, J.R., Wang, A.S.S., Chen, C.H., Jan, K.Y.: Ultrafine titanium dioxide particles in the absence of photoactivation can induce oxidative damage to human bronchial epithelial cells. Toxicology **213**, 66–73 (2005). doi:10.1016/j.tox.2005.05.007
45. Sayes, C.M., et al.: Correlating nanoscale titania structure with toxicity: a cytotoxicity and inflammatory response study with human dermal fibroblasts and human lung epithelial cells. Toxicol. Sci. **92**, 174–185 (2006). doi:10.1093/toxsci/kfj197
46. Zhu, S.Q., Oberdorster, E., Haasch, M.L.: Toxicity of an engineered nanoparticle (fullerene, C-60) in two aquatic species. Daphnia and fathead minnow. Mar. Environ. Res. **62**, S5–S9 (2006). doi:10.1016/j.marenvres.2006.04.059
47. Pitt, M.L., et al.: In vitro correlate of immunity in a rabbit model of inhalational anthrax. Vaccine **19**, 4768–4773 (2001)
48. Zaucha, G.M., Pitt, L.M., Estep, J., Ivins, B.E., Friedlander, A.M.: The pathology of experimental anthrax in rabbits exposed by inhalation and subcutaneous inoculation. Arch. Pathol. Lab. Med. **122**, 982–992 (1998)
49. Roy, C.J., et al.: Human leukocyte antigen-DQ8 transgenic mice: a model to examine the toxicity of aerosolized staphylococcal enterotoxin B. Infect. Immun. **73**, 2452–2460 (2005)
50. LeClaire, R.D., et al.: Potentiation of inhaled staphylococcal enterotoxin B-induced toxicity by lipopolysaccharide in mice. Toxicol. Pathol. **24**, 619–626 (1996)
51. Carter, N.J., Curran, M.P.: Live attenuated influenza vaccine (FluMist(R); Fluenz): a review of its use in the prevention of seasonal influenza in children and adults. Drugs **71**, 1591–1622 (2011). doi:10.2165/11206860-000000000-00000
52. Dhere, R., et al.: A pandemic influenza vaccine in India: from strain to sale within 12 months. Vaccine **29**(Suppl 1), A16–A21 (2011). doi:10.1016/j.vaccine.2011.04.119
53. Reiss, C.S., Plakhov, I.V., Komatsu, T.: Viral replication in olfactory receptor neurons and entry into the olfactory bulb and brain. Ann. N. Y. Acad. Sci. **855**, 751–761 (1998)
54. Mutsch, M., et al.: Use of the inactivated intranasal influenza vaccine and the risk of Bell's palsy in Switzerland. N. Engl. J. Med. **350**, 896–903 (2004). doi:10.1056/NEJMoa030595
55. van Ginkel, F.W., et al.: Enterotoxin-based mucosal adjuvants alter antigen trafficking and induce inflammatory responses in the nasal tract. Infect. Immun. **73**, 6892–6902 (2005). doi:10.1128/IAI.73.10.6892-6902.2005
56. Brandtzaeg, P.: Induction of secretory immunity and memory at mucosal surfaces. Vaccine **25**, 5467–5484 (2007). doi:10.1016/j.vaccine.2006.12.001
57. Gibbons, D.L., Spencer, J.: Mouse and human intestinal immunity: same ballpark, different players; different rules, same score. Mucosal Immunol. **4**, 148–157 (2011). doi:10.1038/mi.2010.85
58. Bemark, M., Boysen, P., Lycke, N.Y.: Induction of gut IgA production through T cell-dependent and T cell-independent pathways. Ann. N. Y. Acad. Sci. **1247**, 97–116 (2012). doi:10.1111/j.1749-6632.2011.06378.x
59. Slack, E., Balmer, M.L., Fritz, J.H., Hapfelmeier, S.: Functional flexibility of intestinal IgA – broadening the fine line. Front. Immunol. **3**, 100 (2012). doi:10.3389/fimmu.2012.00100
60. Rol, N., Favre, L., Benyacoub, J., Corthesy, B.: The role of secretory immunoglobulin A in the natural sensing of commensal bacteria by mouse Peyer's patch dendritic cells. J. Biol. Chem. **287**, 40074–40082 (2012). doi:10.1074/jbc.M112.405001
61. Pabst, O.: New concepts in the generation and functions of IgA. Nat. Rev. Immunol. **12**, 821–832 (2012). doi:10.1038/nri3322
62. Kett, K., Brandtzaeg, P., Radl, J., Haaijman, J.J.: Different subclass distribution of IgA-producing cells in human lymphoid organs and various secretory tissues. J. Immunol. **136**, 3631–3635 (1986)
63. Israel, E.J., et al.: Expression of the neonatal Fc receptor, FcRn, on human intestinal epithelial cells. Immunology **92**, 69–74 (1997)
64. Yoshida, M., et al.: Human neonatal Fc receptor mediates transport of IgG into luminal secretions for delivery of antigens to mucosal dendritic cells. Immunity **20**, 769–783 (2004). doi:10.1016/j.immuni.2004.05.007
65. Devriendt, B., De Geest, B.G., Goddeeris, B.M., Cox, E.: Crossing the barrier: targeting epithelial receptors for enhanced oral vaccine delivery. J. Control. Release: Off. J. Control. Release Soc. **160**, 431–439 (2012). doi:10.1016/j.jconrel.2012.02.006
66. Quiding-Jarbrink, M., et al.: Differential expression of tissue-specific adhesion molecules on human circulating antibody-forming cells after systemic, enteric, and nasal immunizations. A molecular basis for the compartmentalization of effector B cell responses. J. Clin. Invest. **99**, 1281–1286 (1997). doi:10.1172/JCI119286
67. Saurer, L., Mueller, C.: T cell-mediated immunoregulation in the gastrointestinal tract. Allergy **64**, 505–519 (2009). doi:10.1111/j.1398-9995.2009.01965.x

68. Mucida, D.: T-helping colitis. Gastroenterology **141**, 801–805 (2011). doi:10.1053/j.gastro.2011.07.023
69. McArthur, M.A., Sztein, M.B.: Heterogeneity of multifunctional IL-17A producing S. Typhi-specific CD8+ T cells in volunteers following Ty21a typhoid immunization. PLoS One **7**, e38408 (2012). doi:10.1371/journal.pone.0038408
70. Plotkin, S.A.: Correlates of protection induced by vaccination. Clin. Vaccine Immunol. **17**, 1055–1065 (2010). doi:10.1128/CVI.00131-10
71. Ilan, Y.: Oral tolerance: can we make it work? Hum. Immunol. **70**, 768–776 (2009). doi:10.1016/j.humimm.2009.06.018
72. Tsuji, N.M., Kosaka, A.: Oral tolerance: intestinal homeostasis and antigen-specific regulatory T cells. Trends Immunol. **29**, 532–540 (2008). doi:10.1016/j.it.2008.09.002
73. Ruiz-Palacios, G.M., et al.: Safety and efficacy of an attenuated vaccine against severe rotavirus gastroenteritis. N. Engl. J. Med. **354**, 11–22 (2006). doi:10.1056/NEJMoa052434
74. Vesikari, T., et al.: Safety and efficacy of a pentavalent human-bovine (WC3) reassortant rotavirus vaccine. N. Engl. J. Med. **354**, 23–33 (2006). doi:10.1056/NEJMoa052664
75. Levine, M.M., et al.: Safety, immunogenicity, and efficacy of recombinant live oral cholera vaccines, CVD 103 and CVD 103-HgR. Lancet **2**, 467–470 (1988)
76. Germanier, R., Fuer, E.: Isolation and characterization of Gal E mutant Ty 21a of Salmonella typhi: a candidate strain for a live, oral typhoid vaccine. J. Infect. Dis. **131**, 553–558 (1975)
77. Clemens, J.D., et al.: Field trial of oral cholera vaccines in Bangladesh: evaluation of anti-bacterial and anti-toxic breast-milk immunity in response to ingestion of the vaccines. Vaccine **8**, 469–472 (1990)
78. Armah, G.E., et al.: Efficacy of pentavalent rotavirus vaccine against severe rotavirus gastroenteritis in infants in developing countries in sub-Saharan Africa: a randomised, double-blind, placebo-controlled trial. Lancet **376**, 606–614 (2010). doi:10.1016/S0140-6736(10)60889-6
79. Sabin, A.B.: Oral poliovirus vaccine: history of its development and use and current challenge to eliminate poliomyelitis from the world. J. Infect. Dis. **151**, 420–436 (1985)
80. Heaton, P.M., Goveia, M.G., Miller, J.M., Offit, P., Clark, H.F.: Development of a pentavalent rotavirus vaccine against prevalent serotypes of rotavirus gastroenteritis. J. Infect. Dis. **192**(Suppl 1), S17–S21 (2005). doi:10.1086/431500
81. Vesikari, T., et al.: Efficacy of human rotavirus vaccine against rotavirus gastroenteritis during the first 2 years of life in European infants: randomised, double-blind controlled study. Lancet **370**, 1757–1763 (2007). doi:10.1016/S0140-6736(07)61744-9
82. Desai, S.N., Clemens, J.D.: An overview of cholera vaccines and their public health implications. Curr. Opin. Pediatr. **24**, 85–91 (2012). doi:10.1097/MOP.0b013e32834eb625
83. Paul, Y.: Why polio has not been eradicated in India despite many remedial interventions? Vaccine **27**, 3700–3703 (2009). doi:10.1016/j.vaccine.2009.03.078
84. Grassly, N.C., et al.: New strategies for the elimination of polio from India. Science **314**, 1150–1153 (2006). doi:10.1126/science.1130388
85. Glass, R.I., et al.: Rotavirus vaccines: current prospects and future challenges. Lancet **368**, 323–332 (2006). doi:10.1016/S0140-6736(06)68815-6
86. Vesikari, T., et al.: Efficacy of a pentavalent rotavirus vaccine in reducing rotavirus-associated health care utilization across three regions (11 countries). Int. J. Infect. Dis.: IJID: Off. Publ. Int. Soc. Infect. Dis. **11**(Suppl 2), S29–S35 (2007). doi:10.1016/S1201-9712(07)60019-8
87. Breiman, R.F., et al.: Analyses of health outcomes from the 5 sites participating in the Africa and Asia clinical efficacy trials of the oral pentavalent rotavirus vaccine. Vaccine **30**(Suppl 1), A24–A29 (2012). doi:10.1016/j.vaccine.2011.08.124
88. Ciarlet, M., Schodel, F.: Development of a rotavirus vaccine: clinical safety, immunogenicity, and efficacy of the pentavalent rotavirus vaccine. RotaTeq. Vaccine **27**(Suppl 6), G72–G81 (2009). doi:10.1016/j.vaccine.2009.09.107
89. Zaman, K., et al.: Efficacy of pentavalent rotavirus vaccine against severe rotavirus gastroenteritis in infants in developing countries in Asia: a randomised, double-blind, placebo-controlled trial. Lancet **376**, 615–623 (2010). doi:10.1016/S0140-6736(10)60755-6
90. Harris, J.B., LaRocque, R.C., Qadri, F., Ryan, E.T., Calderwood, S.B.: Cholera. Lancet **379**, 2466–2476 (2012). doi:10.1016/S0140-6736(12)60436-X
91. Levine, M.M., et al.: Duration of infection-derived immunity to cholera. J. Infect. Dis. **143**, 818–820 (1981)
92. Patel, S.M., et al.: Memory B cell responses to Vibrio cholerae O1 lipopolysaccharide are associated with protection against infection from household contacts of patients with cholera in Bangladesh. Clin. Vaccine Immunol. **19**, 842–848 (2012). doi:10.1128/CVI.00037-12
93. Alam, M.M., et al.: Antigen-specific memory B-cell responses in Bangladeshi adults after one- or two-dose oral killed cholera vaccination and comparison with responses in patients with naturally acquired cholera. Clin. Vaccine Immunol. **18**, 844–850 (2011). doi:10.1128/CVI.00562-10
94. Ali, M., Emch, M., Park, J.K., Yunus, M., Clemens, J.: Natural cholera infection-derived immunity in an endemic setting. J. Infect. Dis. **204**, 912–918 (2011). doi:10.1093/infdis/jir416
95. Ochiai, R.L., et al.: A study of typhoid fever in five Asian countries: disease burden and implications for controls. Bull. World Health Organ. **86**, 260–268 (2008)
96. Charles, R.C., et al.: Characterization of anti-Salmonella enterica serotype Typhi antibody responses in bacteremic Bangladeshi patients by an immunoaffinity proteomics-based technology. Clin. Vaccine Immunol. **17**, 1188–1195 (2010). doi:10.1128/CVI.00104-10
97. D'Amelio, R., et al.: Comparative analysis of immunological responses to oral (Ty21a) and parenteral (TAB) typhoid vaccines. Infect. Immun. **56**, 2731–2735 (1988)
98. Qadri, F., Bhuiyan, T.R., Sack, D.A., Svennerholm, A.M.: Immune responses and protection in children in developing countries induced by oral vaccines. Vaccine **31**, 452–460 (2013). doi:10.1016/j.vaccine.2012.11.012
99. Kau, A.L., Ahern, P.P., Griffin, N.W., Goodman, A.L., Gordon, J.I.: Human nutrition, the gut microbiome and the immune system. Nature **474**, 327–336 (2011). doi:10.1038/nature10213
100. Lagos, R., et al.: Effect of small bowel bacterial overgrowth on the immunogenicity of single-dose live oral cholera vaccine CVD 103-HgR. J. Infect. Dis. **180**, 1709–1712 (1999). doi:10.1086/315051
101. Albert, M.J., et al.: Supplementation with zinc, but not vitamin A, improves seroconversion to vibriocidal antibody in children given an oral cholera vaccine. J. Infect. Dis. **187**, 909–913 (2003). doi:10.1086/368132
102. Ahmed, T., Svennerholm, A.M., Al Tarique, A., Sultana, G.N., Qadri, F.: Enhanced immunogenicity of an oral inactivated cholera vaccine in infants in Bangladesh obtained by zinc supplementation and by temporary withholding breast-feeding. Vaccine **27**, 1433–1439 (2009). doi:10.1016/j.vaccine.2008.12.036
103. Isolauri, E., Joensuu, J., Suomalainen, H., Luomala, M., Vesikari, T.: Improved immunogenicity of oral D x RRV reassortant rotavirus vaccine by Lactobacillus casei GG. Vaccine **13**, 310–312 (1995)
104. Waggie, Z., et al.: Randomized trial of type 1 and type 3 oral monovalent poliovirus vaccines in newborns in Africa. J. Infect. Dis. **205**, 228–236 (2012). doi:10.1093/infdis/jir721

105. Patel, M., Steele, A.D., Parashar, U.D.: Influence of oral polio vaccines on performance of the monovalent and pentavalent rotavirus vaccines. Vaccine **30**(Suppl 1), A30–A35 (2012). doi:10.1016/j.vaccine.2011.11.093
106. Overbeck, S., Rink, L., Haase, H.: Modulating the immune response by oral zinc supplementation: a single approach for multiple diseases. Arch. Immunol. Ther. Exp. (Warsz.) **56**, 15–30 (2008). doi:10.1007/s00005-008-0003-8
107. Kaufman, D.R., et al.: Vitamin A deficiency impairs vaccine-elicited gastrointestinal immunity. J. Immunol. **187**, 1877–1883 (2011). doi:10.4049/jimmunol.1101248
108. Bahl, R., et al.: Effect of vitamin A administered at Expanded Program on Immunization contacts on antibody response to oral polio vaccine. Eur. J. Clin. Nutr. **56**, 321–325 (2002). doi:10.1038/sj.ejcn.1601325
109. Walker, A.: Breast milk as the gold standard for protective nutrients. J. Pediatr. **156**, S3–S7 (2010). doi:10.1016/j.jpeds.2009.11.021
110. Goveia, M.G., DiNubile, M.J., Dallas, M.J., Heaton, P.M., Kuter, B.J.: Efficacy of pentavalent human-bovine (WC3) reassortant rotavirus vaccine based on breastfeeding frequency. Pediatr. Infect. Dis. J. **27**, 656–658 (2008). doi:10.1097/INF.0b013e318168d29e
111. Moon, S.S., et al.: Inhibitory effect of breast milk on infectivity of live oral rotavirus vaccines. Pediatr. Infect. Dis. J. **29**, 919–923 (2010). doi:10.1097/INF.0b013e3181e232ea
112. Yatsunenko, T., et al.: Human gut microbiome viewed across age and geography. Nature **486**, 222–227 (2012). doi:10.1038/nature11053
113. Turnbaugh, P.J., et al.: A core gut microbiome in obese and lean twins. Nature **457**, 480–484 (2009). doi:10.1038/nature07540
114. Bjorksten, B.: Diverse microbial exposure – consequences for vaccine development. Vaccine **30**, 4336–4340 (2012). doi:10.1016/j.vaccine.2011.10.074
115. Kirkpatrick, B.D., et al.: The novel oral typhoid vaccine M01ZH09 is well tolerated and highly immunogenic in 2 vaccine presentations. J. Infect. Dis. **192**, 360–366 (2005). doi:10.1086/431605
116. Levine, M.M., Kotloff, K.L., Barry, E.M., Pasetti, M.F., Sztein, M.B.: Clinical trials of Shigella vaccines: two steps forward and one step back on a long, hard road. Nat. Rev. Microbiol. **5**, 540–553 (2007). doi:10.1038/nrmicro1662
117. Mel, D.M., Terzin, A.L., Vuksic, L.: Studies on vaccination against bacillary dysentery. 3. Effective oral immunization against Shigella flexneri 2a in a field trial. Bull. World Health Organ. **32**, 647–655 (1965)
118. Herbst-Kralovetz, M., Mason, H.S., Chen, Q.: Norwalk virus-like particles as vaccines. Expert Rev. Vaccines **9**, 299–307 (2010). doi:10.1586/erv.09.163
119. Norton, E.B., Lawson, L.B., Freytag, L.C., Clements, J.D.: Characterization of a mutant Escherichia coli heat-labile toxin, LT(R192G/L211A), as a safe and effective oral adjuvant. Clin. Vaccine Immunol. **18**, 546–551 (2011). doi:10.1128/CVI.00538-10
120. Brandtzaeg, P.: Food allergy: separating the science from the mythology. Nat. Rev. Gastroenterol. Hepatol. **7**, 380–400 (2010). doi:10.1038/nrgastro.2010.80
121. Azevedo, M.S., et al.: An oral versus intranasal prime/boost regimen using attenuated human rotavirus or VP2 and VP6 virus-like particles with immunostimulating complexes influences protection and antibody-secreting cell responses to rotavirus in a neonatal gnotobiotic pig model. Clin. Vaccine Immunol. **17**, 420–428 (2010). doi:10.1128/CVI.00395-09
122. Schoub, B.D., Mphahlele, M.J., Ngcobo, N.J., Hoosen, A.A., Meheus, A.: Introducing new vaccines into the South African national immunisation programme – a case study. Vaccine **30**(Suppl 3), C1–C2 (2012). doi:10.1016/j.vaccine.2012.06.094
123. Gerner, R.R., Moschen, A.R., Tilg, H.: Targeting T and B lymphocytes in inflammatory bowel diseases: lessons from clinical trials. Dig. Dis. **31**, 328–335 (2013). doi:10.1159/000354687
124. Conroy, M.E., Shi, H.N., Walker, W.A.: The long-term health effects of neonatal microbial flora. Curr. Opin. Allergy Clin. Immunol. **9**, 197–201 (2009). doi:10.1097/ACI.0b013e32832b3f1d
125. Kunisawa, J., Nochi, T., Kiyono, H.: Immunological commonalities and distinctions between airway and digestive immunity. Trends Immunol. **29**, 505–513 (2008). doi:10.1016/j.it.2008.07.008
126. Hla, T., et al.: Sphingosine-1-phosphate signaling via the EDG-1 family of G-protein-coupled receptors. Ann. N. Y. Acad. Sci. **905**, 16–24 (2000)
127. Mayo, S., Pagano, R.E.: Pathways of clathrin-independent endocytosis. Nat. Rev. Mol. Cell Biol. **8**, 603–612 (2007). doi:10.1038/nrm2216, Nature Publishing Group

Pediatric Immunology

4

Contents

4.1 Immunity of the Newborn[1]

Newborn's immune system is not nearly as effective as an adult's or even an older child's, and it takes many months before a newborn can fight off infection as well as someone whose immune system is fully matured. In the meantime, pregnant mothers pass immunoglobulin antibodies from their bloodstream, through the placenta, and to the fetus. These antibodies are an essential part of the fetus's immune system. Passive transfer of maternal antibodies occurs after the 28th week of gestation. Premature infants of less than 28 weeks gestation are not expected to have significant amounts of maternal antibody and are especially vulnerable to serious bacterial infection, as well as some viral and fungal infections. The fetal immune system develops in a sterile and protected environment and therefore lacks antigenic experience.

The immunologic competence of the neonate is mainly based on components of the innate and antigen-independent immune system on. The education of the newborn's acquired immune system rapidly progresses in the first three months of life by contact with the microbial world (Fig. 4.1).

The cells of the acquired immune system mature and gain experience with antigens. During this period of education, the success of vaccination in the early life is limited due to this weakness of the newborn's immune system [1, 2].

[1]Paediatric immunology and vaccinology by *Sofia Ygberg and Anna Nilsson* in Molecular Vaccines – From Prophylaxis to Therapy, Volume 1, Springer-Verlag Wien, 2013, Ed. Matthias Giese.

M. Giese, *Introduction to Molecular Vaccinology*, DOI 10.1007/978-3-319-25832-4_4

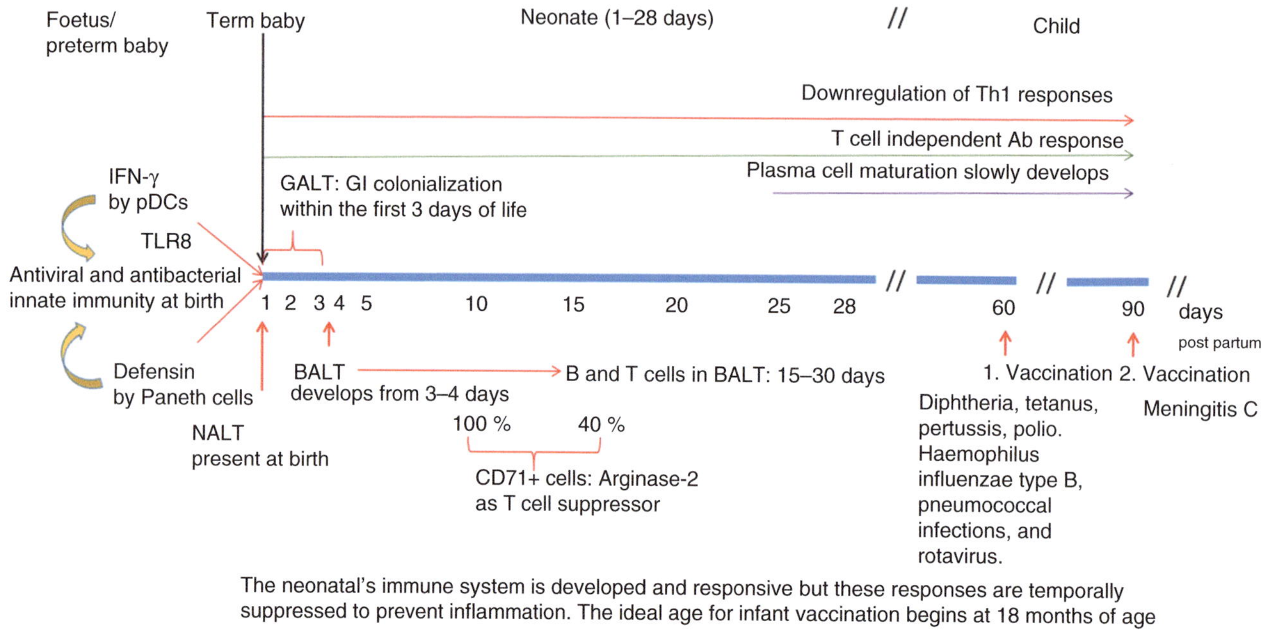

Fig. 4.1 The neonate's immune system is developed and responsive by birth, but Th1 responses are temporally suppressed to prevent inflammation. Within the first 12 months of life, the antibody production is T cell independent and develops slowly. During this critical neonatal period, antiviral and antibacterial components (INF-γ or defensin) of the innate immunity protect the newborn against infectious diseases. Also TLR8 is active, whereas the other TLRs are still in a kind of waiting position. CD71+ erythroid cells produce arginase-2 which has been shown to exert strongly immunosuppressive effects on T cells. The neonatal period is characterized by a downregulation of inflammation processes with the risk of infection. The ideal age for vaccination begins at 18 months of age (Figure by M. Giese Heidelberg/Germany)

4.2 Neonatal and Child Infections

According to WHO (Millennium Development Goal 4, MDG 4), more than one third of all child deaths occur within the first month of life, mainly in developing countries, especially in Africa and South Asia: every year, nearly 41 % of all under-five child deaths are among newborn infants, babies in their first 28 days of life or the neonatal period. Three quarters of all newborn deaths occur in the first week of life. A child's risk of death in the first 4 weeks of life is nearly 15 times greater than any other time before his or her first birthday. One major cause of newborn and child death worldwide, and not only in developing countries, are infectious diseases (overall 36 %).

Generally, at 2 months of age, the infant vaccine regime begins with immunization against diphtheria, tetanus, pertussis, polio, *Haemophilus influenzae* type B, pneumococcal infections, and rotavirus. One month later, vaccination against meningitis C is routinely offered. Booster immunization will follow according to a stringent schedule. Vaccinations against measles, rubella, and mumps virus begin at 11 months of age.

4.3 Intestinal Microflora in Early Infancy

The gastrointestinal immune system is immature at birth. The immunoregulatory network and the epithelial barrier are poorly developed. Therefore, the neonatal period (the first 28 days after birth) is very critical, both with regard to infections and priming for allergic diseases. For full maturation of the gastrointestinal (GI) mucosal immunity, exogenous stimuli of gut microbes are absolutely required. Studies with gnotobiotic germ-free mice demonstrated that these animals had an underdeveloped immune system, at mucosal surfaces and systematically. Reconstitution with microbiota completely restores immune development. The mucosal barrier may be inadequate up to 2 years of age.

The intestinal microbiota is an essential force in the appropriate development not only of mucosal but also of systemic innate and adaptive immunity, B cell development, as well as T cell development [3]. The microbial colonization of mucosal surfaces begins within minutes by passage of the neonate through the birth canal. The bacterial density reaches maximal levels already after 24–72 h [4]. The bacteria originate mainly from the mother: *Escherichia coli, Streptococci, Clostridium, Bacteroides, Lactobacilli, especially Bifidobacterium bifidum*. This gut colonization is stimulated by complex carbohydrates of breast milk.

Delivery Mode. The colonization of the gut is also influenced by the delivery mode, vaginal delivery vs. caesarian section. Caesarian-section-born infants have a different colonization pattern compared to vaginal delivery-born babies. The gut flora of children born by caesarian section has fewer *E. coli* and more *enterobacteria* such as *Klebsiella* and *Enterobacter*. These children show also an enhanced production of IL-13 which is associated primarily with the induction of airway disease. Asthma and atopy in childhood of these children are more frequent than in vaginal-born children.

First Postnatal Barrier. All cellular components of the GI immune systems are already developed during the fetal life. Goblet cells, thus present at birth, generate the mucus layer which contains large amounts of antimicrobial peptides as α-defensins produced by Paneth cells. This is the first postnatal epithelial barrier. Additionally, antibodies, essential for survival, are transferred to the newborn via breast milk, secretory IgM and secretory IgA, whereas the amount of IgG in breast milk is very low. The rapid maturation of the newborn's immune system runs in parallel.

At days 10–15 after birth, T cells became more and more antigen specific. Already-activated T cells in the gut at birth are merely a product of maternal antigen exposure during pregnancy. Also at day 10 post partum, IgA-producing mucosa plasma cells are for the first time detectable. Intestinal DCs capture luminal bacteria via their dendrites and present the antigen to mucosal B cells which in response develop IgA-secreting plasma cells. IgA is transcytosed through epithelial cell into the intestinal lumen. The rapid increase within the first year of life reflects the progressive microbial stimulation of GALT.

Arginase. The neonate's immune system is not only highly vulnerable against disseminated infections but also the abrupt transition from an almost sterile in utero setting to colonization with commensal microbes taking the very high risk of excessive inflammation. S. Way and co-workers recently discovered a mechanism in newborn mice and human cord blood how the immune system is temporarily suppressed to avoid an overexuberant response when it first comes into contact with microbes [5].

Neonatal CD71+ erythroid cells express the enzyme arginase-2. Arginase is known for 30 years to be a key player in the mammalian immune system by suppressing T cell functions and other immunocompetent cells [6]. The highest physiological concentration of CD71+ cells is measurable after parturition, at 6–9 days in newborn mice (comparable to human neonates). At the same time, the comparable number of recoverable *Listeria monocytogenes*, experimentally used for infection, is also high. In 15-day-old mice (comparable to the child immune system), the concentration of CD71+ cells is reduced to 40 %, leading to immune activation and a 100-fold lower *L. monocytogenes* infection rate. Taken together, immunosuppressive CD71+ cells are temporally enriched in neonates during this crucial development period and help to safeguard newborn's life.

4.4 Cellular Components of Innate and Adaptive Immunity

A major disadvantage for the neonatal immune system is, independent of species, that most B and T cells are naive. Although the majority of cells and soluble factors appear early in fetal life, their numbers and relative ratio and activation status differ from adults [7]. There is a lack of knowledge in human infants since the majority of studies in neonatal immunology have been generated in rodent models. It is difficult to translate these findings to humans since newborn mice are underdeveloped compared to human infants [8]. The studies of cells isolated from umbilical cord blood have provided new insight, but these data may not be representative of the circulating cells in the neonatal immune system. Data obtained from cord blood should therefore be combined with data acquired from infants [9].

4.4.1 Neonatal and Childhood Antigen-Presenting Cells

Monocytes and dendritic cells (DCs) function as antigen-presenting cells and are key players in innate immunity but also responsible for initiation of adaptive immune responses. Two subtypes of DCs are identified in peripheral blood: the myeloid DCs (mDCs) and the plasmacytoid DCs (pDCs).

The mDC is the main antigen-presenting cell and plays a crucial role in B cell differentiation by the release of cytokines such as IL-12, IL-6, BAFF, and APRIL, which drive the formation of antibody-producing B cells. On the other hand, pDCs produce interferons and thereby play a vital role in antiviral immunity [10].

There are age-associated differences in the proportion of DCs in peripheral blood in children, where pDC numbers are much higher in infants than in older children, probably reflecting their importance for protection against viral illness in early life before protective adaptive immune responses have been initiated [11]. However, that comes at the cost of less efficient B cell activation early in life.

Cord Blood. Several studies on cord blood DCs have confirmed an immature phenotype with low, or no basal expression of CD40, co-stimulatory molecules CD80/CD86, or MHC class II molecules [12–14]. Functionally, this translates into suboptimal human neonatal DC responses to most stimuli [15]. In addition, the importance of the TLR pathway on DCs for induction of adaptive immune responses is apparent and well established. Despite comparable expression of TLRs on cord blood DCs and adult cells, the capacity of cord blood DCs to respond to TLR agonists is also significantly reduced and characterized by low production of the pro-inflammatory Th1 cytokines TNF-α and IFN-α [16, 17]. However, recent data suggests that neonatal TLR-mediated impairments are selective since the TLR8 agonist R848 is able to induce a robust immune response in cord blood DCs comparable to adult cells. This finding has also been confirmed in infant cells and may have important implications for the choice of adjuvants in neonatal vaccine research [18, 19].

The innate responses of monocytes and antigen-presenting cells develop within the first year of life [19, 20]. Phenotypic analysis of peripheral blood monocytes and DCs has shown that circulating DCs acquire an adultlike phenotype around 6 months of age. Cytokine production after TLR stimulation at birth is skewed toward a Th2 response with production of IL-6, IL-8, and IL-10 and low levels of the Th1 polarizing IL-12p70 cytokine [21]. However, the IL-6 levels are comparable to adults already at 3 months of age. For IL-10, the production remains significantly higher also at 12 months of age and the same trend is shown for IL-8 [20].

Thus, small children are impaired in both the maturation of the antigen-presenting cells and the capacity of such cells to respond to bacterial and viral antigens, with the important exception of TLR8. Using TLR8 ligands as vaccine adjuvants may represent a window of opportunity.

4.4.2 Neonatal and Childhood T Cells

The peripheral blood T-lymphocyte subsets in infants differ from that of adults. At birth, there is a gradual increase in the absolute number of CD3+ T lymphocytes and from the age of 2 years a decrease to levels similar to adults [22]. Helper CD4+T cells and cytotoxic CD8+ T cells also increase in the first months of life and decline after 9–15 months of age [23]. Analysis by flow cytometry has revealed several CD4+ memory cell populations in blood, where only the central memory T cell population is present at birth. As a result of antigenic stimulation, effector memory helper T cells increase during the first year to levels comparable to adults and remain stable during childhood.

The recently described population of CXCR5+ memory T cells, also defined as follicular helper T cells, is absent at birth but increase in number during the first year of life in parallel to the increase in serum IgA and IgG [23]. Follicular helper T cells were first described as cells able to efficiently support the differentiation of switched B cells in secondary lymphoid organs with the subsequent production of IgA and IgG [24]. The absolute numbers of regulatory T cells (Treg) increase the first month of life similar to CD4+ memory T cells and remain stable thereafter. Neonatal Treg exert potent immunosuppressive activities and suppress antigen-specific T cell proliferation and IFN-γ production [25] which may modulate the development of a memory CD4+ T cell pool later in life [26].

Intrinsic defects in T cell immunity have been described for neonatal T cells. A key feature of signaling via TCR-CD3 on naive CD4+ T cells is the upregulation of CD40 ligand on the cell surface. Neonatal CD4+T cells have reduced capacity to express CD40 ligand after TCR-CD3 activation, which in turn negatively affect antibody production, Ig switch, and memory B cell generation [27]. Helper T cell responses after immunizations in newborns have been investigated in many contexts [1], and several factors (antigen dose; adjuvant, routes of immunization) influence whether a predominantly Th1 or Th2 response will be elicited. A majority of current childhood vaccines elicit a predominantly Th2 biased response with the exception of BCG and whole-cell pertussis vaccines [28].

So, the T cell responses early in life are skewed toward a Th2 response, and neonatal helper T cells have reduced capacity to support B cell differentiation and antibody production.

4.4.3 Neonatal and Childhood B Cells

Several studies show age-dependent developmental changes in peripheral blood B cell subsets during the first 5 years of life with a significant decrease in total B cells with age. Most striking is the shift from a predominantly naive and transitional blood B cell pool during infancy to an increase of the memory B cell fraction in the older child and adult. The transitional B cells are increased in infants compared to adults, which may bridge the gap between innate and adaptive immunity early in life. Transitional B cells produce IgM upon toll-like receptor 9 stimulation and thus may be an important mechanism for a first-line defense against bacteria at birth [29]. The expansion of the memory B cell pool is most evident during the first year of life, where after the absolute number is stable over time. Taken together, these findings suggest that the decrease in total B cells with age is mainly related to a reduction in the output from the bone marrow (BM) of transitional and naive cells [30, 31].

Using CD27 as a surrogate marker of human memory B cells together with the surface expression of IgD, several memory B cell populations have been characterized. Classical switched memory B cells increase during infancy and reach a peak between 5 and 10 years of age [31, 32]. Differentiation of classical switched memory B cells occurs in the germinal center (GC) of secondary lymphoid organs; immunohistochemistry studies show that GCs are absent at birth and gradually develop to adult size between 12 and 24 months of life [33]. Interestingly, gut colonization of *Escherichia coli* promotes the early development (0–4 months) of the CD27+ memory pool in infants [34]. The IgM-memory subset appears gradually in circulation from around birth and reaches adult levels at 2 years of age [35]. Several studies have shown that IgM-memory B cells confer protection against *Streptococcus pneumoniae*, both after infection and immunization [36].

Less is known on the terminally differentiated plasma cell pool in infants and children. In preschool children, the plasma cell compartment is similar in size as reported for adults [37]. However, in the mouse model of KLH-NP immunization, it has been shown that survival of plasma cells is impaired in neonatal mice compared to adults [38]. The supportive network of BM stromal cells was less capable of producing plasma cell survival factors in neonatal mice compared to adults.

In summary, postnatal maturation of the B cell compartment occurs in the presence of antigenic stimulation by microbes and also requires maturation of lymphoid organs and the bone marrow (Fig. 4.2).

4.5 Quality of Antibody Responses in Infants

During fetal and early neonatal ontogeny, the peripheral B cell population is much less diverse than that of adults. Early studies showed that the B cell repertoire expressed early in life is skewed toward specific V_H genes and that early neonatal cells lack molecular mechanisms utilized by adult cells for diversification [39]. It is also known that in vivo antibody responses are of lower affinity and restricted heterogeneity compared to adults.

One important difference in outcome of B cell activation is that neonatal B cells produce less amounts of antibodies than adults after antigen-specific activation [40]. The differences in Ab secretion could be due to impaired antigen presentation by DCs or macrophages as well as suboptimal secretion of cytokines by T cells. However, there are also intrinsic B cell differences in that neonatal B cells show little or no proliferation after BCR cross-linking [41] even though signal transduction occurs upon Ig ligation [42]. It has been demonstrated that neonatal B cells are more prone to tolerance induction and/or apoptosis after BCR ligation. Neonatal B cells also express less MHC class II and the co-stimulatory molecules CD80/CD86 are not upregulated after BCR triggering [43]. While these impairments may render neonatal B cells hyporesponsive, CD40 ligation and IL-4 lead to B cell activation and proliferation allowing B cell differentiation. Thus, in the presence of T helper mechanisms, the neonatal B cell response is adequate, although more stimulatory signals may be needed to achieve similar outcomes as for adult B cells [39].

Somatic Hypermutation (SHM). SHM occurs predominantly in germinal centers of the spleen or lymph node and is essential to diversify and improve the antibody formation as it leads to selection of antibodies with high affinity [44]. This process is dependent on the enzyme activation-induced deaminase (AID), which inserts point mutations into the Ig heavy and light chain genes and thus plays an essential role in repertoire diversification and affinity maturation [45]. Data on SHM in human infants are rare, but one early study reported SHM in IgG and IgA heavy chain transcripts in cord blood [46]. In peripheral blood of newborns, few or no mutations could be detected when sequencing the V_H6 gene, but in older infants (10–60 days), more mutations were found in the same locus [47]. By 8 months of age, the range of mutations reached adult levels, and there were signs of repertoire selection [48].

So, neonatal B cells are less responsive to BCR ligation and more prone to apoptosis or tolerance induction. Antibody maturation is limited. The responses to the majority of antigens, T cell-dependent antigens, will be less efficient due to both T and B cell inabilities (Fig. 4.2).

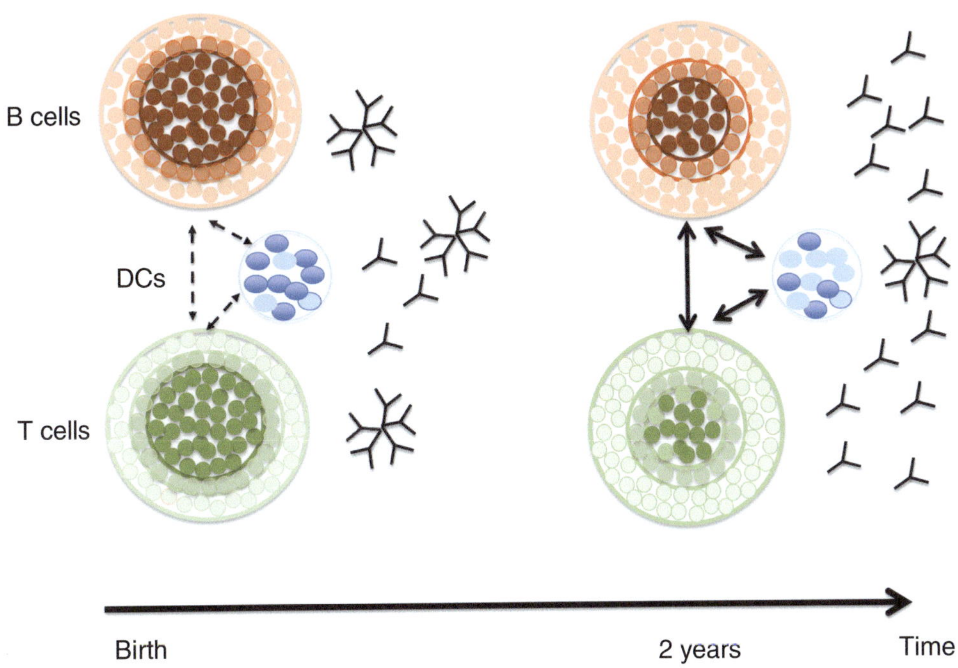

Fig. 4.2 Maturation of peripheral blood cell populations involved in adaptive immune responses occurs during the first 2 years in children. At birth, translational (*orange*) and naive B cells (*dark orange*) are most abundant and the T cell compartment is dominated by naive T cells (*dark green*). After stimulation by environmental antigens, the memory B cell (*pale orange*), memory CD4 T cell (*pale green*), and follicular T cell (*green*) pool increase. Accordingly, the interactions between DCs, B cell, and T cells increase and the antibody response matures with the production of IgG and IgA. Dendritic cells (DCs) at birth are predominantly plasmacytoid DCs (*blue*), but the myeloid DCs (*pale blue*) increase after 1 year

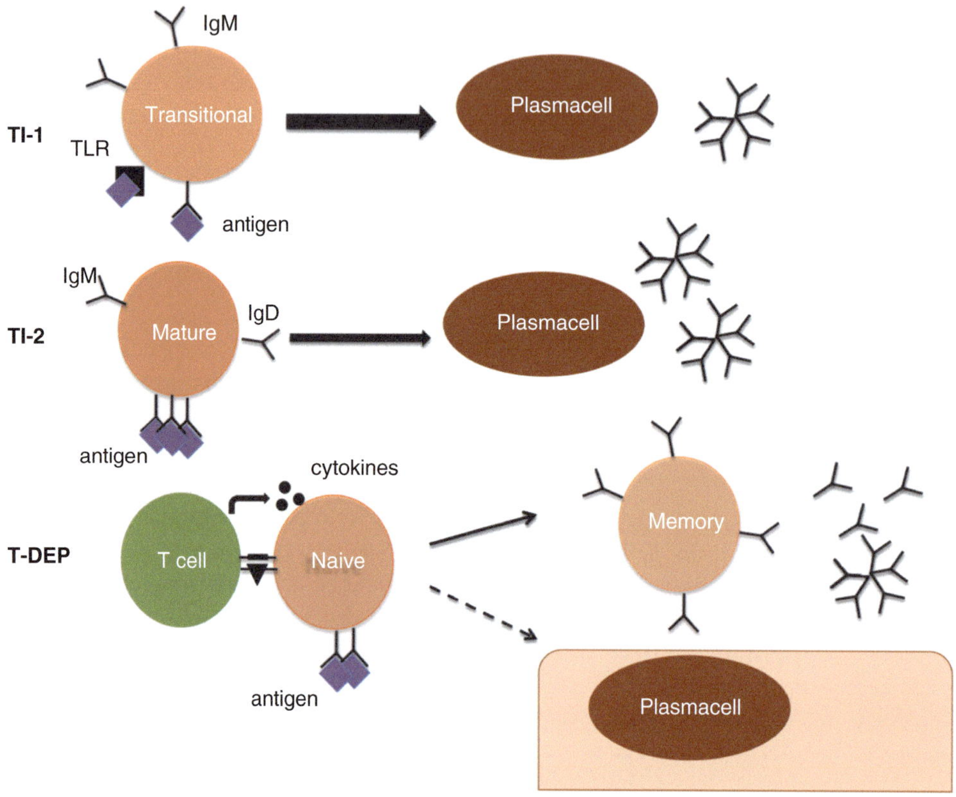

Fig. 4.3 A schematic figure on adaptive immune responses in young children. At birth, translational B cells respond to certain T-independent antigens (TI-1) with the formation of short-lived plasma cells that mainly produce IgM as a first-line defense. IgM+ mature B cells are also able to respond to T cell-independent antigens (TI-2) which cross-link several BCRs through binding of repetitive antigenic structures. The response to T-dependent antigens is not present at birth but mature during the first 2 years. The production of switched memory B cells and homing of plasma cells to the bone marrow are therefore impaired in the infant

For type 1 T cell independent antigens, which themselves can activate immature B cells, these are partially hampered by lack of TLR and BCR signaling (Fig. 4.3). Type 2 T cell independent antigens, which are repetitive structures that can cross-link BCR by multiple binding on mature B cells. Therefore, antibody responses are very limited in young children, both due to few mature B cells but also poor BCR function. Children hence respond poorly to vaccines consisting of such antigens (polysaccharide vaccines).

4.6 Soluble Factors in Neonatal Blood Affecting Adaptive Immune Responses

Although most components of the immune system appear during fetal development, the concentrations of soluble components can differ markedly from those of adults. In particular, the plasma complement proteins and their activity are low in infants. The complement system is an important part of innate immunity, but it may also impact on adaptive immune responses; it enhances the effects of specific immunoglobulins; it primes antigen-presenting cells and aid their maturation; and finally, it enhances the antigen-driven maturation of antibody responses by B lymphocytes. The level of classical complement components in newborns is decreased compared to adult levels, which probably contribute to the deficit in early adaptive immune responses [49]. During the first 6 months of life, there is an evolution toward adult levels for several of the complement proteins [50].

In recent years, neonatal plasma has been shown to contain other molecules with immunomodulatory functions mainly affecting the outcome of TLR activation on antigen-presenting cells. Adenosine, an endogenous purine metabolite, selectively inhibits TNF-α production from TLR2-activated monocytes while IL-6 production is preserved. Thus, adenosine contributes to the Th2-polarizing properties of neonatal plasma [51]. In addition, yet unidentified factors in neonatal plasma have the capacity to polarize TLR4-mediated cytokine responses with low IL-12p70 production and high IL-10 production thus mediating immunosuppression during the first month of life [52].

The influence of maternal antibodies on adaptive immune responses is debated. Potential mechanisms by which maternal antibodies could affect infant vaccine responses include specific masking of infant B cell epitopes by maternal antibodies and the uptake of maternal antibodies: antigen complexes by APC [53]. Abundant data in the literature favors these models and it also fits well with the observation that maternal antibodies lack the capacity to interfere with infant T cell priming in vivo. This issue will be discussed more below.

4.7 Current Global Pediatric Vaccines

More than half of the children that die under the age of five worldwide do so because of an infectious disease. Many of these diseases are vaccine preventable and WHO estimates that around 1.5 million children below the age of 5 died in 2008 in such diseases. *S. pneumoniae* (pneumococcal) infections and *rotavirus* infections are leading causes, followed by infections caused by *Haemophilus influenzae B* (HIB), *Bordetella pertussis* (pertussis), measles virus, and *Clostridium tetani* infection in the neonatal period (neonatal tetanus).

The vaccine schedules used in the world differ due to economic issues and the endemic infection situation of the region. The goals from WHO are focused on reaching a 90 % vaccine coverage rate of each country national policy. In almost all parts of the world, these include vaccinations against diphtheria, tetanus, pertussis, and polio, which have led to a drastic reduction in the incidence the past 30 years. Neonatal tetanus is still quite prevalent, mostly due to low vaccine coverage rates in mothers, hence less antibodies are transferred in utero.

The MMR vaccine (measles, mumps, rubella) is used in Europe, America, Australia, and some Eastern Mediterranean countries, whereas the plain measles vaccine is used in most African countries and Southeast Asia. The measles vaccination coverage is 85 % worldwide; however, the coverage is poor in mid- and southern-Africa. Furthermore, the introduction of the *pneumococcus* vaccine is recently established in Europe, North America, Australia, and many African- and South America countries. Vaccines against HIB are also becoming very prevalent worldwide, but only recently, thus less than half of the world population was protected in 2010, though this number is likely to rise. The introduction of the varicella vaccine has been less successful, and it is primarily used in America but also in other countries for risk groups.

In the coming years, the rotavirus vaccines will be introduced with a focus on African countries but also in America, Europe, and Eastern Mediterranean areas. Vaccines against local endemic infections including *Neisseria meningitidis* (*meningococcus*), Japanese encephalitis, *Mycobacterium tuberculosis*, hepatitis, rabies, *Salmonella typhi* (typhoid fever), and yellow fever may also be included in childhood vaccination schedules. In the older children, utilization of the human papillomavirus (HPV) vaccine, reducing cervical cancer, is increasing in all parts of the world, with the exception of the East Mediterranean countries.

4.8 Vaccine Side Effects

Side effects of vaccinations are a debated field. Immediate reactions, such as allergy [54] and local reactions, such as swelling, sourness, and pain at the site of injection, are easily measured and described. In addition, common early systemic side effects including irritability and fever can be measured on a population basis. Less common side effects, occurring in close proximity to vaccination, are also described. For example, febrile seizures 7–10 days post-MMR vaccination have long been recognized occurring in 1 of 600 doses [55]. Similarly, MMR vaccination associates with a 1/50,000 dose risk of immune thrombocytopenic purpura [56].

When it comes to rare and long-term side effects, the burden of proof is more challenging. Furthermore, such reactions/diseases are often multifactorial. There are basically two approaches to long-term side-effect investigations: either a purely logical hypothesis based on immunological data from the vaccine, or a suspicion from epidemiological data. One example of the first is the effects of childhood vaccination on allergy and atopy. It is known that children who retain the neonatal Th2 profile longer may have an increased likelihood of allergies and that an early Th1-tilted response will decrease incidence of allergy and asthma [21]. Pediatric vaccines that give a predominant Th1 or Th2 response may hence affect development of allergy and atopy. Circumstantial clinical reports suggest such an association for the pertussis vaccine; controlled clinical trials point away from allergy-promoting or allergy-preventing effects [54].

One example of the second type, where epidemiological data has prompted further investigation, comes from the increased frequency of childhood narcolepsy in Scandinavia post-H1N1 influenza vaccinations in 2009. For the group under 11 years, the frequency rose from around 0 cases/100,000 inhabitants to around 3.4/100,000 in 2010. For 11–16-year-olds, it rose from around 1/100,000 to around 8.7/100,000 in 2010 [57]. This occurred almost exclusively in Finland and Sweden and has been attributed to the genetic background and possibly other unknown factors. It has been suggested based on genetic data and the lowered onset age that vaccination brought forward the onset of a disease that normally would have occurred later [57]. In much the same way, the pertussis vaccine has been described as a trigger of severe myoclonic epilepsy (Dravet syndrome) in genetically susceptible individuals. Time for vaccination coincides, however, with characteristic onset time for this disease, and fever (which may be associated with vaccination) is known to trigger first events. Pertussis vaccination does not associate with any altered outcome of disease as compared unvaccinated genetically susceptible individuals [58]. The proposed link between autism spectrum diseases and vaccination (in particular MMR) is hereto not proven [59, 60].

In parallel, data also suggest that you are more likely to have side effects if you are vaccinated early in vaccine campaign. One interpretation of this is that people with underlying disease and/or risk factors are vaccinated early, and such individuals appear more prone to side effects. This was shown for the H1N1 vaccine, where the early cohorts had increased frequencies of Bell's palsy, paresthesia, and inflammatory bowel disease [61].

Finally, it is not only the antigen as such that is important for the side effects but also the formulation. This has been demonstrated by comparing the seizure frequency when giving a combined MMR–varicella (MMRV) vaccination or MMR and varicella (MMR+V) vaccine separately on the same day. Using MMRV, the seizure frequency rises to 1/2300 doses, as compared to MMR+V where the seizure risk is comparable to MMR alone [62].

So when it comes to side effects causing long-term morbidity, these are linked to the onset of a disease that most likely would have occurred in an unvaccinated child as well. Children with underlying disease may be at higher risk of side effects. For the short-term side effects, formulation appears to play a role.

4.9 Vaccination During Pregnancy

Since vaccinations are less efficient in very young children, one way to protect neonates against severe infection is to vaccinate women during pregnancy, utilizing the transmission of antibodies from the mother to the child in utero. This strategy is already in use in some countries, and US health authorities recommend the seasonal trivalent inactivated influenza vaccine and the tetanus/diphtheria/acellular pertussis vaccine to be used during second and third trimester of pregnancy. Furthermore, a number of other killed vaccines are recommended to pregnant risk groups including vaccines against hepatitis A, hepatitis B, meningococcus, and the 23-valent pneumococcus polysaccharide vaccine. Live viral vaccines are contraindicated in pregnant women.

General concerns include the safety and efficacy of maternal–fetal immunization. Safety has been shown using killed vaccines against seasonal as well as H1N1 influenza [63]. Furthermore, similar data are available for the adult-type tetanus, reduced diphtheria toxoids, and acellular pertussis vaccine [64].

Fetal Immunization. For the discussion of efficacy, several aspects have to be taken into consideration. First, whether fetal immunization is efficient in preventing fetal illness, either from the community or from the mother during fetal life or not. In addition, whether there will be negative effects of the passive antibodies transferred on later immunizations of the child. For the efficacy, two types of vaccines will be discussed: the vaccines containing T-dependent antigens and the vaccines containing T-independent antigens. One can assume that T-dependent antigens will be more efficient, as they give rise to antibodies that are more efficiently enriched over the placenta. For T-dependent antigens, such as the influenza vaccine, epidemiological data show that children born to vaccinated mothers have milder influenza-like symptoms and a reduced incidence of verified influenza [65].

For T-independent antigens, the efficacy is less clear. It has been shown that pneumococcal antibodies are transferred in utero, at sufficient levels, postmaternal immunization with the pneumococcal polysaccharide vaccine [66]. These are results for serotype 1 and 5, where only 5 can be really seen as T-independent due to the zwitterionic nature of the serotype 1 polysaccharide [67]. Maternal immunization does in this case interfere with early childhood vaccination (7–17 weeks postpartum), in that vaccination does not increase the amount of specific antibodies, if already present at high concentration. No effect of maternal vaccination was seen on vaccination efficacy at 3 years of age [68]. There is little evidence for a role of these antibodies in preventing disease, and neonatal pneumococcal colonization is not affected [69].

Possible Interference. One argument against fetal immunization is the possible interference with later childhood immunizations. This can be mediated both by the ability of neutralizing antibodies to interfere with specific T cell responses and the ability of neutralizing antibodies to interfere with humoral responses upon immunization. As for T cell responses, these are clearly less prominent, as discussed above, in small children as compared to in adults. The presence of maternal neutralizing antibodies does not affect efficacy of T cell responses, measured as IFN-γ production [53, 70].

When it comes to the humoral response, the situation is more complex. It is clear that lower levels of neutralizing antibodies are produced upon vaccination in children that are still retaining maternal antibodies at the age of 9 months [70] and that at 6 months the ability to produce antibodies upon vaccination is poor in general irrespective of maternal antibodies. The potential interference with childhood immunization at 9 months will then depend of the persistence of maternal antibodies.

Antibodies against different antigens show different half-life in vivo, and antibodies against measles virus and rubella virus persist longer than, for example, antibodies against mumps virus. Mumps antibodies also persist even shorter if the mother has been vaccinated as compared to infected naturally [71]. Furthermore, transport across the placenta will not depend only on subclass, as both IgG1 and IgG2 antibodies against pneumococcus are transferred less well than antibodies of similar subclasses against tetanus [72]. Clearly, the potential interference will have to be judged for each vaccine. Most children that were vaccinated while still immune from the mother, however, have a good response upon second dose vaccination [70]. Some studies have found a slightly higher vaccine failure rate upon second vaccination, where the first early vaccination has failed [73]. If this is a result of the child's intrinsic ability to respond to vaccination, or a result of interference by maternal antibodies, is not known.

Vaccination with killed vaccines, preferentially in third trimester, appears safe, and at least for some vaccines efficient. There are conflicting data on interference with childhood immunizations, but most data point toward little interference. Recommendations will have to be specific for each vaccine, and more studies are required.

4.10 Immunization Responses in Children with Primary or Acquired Immunodeficiency

A growing number of children survive infancy and early childhood despite severe immunodeficiency including transplantation and chemotherapy, primary inherited immunodeficiency disorders, or congenital HIV infection. These children are vulnerable to infections and thus would benefit from effective immunizations. It is also possible that a better understanding of the molecular deficits behind impaired vaccine responses in these patients could contribute to the development of better vaccines.

Common variable immunodeficiency disorder (CVID) affects antibody production and is characterized by low serum concentrations of IgG and IgA and/or IgM and increased susceptibility to respiratory infections with encapsulated bacteria (*H. influenzae*, *S. pneumoniae*). CVID is a heterogeneous disease with several genetic defects involving important molecules for B cell signaling and/or T and B cell interactions. In adult CVID patients, who had switched memory B cells (CD27+) in peripheral blood before immunization, a protective antibody response could be detected against several antigens [74]. Similarly, in a pediatric study, 11/16 children were found to respond to the meningococcal group C polysaccharide vaccine [75]. In addition, vaccine responses against polysaccharide vaccines were associated with the presence of IgM-memory B cells in these patients. A similar study of CVID patients indicates that there is a block in the formation of plasmablasts after immunization against both *Clostridium tetani* and *S. pneumoniae* [76].

Pediatric HIV-1 Infection. Immunization responses in HIV-I infected patients are severely impaired, both in adults and children [77] for the majority of antigens. The introduction of highly active antiretroviral therapy (HAART) has improved vaccination outcome for the majority of patients [78]. Immunization guidelines for this vulnerable pediatric group have recently been published [79]. Vaccination is safe with few side effects, and the only vaccine that is contraindicated as of today is BCG for HIV-1-infected children. However, there are still unresolved questions regarding immunizations in pediatric HIV-1 infection and, in particular, how durable the antibody response in HAART treated children will be compared to healthy individuals.

Re-immunization of children posttransplantation and after chemotherapy is required since the different treatment modalities eradicate protective antibody-mediated memory [80]. As for HIV-1-infected children, most vaccines are safe although revaccination with live vaccines should be postponed 12–24 months after completion of therapy. There is no consensus on the optimal time to start revaccination or how many doses that should be administered to achieve long-lasting protection [81, 82].

4.11 Development of New Pediatric Vaccines

Traditional vaccines often consist of whole-killed viruses, administered by intramuscular injection (i.m.). For some important childhood pathogens, for example, respiratory syncytial virus (RSV), such attempts have failed. The development of an RSV vaccine will be discussed as an example of a novel vaccine strategy in infants. Initial clinical studies using formalin inactivated RSV for administration to small children resulted in disease aggravation upon infection, hospitalization, and in some cases death [83]. This has later been attributed to a devastating Th2 response, resulting in lung pathology. RSV causes a localized respiratory disease, without general viremia, resulting in significant hospitalization, morbidity, and mortality rates. From an immunological perspective, RSV is challenging because of the failure of adaptive immunity to prevent reinfection.

This has been ascribed to the poor quality of the T cell response and the short durability of the antibody response. One hypothesis is that the mucosal immunity is too slow for this rapid virus and that the serum antibodies are present at low levels in the tissue. Finding alternative strategies for RSV vaccination is key. One such way is to deliver the vaccine at mucosal linings such as intranasally (i.n.), instead of i.m. Then immune activation will take place within the mucosa nasal-associated lymphoid tissue (NALT) with activation of microfold epithelial cells (M cells) and subsequently underlying antigen-presenting cells such as DCs. This will induce both local IgA and systemic IgG.

Depending on which route that is used, different local immunity will result. For example, using i.n. administration, immunity in the upper respiratory tract and the cervicovaginal tract will prevail, whereas oral administration will induce IgA production mostly in the small intestine and in the mammary glands. Experiments using live-killed RSV nanoemulsions for i.n. administration in mice have shown an IgA response in the lung as well as protective capacity [84]. Current most promising results come from clinical phase II trials where live-attenuated RSV strains have been given i.n [83]. Still, RSV vaccine development suffers from the initial failures, and no good vaccine is yet available. Results are to be awaited from clinical studies of naked DNA and vector-expressed DNA vaccines in the pediatric population.

Development of new vaccines also includes the introduction of adjuvants with enhanced immune stimulatory capacity to compensate for low intrinsic immunogenicity of antigens [85]. Novel adjuvants aim at optimizing B cell responses and generating appropriate T cell responses, which could be of particular importance in childhood vaccines. One of new adjuvants is the TLR4 agonist monophosphoryl lipid A (MPL) which of to date is licensed or in phase III clinical trials [86]. MPL, when combined with alum, acts on DCs and promotes INF-γ production and thus overcomes the Th2-biased response associated with alum. It is now licensed in a human papillomavirus (HPV)-16/18 vaccine and has been shown to induce long-lasting B cell memory and persistent antibodies [87]. In children immunized at 1–4 years of age against *Plasmodium falciparum*, an MPL-containing adjuvant induced high antiparasite antibodies with long-term protection against clinical disease as a result [88]. An additional potential new adjuvant, the nontoxic mutant of heat-labile enterotoxin (LT) of *E. coli (LTK63)*, was shown to overcome delayed maturation of follicular DCs and thus induce germinal centers when given parentally in mice together with a polysaccharide conjugate vaccine [89]. In addition to an improved B cell response, LTK63 upon binding to macrophages induces a balanced Th1/Th2 cytokine production as well as cytotoxic T cell responses [90].

So, the development of new efficient vaccines to be administered early in life may take advantage of novel adjuvants to circumvent the hyporesponsiveness of neonatal adaptive immunity.

4.12 Challenges to Early Life Vaccines

Many infant vaccines require several booster immunizations, and yet there is still inadequate protection from some of these diseases. This is partly due to the limited infant immunology as discussed before. *The ideal age for infant vaccination begins at 18 months of age.* The functional development of the immune system seems to be finished with roughly 24 months of age. Of course, every contact with a new antigen means a new education. In this way, life is not only an adventure; it's a lifelong learning for the immune system.

Maternal Antibodies. The uptake of maternal sIgA antibodies from breast milk via the neonatal gut mucosa is negligible and does not influence the T cell activation. However, the presence of maternal antibodies can inhibit the development of infant humoral immune response to vaccines. Inhibition of measles vaccine by maternal antibodies is well documented and can last until the infant is up to 12 months [91]. This is why measles vaccination is generally deferred until 9–12 months of age. The same situation with interfering maternal antibodies is described for some other infant vaccines. Maternally acquired antibody levels wane over the first 6 months of life and are usually absent by 1 year of age.

B Cell Memory. Inadequate adaptive immunity is also documented for the generation of B cell memory. The neonatal B cell repertoire is still underdeveloped due to inadequate B cell receptor (BCR) signaling and lower levels of MHC class II expression. Neonates and young children produce lower vaccine-specific IgG serum titers than older children. The antibody responses are delayed in onset, are of shorter duration, and are of lower affinity.

T Cell Memory. CD8+ T cells in neonates do their job like in adults. The situation for CD4+ T cells is quite different. Compared to adults, neonatal CD4+ T cell response is toward to Th2 response, characterized by the production of IL-4, IL-5, and IL-10. The generation of memory CD4+ T cells in neonates is also poor, especially due to a defect in the TCR signaling pathway.

Immunosuppression. Treg cells are a subpopulation of T cells, formerly known as suppressor T cells, and are necessary to control and downregulate T effector cells. High levels of naturally occurring Treg cells (CD4+, CD25+++, and Foxp3+) are present in utero and decline to adult levels by birth. Treg-mediated suppression of T cells, B cells, monocytes, macrophages, and eosinophils are performed by the production of soluble factors such as IL-10, TGF-β, and IL-35. In addition, Treg cells also produce high levels of adenosine (see also: Sect. 4.3) [92].

Antigen Presenting Cells. Deficiencies in numbers of DCs and their functional incompetence are another limiting factor to generate T cell memory responses. The maturation of naive T cells into effector and memory cells is also dependent from the cytokine milieu provided by matured DCs as result of TLR-mediated DC activation. A low T cell vaccine response in neonate and young children is linked to a diminished production of specific cytokines because DCs cannot fully respond to TLR stimulation in early life due to diminished signaling pathways [93, 94].

Adjuvants. Some adjuvants might be able to increase neonatal response. Agents used in neonatal mice are often potent immunomodulators with the risk to lead to inflammation. Thus, IL-12 treatment enhances Th1 responses but causes toxicity or death at higher concentrations [95]. Artificial enhancement of immune responses to an antigen by adjuvants in early life can also lead to bystander effects on unrelated antigens, namely, tolerance to those antigens [96].

Polysaccharide Vaccines. Polysaccharide antigen molecules are often small, are not very immunogenic, and tend not to be effective in infants and young children (under 18–24 months). These antigens activate B cells without help by T cells (T cell independent) and are characterized by a lack of immunologic memory. Polysaccharide vaccines induce only a slow immune response, with antibody levels rising slowly, and a short-term immunity.

Conclusions. Taken together, the earlier in life that children are vaccinated, the poorer the immune response due to the limited functional capacity of the neonatal immune system. Although the neonatal immune system lacks memory of prior antigen exposure, it provides an innate defense, even if restricted, against bacteria, viruses, fungi, and parasites. The colonization of the gut and the antigen exposure is necessary to induce the education of the acquired immune system. Acquired immunity in neonates is matured but needs training. Neonatal lymphocytes are predominantly naive and have a "resting" phenotype, but neonatal lymphocytes don't display any immune dysfunction. The neonatal CD4+ Th1/Th2 imbalance is only a bias toward Th2 response due to suppression of excessive inflammation. At birth, CD8+ T cells fully work, but the function seems to be dependent on the nature and dose of antigen that is emphasized by booster vaccinations (Fig. 4.4).

Neonates are competent to mount mature immune responses [97]; simply, the smaller size of immunocompetent cells and the strong control and regulation by Treg cells during the early life could account for the difference between neonates and adult.

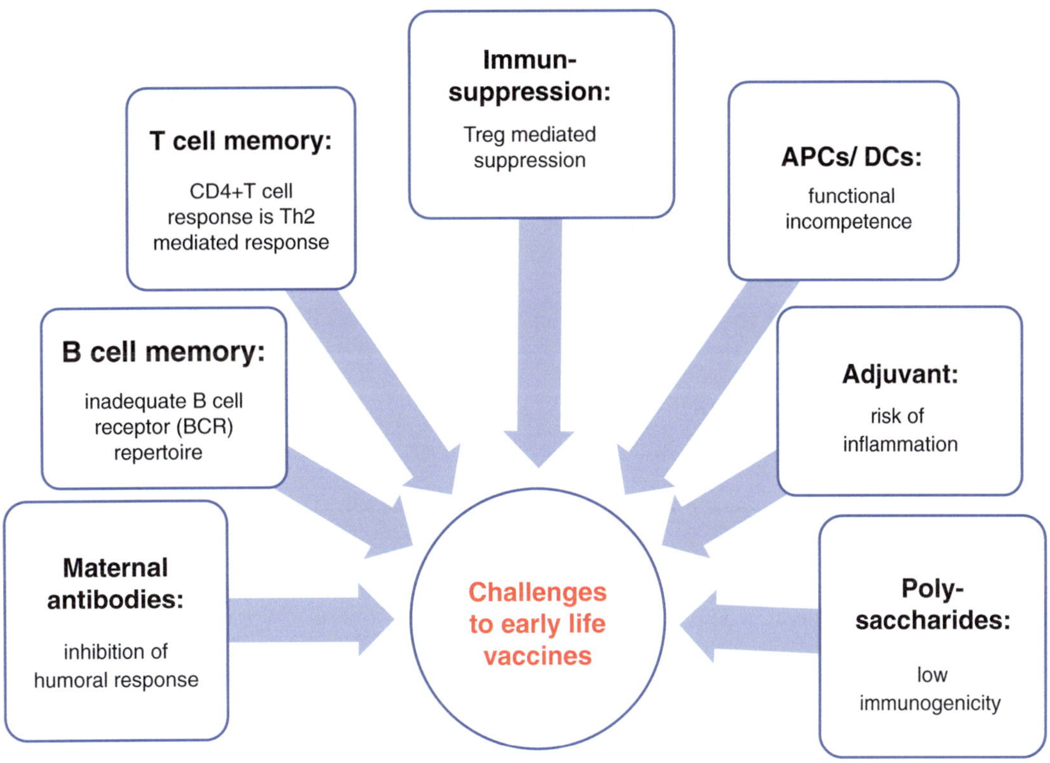

Fig. 4.4 Many infant vaccines require several booster immunizations, and yet there is still inadequate protection from some of these diseases. This is partly due to the limited infant immunology. Only with 12 months post partum a T cell-dependent antibody response develops. The ideal age for infant vaccination begins at 18 months of age. The functional development of the immune system seems to be finished with roughly 24 months of age. Of course, every contact with a new antigen means a new education. In this way, life is not only an adventure; it's a lifelong learning for the immune system (Figure by M. Giese Heidelberg/Germany)

References

1. Wood, N., Siegrist, C.A.: Neonatal immunization: where do we stand? Curr. Opin. Infect. Dis. 24, 190–195 (2011). doi:10.1097/QCO.0b013e328345d563
2. Adkins, B., Leclerc, C., Marshall-Clarke, S.: Neonatal adaptive immunity comes of age. Nat. Rev. Immunol. 4, 553–564 (2004). doi:10.1038/nri1394
3. Dimmitt, R.A., et al.: Role of postnatal acquisition of the intestinal microbiome in the early development of immune function. J. Pediatr. Gastroenterol. Nutr. 51, 262–273 (2010). doi:10.1097/MPG.0b013e3181e1a114
4. Scholtens, P.A., Oozeer, R., Martin, R., Amor, K.B., Knol, J.: The early settlers: intestinal microbiology in early life. Annu. Rev. Food Sci. Technol. 3, 425–447 (2012). doi:10.1146/annurev-food-022811-101120
5. Elahi, S., et al.: Immunosuppressive CD71+ erythroid cells compromise neonatal host defence against infection. Nature 504, 158–162 (2013). doi:10.1038/nature12675
6. Kung, J.T., Brooks, S.B., Jakway, J.P., Leonard, L.L., Talmage, D.W.: Suppression of in vitro cytotoxic response by macrophages due to induced arginase. J. Exp. Med. 146, 665–672 (1977)
7. Ygberg, S., Nilsson, A.: The developing immune system – from foetus to toddler. Acta Paediatr. 101, 120–127 (2012). doi:10.1111/j.1651-2227.2011.02494.x
8. Siegrist, C.A.: Neonatal and early life vaccinology. Vaccine 19, 3331–3346 (2001)
9. Hodgins, D.C., Shewen, P.E.: Vaccination of neonates: problem and issues. Vaccine **30**, 1541–1559 (2012). doi:10.1016/j.vaccine.2011.12.047
10. Ueno, H., et al.: Dendritic cell subsets in health and disease. Immunol. Rev. **219**, 118–142 (2007). doi:10.1111/j.1600-065X.2007.00551.x
11. Teig, N., Moses, D., Gieseler, S., Schauer, U.: Age-related changes in human blood dendritic cell subpopulations. Scand. J. Immunol. **55**, 453–457 (2002)
12. Sorg, R.V., Kogler, G., Wernet, P.: Identification of cord blood dendritic cells as an immature CD11c- population. Blood **93**, 2302–2307 (1999)
13. Jones, C.A., Holloway, J.A., Warner, J.O.: Fetal immune responsiveness and routes of allergic sensitization. Pediatr. Allergy Immunol. **13**(Suppl 15), 19–22 (2002)
14. Liu, E., Tu, W., Law, H.K., Lau, Y.L.: Decreased yield, phenotypic expression and function of immature monocyte-derived dendritic cells in cord blood. Br. J. Haematol. **113**, 240–246 (2001)
15. Langrish, C.L., Buddle, J.C., Thrasher, A.J., Goldblatt, D.: Neonatal dendritic cells are intrinsically biased against Th-1 immune responses. Clin. Exp. Immunol. **128**, 118–123 (2002)
16. De Wit, D., et al.: Impaired responses to toll-like receptor 4 and toll-like receptor 3 ligands in human cord blood. J. Autoimmun. **21**, 277–281 (2003)
17. De Wit, D., et al.: Blood plasmacytoid dendritic cell responses to CpG oligodeoxynucleotides are impaired in human newborns. Blood **103**, 1030–1032 (2004). doi:10.1182/blood-2003-04-1216
18. Levy, O., et al.: Selective impairment of TLR-mediated innate immunity in human newborns: neonatal blood plasma reduces monocyte TNF-alpha induction by bacterial lipopeptides, lipopolysaccharide, and imiquimod, but preserves the response to R-848. J. Immunol. **173**, 4627–4634 (2004)
19. Burl, S., et al.: Age-dependent maturation of Toll-like receptor-mediated cytokine responses in Gambian infants. PLoS One **6**, e18185 (2011). doi:10.1371/journal.pone.0018185
20. Nguyen, M., et al.: Acquisition of adult-like TLR4 and TLR9 responses during the first year of life. PLoS One **5**, e10407 (2010). doi:10.1371/journal.pone.0010407
21. Belderbos, M.E., et al.: Skewed pattern of Toll-like receptor 4-mediated cytokine production in human neonatal blood: low LPS-induced IL-12p70 and high IL-10 persist throughout the first month of life. Clin. Immunol. **133**, 228–237 (2009). doi:10.1016/j.clim.2009.07.003
22. de Vries, E., et al.: Longitudinal survey of lymphocyte subpopulations in the first year of life. Pediatr. Res. **47**, 528–537 (2000)
23. Schatorje, E.J., et al.: Pediatric reference values for the peripheral T-cell compartment. Scand. J. Immunol. **75**(4), 436–444 (2011). doi:10.1111/j.1365-3083.2011.02671.x
24. Schaerli, P., et al.: CXC chemokine receptor 5 expression defines follicular homing T cells with B cell helper function. J. Exp. Med. **192**, 1553–1562 (2000)
25. Wing, K., et al.: CD4+ CD25+ FOXP3+ regulatory T cells from human thymus and cord blood suppress antigen-specific T cell responses. Immunology **115**, 516–525 (2005). doi:10.1111/j.1365-2567.2005.02186.x
26. Rabe, H., et al.: Higher proportions of circulating FOXP3+ and CTLA-4+ regulatory T cells are associated with lower fractions of memory CD4+ T cells in infants. J. Leukoc. Biol. **90**, 1133–1140 (2011). doi:10.1189/jlb.0511244
27. Jullien, P., et al.: Decreased CD154 expression by neonatal CD4+ T cells is due to limitations in both proximal and distal events of T cell activation. Int. Immunol. **15**, 1461–1472 (2003)
28. Fadel, S., Sarzotti, M.: Cellular immune responses in neonates. Int. Rev. Immunol. **19**, 173–193 (2000)
29. Capolunghi, F., et al.: CpG drives human transitional B cells to terminal differentiation and production of natural antibodies. J. Immunol. **180**, 800–808 (2008)
30. Morbach, H., Eichhorn, E.M., Liese, J.G., Girschick, H.J.: Reference values for B cell subpopulations from infancy to adulthood. Clin. Exp. Immunol. **162**, 271–279 (2010). doi:10.1111/j.1365-2249.2010.04206.x
31. Smet, J., Mascart, F., Schandene, L.: Are the reference values of B cell subpopulations used in adults for classification of common variable immunodeficiencies appropriate for children? Clin. Immunol. **138**, 266–273 (2011). doi:10.1016/j.clim.2010.12.001
32. Huck, K., et al.: Memory B-cells in healthy and antibody-deficient children. Clin. Immunol. **131**, 50–59 (2009). doi:10.1016/j.clim.2008.11.008
33. Kruschinski, C., Zidan, M., Debertin, A.S., von Horsten, S., Pabst, R.: Age-dependent development of the splenic marginal zone in human infants is associated with different causes of death. Hum. Pathol. **35**, 113–121 (2004)
34. Lundell, A.C., et al.: Infant B cell memory differentiation and early gut bacterial colonization. J. Immunol. **188**, 4315–4322 (2012). doi:10.4049/jimmunol.1103223
35. Weller, S., et al.: Human blood IgM "memory" B cells are circulating splenic marginal zone B cells harboring a prediversified immunoglobulin repertoire. Blood **104**, 3647–3654 (2004). doi:10.1182/blood-2004-01-0346
36. Kruetzmann, S., et al.: Human immunoglobulin M memory B cells controlling Streptococcus pneumoniae infections are generated in the spleen. J. Exp. Med. **197**, 939–945 (2003). doi:10.1084/jem.20022020
37. Nilsson, A., et al.: Current chemotherapy protocols for childhood acute lymphoblastic leukemia induce loss of humoral immunity to viral vaccination antigens. Pediatrics **109**, e91 (2002)
38. Pihlgren, M., et al.: Reduced ability of neonatal and early-life bone marrow stromal cells to support plasmablast survival. J. Immunol. **176**, 165–172 (2006)
39. Press, J.L.: Neonatal immunity and somatic mutation. Int. Rev. Immunol. **19**, 265–287 (2000)
40. Siegrist, C.A.: The challenges of vaccine responses in early life: selected examples. J. Comp. Pathol. **137**(Suppl 1), S4–S9 (2007). doi:10.1016/j.jcpa.2007.04.004
41. Tasker, L., Marshall-Clarke, S.: Immature B cells from neonatal mice show a selective inability to up-regulate MHC class II expression in response to antigen receptor ligation. Int. Immunol. **9**, 475–484 (1997)
42. Chang, T.L., Capraro, G., Kleinman, R.E., Abbas, A.K.: Anergy in immature B lymphocytes. Differential responses to

receptor-mediated stimulation and T helper cells. J. Immunol. **147**, 750–756 (1991)
43. Marshall-Clarke, S., Reen, D., Tasker, L., Hassan, J.: Neonatal immunity: how well has it grown up? Immunol. Today **21**, 35–41 (2000)
44. McHeyzer-Williams, L.J., McHeyzer-Williams, M.G.: Antigen-specific memory B cell development. Annu. Rev. Immunol. **23**, 487–513 (2005). doi:10.1146/annurev.immunol.23.021704.115732
45. Pan-Hammarstrom, Q., Zhao, Y., Hammarstrom, L.: Class switch recombination: a comparison between mouse and human. Adv. Immunol. **93**, 1–61 (2007). doi:10.1016/S0065-2776(06)93001-6
46. Mortari, F., Wang, J.Y., Schroeder Jr., H.W.: Human cord blood antibody repertoire. Mixed population of VH gene segments and CDR3 distribution in the expressed C alpha and C gamma repertoires. J. Immunol. **150**, 1348–1357 (1993)
47. Ridings, J., et al.: Somatic hypermutation of immunoglobulin genes in human neonates. Clin. Exp. Immunol. **108**, 366–374 (1997)
48. Ridings, J., Dinan, L., Williams, R., Roberton, D., Zola, H.: Somatic mutation of immunoglobulin V(H)6 genes in human infants. Clin. Exp. Immunol. **114**, 33–39 (1998)
49. McGreal, E.P., Hearne, K., Spiller, O.B.: Off to a slow start: under-development of the complement system in term newborns is more substantial following premature birth. Immunobiology **217**, 176–186 (2012). doi:10.1016/j.imbio.2011.07.027
50. Davis, C.A., Vallota, E.H., Forristal, J.: Serum complement levels in infancy: age related changes. Pediatr. Res. **13**, 1043–1046 (1979)
51. Levy, O., et al.: The adenosine system selectively inhibits TLR-mediated TNF-alpha production in the human newborn. J. Immunol. **177**, 1956–1966 (2006)
52. Belderbos, M.E., et al.: Neonatal plasma polarizes TLR4-mediated cytokine responses towards low IL-12p70 and high IL-10 production via distinct factors. PLoS One **7**, e33419 (2012). doi:10.1371/journal.pone.0033419
53. Siegrist, C.A.: Mechanisms by which maternal antibodies influence infant vaccine responses: review of hypotheses and definition of main determinants. Vaccine **21**, 3406–3412 (2003)
54. Gruber, C., Nilsson, L., Bjorksten, B.: Do early childhood immunizations influence the development of atopy and do they cause allergic reactions? Pediatr. Allergy Immunol. **12**, 296–311 (2001)
55. Klein, N.P., et al.: Measles-mumps-rubella-varicella combination vaccine and the risk of febrile seizures. Pediatrics **126**, e1–e8 (2010). doi:10.1542/peds.2010-0665
56. O'Leary, S.T., et al.: The risk of immune thrombocytopenic purpura after vaccination in children and adolescents. Pediatrics **129**, 248–255 (2012). doi:10.1542/peds.2011-1111
57. Partinen, M., et al.: Increased incidence and clinical picture of childhood narcolepsy following the 2009 H1N1 pandemic vaccination campaign in Finland. PLoS One **7**, e33723 (2012). doi:10.1371/journal.pone.0033723
58. McIntosh, A.M., et al.: Effects of vaccination on onset and outcome of Dravet syndrome: a retrospective study. Lancet Neurol. **9**, 592–598 (2010). doi:10.1016/S1474-4422(10)70107-1
59. Uno, Y., Uchiyama, T., Kurosawa, M., Aleksic, B., Ozaki, N.: The combined measles, mumps, and rubella vaccines and the total number of vaccines are not associated with development of autism spectrum disorder: the first case-control study in Asia. Vaccine **30**, 4292–4298 (2012). doi:10.1016/j.vaccine.2012.01.093
60. Demicheli, V., Rivetti, A., Debalini, M.G., Di Pietrantonj, C.: Vaccines for measles, mumps and rubella in children. Cochrane Database Syst. Rev. **2**, CD004407 (2012). doi:10.1002/14651858.CD004407.pub3
61. Bardage, C., et al.: Neurological and autoimmune disorders after vaccination against pandemic influenza A (H1N1) with a monovalent adjuvanted vaccine: population based cohort study in Stockholm, Sweden. BMJ **343**, d5956 (2011). doi:10.1136/bmj.d5956
62. Klein, N.P., et al.: Measles-containing vaccines and febrile seizures in children age 4 to 6 years. Pediatrics **129**, 809–814 (2012). doi:10.1542/peds.2011-3198
63. Oppermann, M., et al.: A(H1N1)v2009: a controlled observational prospective cohort study on vaccine safety in pregnancy. Vaccine **30**, 4445–4452 (2012). doi:10.1016/j.vaccine.2012.04.081
64. Fortner, K.B., Kuller, J.A., Rhee, E.J., Edwards, K.M.: Influenza and tetanus, diphtheria, and acellular pertussis vaccinations during pregnancy. Obstet. Gynecol. Surv. **67**, 251–257 (2012). doi:10.1097/OGX.0b013e3182524cee
65. Eick, A.A., et al.: Maternal influenza vaccination and effect on influenza virus infection in young infants. Arch. Pediatr. Adolesc. Med. **165**, 104–111 (2011). doi:10.1001/archpediatrics.2010.192
66. Quiambao, B.P., et al.: Immunogenicity and reactogenicity of 23-valent pneumococcal polysaccharide vaccine among pregnant Filipino women and placental transfer of antibodies. Vaccine **25**, 4470–4477 (2007). doi:10.1016/j.vaccine.2007.03.021
67. Groneck, L., et al.: Oligoclonal CD4+ T cells promote host memory immune responses to Zwitterionic polysaccharide of Streptococcus pneumoniae. Infect. Immun. **77**, 3705–3712 (2009). doi:10.1128/IAI.01492-08
68. Holmlund, E., Nohynek, H., Quiambao, B., Ollgren, J., Kayhty, H.: Mother-infant vaccination with pneumococcal polysaccharide vaccine: persistence of maternal antibodies and responses of infants to vaccination. Vaccine **29**, 4565–4575 (2011). doi:10.1016/j.vaccine.2011.04.068
69. Lopes, C.R., et al.: Ineffectiveness for infants of immunization of mothers with pneumococcal capsular polysaccharide vaccine during pregnancy. Braz. J. Infect. Dis. **13**, 104–106 (2009)
70. Gans, H., et al.: Measles and mumps vaccination as a model to investigate the developing immune system: passive and active immunity during the first year of life. Vaccine **21**, 3398–3405 (2003)
71. Leuridan, E., Goeyvaerts, N., Hens, N., Hutse, V., Van Damme, P.: Maternal mumps antibodies in a cohort of children up to the age of 1 year. Eur. J. Pediatr. **171**, 1167–1173 (2012). doi:10.1007/s00431-012-1691-y
72. Shahid, N.S., et al.: Serum, breast milk, and infant antibody after maternal immunization with pneumococcal vaccine. Lancet **346**, 1252–1257 (1995)
73. Redd, S.C., et al.: Comparison of vaccination with measles-mumps-rubella vaccine at 9, 12, and 15 months of age. J. Infect. Dis. **189**(Suppl 1), S116–S122 (2004). doi:10.1086/378691
74. Goldacker, S., et al.: Active vaccination in patients with common variable immunodeficiency (CVID). Clin. Immunol. **124**, 294–303 (2007). doi:10.1016/j.clim.2007.04.011
75. Rezaei, N., et al.: Serum bactericidal antibody response to serogroup C polysaccharide meningococcal vaccination in children with primary antibody deficiencies. Vaccine **25**, 5308–5314 (2007). doi:10.1016/j.vaccine.2007.05.021
76. Chovancova, Z., Vlkova, M., Litzman, J., Lokaj, J., Thon, V.: Antibody forming cells and plasmablasts in peripheral blood in CVID patients after vaccination. Vaccine **29**, 4142–4150 (2011). doi:10.1016/j.vaccine.2011.03.087
77. Cagigi, A., Nilsson, A., Pensieroso, S., Chiodi, F.: Dysfunctional B-cell responses during HIV-1 infection: implication for influenza vaccination and highly active antiretroviral therapy. Lancet Infect. Dis. **10**, 499–503 (2010). doi:10.1016/S1473-3099(10)70117-1
78. Sutcliffe, C.G., Moss, W.J.: Do children infected with HIV receiving HAART need to be revaccinated? Lancet Infect. Dis. **10**, 630–642 (2010). doi:10.1016/S1473-3099(10)70116-X
79. Menson, E.N., et al.: Guidance on vaccination of HIV-infected children in Europe. HIV Med. **13**, 333–336; e1–e14 (2012). doi:10.1111/j.1468-1293.2011.00982.x
80. Patel, S.R., Chisholm, J.C., Heath, P.T.: Vaccinations in children treated with standard-dose cancer therapy or hematopoietic stem

cell transplantation. Pediatr. Clin. North Am. **55**, 169–186, xi (2008). doi:10.1016/j.pcl.2007.10.012

81. Brodtman, D.H., Rosenthal, D.W., Redner, A., Lanzkowsky, P., Bonagura, V.R.: Immunodeficiency in children with acute lymphoblastic leukemia after completion of modern aggressive chemotherapeutic regimens. J. Pediatr. **146**, 654–661 (2005). doi:10.1016/j.jpeds.2004.12.043
82. Lehrnbecher, T., et al.: Revaccination of children after completion of standard chemotherapy for acute lymphoblastic leukaemia: a pilot study comparing different schedules. Br. J. Haematol. **152**, 754–757 (2011). doi:10.1111/j.1365-2141.2010.08522.x
83. Graham, B.S.: Biological challenges and technological opportunities for respiratory syncytial virus vaccine development. Immunol. Rev. **239**, 149–166 (2011). doi:10.1111/j.1600-065X.2010.00972.x
84. Lindell, D.M., et al.: A novel inactivated intranasal respiratory syncytial virus vaccine promotes viral clearance without Th2 associated vaccine-enhanced disease. PLoS One **6**, e21823 (2011). doi:10.1371/journal.pone.0021823
85. Mastelic, B., et al.: Mode of action of adjuvants: implications for vaccine safety and design. Biologicals **38**, 594–601 (2010). doi:10.1016/j.biologicals.2010.06.002
86. Garcon, N., Segal, L., Tavares, F., Van Mechelen, M.: The safety evaluation of adjuvants during vaccine development: the AS04 experience. Vaccine **29**, 4453–4459 (2011). doi:10.1016/j.vaccine.2011.04.046
87. Giannini, S.L., et al.: Enhanced humoral and memory B cellular immunity using HPV16/18 L1 VLP vaccine formulated with the MPL/aluminium salt combination (AS04) compared to aluminium salt only. Vaccine **24**, 5937–5949 (2006). doi:10.1016/j.vaccine.2006.06.005
88. Sacarlal, J., et al.: Long-term safety and efficacy of the RTS, S/AS02A malaria vaccine in Mozambican children. J. Infect. Dis. **200**, 329–336 (2009). doi:10.1086/600119
89. Bjarnarson, S.P., Adarna, B.C., Benonisson, H., Del Giudice, G., Jonsdottir, I.: The adjuvant LT-K63 can restore delayed maturation of follicular dendritic cells and poor persistence of both protein- and polysaccharide-specific antibody-secreting cells in neonatal mice. J. Immunol. **189**, 1265–1273 (2012). doi:10.4049/jimmunol.1200761
90. da Hora, V.P., Conceicao, F.R., Dellagostin, O.A., Doolan, D.L.: Non-toxic derivatives of LT as potent adjuvants. Vaccine **29**, 1538–1544 (2011). doi:10.1016/j.vaccine.2010.11.091
91. Naniche, D.: Human immunology of measles virus infection. Curr. Top. Microbiol. Immunol. **330**, 151–171 (2009)
92. Ndure, J., Flanagan, K.L.: Targeting regulatory T cells to improve vaccine immunogenicity in early life. Front. Microbiol. **5**, 477 (2014). doi:10.3389/fmicb.2014.00477
93. Basha, S., Surendran, N., Pichichero, M.: Immune responses in neonates. Expert Rev. Clin. Immunol. **10**, 1171–1184 (2014). doi:10.1586/1744666X.2014.942288
94. Flanagan, K.L., Burl, S., Lohman-Payne, B.L., Plebanski, M.: The challenge of assessing infant vaccine responses in resource-poor settings. Expert Rev. Vaccines **9**, 665–674 (2010). doi:10.1586/erv.10.41
95. Arulanandam, B.P., Van Cleave, V.H., Metzger, D.W.: IL-12 is a potent neonatal vaccine adjuvant. Eur. J. Immunol. **29**, 256–264 (1999). doi:10.1002/(SICI)1521-4141(199901)29:01<256::AID-IMMU256>3.0.CO;2-G
96. Henderson, R.A., Watkins, S.C., Flynn, J.L.: Activation of human dendritic cells following infection with Mycobacterium tuberculosis. J. Immunol. **159**, 635–643 (1997)
97. Vekemans, J., et al.: Neonatal bacillus Calmette-Guerin vaccination induces adult-like IFN-gamma production by CD4+ T lymphocytes. Eur. J. Immunol. **31**, 1531–1535 (2001). doi:10.1002/1521-4141(200105)31:5<1531::AID-IMMU1531>3.0.CO;2-1

Elderly Immunology

5

Contents

5.1 Immunosenescence and Vaccination

The immune system is one function of the body profoundly affected by aging. The reduced efficacy of vaccines in the elderly (>65 years) is generally attributed to immunosenescence [1–3]. It involves both the host's capacity to respond to infections and the development of long-term immune memory, especially by vaccination. The decline in age-associated immune function on molecular, cellular, and organismal changes is common to most if not all vertebrates; it is an evolutionary ubiquitous process which runs in only one direction – a way of no return. Most of the parameters affected by immunosenescence appear to be under genetic control (Fig. 5.1).

Consequently, older adults are more susceptible to infectious diseases. Age-associated immune changes take place in the innate and acquired immune systems and affect not only lymphocytes but also myeloid cells with a change in pro-inflammatory cytokines.

The functional decline that characterizes aging begins after sexual maturity. This occurs at age 13, as in humans; age 5, as in monkeys; or at less than 2 months, as in mice.

According to the evolutionary theory of aging, the genetic program is optimized for reproduction. In all vertebrates the emphasis of genomes is on reproduction, not post-reproductive survival, and therefore aging is an irreversible biological process.

Of note to underline that immunosenescence is not only restricted to aging. During chronic infections certain pathogens, such as CMV and HIV, remodel the immune system toward aged T cells [4, 5]. Chronic antigen stimulation like in chronic infections is the major trigger of immunosenescence.

Loss of Immunosurveillance. A depressed immune system loses also its ability for surveillance with the possibility of cancer development. Chronic HBV infection is a leading cause of hepatocellular carcinoma (HCC) and a major contributing factor to liver cirrhosis. The same is probable for cervix carcinoma. Here, again, the chronic antigen

M. Giese, *Introduction to Molecular Vaccinology*, DOI 10.1007/978-3-319-25832-4_5

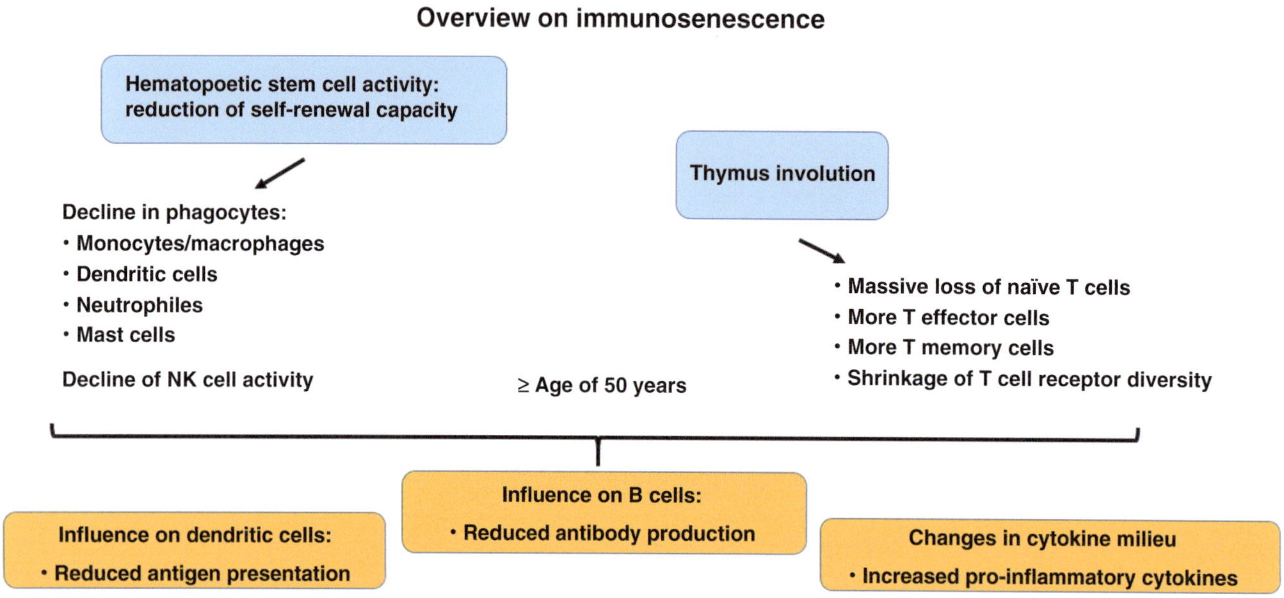

Fig. 5.1 The reduced efficacy of vaccines in the elderly is generally attributed to immunosenescence. Age-associated immune changes take place in the innate and acquired immune systems and affect not only lymphocytes but also myeloid cells with a change in pro-inflammatory cytokines. The decline in age-associated immune function on molecular, cellular, and organismal changes is common to most if not all vertebrates. The functional decline that characterizes aging begins after sexual maturity. Thymus involution begins with the puberty by the early teens

stimulation with human papilloma virus (HPV) could lead after years to immunosenescence, and the development of carcinoma would be a causal consequence of a depressed immune system rather than the direct molecular involvement of papilloma virus. We now know that it typically takes many years for an HPV infection, even if persistent, to cause cervical cancer. The typical time course of the infection begins with HPV acquisition in adolescence and early adulthood, around 17–25 years of age, and cancer arises around 45–60.

HPV and other oncoviruses should be discussed against this background of immunosenescence. Only the chronic antigen stimulation results in a continuous overproduction of pro-inflammatory cytokines and is responsible for the loss of immunosurveillance.

Escape from immunosurveillance is considered a cancer hallmark. Therefore HPV would be a major contributing factor to cervix carcinoma among other factors but not the only cause [6]. The vaccination against HPV can prevent the development of a chronic infection. It is an antiviral vaccine but also a cancer vaccine? There are no clinical data demonstrating this effect.

5.2 Malnutrition

There is also an interface between malnutrition, premature T cell senescence, and susceptibility to infections. Chronic hunger may modulate the immune system through T cell repertoire. Hunger also influences the telomere length of CD8+ T cells, resulting in a shortening [7]. Telomeres are protective structures that cap the end of all eukaryotic chromosomes. Chronic hunger in early life dramatically impacts the programming of the young thymus, a very crucial phase, having long-term effects on T cell development. Zinc is an essential mineral for the immune system and a zinc deficiency results in thymic atrophy [8]. Zinc deficiency in humans is now known to be an important malnutrition problem worldwide. It is more prevalent in areas of high cereal and low animal food consumption. It is suggested that the nutritional disturbance predisposes this population to infections. Malnutrition is one important reason for the loss of efficacy of oral vaccines in the Third World.

5.3 T Cells

Beginning with the puberty by the early teens, and directed by circulating sex hormones, the thymus undergoes involution: Thymic epithelial cells (TEC) (niche for lymphocyte development) are primarily replaced with fat cells, 3 % per year during adulthood [9]. Size and function dramatically decline. The generation and the export of naïve T cells decrease [10]. The thymic epithelial tissue shrinks to 10 % by the age of 70 years.

A loss of crucial cytokines essential for thymopoiesis and also produced by these epithelial cells, such as IL-1, IL-3, IL-6, and IL-7 and transforming growth factor beta (TGF-β). IL-7 is known as survival cytokine for the devel-

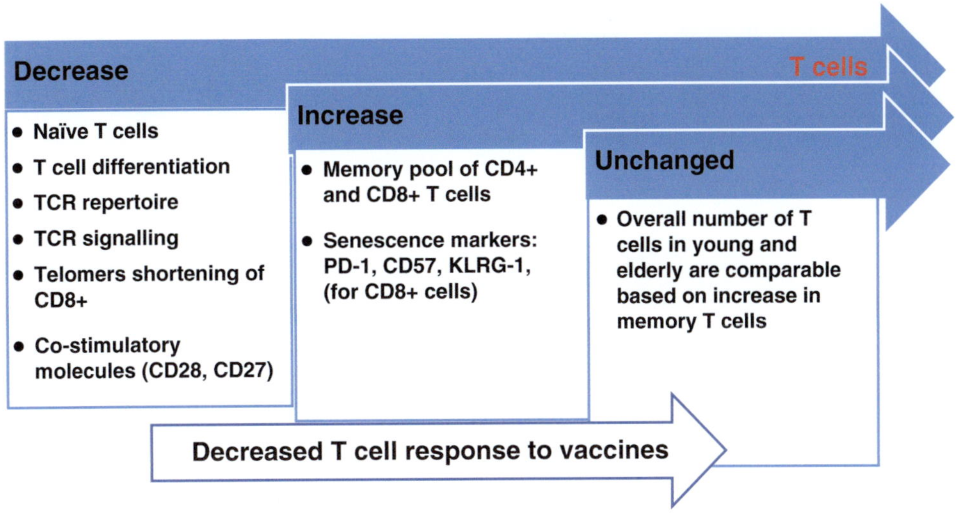

Fig. 5.2 The age-related changes in the T cell life comprise quantitative and qualitative alterations and lead to a reduced immune responsiveness to vaccines

opment and homeostasis of T cells [11]. The naïve T cell immunity is waning with the age and diminishes responsiveness to novel antigens during elderly life. The decreased production of naïve T cells is followed by a diminished response of TCR signaling (NF-kB, MAPK), leading to a blunted T cell proliferation to antigen stimulation [12] and reduced T cell differentiation [13]. This is in contrast to the memory pool of CD4+ and CD8+ T cells, induced at an early age, that can persist for a lifetime of an individual [14]. More than this, the loss of naïve T cells leads to a memory T cell clonal expansion so that the overall number of T cells in the young and elderly is comparable [15]. The increase of memory T cells could be explained by a long-lasting antigen contact of the elderly. However, this expansion is associated with an age-dependent dramatic loss of TCR repertoire [16].

Replicative Senescence. Another drawback is the telomere shortening of senescent CD8+ T cells, called replicative senescence. It does not affect only the replicative potential but also significantly antiviral effector functions, such as IFN-γ production or antigen-specific cytotoxicity [17, 18]. Old T cells lack important co-stimulatory molecules such as CD28 and CD27 but highly express senescence markers PD-1, CD57, and KLRG-1. This counts to a lesser extent for CD4+ T cells but especially for CD8+ T cells which develop the most functional defects.

Thus, the age-related changes in the T cell life comprise quantitative and qualitative alterations and leads to a reduced immune responsiveness. The massive shrinkage of naïve T cells is measurable at ages as early as 40–50 years. Changes after the age of 50 years have received particular attention because of their clinical impact on the limited efficacy of vaccines (Fig. 5.2).

5.4 B Cells

Most results on age-related changes in the B lymphopoiesis come from mouse models. But recently studies in humans share some common mechanistic features and similarities. Mouse hematopoietic aging is a reasonable model of human hematopoietic aging [19].

The decline of high-affinity antibodies results partially from defects in T cells. Beside extrinsic factors/microenvironmental factors influencing B cell functions, important intrinsic changes in senescent B cells occur [20].

Hematopoietic Stem Cells. The human B cell number in the periphery (blood, spleen, lymph nodes) declines moderately with aging or not [21, 22]. But the peripheral B cell repertoire in elderly is less diverse, correlating with poor health status [23]. The B lymphopoiesis is limited by a loss of naïve follicular B cells.

All blood cell lineages, lymphoid (T and B cells) and myeloid (polymorphonuclear cells, monocytes/macrophages), are continuously generated from hematopoietic stem cells (HSCs) in the bone marrow that can self-renew and are critical for maintaining cellular homeostasis throughout life (Fig. 5.3). One dramatic change in the HSC compartment is the shift toward production of myeloid progenitors at the expense of lymphoid progenitors [24–26]. Changes on gene transcription level but also epigenetic changes are responsible for these alterations [27].

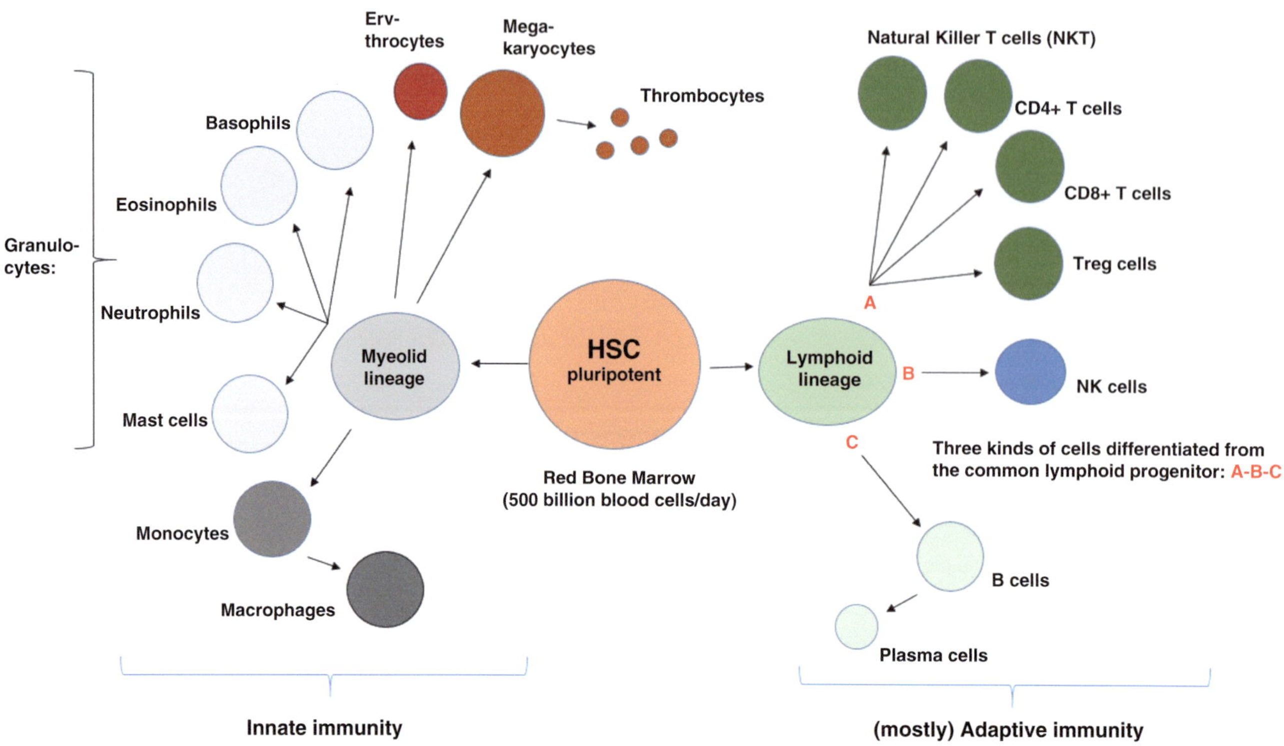

Fig. 5.3 Pluripotent hematopoietic stem cells as origin of immune cells. All blood cell lineages, lymphoid (T and B cells) and myeloid (granulocytes [polymorphonuclear] cells, monocytes/macrophages, erythrocytes, megakaryocytes, and thrombocytes), are continuously generated from hematopoietic stem cells (HSCs) in the bone marrow

Class Switch Recombination. Intrinsic changes are shown in murine and human B cells in vitro. Old B cells show an impaired ability to undergo immunoglobulin class switch recombination (CSR) measured by a reduced antibody production. Activation-induced cytidine deaminase (AID) is essential for immunoglobulin (Ig) gene CSR and somatic hypermutation (SHM). The AID expression in elderly B cells is significantly reduced compared to young due to the impaired transcription factor E47 [20] (Fig. 5.4).

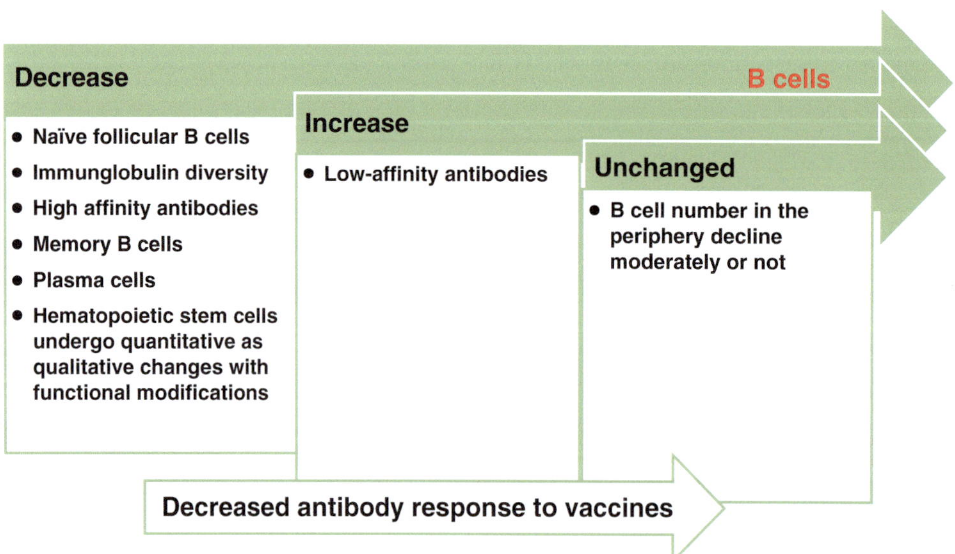

Fig. 5.4 The age-related changes in the B cell life comprise quantitative and qualitative alterations and lead to a reduced immune responsiveness to vaccines

5.5 Dendritic Cells

DCs are the most potent APCs and target for cell-based vaccines. There is an age-related reduction of Langerhans cells (LCs) in the skin, resulting in a reduced immunosurveillance [28]. Murine aging LCs has the same ability to migrate to LNs as young LCs; however, step by step, they lose their capacity to stimulate T cells [29], what should be considered for application of vaccine patches in elderly. DCs from older individuals showed significantly lower production of type I interferon compared to younger individuals that may contribute to a weakened antiviral response and higher susceptibility to viral infections in aging.

The number and the functions of plasmacytoid DCs (pDCs), present in the peripheral blood and in secondary lymphoid organs, are changed in elderly, in contrast to unchanged number of myeloid DCs [30]. Impaired pDCs show a reduced ability for antigen presentation to CD4+ and CD8+ T cells with lack of induction of cytotoxicity in CD8+ cells. In addition, aged pDCs secrete lesser IFN than young pDCs, resulting in a loss of antiviral activities [31]. The reactivity of DCs to self-antigens is increased and can cause autoimmunity [32, 33].

5.6 Toll-Like Receptors

TLRs are expressed by DCs, monocytes, NK cells, B and T cells, and others. In contrast, no significant differences in TLR expression were observed between young and aged macrophages in mice and in humans [34]. Recently it was shown that not only the expression of some TLRs on DCs is reduced but especially the TLR signaling pathways in elderly individuals which correlates with a diminished vaccine responsiveness [35, 36].

The dysregulation of TLR signaling is observed, e.g., of a decreased signaling activity of phosphor-inositol 3 (PI3)-kinase leading to decreased phosphorylation of AKT (a protein kinase B that plays a key role in multiple cellular processes such as cell proliferation, transcription, and cell migration). Parallel to this an increase of phosphorylation of the p38 mitogen-activated protein kinase which inhibits TLR signaling is measurable.

Additionally an age-related reduction in the levels of major signaling adaptors for TLRs, such as MAPK, NF-kB, or MyD88, was observed [37, 38]. The massive shrinkage of aging immune responses is illustrated in Fig. 5.5.

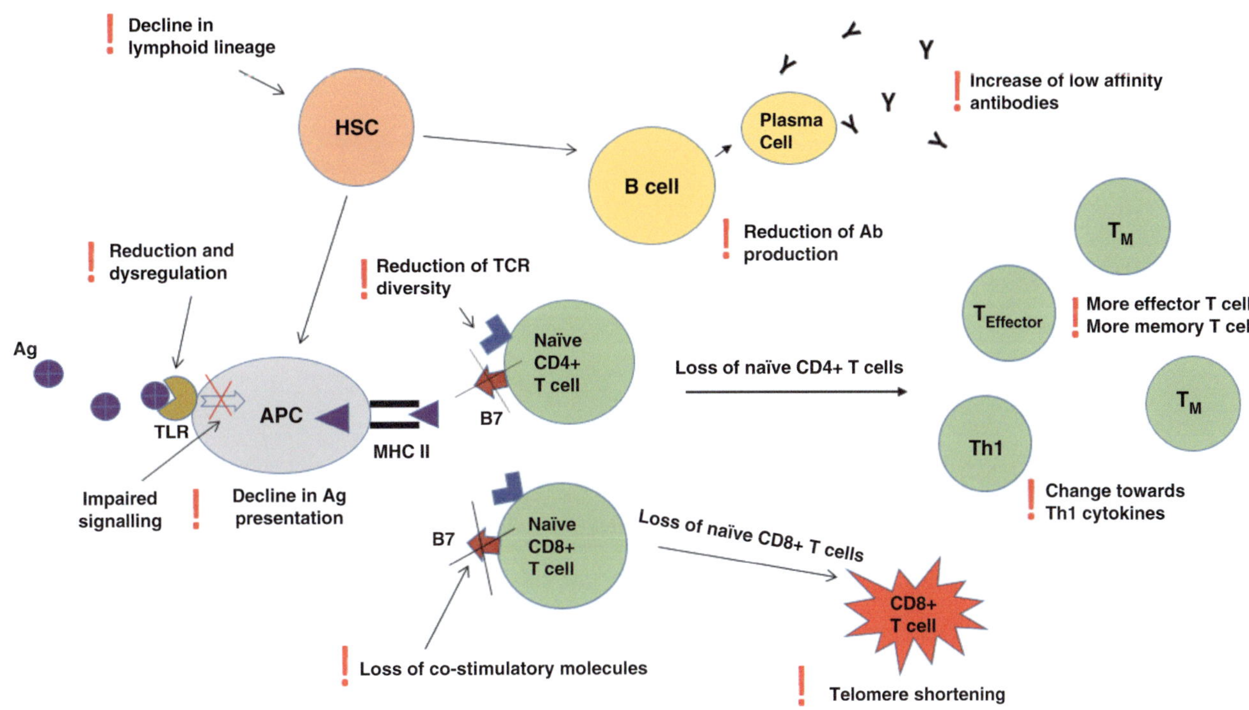

Fig. 5.5 Shrinkage of aging immune responses. Immunosenescence is a multicell and multifactorial process in the innate and acquired system. Age-associated immune changes take place in the innate and acquired immune systems and affect not only lymphocytes but also myeloid cells with a change in pro-inflammatory cytokines. The most important aging processes are marked by ! According to the evolutionary theory of aging, the genetic program is optimized for reproduction. In all vertebrates the emphasis of genomes is on reproduction, not post-reproductive survival, and therefore aging is an irreversible biological process (*TLR* Toll-like receptor, *TCT* T cell receptor, *Ag* antigen, *HSC* hematopoetic stem cell, *APC* antigen-presenting cell, *B7* co-stimulatory molecule)

5.7 Inflammaging

The upregulation of certain cytokines, such as IFN-α, TNF-α, and IL-6, but also C-reactive protein (CRP) in elderly individuals with persistent low-grade innate immune activation is collectively called inflammaging and probably provoked by a continuous overload of antigens and stressors [39]. Other studies explain that inflammaging is partially independent of such immunostimulants and rather dependent on the microenvironment, such as a diminished cross talk between tissue-specific cytokine-producing cells [40].

Generally, the age-related inflammatory activity is composed of local events and systemic activation of both the innate and adaptive immune system. Such asymptomatic chronic inflammatory response could build up with time and gradually causes tissue damage. Various cell types are involved in the continuous overproduction of pro-inflammatory cytokines, such as T cells, DCs, macrophages, and endothelial cells, and raise the risk to come down with age-associated disorders [41]. Table 5.1 summarizes some important key features of immunosenescence.

Current research suggests that a large number of miRNAs (see also Chap. 1 for miRNAs) are differentially expressed during cell aging. Other lines of evidence indicate that several miRNAs likely share in "inflammaging," an aging-related state characterized by systemic chronic inflammation that in turn provides a biological background favoring susceptibility to age-related diseases and disabilities (Fig. 5.6).

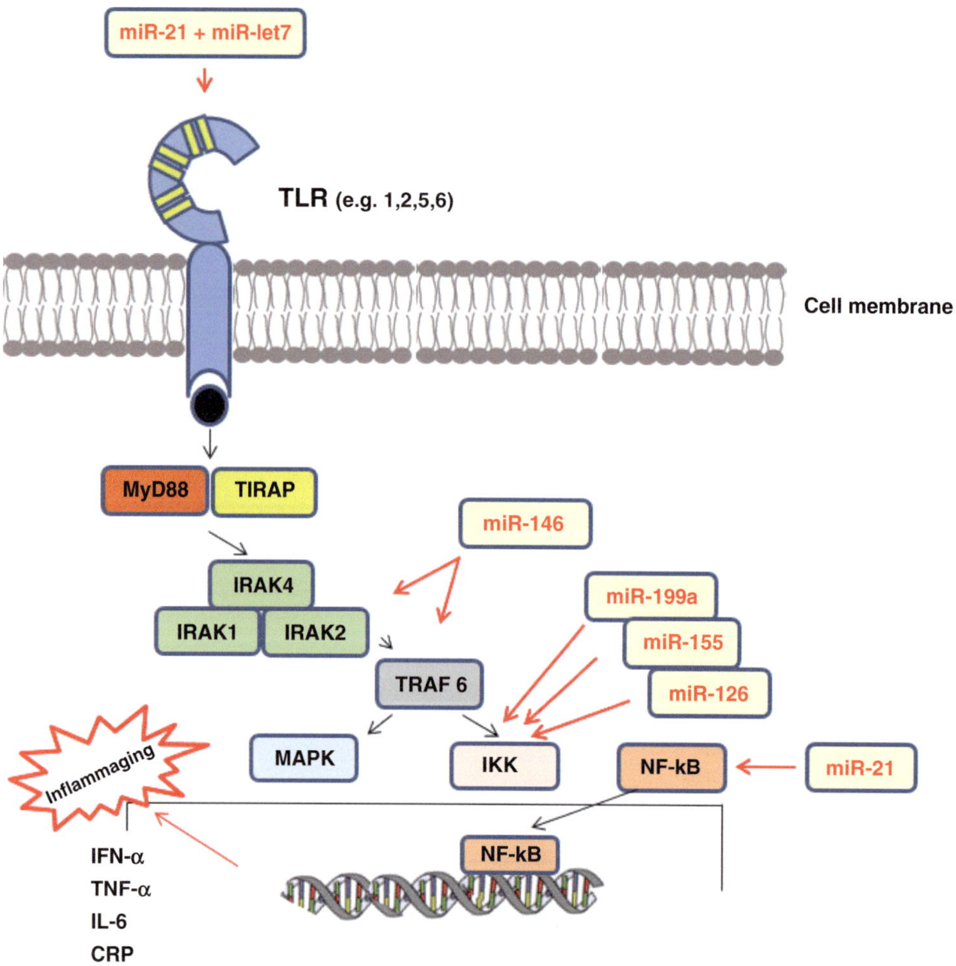

Fig. 5.6 MicroRNA (miRs) modulating TLRs pathways. The miRNA property to finely tune gene expression makes them right for immune system regulation. MiRNAs can modulate TLR signaling mainly by three different mechanisms: (*1*) miRNAs can directly target components of the TLR signaling system (like miR-21), (*2*) miRNA expression can be directly regulated by TLRs pathway activation, and (3) miRNAs can directly activate the RNA-sensing TLRs, like TLR-8, in humans. During aging TLR signaling is modulated by miRNAs leading to an impaired miRNAs/TLR signaling interaction in immune system cells with induction of pro-inflammatory cytokines (*IFN-α, TNF-α, IL-6, CRP*) and related cells, i.e., endothelial cells and adipocytes, thus contributing to inflammaging (Modulated version after Fabiola Olivieri [42])

Table 5.1 Some key features of immunosenescence

Aged cell type	Dysfunction	Consequence
CD4+ T cell	Reduced IL-2 production	Reduced support for B cells
	Reduced cognate helper activity	
CD8+ T cell	Suboptimal signaling pathways	Reduced CTL activity
	Replicative senescence	
	Reduced differentiation	
	Loss of TCR repertoire	
B cell	Loss of naïve follicular B cells	Decreased diversity of antibody response
	Reduced number of GCs	
	Reduced B cell differentiation	
	Reduced Ig class switch	
Plasma cell	Accumulation of antigen-experienced old cells in the bone marrow	Reduced antibody production
		Loss of high affinity
DCs	Impaired TLR signaling	Decreased T cell immunity
	Increased reactivity to self	Loss of self-tolerance, autoimmunity
	Overproduction of cytokines	Chronic inflammation
Inflammaging	Increased secretion of pro-inflammatory cytokines by various cell types (IFN-α, TNF-α, IL-6, CRP)	Atherogenic profile related to age-associated disorders (e.g., atherosclerosis)

5.8 The Impact of Zinc During Aging

Zinc essentiality was first established in 1961 for humans [43].

Zinc (Zn) is known to be an essential trace element and known to have a regulatory role in the immune system. Zn deficiency in aged persons induces oxidative stress and subsequently influences oxidant-sensitive transcription factors that can affect cell function and proliferation and differentiation of the cells of different organs and systems and, in particular, cells of the immune system [44].

Zip10. Zn deficiency affects monocytes and polymorphonuclear, natural killer, T, and B cells. Chronic Zn deficiency increases inflammation. During chronic deficiency, the production of pro-inflammatory cytokines increases and contributes to inflammaging. Zn transporters and metallothioneins regulate Zn concentration and distribution in individual cells. Deficiency of the Zn transporter Zip10 in mature B cells causes attenuation of both T cell dependent and independent immune responses [45]. Inadequate dietary intake of absorbable zinc is the primary cause of zinc deficiency in most situations.

Clinical diagnosis of marginal Zn deficiency in humans remains problematic.

5.9 Mucosal Immunosenescence

Influenza virus and *Streptococcus pneumoniae* are two major pathogens responsible for morbidity and mortality in the elderly. The increased risk of the elderly especially for pneumococcal pneumonia is independent from health status and access to high-quality health care. In high-income countries, mortality to *S. pneumoniae* in the elderly ranges from 15 to 30 % [46].

Since both pathogens enter the host via the mucosa, the increased risk of those infectious diseases in the elderly has been attributed to mucosal immunosenescence. Despite recent findings within the mucosal immune system, only limited results are available in terms of mucosal immunosenescence. Also, most results are generated in small animal models, mice or rats, a further limitation, because rodents have a limited predictive value in context of mucosal vaccine studies: human and mice differ more from each other in physiology, nasal and intestinal architecture, and molecular immune reactions than pig and human or horse and human.

The mucosa, both in the nasopharyngeal (NALT) and in the gastrointestinal (GALT) tract, can be anatomically and functionally divided in an induction and an effector site. NALT and GALT are lined with a monolayer of epithelium containing (microfold) M cells. The subepithelium is enriched in antigen-presenting cells (APC), especially dendritic cells. Underneath this APC subepithelium lies a distinct B cell zone with germinal centers and a separate T cell zone. The mucosal inductive sites in the NALT include the Waldeyer's ring of tonsils and adenoids and the Peyer's patches for GALT. The effector side both of NALT and of GALT is characterized by the lamina propria (LP). Plasma cells within the LP produce the secretory antigen-specific IgA antibodies. And also CTLs, primed at mucosal inductive sites, exhibit their actual function at mucosal effector sites.

Age-associated changes occur to both sites of the mucosal immunity, the inductive and the effector site. The natural immunosenescence of GALT occurs at distinct times and in a distinct manner compared to the immunosenescence of NALT. Signs of mucosal senescence first appear in the gut immune system. NALT remains for a long time intact during aging, and age-associated changes occur step by step. Nasal immunity shows a slower decline in function with age [47]. From this result it seems obviously that nasal vaccination might be preferable over oral vaccination in the elderly.

5.9.1 Age-Associated Changes in the Gut

The first evidence of a dysregulation in the GI tract of the elderly could be evaluated by measuring the sIgA secretion into the lumen. The results in total IgA synthesis from aged mice, rats, and human show no difference between young and old. But the impairment is measurable on the level of specificity. Antigen-specific IgA responses are clearly diminished, and the induction of oral tolerance to new antigens was impaired in old individuals. This leads to the next defect.

Human microbiome analyses have revealed significant changes in the microbiota in the elderly [48]. Data have shown that bifidobacteria significantly decrease, whereas lactobacilli, coliforms, enterococci, and *Clostridium perfringens* are increased. Whether these age-related differences in the compositions of the gut microbiota are the cause of increased inflammation in the elderly or a consequence of the systemic inflammatory process is still open. A direct evidence that inflammaging is the consequence of age-associated changes in the gut is not given.

M cells are responsible for transcytosis of antigens from the gut lumen across the follicle-associated epithelium (FAE) into the GALT and are the main target for many mucosal vaccines. Under normal health condition, only 10 % of the cells within FAE are M cells. Using a mouse model, it was shown that there is a dramatic decline in the density of mature M cells in aged mice [49]. The impaired transcription factor Spi-B could be identified as one mechanism behind the aging process of M cells. Taken these results together, the efficacy of M cell targeted vaccines may be significantly reduced in the elderly [50].

5.9.2 Age-Associated Changes in the Nose

Antigen-specific IgA responses against ovalbumin OVA plus naïve cholera toxin (nCT) as adjuvant were measured in aged rats (>24 months of age) using the oral or the nasal route for application and compared to young rats (3–6 months of age). The same experiments were performed with aged and young mice. In all studies, oral vaccination showed a diminished impaired IgA production and specificity compared to the young animals. There was no change of the IgA production and specificity between young and old after nasal vaccination.

Nasal but not oral immunization induced normal levels of IgA in 1-year-old mice, suggesting that aging occurs more slowly in NALT than in GALT immune system. The mechanisms behind these different aging processes are still unknown.

M cells are also found in NALT's FAE, but there is no report describing a change in the density of mature M cells with aging.

5.10 Challenges to Elderly Life Vaccines

The proportion of the world's population over 60 years will increase to 22 % by 2050 or, in absolute number, 2 billion people aged 60 years and older (according to WHO estimates, March 2012). Vaccination of elderly is recommended especially against infections with influenza virus or pneumococcal infections. Travelers' vaccines against (sub)tropical pathogens, such as typhoid or yellow fever, are recommended due to the mobility of elderly travelers.

Immunosenescence is a multicell and multifactorial process in the innate and acquired system: a multiple decline of major immune functions. This includes also the immunodominance: one epitope is dominant and trigger the response; all other epitopes are subdominant and do not mount for an effective response. Aged individuals have a diminished ability for immunodominance, resulting in a weak and more diffuse immune response [51] (see Chap. 6). Several intrinsic defects could be identified.

Some apparent extrinsic factors are described for immunosenescence. But little is known on the deep influence of the tissue-specific microenvironments on immune cells. Every in vitro experimental design fails to imitate this specific natural niche in vivo.

Is there an early key event synchronizing all other alterations? Are aging HSCs the door opener to understand the process of immunosenescence? Or is the thymic atrophy the pacemaker? Figure 5.7 illustrates the major challenges to elderly life vaccines.

Several vaccine developments for elderly focus on increased antigen dosages [52], novel adjuvant strategies [53], shortened intervals, vector-driven vaccines, change of application routes [54], or the rejuvenation of the thymus by growth hormones and cytokines [55, 56]. All these strategies have been of limited benefit.

Can such approaches circumvent the decreased ability of HSCs to replenish the follicular B cell compartment, the impaired

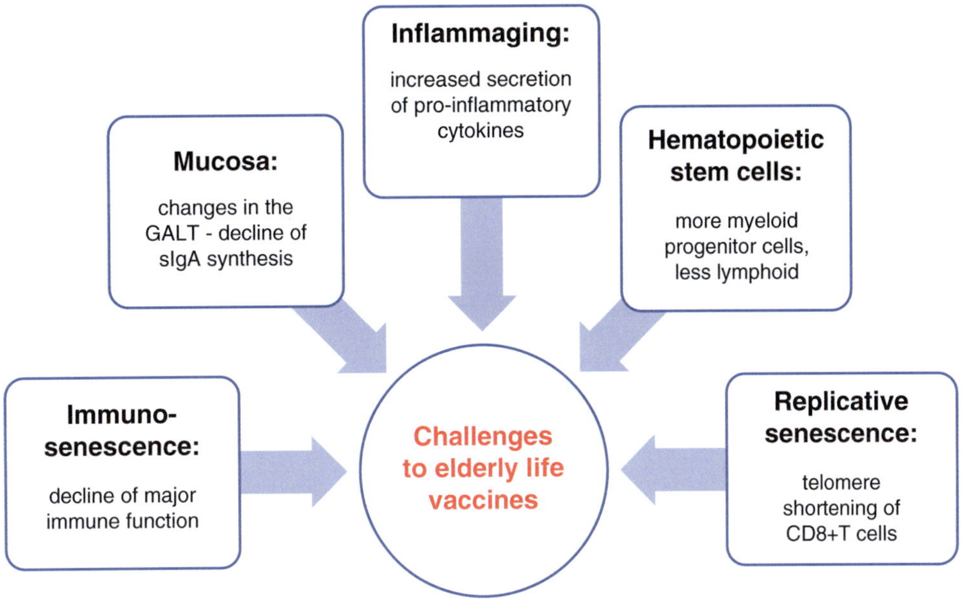

Fig. 5.7 Immunosenescence is a multicell and multifactorial process in the innate and acquired system. The functional decline that characterizes aging begins after sexual maturity. This occurs at age 13, as in humans, and age 5, as in monkeys. Aging is an evolutionary ubiquitous process which runs in only one direction – a way of no return. Most of the parameters affected by immunosenescence appear to be under genetic control

immunoglobulin class switch, loss of high-affinity antibodies, reduced capacity for novel antigens, loss of naïve T cells, replicative senescence, loss of TCR repertoire, impaired TLR signaling, decline of transcription factors or shortening of telomere lengths of leucocytes, etc.? It would be squaring the circle.

The best vaccines for the elderly is to start the vaccination regime before aging is coming.

What can be done? Novel (conjugate) vaccines with a broad antigenic, multivalent spectrum, e.g., influenza, pneumococcal infection should be developed, including a strong complete long-lived memory B cell and memory T cell response with generating robust CTL activities. A prime-boost regime with repeated booster vaccinations during adulthood before the age 40 should be established. This expanded education of the immune system in young age is a solid basis for a recall and also powerful immunological background against novel antigens in old age.

References

1. Wong, K.L., et al.: Gene expression profiling reveals the defining features of the classical, intermediate, and nonclassical human monocyte subsets. Blood **118**, e16–e31 (2011). doi:10.1182/blood-2010-12-326355
2. McElhaney, J.E., Effros, R.B.: Immunosenescence: what does it mean to health outcomes in older adults? Curr. Opin. Immunol. **21**, 418–424 (2009). doi:10.1016/j.coi.2009.05.023
3. Cicin-Sain, L., et al.: Loss of naive T cells and repertoire constriction predict poor response to vaccination in old primates. J. Immunol. **184**, 6739–6745 (2010). doi:10.4049/jimmunol.0904193
4. Appay, V., et al.: Old age and anti-cytomegalovirus immunity are associated with altered T-cell reconstitution in HIV-1-infected patients. AIDS **25**, 1813–1822 (2011). doi:10.1097/QAD.0b013e32834640e6
5. Miles, D.J., et al.: Cytomegalovirus infection in Gambian infants leads to profound CD8 T-cell differentiation. J. Virol. **81**, 5766–5776 (2007). doi:10.1128/JVI.00052-07
6. Hanahan, D., Weinberg, R.A.: Hallmarks of cancer: the next generation. Cell **144**(5), 646–674 (2011). doi:10.1016/j.cell.2011.02.013
7. Ngom, P.T., et al.: Thymic function and T cell parameters in a natural human experimental model of seasonal infectious diseases and nutritional burden. J. Biomed. Sci. **18**, 41 (2011). doi:10.1186/1423-0127-18-41
8. Jones, K.D., Berkley, J.A., Warner, J.O.: Perinatal nutrition and immunity to infection. Pediatr. Allergy Immunol. **21**, 564–576 (2010). doi:10.1111/j.1399-3038.2010.01002.x
9. Taub, D.D., Longo, D.L.: Insights into thymic aging and regeneration. Immunol. Rev. **205**, 72–93 (2005). doi:10.1111/j.0105-2896.2005.00275.x
10. Simpson, J.G., Gray, E.S., Beck, J.S.: Age involution in the normal human adult thymus. Clin. Exp. Immunol. **19**, 261–265 (1975)
11. Plum, J., De Smedt, M., Leclercq, G., Verhasselt, B., Vandekerckhove, B.: Interleukin-7 is a critical growth factor in early human T-cell development. Blood **88**, 4239–4245 (1996)
12. Linton, P.J., Dorshkind, K.: Age-related changes in lymphocyte development and function. Nat. Immunol. **5**, 133–139 (2004). doi:10.1038/ni1033
13. Gillis, S., Kozak, R., Durante, M., Weksler, M.E.: Immunological studies of aging. Decreased production of and response to T cell growth factor by lymphocytes from aged humans. J. Clin. Invest. **67**, 937–942 (1981)
14. Kedzierska, K., Valkenburg, S.A., Doherty, P.C., Davenport, M.P., Venturi, V.: Use it or lose it: establishment and persistence of T cell memory. Front. Immunol. **3**, 357 (2012). doi:10.3389/fimmu.2012.00357

15. Posnett, D.N., Sinha, R., Kabak, S., Russo, C.: Clonal populations of T cells in normal elderly humans: the T cell equivalent to "benign monoclonal gammapathy". J. Exp. Med. **179**, 609–618 (1994)
16. Messaoudi, I., Lemaoult, J., Guevara-Patino, J.A., Metzner, B.M., Nikolich-Zugich, J.: Age-related CD8 T cell clonal expansions constrict CD8 T cell repertoire and have the potential to impair immune defense. J. Exp. Med. **200**, 1347–1358 (2004). doi:10.1084/jem.20040437
17. Effros, R.B., Dagarag, M., Spaulding, C., Man, J.: The role of CD8+ T-cell replicative senescence in human aging. Immunol. Rev. **205**, 147–157 (2005). doi:10.1111/j.0105-2896.2005.00259.x
18. Dock, J.N., Effros, R.B.: Role of CD8 T cell replicative senescence in human aging and in HIV-mediated immunosenescence. Aging Dis. **2**, 382–397 (2011)
19. Pang, W.W., et al.: Human bone marrow hematopoietic stem cells are increased in frequency and myeloid-biased with age. Proc. Natl. Acad. Sci. U. S. A. **108**, 20012–20017 (2011). doi:10.1073/pnas.1116110108
20. Frasca, D., Diaz, A., Romero, M., Landin, A.M., Blomberg, B.B.: Age effects on B cells and humoral immunity in humans. Ageing Res. Rev. **10**, 330–335 (2011). doi:10.1016/j.arr.2010.08.004
21. McKenna, R.W., Washington, L.T., Aquino, D.B., Picker, L.J., Kroft, S.H.: Immunophenotypic analysis of hematogones (B-lymphocyte precursors) in 662 consecutive bone marrow specimens by 4-color flow cytometry. Blood **98**, 2498–2507 (2001)
22. Rossi, M.I., et al.: B lymphopoiesis is active throughout human life, but there are developmental age-related changes. Blood **101**, 576–584 (2003). doi:10.1182/blood-2002-03-0896
23. Gibson, K.L., et al.: B-cell diversity decreases in old age and is correlated with poor health status. Aging Cell **8**, 18–25 (2009). doi:10.1111/j.1474-9726.2008.00443.x
24. Cho, R.H., Sieburg, H.B., Muller-Sieburg, C.E.: A new mechanism for the aging of hematopoietic stem cells: aging changes the clonal composition of the stem cell compartment but not individual stem cells. Blood **111**, 5553–5561 (2008). doi:10.1182/blood-2007-11-123547
25. Rossi, D.J., et al.: Cell intrinsic alterations underlie hematopoietic stem cell aging. Proc. Natl. Acad. Sci. U. S. A. **102**, 9194–9199 (2005). doi:10.1073/pnas.0503280102
26. Kuranda, K., et al.: Age-related changes in human hematopoietic stem/progenitor cells. Aging Cell **10**, 542–546 (2011). doi:10.1111/j.1474-9726.2011.00675.x
27. Schroeder, T.: Hematopoietic stem cell heterogeneity: subtypes, not unpredictable behavior. Cell Stem Cell **6**, 203–207 (2010). doi:10.1016/j.stem.2010.02.006
28. Sunderkotter, C., Kalden, H., Luger, T.A.: Aging and the skin immune system. Arch. Dermatol. **133**, 1256–1262 (1997)
29. Xu, Y.P., et al.: Aging affects epidermal Langerhans cell development and function and alters their miRNA gene expression profile. Aging (Albany NY) **4**, 742–754 (2012)
30. Jing, Y., et al.: Aging is associated with a numerical and functional decline in plasmacytoid dendritic cells, whereas myeloid dendritic cells are relatively unaltered in human peripheral blood. Hum. Immunol. **70**, 777–784 (2009). doi:10.1016/j.humimm.2009.07.005
31. Sridharan, A., et al.: Age-associated impaired plasmacytoid dendritic cell functions lead to decreased CD4 and CD8 T cell immunity. Age (Dordr.) **33**, 363–376 (2011). doi:10.1007/s11357-010-9191-3
32. Agrawal, A., Sridharan, A., Prakash, S., Agrawal, H.: Dendritic cells and aging: consequences for autoimmunity. Expert Rev. Clin. Immunol. **8**, 73–80 (2012). doi:10.1586/eci.11.77
33. Agrawal, A., Tay, J., Ton, S., Agrawal, S., Gupta, S.: Increased reactivity of dendritic cells from aged subjects to self-antigen, the human DNA. J. Immunol. **182**, 1138–1145 (2009)
34. Hajishengallis, G.: Too old to fight? Aging and its toll on innate immunity. Mol. Oral Microbiol. **25**, 25–37 (2010). doi:10.1111/j.2041-1014.2009.00562.x
35. Qian, F., et al.: Impaired interferon signaling in dendritic cells from older donors infected in vitro with West Nile virus. J. Infect. Dis. **203**, 1415–1424 (2011). doi:10.1093/infdis/jir048
36. Renshaw, M., et al.: Cutting edge: impaired Toll-like receptor expression and function in aging. J. Immunol. **169**, 4697–4701 (2002)
37. Medzhitov, R.: Recognition of microorganisms and activation of the immune response. Nature **449**, 819–826 (2007). doi:10.1038/nature06246
38. Gomez, C.R., Nomellini, V., Faunce, D.E., Kovacs, E.J.: Innate immunity and aging. Exp. Gerontol. **43**, 718–728 (2008). doi:10.1016/j.exger.2008.05.016
39. Franceschi, C., et al.: Inflamm-aging. An evolutionary perspective on immunosenescence. Ann. N. Y. Acad. Sci. **908**, 244–254 (2000)
40. Salvioli, S., et al.: Immune system, cell senescence, aging and longevity – Inflamm-aging reappraised. Curr. Pharm. Des. **19**(9), 1675–1679 (2013)
41. Bruunsgaard, H., Pedersen, M., Pedersen, B.K.: Aging and proinflammatory cytokines. Curr. Opin. Hematol. **8**, 131–136 (2001)
42. Olivieri, F., et al.: Toll like receptor signaling in "inflammaging": microRNA as new players. Immun. Ageing **10**(1), 11 (2013). doi:10.1186/1742-4933-10-11
43. King, J.C., Cousins, R.J.: Zinc. In: Shils, M.E., Shike, M., Ross, A.C., Caballero, B., Cousins, R.J. (eds.) Modern nutrition in health and disease, 10th edn, pp. 271–285. Lippincott Williams and Wilkins, Baltimore (2006)
44. Hojyo, S., et al.: Zinc transporter SLC39A10/ZIP10 controls humoral immunity by modulating B-cell receptor signal strength. Natl. Acad. Sci. U. S. A. **111**(32), 11786–11791 (2014). doi:10.1073/pnas.1323557111
45. Bonaventura, P., Benedetti, G., Albarede, F., Miossec, P.: Zinc and its role in immunity and inflammation. Autoimmun. Rev. **14**(4), 277–285 (2015)
46. Janssens, J.P., Krause, K.H.: Pneumonia in the very old. Lancet Infect. Dis. **4**, 112–124 (2004). doi:10.1016/S1473-3099(04)00931-4
47. Fujihashi, K., Kiyono, H.: Mucosal immunosenescence: new developments and vaccines to control infectious diseases. Trends Immunol. **30**, 334–343 (2009). doi:10.1016/j.it.2009.04.004
48. Woodmansey, E.J.: Intestinal bacteria and ageing. J. Appl. Microbiol. **102**, 1178–1186 (2007). doi:10.1111/j.1365-2672.2007.03400.x
49. Mabbott, N.A., et al.: Aging and the mucosal immune system in the intestine. Biogerontology (2014). doi:10.1007/s10522-014-9498-z
50. Misumi, S., et al.: Targeted delivery of immunogen to primate m cells with tetragalloyl lysine dendrimer. J. Immunol. **182**, 6061–6070 (2009). doi:10.4049/jimmunol.0802928
51. Akram, A., Inman, R.D.: Immunodominance: a pivotal principle in host response to viral infections. Clin. Immunol. **143**, 99–115 (2012). doi:10.1016/j.clim.2012.01.015
52. Keitel, W.A., et al.: Safety of high doses of influenza vaccine and effect on antibody responses in elderly persons. Arch. Intern. Med. **166**, 1121–1127 (2006). doi:10.1001/archinte.166.10.1121
53. Vandepapeliere, P., et al.: Vaccine adjuvant systems containing monophosphoryl lipid A and QS21 induce strong and persistent

humoral and T cell responses against hepatitis B surface antigen in healthy adult volunteers. Vaccine **26**, 1375–1386 (2008). doi:10.1016/j.vaccine.2007.12.038

54. Hutt, H.J., Bennerscheidt, P., Thiel, B., Arand, M.: Immunosenescence and vaccinations in the elderly. Med. Klin. (Munich) **105**, 802–807 (2010). doi:10.1007/s00063-010-1137-0
55. Taub, D.D., Murphy, W.J., Longo, D.L.: Rejuvenation of the aging thymus: growth hormone-mediated and ghrelin-mediated signaling pathways. Curr. Opin. Pharmacol. **10**, 408–424 (2010). doi:10.1016/j.coph.2010.04.015
56. Aspinall, R.: T cell development, ageing and Interleukin-7. Mech. Ageing Dev. **127**, 572–578 (2006). doi:10.1016/j.mad.2006.01.016

Part II

Vaccine Design

6 Antigens and Epitopes

Contents

6.1 From Empirical Approaches to Epitopes

The original scientific strategy behind vaccinology has historically been to "isolate, inactivate, and inject," first invoked by Louis Pasteur. Subsequently, this empirical approach dominated the vaccine development over 80 years. The recombinant DNA technology arised, and in 1980 the first recombinant vaccine against hepatitis B virus was presented. With MenACWY in 1990, a quadrivalent meningococcal meningitis vaccine, in which the capsular polysaccharides from *Neisseria meningitidis* serogroups A, C, W, and Y are conjugated to the diphtheria toxin mutant CRM197, the first glycoconjugate vaccine, was approved. Finally, MenB, meningococcal B vaccine, was the first genome-derived vaccine in 2010 developed by reverse vaccinology. Table 6.1 highlights these technological progresses.

Immunodominance. Protein antigens typically contain multiple epitopes capable of binding MHC I or II molecules, but T cell responses are limited to only a small number of these determinants in each individual. This ability to focus only on some selected epitopes out of many is called immunodominance: one epitope is dominant and triggers the response, and all other epitopes are subdominant and don't mount for an effective response. A vaccine that induces responses against subdominant epitopes will be less protective than a vaccine that induces a robust immunodominant response.

Immunodominance is evident for both antibody-mediated immunity and cell-mediated immunity [1]. The impact of immunodominance is the potential to generate the strongest immune response against a certain pathogen, virus or bacteria, thus eliminating the pathogen fast and effectively. A drawback of this privileged immune response could be the mutation of the immunodominant epitope, as described for some viruses, thus allowing for instance HIV to avoid the adaptive immune response when reintroduced from latency.

M. Giese, *Introduction to Molecular Vaccinology*, DOI 10.1007/978-3-319-25832-4_6

Table 6.1 From empirical approaches toward epitope prediction and reverse vaccinology

1885 - 1950	• **Empirical Approach:** Diphtheria, Tetanus, Polio, Rabies, Bacillus Calmette–Guérin (BCG)
1980	• **Recombinant DNA:** Hepatitis B, Papillomavirus, Lymeborreliosis
1990	• **Glycoconjugation:** Meningococcal meningitis serogroups A, C, W, and Y (MenACWY), Haemophilus influenzae Typ b (Hib), Pneumonia, S.aureus
2010	• **Reverse Vaccinology:** Meningococcal B (MenB), Group A Streptococcal (GAS), Guillain-Barré syndrome (GBS)

The immunological focus on only a manageable amount of epitopes corresponds to the limited capacity of dendritic cells, the major APC, to express MHC molecules for antigen presentation. Only three to six different types of MHC molecules are on the surface of DCs. Therefore, only the most effective epitopes are bound. The mechanisms of T cell immunodominance are poorly understood. The mechanism of B cell immunodominance focuses on the affinity of epitope binding to the B cell receptor.

T and B cell Epitopes. They differ fundamentally in the way they are recognized by the immune system. T cell epitopes are parts of internalized and processed protein antigens that are presented to T lymphocytes in association with MHC molecules. B cell epitopes are recognized as three-dimensional structures on the surface of native antigens. Both immunodominant T and B cell epitopes are potential vaccine candidates.

Antigenicity and Immunogenicity. Neither antigenicity nor immunogenicity is an inherent characteristic of an epitope or generally of an antigen. Antigenicity is defined only by the antibody–antigen interaction: the antibody makes the antigen. Immunogenicity encompasses the specific environment of an encountering antigen: rabbit albumin is not immunogenic in rabbits but in other species.

6.2 T Cell Epitopes

T cell epitopes (TCEs) presented by MHC class I molecules are typically peptides between 8 and 11 amino acids in length, whereas MHC class II molecules present longer peptides, 12–26 amino acids (aa) in length with a core peptide of 9 aa. This core peptide must fit into the MHC pockets. In contrast to the MHC I pocket, the peptide-binding groove of MHC class II molecules is not closed at the ends and therefore accommodates peptides of varying lengths. Within the pocket, several peptide side chains, typically the residues at positions 1, 4, 6, and 9, interact with MHC peptides (Fig. 6.1). Short peptides of 8–10 aa do not stimulate CD4+ T cells. Ideal peptides are typically 12–20 aa long. T cells recognize linear (continuous) epitopes, in contrast to B cells.

T Cell Based Vaccines. In contrast to antibodies, T cells often recognize epitopes that are located in highly conserved

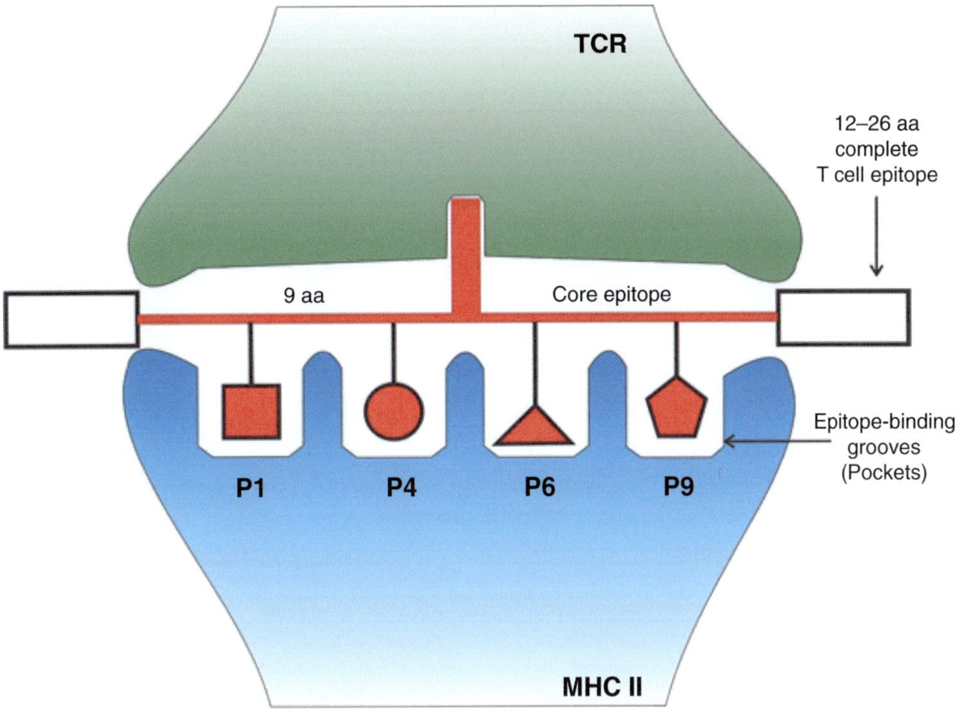

Fig. 6.1 T cell epitopes (TCEs) presented by MHC class II molecules are typically peptides between 12 and 26 amino acids in length, with a core peptide of 9 aa. This core peptide must fit into the MHC-pockets P1, P4, P6, and P9, epitope-binding grooves. MHC II, in contrast to MHC I, can bind variable peptide lengths. Within the pockets, several peptide side chains, typically the residues at positions 1, 4, 6, and 9, interact with MHC peptides. In contrast to the MHC I pocket, the peptide-binding groove of MHC class II molecules is not closed at the ends and therefore accommodates peptides of varying lengths

regions of pathogen-derived proteins. Thus, vaccines targeting T cell epitopes (T cell-based vaccines) could create cross-protecting against a wide range of strains of the same pathogen. Strong evidences for a CD8+ T cell-mediated protection is given by some live attenuated vaccines, such as against polio, mumps, and small pox [2]. T cell-based vaccines are also necessary for those infections against which neutralizing antibody-based vaccines are not effective enough.

The classical experimental approach to identify T cell epitopes is to synthesize a library with overlapping peptides, usually 15-mers, spanning the full length of the target antigen, and test for T cell immunogenicity, e.g., by peptide–MHC binding assay. These cellular tests must be performed for each synthesized peptide and are very costly and time consuming.

First algorithms for the prediction of T cell epitopes were already developed in the 1980s.

6.3 B Cell Epitopes

B cell receptors (BCRs) and soluble antibodies recognize B cell epitopes (BCEs), which can be soluble antigen molecules present in the extracellular fluid, intact, small chemical compounds or components of larger macromolecules such as nucleotides, lipids, glycans, and proteins. B cell antigens include components of bacterial cell wall or antigens containing highly repetitious molecules (e.g., bacterial flagellin).

B cells can pluck antigens from APC such as macrophages and DCs. The bound antigens are endocytosed into the B cell, digested into fragments which are then displayed at the cell surface nestled inside a class II MHC molecule for presenting to T helper cells. T helper cells bind to B cells and stimulate their activation by secretion of interleukins. Antibodies are soluble B cell receptors (BCRs) (Fig. 6.2). B cells can be activated in a T cell-dependent (TD) or T cell-independent (TI) manner.

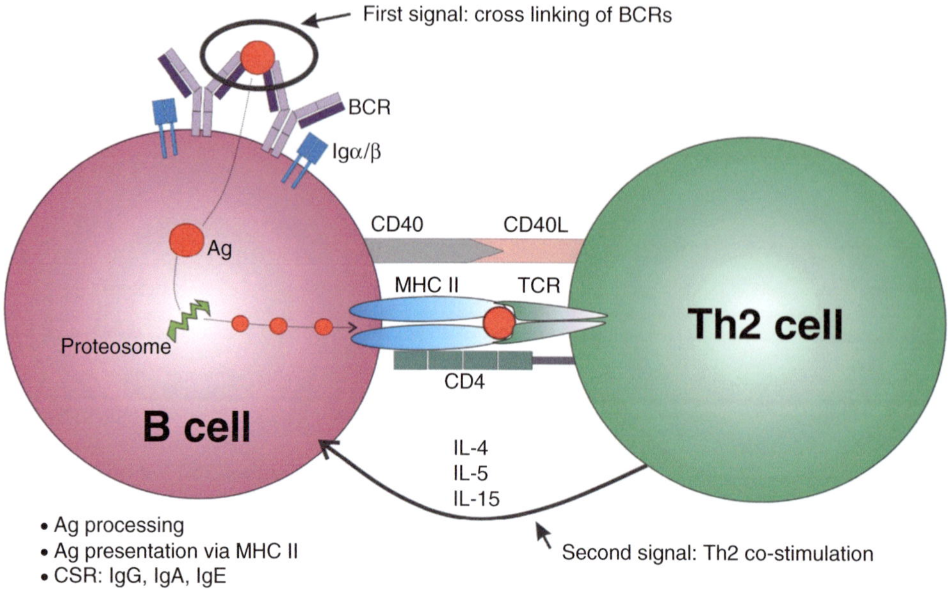

Fig. 6.2 B cell activation in a T cell-dependent manner. Two signals are necessary: the first is the cross-linking of the BCRs by antigen, and the second signal is the co-stimulation of cytokines such as IL-4, 5, and 15 by Th2 cells. The bound antigens (*Ag*) are endocytosed into the B cell and processed and Ag-fragments are then displayed at the cell surface nestled inside a class II MHC molecule for presenting to T helper cells in combination with co-stimulatory molecules CD40 and CD40L. The class switch recombination (*CSR*) results in a change from IgM to other immunoglobulin classes. The disulfide-linked heterodimer Igα/β is part of the B cell receptor and involved in signaling pathways for activation and differentiation. *BCR* B cell receptor, *TCR* T cell receptor

T Dependent Antigens. B cell antigens that require co-stimulation by a helper T cell for B cell activation are *T dependent (TD)* and are usually proteins. The activated B cell clonally proliferates (clonal selection) to produce a population of plasma cells and memory cells, which all recognize the same antigen (Fig. 6.2).

T Independent Antigens. B cells can also be activated in a T cell-independent manner without co-stimulation by helper T cells. T-independent (TI) antigens that stimulate B cells directly are not processed and presented via MHC proteins and hence cannot be recognized by helper T cells. Most TI antigens are polyvalent, with multiple identical epitopes. Such polyvalent antigens may induce cross-linking of surface IgM molecules on B cells.

There are two classes of TI antigens: TI-1 is lipopolysaccharide (LPS) (Fig. 6.3a) and TI-2 antigens are polysaccharides, glycolipids, and nucleic acids (Fig. 6.3b). TI-1 antigens can directly stimulate B cells without requirement of any other cell. At low concentration, bacterial LPS stimulates specific IgM antibody production but don't generate as strong a response (no memory cells, IgM is the only antibody class produced, and the immunity doesn't last long).

Polyclonal Activation

T-independent antigens are subdivided into Type 1 and Type 2 based on their ability to polyclonally activate B cells. Type 1 T-independent antigens are polyclonal activators while Type 2 are not.

Length of B Cell Epitopes. Protein-based BCEs are either conformational (discontinuous) epitopes or linear epitopes. Linear B cell epitopes typically vary from 5 to 20 amino acids in length. Only a few epitopes have length of more than 40 residues. The main common feature of BCEs is accessibility on the surface of the antigen.

A conformational epitope is composed of discontinuous sections of the antigen's amino acid sequence. These epitopes interact with the paratope of the antibody based on the 3D surface features and shape or tertiary structure of the antigen. This makes B cell epitopes more difficult to identify than T cell epitopes, which are only determined by their amino acid sequence (see also Chap. 1). Conformational epitopes are thought to form the majority of strong antibody-binding epitopes on most proteins.

B cell epitope mapping is an integral part in the development of subunit vaccines in which immunogenic regions of protein is used instead of complete pathogen or antigen.

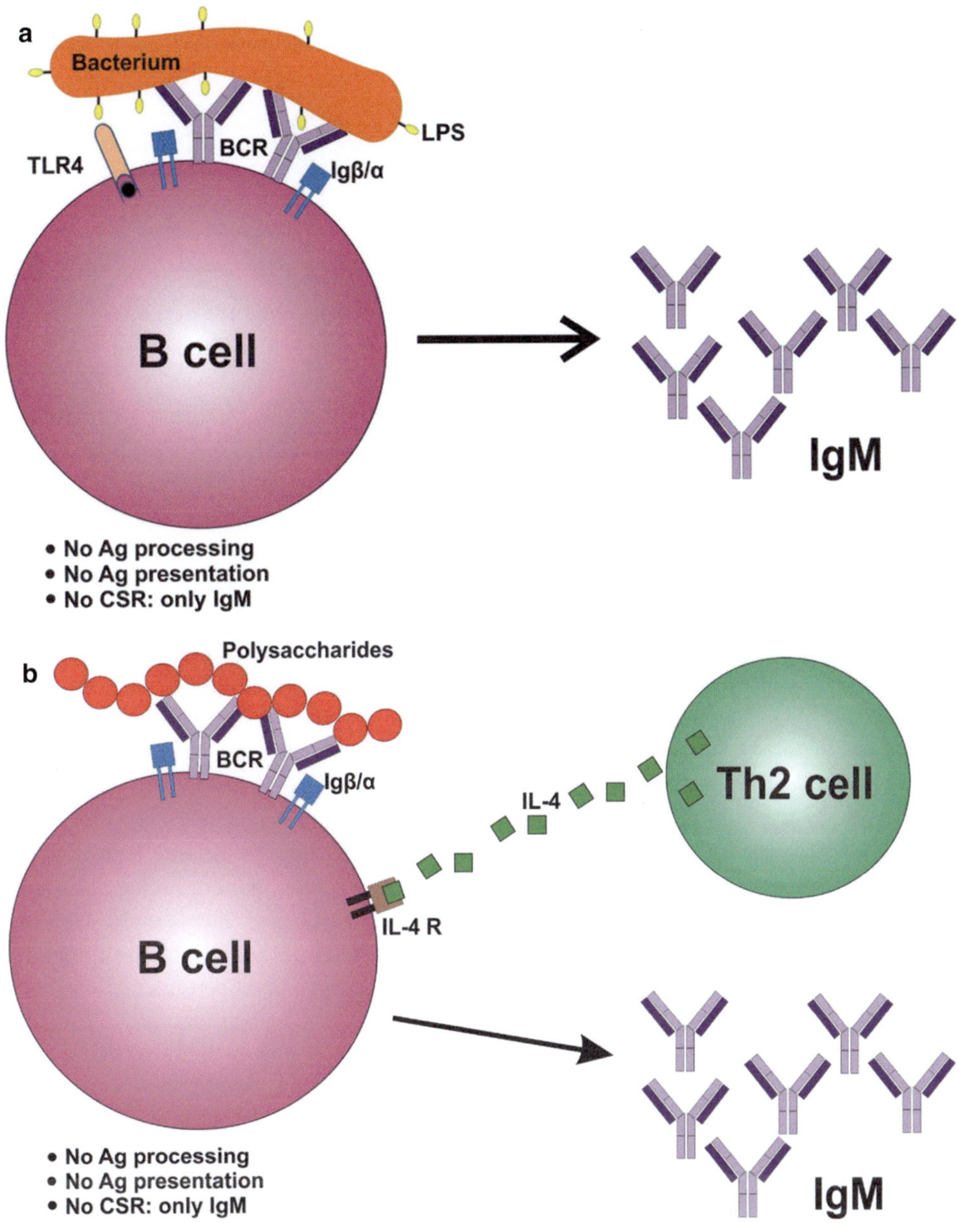

Fig. 6.3 (**a**) Type 1 T cell-independent B cell activation. Antigens are not endocytosed, not processed, and not presented and there is no class switch recombination (*CSR*). The resulting activated B cell is restricted to IgM antibodies that are specific to the TLR-binding antigen (here bacterial *LPS* via *TLR4*). BCR (*IgM*) binds a TI-1 antigen such as LPS, leading to cross-link of BCRs. LPS is directly mitogenic for the B cells (polyclonal activation). (**b**) Type 2 T cell-independent B cell activation. BCR binds a TI-2 antigen, such as bacterial polysaccharide, which has repeating, identical epitopes. A nearby activated Th2 cell is secreting cytokines such as IL-4, which stimulate the B cell via IL-4 receptor (*IL-4R*) activation to divide and produce antibodies. Antigens are not endocytosed, not processed, and not presented and there is no class switch recombination (*CSR*). The resulting activated B cell is restricted to IgM antibodies

Antibodies against specific epitopes perform various functions such as neutralization, compliment activation, phagocytosis, or cell-mediated cytotoxicity. BCEs can be found in all immunoglobulin subclasses, IgG, IgE, IgM, IgΛ, and IgD. The class of the antibody could be determined by the sequence of the epitope. In other words, the composition of the sequence can be used to discriminate epitopes of different classes. Thus for a better vaccine design, it is possible to predict class-specific BCEs with appropriate antibody effector function.

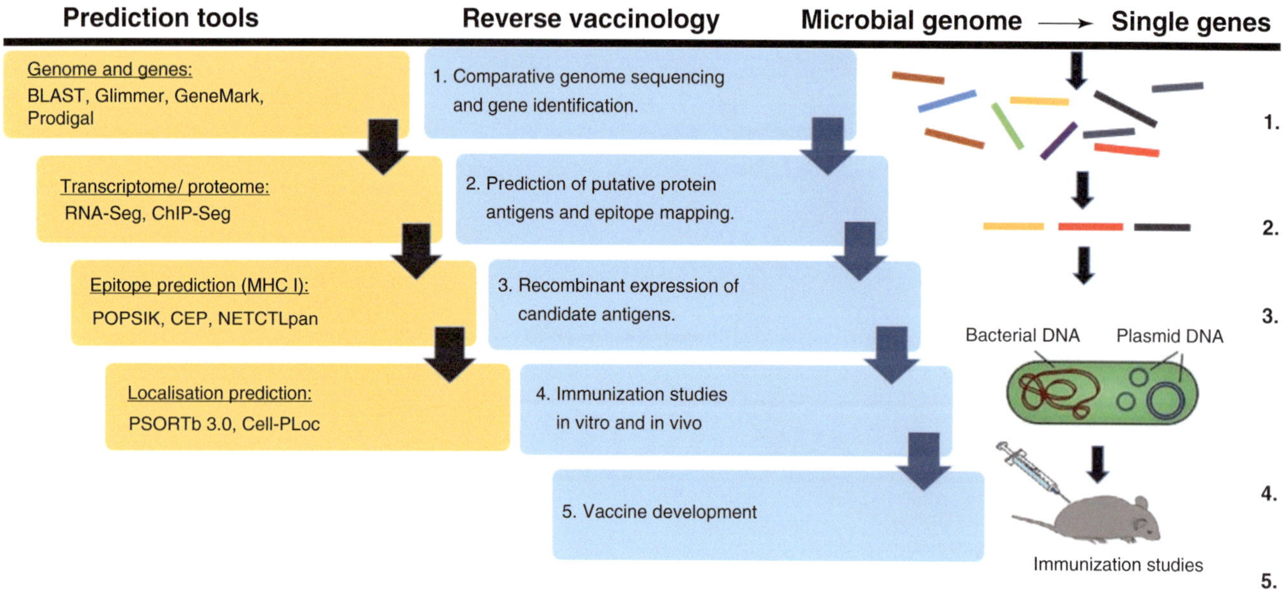

Fig. 6.4 The exclusive goal of reverse vaccinology is to discover novel antigens and to predict epitopes for B and T cell responses. This approach focuses on isolated genes of microbial organisms. The entire process can be divided roughly in five major activities. The first 2 steps are dry experiments (in silico). Several bioinformatical prediction tools are used alone or in combination for genome, gene, and proteome analyses. A complete list of different prediction tools is summarized in Table 6.2 (Figure by M.Giese Heidelberg/Germany)

6.4 In Silico Tools for Epitope Prediction[1]

Modern vaccine research and development is technically assisted by bioinformatics tools: Large DNA genomes are automatically sequenced and RNA analyses have been used with great success to study between-subject differences in immune responses to a pathogen or a candidate vaccine. High-throughput mass spectrometry is accelerating membrane protein analysis, and also a vast amount of protein subcellular localization predictors are freely available. Figure 6.4 summarizes available bioinformatics tools for prediction in vaccine research and development.

6.4.1 Gene Prediction and Annotation

Pathogens for which vaccines are required range from viruses, prokaryotic bacteria, eukaryotic intracellular endoparasites (such as *Plasmodium* causing malaria) and extracellular parasites (such as helminths) to ectoparasites (such as ticks and mites). Each of these has its own unique biology and effect on the host immune system which must be understood if a successful vaccine is to be developed.

[1]Considerations for vaccine design in the post-genomic era by *Christine Maritz-Olivier and Sabine Richards* in Molecular Vaccines – From Prophylaxis to Therapy, Volume 2, Springer-Verlag Wien, 2013, Ed. Matthias Giese.

The ability to obtain genomic DNA sequence information within a short time frame and at an affordable price is without doubt shaping modern biology. In the field of vaccinology, genomes hold the key to understanding pathogen genes, the host immune genes and the interplay between genes involved in host–pathogen interactions during infection and vaccination. Next-generation sequencing has been used with great success to gain insight into detection of both pathogen and host genetic variation, evidence of selection pressures, immune escape mechanisms, vaccine safety, the diversity of T and B cell repertoires, immune regulation, and assessment of the quality of vaccine stocks [3].

Pan-genomic Analyses and MenB. It is nowadays becoming routine to start analyses with more than one genome of closely related organisms. This allows for the identification of immunogenic and conserved antigens suitable for use in a combinatorial vaccine that offers protection against genetically diverse strains.

The best example is that of the Bexsero vaccine containing four immunogenic and conserved antigens, protecting against 77 % of more than 800 genetically diverse disease-causing MenB strains. Comparative studies on eight gram-positive pathogenic *Streptococcus agalactiae* genomes revealed both a core genome and a dispensable genome. Interestingly, the proteins found to be protective did not all originate from the core genome. In contrast, only one core genome antigen and three dispensable genome antigens were found to be protective in combination against a large panel of strains [4].

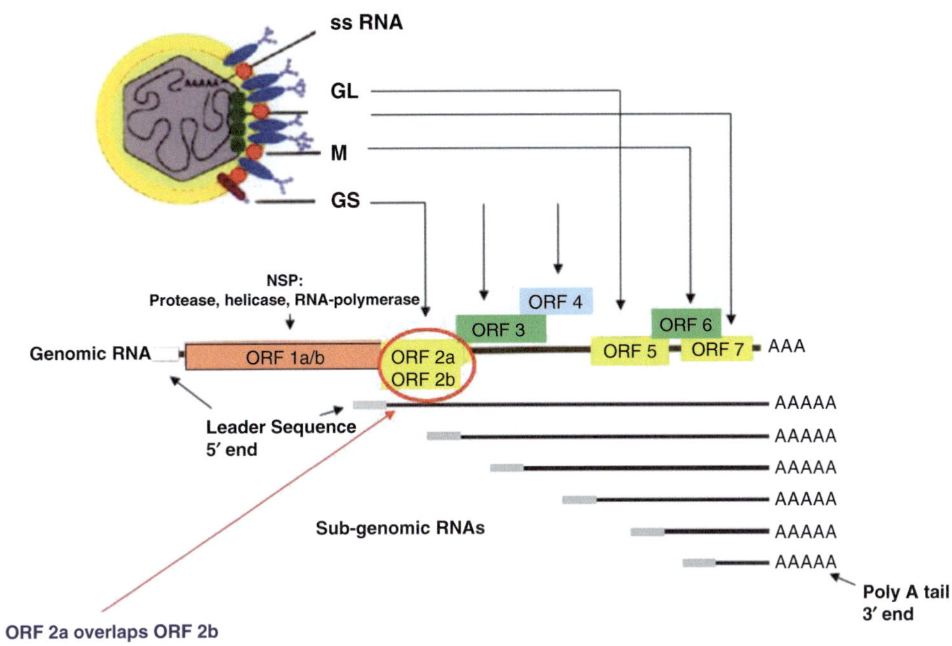

Fig. 6.5 Equine arteritis virus (EAV) has a small 13–16 kb positive-sense RNA genome EAV's seven structural proteins are encoded by a set of partially overlapping genes in the genomic 3'proximal region. The subgenomic mRNAs are functionally monocistronic with the exception for a bicistronic mRNA encoding the E and GP2 proteins. Their genes and transcripts are overlapping (*GL* large glycoprotein, *M* matrix protein, *GS* small glycoprotein) (Figure by M.Giese Heidelberg/Germany)

Subtractive Genomics. Between pathogenic and non-pathogenic strains, it has been used with great success for the identification of the ECOK I-3385 antigen from pathogenic *Escherichia coli*.

BLAST. In this post-genomic era, genome sequence assembly and gene prediction remains a bottleneck, especially for complex eukaryotic pathogens lacking gene scaffolds. Subsequent gene and open reading frame (ORF) prediction is one of the most fundamental and important steps in genome analysis having major implications for any downstream analysis. One method for the identification of ORFs is BLAST [5]. Otherwise, ab initio gene prediction can be performed utilizing mathematical models if no other evidence of a gene is present [6]. A number of programs optimized for prokaryotic ORF predictions are available, such as Glimmer [7], GeneMark.hmm [8], and Prodigal [9]. Pipelines providing increased accuracy of gene prediction by evaluating gene models of prokaryotes and detecting anomalies are also coming of age [10].

Overlapping Transcripts. In eukaryotes, this is not a trivial process, as recent observation from the ENCODE project revealed that genes have overlapping transcripts as well as transcription from both DNA strands [11]. Furthermore, mathematical models are trained on organism-specific genomic traits often using classic model organisms such as *Drosophila melanogaster*. The accuracy of these predictions is then dependent on how distantly the organism of interest is related to these eukaryotes. Some gene predictors can also be trained using pipelines such as MAKER [12]. Other programs are capable of incorporating external evidence (such as EST and RNA-Seq data) into an ab initio approach for the improvement of prediction.

Such software includes AUGUSTUS [13] and GNOMON (http://0-www.ncbi.nlm.nih.gov.innopac.up.ac.za/genome/guide/gnomon.shtml).

Other strategies, such as SAGE libraries tag-to-gene mapping (mapping tags to a genome via BLAST and then mapping tags to their genes using a data-driven probability distribution), were required to obtain insight into the *Leishmania* genome structure and transcription [14].

Overlapping in RNA Viruses. A simple example for overlapping viral transcripts is the genome of equine arteritis virus (EAV) with a small 13–16 kb positive-sense RNA genome (Fig. 6.5). EAV's seven structural proteins are encoded by a set of partially overlapping genes in the genomic 3'proximal region. The subgenomic mRNAs are functionally monocistronic with the exception for a bicistronic mRNA encoding the E and GP2 proteins. Their genes and transcripts are overlapping. Overlapping coding sequences are particularly common in RNA viruses and are difficult to detect, especially when this sequences are short. Overlapping transcripts are of interest because this region is often conserved and thus a vaccine candidate.

Annotation. Gene annotation is the process of attaching biological information to DNA sequences. Subsequent functional annotation (biochemical and biological functions; protein interactions and regulations) of a gene product is also not a trivial process. Homology searches using BLAST [15] and BLAST-based algorithms have proved successful, while many online databases provide tools and information for annotation, e.g., PIR [16], Pfam [17], SWISS-PROT [18], Uni-Prot [19], COG [20], and others. Unfortunately most of these approaches rely on the availability of accurately characterized protein information. In addition, functional similarity cannot always be inferred from homology, and additional information is required to increase confidence in functional predictions [17].

Gene Ontology (GO) [21] is used very widely and successfully but can be limited by a dependence on un-curated, experimentally unverified, and computationally derived annotations [22]. One alternative that is increasingly being incorporated is the use of protein–protein interactions to predict and identify functional relationships. A main limitation is the absence of protein interaction data [23], though the geometric relationship in the alignment of predicted secondary structural elements could be used to model and evaluate putative structural interactions for functional predictions [24]. Combinations of data, such as protein sequence, gene expression, and protein–interaction data, could be amalgamated to infer and confirm functional annotation predictions [25].

6.4.2 Transcriptome and Proteome Analyses

A transcriptome is the set of all RNA molecules, including mRNA, rRNA, tRNA, and other noncoding RNAs transcribed in one cell.

Transcriptome analyses provide researchers with clues regarding rare transcripts, alternate splicing, copy number variation, sequence variation, regulatory mechanisms, and biochemical pathways involved in cellular function. *RNA-Seq* is the choice of technique in the post-genomic era for obtaining large transcriptome datasets, as it has been estimated to detect 25 % more transcripts than conventional DNA microarrays. *To date, RNA-Seq and conventional transcriptome profiling have been used with great success to study between-subject differences in immune responses* to a pathogen or a candidate vaccine, the role of miRNAs in regulating mRNA expression, epigenetic responses to viral vaccines, understanding of molecular processes and survival mechanisms (e.g., the heartworm *Dirofilaria immitis* for identification of vaccine and drug targets [26]), identification of additional surface-expressed vaccine candidates (e.g., *Neisseria meningitidis* [27]), and identification of expressed surface and secreted proteins in complex pathogens (e.g., the apicomplexan parasite *Eimeria tenella* [28] and the ectoparasitic cattle tick, *R. microplus* [29]) which can now be exploited as vaccine candidates.

Proteome. A proteome represent the complete protein complement expressed by a cell, allowing a more direct measure of cellular response than nucleic acid-based analyses and insight into posttranscriptional modifications.

Typically proteomes were evaluated by *two-dimensional electrophoresis*, but this presented with the obstacle that few hydrophobic proteins were recovered for downstream analyses. Nowadays high-throughput *mass spectrometry is accelerating membrane protein* analysis [30] and revealing the presence of plasma membrane proteins that are unknown in databases despite extensive genome sequencing. Proteome analysis is vital to overcoming the limitations of in silico localization prediction software. As surface-exposed proteins are mostly targeted during vaccination, surfaceome analyses have received quite a bit of attention. Novel approaches include analysis of membrane proteins using "shaving," whereby cells are treated with proteases and the resulting peptides analyzed by LC-MS-MS and advanced mass spectrometry-based identification of viral peptides from high- or low-responder-associated MHC molecules as candidate antigens [31].

To date, proteomics provided insight into the neglected malaria parasite *Plasmodium vivax* which identified 153 proteins that show no homology to previously identified products as well as 29 new proteins [32] and insight into the pathogen biology, genes, and metabolic pathways of *Trypanosoma cruzi* [33] as well as providing a platform for the development of epitope-driven vaccines and structural proteomics in *Mycobacterium tuberculosis* [34]. The availability of host proteome data, and its integration with other "-omic" data (predominantly transcriptome data), is vital to the success of future vaccines. A glossary relevant to the multidisciplinary fields of vaccine development in the post-genomic era is presented in Table 6.2.

ChIP-Seq Technology. This data provides insight into the differentiation of immune cells and their roles in inflammation and immunity, cellular localization of proteins, and signaling pathways of the immune system [36]. Large-scale studies into T cell receptor diversity were made possible with next-generation sequencing and have since provided insight into the role

Table 6.2 Glossary relevant to the multidisciplinary fields of vaccine development in the post-genomic era

Term	Published definition/*popular explanation*	Reference
Immunogenetics	Genetic analysis of the immune system/*the study of genes involved in the immune system*	[106]
Immunogenomics	Genomics technology combined with immunology/*the study of sets of genes and their expression profile involved in immune responses*	[107, 108]
Systems biology	Systems biology aims to understand quantitatively how properties of biological systems can be understood as functions of the characteristics of and interactions between their macromolecular components/*the study of the complete system of organisms including all interactions between biological elements and their surrounding environment*	[109]
Immunoproteomics	Defines the subset of proteins that induce an immune response (immunoproteome)/*the study of all proteins involved in the immune response and their identification and function*	[110]
Vaccinomics	The term refers to immunogenetics and immunogenomics as applied to vaccine immune responses and the mechanisms underlying heterogeneity in both the pathogen and the host response to vaccination/*an integrative approach incorporating immunogenetics and immunogenomics for the study of immune responses to vaccines or pathogens*	[111]
Reverse vaccinology	Genomic-based approaches to vaccine development/*the methodology of vaccine development based on genomic information of organisms*	[62]
Immunotherapy	The complex network of interactions between immune cells during manipulation of the host immune system/*treatment of disease by inducing, enhancing, or suppressing an immune response*	[35]

of rearrangement of segments (predominantly in the VDJ region) in the TCR gene and how this brings about the vast repertoire of antigen-specific T cells. This also expanded into B cell studies with the identification of 14 new allelic variants in the human heavy-chain immunoglobulin variable regions as well as improved understanding of vaccines targeting dendritic cell subsets [37]. *ChIP-Seq technology has also been used with success to provide insight into the transcription factors involved in the development of B- and T cell responses.*

Personalized Vaccines. Findings on the role of polymorphisms in the genome of immune cell insight into the heterogeneity of responses against vaccines are fast expanding and paving the way forward to personalized vaccines [38]. Evidence for genetic host polymorphisms in determining responses against vaccines in humans was provided by the classical studies of Jacobson and colleagues as well as Tan and colleagues in which monozygotic and dizygotic twin pairs were evaluated in response to the MMR, hepatitis B, oral polio, tetanus toxoid, and diphtheria vaccines.

Polymorphisms. Subsequently, a number of polymorphisms (predominantly SNPs) in the human leukocyte antigen (HLA) genes and their contribution to vaccine immunity toward MMR and rubella have been published (reviewed in [38]). Such linkages remain to be elucidated for other vaccines but are currently limited by the vast amount of data required for large-scale genome-wide linkage studies. Polymorphisms in non-HLA genes such as SNPs in cytokines and cytokine receptors, Toll-like receptors, signaling molecules, vitamin A and D receptors, antiviral effectors, and genes associated with innate and adaptive immunity have also been published for rubella and a number of adjuvants and how these affect vaccine efficacy [38].

6.4.3 Vaccinomics and the Immune Response Network

Upon infection, pathogens activate a great number of immune triggers in both innate and adaptive immune responses, mediating protective immunity, and the progression to long-lived protection against the pathogen [39]. This has been termed "the immune response network theory," which aims to integrate environmental, host and pathogen, or vaccination factors. Our ability to understand the gene players involved in infection and vaccination and how they correlate to protective immunity will provide essential insights for improved vaccine development (Fig. 6.6).

The latter is clearly stated by Bernstein and colleagues as "Future vaccines will focus not only on the identification of a single correlate (or multiple, independent correlates), but on the identification of multifactorial signatures associated with immune protection (i.e. pathogen, host and interacting

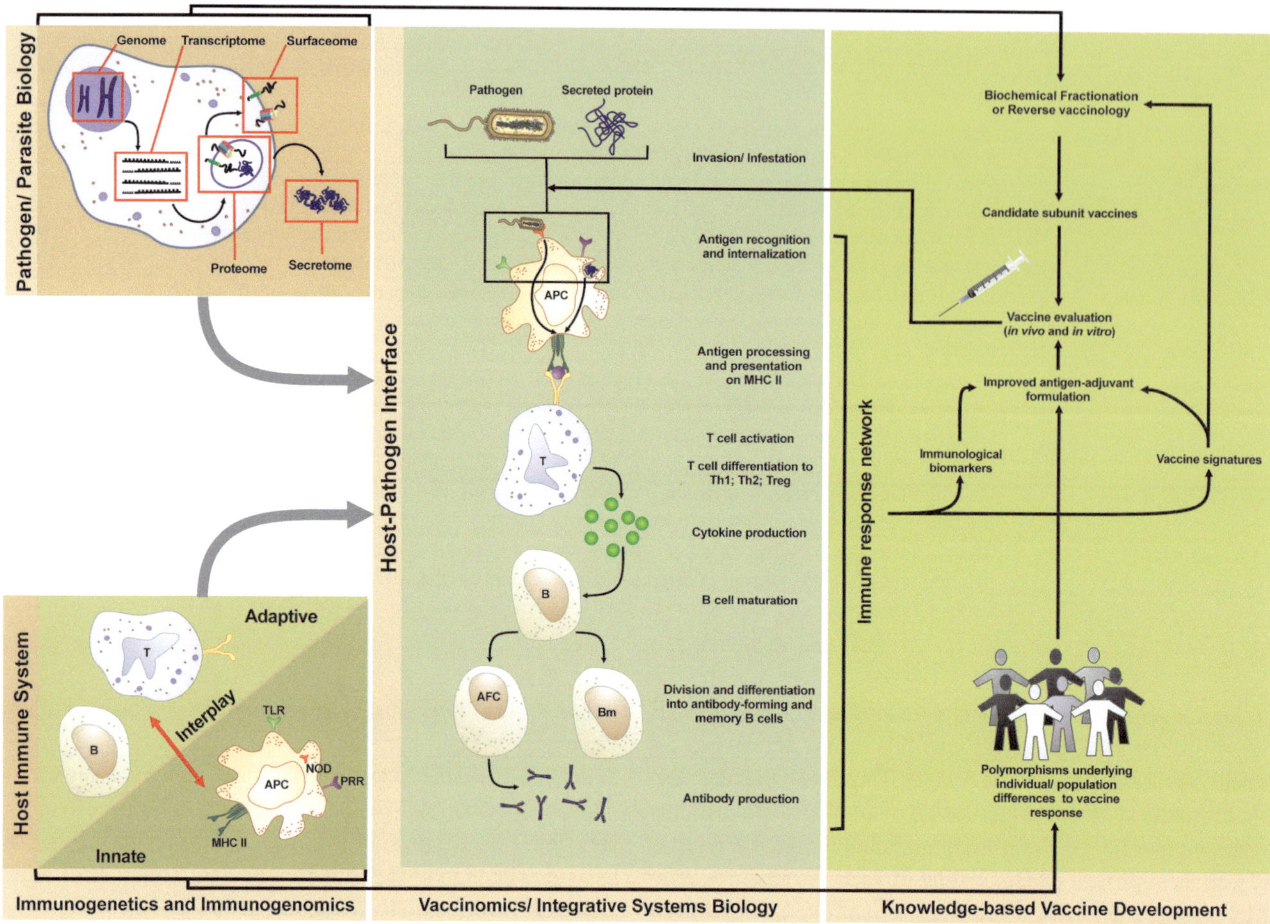

Fig. 6.6 Considerations for vaccine development. An in-depth understanding of the parasite/pathogen biology as well as the host immune system is required to fully comprehend the processes underlying infection and development of protective immunity. This is achieved by the combination of genomic, transcriptome and proteome data which in turn drives reverse vaccinology approaches and subunit vaccine development. Integrative systems biology approaches provide insight into the complex networks underlying infection and the development of protective immunity. By linking polymorphisms to heterogeneities observed in responses to vaccines and survival/virulence of pathogens, insight is gained for the development of improved vaccines. Abbreviations corresponds to T cell receptor (TLR), nuclear-binding oligomerization domain (NOD)-containing proteins, pathogen recognition receptor (PRR), major histocompatibility complex II (MHC), antigen-presenting cell (APC), T-helper type 1 and 2 or tolerance response (*Th1*, *Th2* or *T-reg*, respectively), B cell (*B*), antibody-forming cell (*AFC*), and memory B cells (*Bm*)

signatures)" [39], paving the way forward to the ultimate goal of universal vaccine signatures.

Vaccinomics was first described by Poland in 2007 as the application of immunogenetics and immunogenomics, which is the study of genetic and epigenetic determinants and pathways relevant to vaccine-induced responses. In 2011 it was expanded to include the mechanisms underlying heterogeneity in both the pathogen and the host response to vaccination, which aims at providing insight into the observed variability in response to vaccination [40].

Integrative approaches have been used successfully to provide insight into future vaccines. For microbial biology, this has been excellently reviewed by Zhang et al. [41]. Other examples include simultaneous analysis of host and pathogen transcriptomes in high and low antibody responders to rubella, smallpox, and influenza vaccines as well as integrating genotypes/haplotypes and phenotypes for measles, mumps, rubella, influenza, and smallpox vaccines. The combination of genome-wide expression data with interactome (yeast two-hybrid) data in influenza infection resulted in the identification of novel viral genes regulating interferon production and viral replication. It has also been used in understanding T cell responses to yellow fever vaccination (identifying signatures of neutralizing antibody responses and two additional signatures of CD8$^+$ T cells) as well as identifying two distinct IFN responses by neutrophils in tuberculosis patients [40].

MAGE-A3 Peptide Vaccine. Global transcriptional profiling of patients receiving the MAGE-A3 peptide vaccine for non-small-cell lung cancer revealed signatures correlating with responsiveness to treatment [35]. Immunogenetics studies focusing on the host OAS gene family and West Nile virus (WNV) revealed that polymorphisms in OASL was linked to susceptibility in WNV infection and that therapeutic agents/adjuvants capable of inducting OAS1 activity could enhance WNV vaccine efficacy [40]. Integrated transcriptome studies in zebra fish vaccinated with *Edwardsiella tarda* live attenuated vaccines revealed pathways involved in antigen processing and acute-phase responses which provided insight into the mechanisms underlying zebra fish immune responses and directions for improved vaccines. Interestingly, they found that MHC I pathways were upregulated and MHC II pathways were downregulated during vaccination [42].

In another study, gene expression profiling of dendritic cells in the presence of *Staphylococcus aureus* revealed a unique role for the inflammatory process and T-helper-cell polarization as well as 204 differentially expressed genes between susceptible and resistant animals, providing explanations for the difference in susceptibility towards *S. aureus* infection [43]. Genome-wide digital gene expression (DGE) was successfully used to study the host response to the zoonotic pathogen, *Brucella melitensis*.

An in-depth understanding of the parasite/pathogen biology as well as the host immune system is required to fully comprehend the processes underlying infection and development of protective immunity. This is achieved by the combination of genomic, transcriptome and proteome data which in turn drives reverse vaccinology approaches and subunit vaccine development. Integrative systems biology approaches provide insight into the complex networks underlying infection and the development of protective immunity. By linking polymorphisms to heterogeneities observed in responses to vaccines and survival/virulence of pathogens, insight is gained for the development of improved vaccines. Abbreviations correspond to T cell receptor (TLR), nuclear-binding oligomerization domain (NOD)-containing proteins, pathogen recognition receptor (PRR), major histocompatibility complex II (MHC), antigen-presenting cell (APC), T-helper type 1 and 2 or tolerance response (Th1, Th2, or T-reg, respectively), B cell (B), antibody-forming cell (AFC), and memory B cells (Bm).

This study revealed, among others, a strong role for macrophages during infection and the induction of anti-inflammatory and antiapoptotic factors in the survival of strains with differing virulence, directing research into development of new attenuated vaccines with enhanced efficacy [44].

Bottleneck in Systems Biology. To accomplish insight into the complex traits underlying immunity and vaccine reactivity, an integrated systems biology approach that combines different "omics" datasets with powerful analytical tools, providing scoring and correlation between datasets, is required [40]. This remains a serious bottleneck in a systems biology approach to vaccine design, but the field is expanding rapidly. Several good reviews on in silico tools to combine "omics" data have been published [41, 45–47].

RefDIC, Booly, PARE. To date, software packages and databases for integration of "omics" data include RefDIC [48] (the reference genomics database of immune cells which combines transcriptome, proteome, and immunogenetic data), IIDB [49] (the innate immune database), WIBL [50] (workbench for integrative biological learning), a guided clustering package for use in R [51] (integration of microarray, genome-wide chromatin immunoprecipitation and cell perturbation assays), and EchoBasE [52] (for *E. coli*).

Several public available databases such as integrOmics [53], bioPIXIE [47] (currently optimized for yeast biological processes), VESPA [54] (integration of genomic, transcriptome and proteome data from prokaryotes), openBIS [55] (integration of next-generation sequencing, metabolomics, and proteomics), GPS-Prot [56] (integration of HIV–human interaction networks, in the process of being extended to other host–pathogen systems), Booly [57], and PARE [58] are also available.

VRC01 Antibody and HIV-1. Finally, structural biology has started to provide insight into how the VRC01 antibody neutralizes some 90 % of HIV-1 strains, indicating a vast diversity in neutralizing antibodies directed against autologous HIV envelope sequences across many vaccine recipients and infected individuals [3]. Structural vaccinology incorporates structural biology with vaccinology and can be used for the improvement of vaccine design. As neutralizing antibodies need to recognize specific antigen architectures, the identification of these regions using high-resolution structural analysis is important. By keeping these neutralizing architectures intact, while changing other regions to make an antigen more stable, cost-effective, and eliminate variable regions, vaccines can be improved.

Furthermore, the knowledge about the structure of certain antigenic regions will allow the improvement of our understanding of immunogenicity and immunodominance, thus helping with future vaccine design [59]. The structural vaccinology approach was followed in several studies, for example, constructing a chimeric protein as vaccine against

Group B *Streptococcus* [60]. Some proteins of these microbes have evolved to contain antigenic regions with non-similar properties in different isolates, however, with the same functional properties, thus helping evade the host immune system. Therefore, Nuccitelli et al. constructed a chimeric protein containing the domains of six antigenic variants, resulting in protection against all six tested isolates [60].

6.5 Reverse Vaccinology

Reverse vaccinology is a process whereby genome and transcriptome sequences are analyzed by bioinformatics tools to identify potentially protective secreted and surface-displayed antigenic proteins. These proteins are then expressed and used to immunize a suitable host to validate their immunogenicity and protective abilities before proceeding to production and formulation (Fig. 6.7). A main concern associated with this approach is that vaccinologists have not been able to improve the initial bioinformatics of candidate selection steps, allowing improved prediction of antigenicity and, even more so, their ability to induce protective immunity.

Although reverse vaccinology has been applied to a number of human and animal pathogens, it must be noted that it may not be applicable to all vaccine development projects.

6.5.1 Prediction of Subcellular Localization

Most vaccines require that the antigenic determinants are displayed on the surface of the pathogen as immune factors may be unable to cytoplasmic or inner-membrane proteins [61, 63]. To date, vaccines have targeted an array of surface-displayed adhesins, fimbrial proteins, GPI-anchored antigens, toxins, invasins, and porins [64]. Knowledge on the localization of an antigen additionally provides researchers with clues to the biological function of a protein and its involvement in biological pathways [65].

A vast amount of protein subcellular localization predictors are freely available, and choosing a program suitable for your organism of choice can be challenging. In many cases, a combinatorial approach is required to identify secreted proteins as was the case in the parasitic nematode *Strongyloides ratti* [66].

PSORTb 3.0. The software used for subcellular localization prediction can be divided into two groups. The first uses amino acid sequence for the prediction while the second is annotation based [67]. PSORT, the first computer program based on protein sorting signals was published in 1990. Several improvements have followed, such as the incorporation of machine learning techniques, in order to increase the accuracy of localization prediction in various organisms. The latest version of PSORT, PSORTb 3.0, was published in 2010 and represents one of the most accurate subcellular localization prediction programs for bacteria and can be used for all prokaryotes [68].

Cell-PLoc. A study conducted in 2006 compared several mammalian subcellular localization predictors and determined that no method was sensitive enough to predict the protein localization in both tested datasets accurately. Furthermore, proteins targeted to the secretory pathway were found to be the most difficult to predict [69]. Newer predictors for eukaryotic protein localization include iLoc-Euk, which is the most accurate software taking into account that some proteins can be present at more than one subcellular localizations and even move between these. Other software, such as SherLoc2, includes sequence-based and annotation-based features, phylogenetic profiles, as well as gene ontology terms obtained from the protein sequence [67]. The Cell-PLoc package contains six predictors, Euk-mPLoc, Hum-mPLoc, Plant-PLoc, Gpos-PLoc, Gneg-PLoc, and Virus-PLoc. These predict the subcellular localization of proteins in eukaryotes, human, plants, gram-positive bacteria, gram-negative bacteria, and viruses, respectively, combining different web servers with various approaches [70].

Virus-mPLoc and iLoc-Virus. The subcellular localization of viral proteins in infected cells is of interest as this is directly linked to the health of the host and antiviral drug design [71]. Virus-mPLoc is one of the newer predictors and uses gene ontology, functional domain, as well as evolutionary information. One of the main improvements to previous viral protein localizers is the ability of this program to detect proteins which can be found at multiple localizations [72]. Another web-based software with allegedly improved features is iLoc-Virus [71].

Most proteins are synthesized in the cytosol following sorting to different organelles based on N-terminal sorting signals [73]. For the use in a reverse vaccinology, signal peptides are of interest as these are responsible for the transport of proteins through the secretory pathway in both pro- and eukaryotes, thus, able to result in a localization on or outside the cell surface [74].

SignalP 4.0. A study conducted in 2009 identified SignalP 3.0 as the most accurate predictor compared to 11 others, followed by rapid prediction of signal peptides (RPSP) [75]. Viruses require the host cell machinery for replication and protein synthesis and thus often contain eukaryotic targeting signals and functional domains in order to exploit the host localization mechanisms [76]. Therefore, appropriate

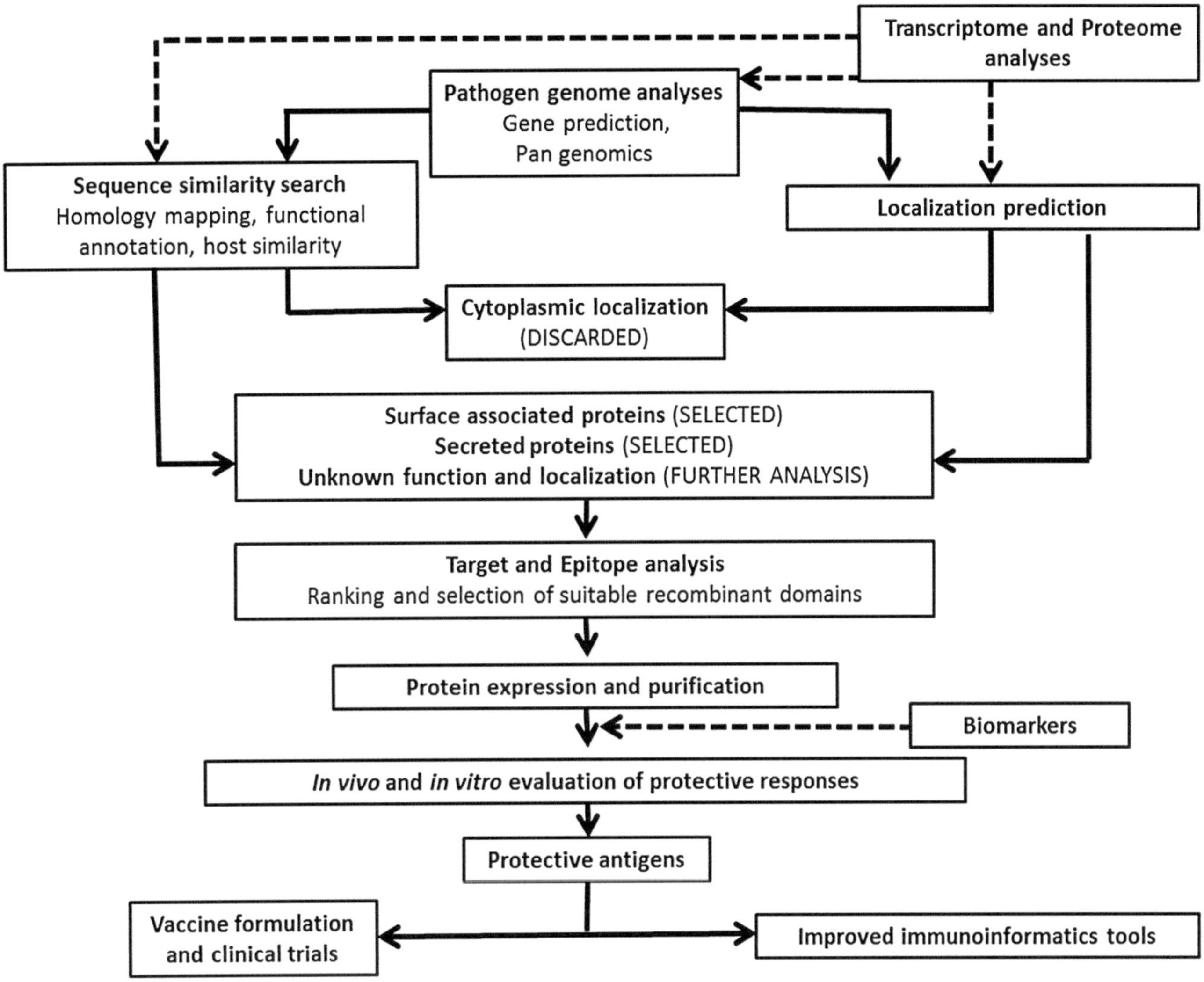

Fig. 6.7 Strategy for the identification of vaccine candidates using a reverse vaccinology approach (Adapted from [112, 113]). The process starts with the analysis of the transcriptome and the proteome of a parasite/pathogen from which predicted surface-associated and secreted proteins are identified following localization prediction and sequence similarity searches. Homology mapping of neutralizing antibodies, functional annotation, and host similarity searches for the prevention of autoimmunity follows. Identified targets may be ranked and used to predict epitopes and suitable recombinant domains and analyze B- and T cell epitope variability. The chosen proteins then have to be expressed and purified followed by evaluation of immune responses using biomarker information if available. Protective antigens can then be used for vaccine formulation and clinical trials and the obtained data can be used to improve available immunoinformatics tools

eukaryotic subcellular localization predictors can be used. Both signal peptides and transmembrane regions have hydrophobic regions and can thus be misinterpreted by software when they occur in the N-terminal region of a protein [77]. To overcome this obstacle SignalP version 4.0 was trained on datasets differentiating between transmembrane region and signal peptide. SignalP versions 3.0 and 4.0 can be used for eukaryotes and gram-positive and gram-negative bacteria. Other softwares, such as the Phobius web server [78] or SPOCTOPUS [79], are available also taking the difficulty of correct prediction between signal peptide and transmembrane region into account.

Transmembrane Protein Helices. Furthermore, it is important to consider the number of transmembrane helices in a protein. Firstly, if only part of a protein is expressed due to experimental constraints, an extracellular domain should be chosen due to its accessibility to the immune system. Secondly, if complete proteins are expressed, it has to be taken into consideration that proteins containing more than one transmembrane domain have been found to be more difficult to express. *Therefore, if one can choose an antigen from a number of available proteins, preference should be given to single-spanning compared to multi-spanning proteins.*

6.5.2 Prediction of Immunogenicity and Epitopes

The prediction of epitopes remains a crucial step in the screening of pathogen protein-coding sequences before experimental confirmation of immunogenicity. Several computational methods are available to date (reviewed in [80–83]) based on either sequence and/or structure.

Sequence-based approaches assume that a similar amino acid sequence leads to a similar protein structure and function. *The ability to detect B and T cell epitopes also depends on a protein's sequence pattern and physicochemical properties such as flexibility, accessibility, hydrophilicity, and charge* [84]. In a comparative study conducted by Yu and colleagues, the use of sequence and protein motifs was found to be most accurate for the prediction of MHC binding. However, with increasing data volume, software-utilizing machine learning techniques become more precise [85]. Although structure-based predictions are possible with methods like homology modeling, these approaches are relatively new and costly and require the knowledge of the three-dimensional structure of proteins. Therefore, the latter approach is not yet commonly used [86]. The most accurate prediction would include several techniques as the strengths of each method can then be combined.

MHC Binders. The prediction of T cell epitopes can be indirectly predicted by the detection of MHC binders. Due to different conformations of MHC I and MHC II proteins, the will bind different molecules [87, 88].

MHC II, in contrast to MHC I, can bind variable peptide lengths, resulting in MHC II binding predictions to have a much lower accuracy than for MHC I. These predictions are not always accurate as some proteins, even though bound to MHC, do not elicit an immune response. For both MHC classes, ligands can be identified either by using predictions for the binding of the peptide to the MHC complex or by predicting the peptide's processing pathway before binding.

POPISK and NetCTLpan. One of the newest software, POPISK, focuses on the prediction of the MHC I-peptide complex sequence which is recognized by the T cell receptors. This recognition should then result in T cell activation and further immune responses [89]. One of the most accurate predictors for cytotoxic T lymphocyte epitopes is NetCTLpan [90]. However, it is known that many different factors play a role in whether a protein results in an immune response or not. Binding affinity to MHC I, for example, is necessary but not sufficient to result in a T cell response [89]. To therefore be able to fully exploit epitope prediction methods, more knowledge about the complex interplay of all factors involved in the immune system is required.

B Cell Epitopes. The prediction of B cell epitopes is a more difficult task than for T cells. One reason for this is that MHC proteins are highly specific in the molecules they bind while a vast amount of short, linear peptides have the potential to be able to bind to antibodies [87]. Due to the fact that two types of B cell epitopes can be distinguished – continuous and discontinuous – different prediction methods must be applied. Methods identifying continuous B cell epitopes are similar to T cell epitope predictors based on protein properties. In contrast, discontinuous B cell epitope prediction requires the knowledge of the 3D structure of the antigen–antibody complex [86].

Discontinuous B Cell Epitopes. This type of prediction is thus very difficult and current software for this purpose show relatively poor performance. Bioinformatics tools for the prediction of discontinuous B cell epitopes started with the obtainment of residue solvent accessibility (CEP server) [91]. Some of the newer software use a large amount of physiochemical as well as structural–geometrical properties included in a Bayesian analysis [92], consensus scoring from different functions (propensity, conservation, energy, contact, surface planarity, and secondary structure composition) [93], and a logistic regression algorithm using B-factor and accessible surface area as structural features in addition to taking the spatial environment for each residue into consideration [94]. Another approach for the identification of discontinuous B cell epitopes uses a new concept of spatial characteristics of antigen residues (a distance-based feature) and three-dimensional structures [95].

VaxiJen. The use of deep panning combining the strengths of phage display with deep sequencing may aid in our understanding of the humoral response to disease, by mapping polyclonal antisera specificities [96]. For the prediction of protective bacterial, viral, and tumor antigens, an alignment-independent method was published in the form of the VaxiJen server based on an auto-cross covariance method [97]. A method including support vector machine classification showed improved results, thus having potential for the improvement of reverse vaccinology approaches [63]. Protein microarrays can also be used to identify proteins expressed during host infection and for the prediction of protein antigenicity [98, 99].

6.5.3 Reverse Vaccinology Platforms

In an attempt to simplify the reverse vaccinology approach, several platforms have been created. This enables a user to repeat the process as often as required with altered stringency conditions in order obtain less vaccine candidates for further evaluation. NERVE (new enhanced reverse vaccinology environment) is a server used for automated reverse vaccinology analyses [100]. It does have the drawback of being computationally complicated. Several filters are used which allow the prediction of a protein's localization (PSORTb) [101] (required to be non-cytoplasmic) and the identification of adhesins (SPAAN) [102]. Furthermore, the number of transmembrane helices (required to be <2) is identified according to HMMTOP [103]. Similarity searches are done in order to prevent significant similarity to human proteins, identify homology to known antigens, and aid functional annotation.

Vaxign and VaxiJen. Vaxign is a web-based platform that searches for antigens from over 70 pathogenic genomes, identifying protein conservation between genomes and excluding sequences present in nonpathogenic organisms. It includes a number of different programs for the prediction of a protein's subcellular localization, number of transmembrane helices, adhesion probabilities, functional analysis, and immune epitopes (MHC class I and II). Furthermore, the server allows comparison of the input sequences to the host in order to prevent any cross-reactions and consequent harming of the host. Currently, this server only allows the processing of high-throughput data of microbes. Systems allowing insight into eukaryotic organisms are not available to date, but VaxiJen has been able to show impressive prediction accuracy of up to 70–89 % for bacterial, viral, and tumor antigens and 78–97 % accuracy for endoparasitic and fungal antigens [104, 105].

In conclusion, vaccine development has come a long way from trial and error testing of live attenuated pathogens to the development of the first subunit vaccines. In the post-genomic era, the availability of a vast array of "omics" data coupled with the ability to integrate this data, is fast enabling researchers to word towards a multidisciplinary, exciting, yet challenging future for vaccine design. A glossary of software and databases mentioned in this chapter is given in Table 6.3.

Table 6.3 Glossary of software and databases mentioned in this chapter

Name	Description	Reference
BLAST	Similarity searches for various applications	[15]
ORF identification		
Glimmer	Bacteria, archaea, viruses	[7]
GeneMark.hmm	Bacteria	[8]
Prodigal	Prokaryotes	[9]
AUGUSTUS	Eukaryotes	[13]
GNOMON	Eukaryotes	http://0-www.ncbi.nlm.nih.gov.innopac.up.ac.za/genome/guide/gnomon.shtml
MAKER	Eukaryotes, annotation pipeline	[12]
Functional annotation		
PIR	Protein information resource	[16]
Pfam	Protein families database	[17]
SWISS-PROT	Manually annotated and reviewed section of UniProt knowledge base	[18]
Uni-Prot	Knowledge base	[19]
COG	Database	[20]
GO	Database	[21]
Subcellular localization		
PSORT	Bacteria, eukaryotes	[68]
PSORTb v3.0	Prokaryotes	[68]
iLoc-Euk	Eukaryotes	[65]
SherLoc2	Eukaryotes	[67]
Cell-PLoc	Eukaryotes, Prokaryotes, Viruses	[70]
Virus-mPloc	Viruses	[72]
iLoc-Virus	Viruses	[71]
Signal peptide		
SignalP 4.0	Signal peptide prediction	[114]
Phobius	Signal peptide prediction	[78]
SPOCTOPUS	Signal peptide prediction	[79]
Epitopes		
POPISK	MHC-I predictor	[89]
NetCTLpan	CTL predictor	[90]
CEP	Prediction of conformational epitopes	[91]

(continued)

Table 6.3 (continued)

Name	Description	Reference
VaxiJen	Viral, tumor, bacterial protective antigens	[97]
Epitope conservancy tool	Database of conserved epitopes	[115]
Reverse vaccinology platforms		
NERVE	Pipeline	[100]
Vaxign	Pipeline	[116]
Software packages and databases for integration of "omics" data		
RefDIC	Reference genomics database of immune cells	[48]
IIDB	Innate immune database	[49]
WIBL	Workbench for integrative biological learning	[50]
Guided clustering	Combines experimental and clinical data	[51]
EchoBasE	Database for *E. coli*	[52]
integrOmics		[53]
bioPIXIE	Network predictions for *S. cerevisiae*	[47]
VESPA	Genomic annotation of prokaryotes	[54]
openBIS		[55]
GPS-Prot	Platform for integrating host–pathogen interaction data	[56]
Booly	Data integration platform	[57]
PARE	Protein abundance and mRNA expression	[58]
Other		
IRIS	Immune response in silico	[36]
Vaxjo	Curation, storage, and analysis of vaccine adjuvants	[117]

References

1. Berzofsky, J.A.: Immunodominance in T lymphocyte recognition. Immunol. Lett. **8**(2), 83–92 (1988)
2. Dietrich, G., Griot-Wenk, M., Metcalfe, I.C., Lang, A.B., Viret, J.F.: Experience with registered mucosal vaccines. Vaccine **21**(7–8), 678–683 (2003)
3. Luciani, F., Bull, R.A., Lloyd, A.R.: Next generation deep sequencing and vaccine design: today and tomorrow. Trends Biotechnol. **30**, 443–452 (2012)
4. Seib, K.L., Zhao, X., Rappuoli, R.: Developing vaccines in the era of genomics: a decade of reverse vaccinology. Clin. Microbiol. Infect. **18**, 1–8 (2012)
5. Cheng, H., Chan, W.S., Wang, D., Liu, S., Zhou, Y.: Small open reading frames: current prediction techniques and future prospect. Curr. Protein Pept. Sci. **12**, 503–507 (2011)
6. Yandell, M., Ence, D.: A beginner's guide to eukaryotic genome annotation. Nat. Rev. Genet. **13**, 329–342 (2012)
7. Delcher, A.L., Bratke, K.A., Powers, E.C., Salzberg, S.L.: Identifying bacterial genes and endosymbiont DNA with Glimmer. Bioinformatics **23**, 673–679 (2007). doi:10.1093/bioinformatics/btm009
8. Lukashin, A.V., Borodovsky, M.: GeneMark.hmm: new solutions for gene finding. Nucleic Acids Res. **26**, 1107–1115 (1998). doi:10.1093/nar/26.4.1107
9. Hyatt, D., et al.: Prodigal: prokaryotic gene recognition and translation initiation site identification. BMC Bioinf. **11**, 119 (2010)
10. Pinheiro, C.S., et al.: Computational vaccinology: an important strategy to discover new potential *S. mansoni* vaccine candidates. J. Biomed. Biotechnol. **503068**, 2011 (2011). doi:10.1155/2011/503068
11. Ecker, J.R., et al.: Genomics: ENCODE explained. Nature **489**, 52–55 (2012). doi:10.1038/489052a
12. Cantarel, B.L., et al.: MAKER: an easy-to-use annotation pipeline designed for emerging model organism genomes. Genome Res. **18**, 188–196 (2008). doi:10.1101/gr.6743907
13. Keller, O., Kollmar, M., Stanke, M., Waack, S.: A novel hybrid gene prediction method employing protein multiple sequence alignments. Bioinformatics (2011). doi:10.1093/bioinformatics/btr010
14. Smandi, S., et al.: Methodology optimizing SAGE library tag-to-gene mapping: application to Leishmania. BMC Res. Notes **5**, 74 (2012). doi:10.1186/1756-0500-5-74
15. Altschul, S.F., Gish, W., Miller, W., Myers, E.W., Lipman, D.J.: Basic local alignment search tool. J. Mol. Biol. **215**, 403–410 (1990)
16. Barker, W.C., et al.: The protein information resource (PIR). Nucleic Acids Res. **28**, 41–44 (2000)
17. Punta, M., et al.: The Pfam protein families database. Nucleic Acids Res. **40**, D290–D301 (2012). doi:10.1093/nar/gkr1065
18. Boeckmann, B., et al.: The SWISS-PROT protein knowledgebase and its supplement TrEMBL in 2003. Nucleic Acids Res. **31**, 365–370 (2003). doi:10.1093/nar/gkg095
19. Magrane, M., Consortium, U.: UniProt Knowledgebase: a hub of integrated protein data. Database (2011). doi:10.1093/database/bar009 (2011)
20. Tatusov, R.L., Galperin, M.Y., Natale, D.A., Koonin, E.V.: The COG database: a tool for genome-scale analysis of protein functions and evolution. Nucleic Acids Res. **28**, 33–36 (2000). doi:10.1093/nar/28.1.33
21. GeneOntologyConsortium: The Gene Ontology (GO) database and informatics resource. Nucleic Acids Res. **32**, D258–D261 (2004). doi:10.1093/nar/gkh036
22. Yon Rhee, S., Wood, V., Dolinski, K., Draghici, S.: Use and misuse of the gene ontology annotations. Nat. Rev. Genet. **9**, 509–515 (2008)

23. Gomez, A., et al.: Gene ontology function prediction in mollicutes using protein-protein association networks. BMC Syst. Biol. **5**, 49 (2011). doi:10.1186/1752-0509-5-49
24. Zhang, Q.C., et al.: Structure-based prediction of protein-protein interactions on a genome-wide scale. Nature **490**, 556–560 (2012)
25. Wass, M.N., Barton, G., Sternberg, M.J.E.: CombFunc: predicting protein function using heterogeneous data sources. Nucleic Acids Res. **40**, W466–W470 (2012). doi:10.1093/nar/gks489
26. Fu, Y., et al.: Novel insights into the transcriptome of *Dirofilaria immitis*. PLoS One **7**, e41639 (2012). doi:10.1371/journal.pone.0041639
27. Hedman, A.K., Li, M.S., Langford, P.R., Kroll, J.S.: Transcriptional profiling of serogroup B *Neisseria meningitidis* growing in human blood: an approach to vaccine antigen discovery. PLoS One **7**, e39718 (2012). doi:10.1371/journal.pone.0039718
28. Amiruddin, N., et al.: Characterisation of full-length cDNA sequences provides insights into the *Eimeria tenella* transcriptome. BMC Genomics **13**, 21 (2012). doi:10.1186/1471-2164-13-21
29. Maritz-Olivier, C., van Zyl, W., Stutzer, C.: A systematic, functional genomics and reverse vaccinology approach to the identification of vaccine candidates in the cattle tick, *Rhipicephalus microplus*. Ticks Tick Borne Dis. **3**, 179–189 (2012)
30. Savas, J.N., Stein, B.D., Wu, C.C., Yates, J.R.: Mass spectrometry accelerates membrane protein analysis. Trends Biochem. Sci. **36**, 388–396 (2011). doi:10.1016/j.tibs.2011.04.005
31. Haralambieva, I.H., Poland, G.A.: Vaccinomics, predictive vaccinology and the future of vaccine development. Future Microbiol. **5**, 1757–1760 (2010). doi:10.2217/fmb.10.146
32. Acharya, P., et al.: Clinical proteomics of the neglected human malarial parasite *Plasmodium vivax*. PLoS One **6**, e26623 (2011). doi:10.1371/journal.pone.0026623
33. Minning, T.A., Weatherly, D.B., Atwood, J., Orlando, R., Tarleton, R.L.: The steady-state transcriptome of the four major life-cycle stages of *Trypanosoma cruzi*. BMC Genomics **10**, 370 (2009). doi:10.1186/1471-2164-10-370
34. Jagusztyn-Krynicka, E.K., Roszczenko, P., Grabowska, A.: Impact of proteomics on anti-*Mycobacterium tuberculosis* (MTB) vaccine development. Pol. J. Microbiol. **58**, 281–287 (2009)
35. Buonaguro, L., Wang, E., Tornesello, M.L., Buonaguro, F.M., Marincola, F.M.: Systems biology applied to vaccine and immunotherapy development. BMC Syst. Biol. **5**, 146–157 (2011)
36. Abbas, A.R., et al.: Immune response in silico (IRIS): immune-specific genes identified from a compendium of microarray expression data. Genes Immun. **6**, 319–331 (2005). doi:10.1038/sj.gene.6364173
37. Banchereau, J., et al.: Harnessing human dendritic cell subsets to design novel vaccines. Ann. N. Y. Acad. Sci. **1174**, 24–32 (2009). doi:10.1111/j.1749-6632.2009.04999.x
38. Ovsyannikova, I.G., Poland, G.A.: Vaccinomics: current findings, challenges and novel approaches for vaccine development. AAPS J. **13**, 438–444 (2011). doi:10.1208/s12248-011-9281-x
39. Bernstein, A., Pulendran, B., Rappuoli, R.: Systems vaccinomics: the road ahead for vaccinology. OMICS **15**, 529–531 (2011). doi:10.1089/omi.2011.0022
40. Kennedy, R.B., Poland, G.A.: The top five "game changers" in vaccinology: toward rational and directed vaccine development. OMICS **15**, 533–537 (2011). doi:10.1089/omi.2011.0012
41. Zhang, W., Li, F., Nie, L.: Integrating multiple 'omics' analysis for microbial biology: application and methodologies. Microbiology **156**, 287–301 (2010). doi:10.1099/mic.0.034793-0
42. Yang, D., et al.: RNA-seq liver transcriptome analysis reveals an activated MHC-I pathway and an inhibited MHC-II pathway at the early stage of vaccine immunization in zebrafish. BMC Genomics **13**, 319 (2012). doi:10.1186/1471-2164-13-319
43. Toufeer, M., et al.: Gene expression profiling of dendritic cells reveals important mechanisms associated with predisposition to *Staphylococcus* infections. PLoS One **6**, e22147 (2011). doi:10.1371/journal.pone.0022147
44. Wang, F., et al.: Deep-sequencing analysis of the mouse transcriptome response to infection with *Brucella melitensis* strains of differing virulence. PLoS One **6**, e28485 (2011). doi:10.1371/journal.pone.0028485
45. Kaleta, C., de Figueiredo, L.F., Heiland, I., Klamt, S., Schuster, S.: Special issue: integration of OMICs datasets into metabolic pathway analysis. Biosystems **105**, 107–108 (2011). doi:10.1016/j.biosystems.2011.05.008
46. Joyce, A.R., Palsson, B.O.: The model organism as a system: integrating 'omics' data sets. Nat.Rev. Mol. Cell Biol. **7**, 198–210 (2006). doi:10.1038/nrm1857
47. Myers, C.L., Chiriac, C., Troyanskaya, O.G.: Discovering biological networks from diverse functional genomic data. Methods Mol. Biol. **563**, 157–175 (2009). doi:10.1007/978-1-60761-175-2_9
48. Hijikata, A., et al.: Construction of an open-access database that integrates cross-reference information from the transcriptome and proteome of immune cells. Bioinformatics **23**, 2934–2941 (2007). doi:10.1093/bioinformatics/btm430
49. Korb, M., et al.: The Innate Immune Database (IIDB). BMC Immunol. **9**, 7 (2008). doi:10.1186/1471-2172-9-7
50. Lesk, V., Taubert, J., Rawlings, C., Dunbar, S., Muggleton, S.: WIBL: workbench for integrative biological learning. J. Integr. Bioinform. **8**, 156 (2011). doi:10.2390/biecoll-jib-2011-156
51. Maneck, M., Schrader, A., Kube, D., Spang, R.: Genomic data integration using guided clustering. Bioinformatics **27**, 2231–2238 (2011). doi:10.1093/bioinformatics/btr363
52. Misra, R.V., Horler, R.S.P., Reindl, W., Goryanin, I.I., Thomas, G.H.: *Echo*BASE: an integrated post-genomic database for *Escherichia coli*. Nucleic Acids Res. (2005). doi:10.1093/nar/gki028
53. Le Cao, K.A., Gonzalez, I., Dejean, S.: IntegrOmics: an R package to unravel relationships between two omics datasets. Bioinformatics **25**, 2855–2856 (2009). doi:10.1093/bioinformatics/btp515
54. Peterson, E.S., et al.: VESPA: software to facilitate genomic annotation of prokaryotic organisms through integration of proteomic and transcriptomic data. BMC Genomics **13**, 131 (2012). doi:10.1186/1471-2164-13-131
55. Bauch, A., et al.: OpenBIS: a flexible framework for managing and analyzing complex data in biology research. BMC Bioinf. **12**, 468 (2011). doi:10.1186/1471-2105-12-468
56. Fahey, M.E., et al.: GPS-Prot: a web-based visualization platform for integrating host-pathogen interaction data. BMC Bioinf. **12**, 298 (2011). doi:10.1186/1471-2105-12-298
57. Do, L.H., Esteves, F.F., Karten, H.J., Bier, E.: Booly: a new data integration platform. BMC Bioinf. **11**, 513 (2010). doi:10.1186/1471-2105-11-513
58. Yu, E.Z., Burba, A.E.C., Gerstein, M.: PARE: a tool for comparing protein abundance and mRNA expression data. BMC Bioinf. **8**, 309 (2007). doi:10.1186/1471-2105-8-309
59. Dormitzer, P.R., Ulmer, J.B., Rappuoli, R.: Structure-based antigen design: a strategy for next generation vaccines. Trends Biotechnol. **26**, 659–667 (2008)
60. Nuccitelli, A., et al.: Structure-based approach to rationally design a chimeric protein for an effective vaccine against Group B *Streptococcus* infections. Proc. Natl. Acad. Sci. **108**, 10278–10283 (2011). doi:10.1073/pnas.1106590108
61. Rappuoli, R.: Reverse vaccinology. Curr. Opin. Microbiol. **3**, 445–450 (2000)
62. Pizza, M., et al.: Identification of vaccine candidates against serogroup *B. meningococcus* by whole-genome sequencing. Science **287**, 1816–1820 (2000). doi:10.1126/science.287.5459.1816
63. Bowman, B., et al.: Improving reverse vaccinology with a machine learning approach. Vaccine **29**, 8156–8164 (2011)
64. Vivona, S., et al.: Computer-aided biotechnology: from immunoinformatics to reverse vaccinology. Trends Biotechnol. **26**, 190–200 (2008). doi:10.1016/j.tibtech.2007.12.006
65. Chou, K.-C., Wu, Z.-C., Xiao, X.: iLoc-Euk: a multi-label classifier for predicting the subcellular localization of singleplex and

multiplex eukaryotic proteins. PLoS One **6**, e18258 (2011). doi:10.1371/journal.pone.0018258
66. Garg, G., Ranganathan, S.: *In silico* secretome analysis approach for next generation sequencing transcriptomic data. BMC Genomics **12**, 514–524 (2011)
67. Briesemeister, S., et al.: SherLoc2: a high-accuracy hybrid method for predicting subcellular localization of proteins. J. Proteome Res. **8**, 5363–5366 (2009). doi:10.1021/pr900665y
68. Yu, N.Y., et al.: PSORTb 3.0: improved protein subcellular localization prediction with refined localization subcategories and predictive capabilities for all prokaryotes. Bioinformatics **26**, 1608–1615 (2010). doi:10.1093/bioinformatics/btq249
69. Sprenger, J., Fink, J., Teasdale, R.: Evaluation and comparison of mammalian subcellular localization prediction methods. BMC Bioinf. **7**, S3 (2006). doi:10.1186/1471-2105-7-S5-S3
70. Chou, K.-C., Shen, H.-B.: Cell-PLoc: a package of web servers for predicting subcellular localization of proteins in various organisms. Nat. Protoc. **3**, 153–162 (2008)
71. Xiao, X., Wu, Z.-C., Chou, K.-C.: iLoc-Virus: a multi-label learning classifier for identifying the subcellular localization of virus proteins with both single and multiple sites. J. Theor. Biol. **284**, 42–51 (2011)
72. Shen, H.-B., Chou, K.-C.: Virus-mPLoc: a fusion classifier for viral protein subcellular location prediction by incorporating multiple sites. J. Biomol. Struct. Dyn. **28**, 175–186 (2010)
73. Bannai, H., Tamada, Y., Maruyama, O., Nakai, K., Miyano, S.: Extensive feature detection of N-terminal protein sorting signals. Bioinformatics **18**, 298–305 (2002). doi:10.1093/bioinformatics/18.2.298
74. Nielsen, H., Engelbrecht, J., Brunak, S., von Heijne, G.: Identification of prokaryotic and eukaryotic signal peptides and prediction of their cleavage sites. Protein Eng. **10**, 1–6 (1997). doi:10.1093/protein/10.1.1
75. Choo, K.H., Tan, T.W., Ranganathan, S.: A comprehensive assessment of N-terminal signal peptides prediction methods. BMC Bioinf. **10**, S2 (2009). doi:10.1186/1471-2105-10-S15-S2
76. Scott, M.S., Oomen, R., Thomas, D.Y., Hallett, M.T.: Predicting the subcellular localization of viral proteins within a mammalian host cell. J. Virol. **3**, 24 (2006). doi:10.1186/1743-422X-3-24
77. Petersen, T.N., Brunak, S., Von Heijne, G., Nielsen, H.: SignalP 4.0: discriminating signal peptides from transmembrane regions. Nat. Methods **8**, 785–786 (2011). doi:10.1038/nmeth.1701
78. Käll, L., Krogh, A., Sonnhammer, E.: Advantages of combined transmembrane topology and signal peptide prediction – the Phobius web server. Nucleic Acids Res. **35**, W429–W432 (2007). doi:10.1093/nar/gkm256
79. Viklund, H.K., Bernsel, A., Skwark, M., Elofsson, A.: SPOCTOPUS: a combined predictor of signal peptides and membrane protein topology. Bioinformatics **24**, 2928–2929 (2008). doi:10.1093/bioinformatics/btn550
80. Chen, P., Rayner, S., Hu, K.H.: Advances of bioinformatics tools applied in virus epitopes prediction. Virol. Sin. **26**, 1–7 (2011). doi:10.1007/s12250-011-3159-4
81. Flower, D.R. Vaccines data driven prediction of binders, epitopes and immunogenecity. In: Flower, D.R. (eds.). Wiley-Blackwell, Chichester (2008)
82. Iurescia, S., Fioretti, D., Fazio, V.M., Rinaldi, M.: Epitope-driven DNA vaccine design employing immunoinformatics against B cell lymphoma: a biotech's challenge. Biotechnol. Adv. **30**, 372–383 (2012)
83. Sirskyj, D., Diaz-Mitoma, F., Golshani, A., Kumar, A., Azizi, A.: Innovative bioinformatic approaches for developing peptide-based vaccines against hypervariable viruses. Immunol. Cell Biol. **89**, 81–89 (2011). doi:10.1038/icb.2010.65
84. Yang, X., Yu, X.: An introduction to epitope prediction methods and software. Rev. Med. Virol. **19**, 77–96 (2009)
85. Yu, K., Petrovsky, N., Schönbach, C., Koh, J., Brusic, V.: Methods for prediction of peptide binding to MHC molecules: a comparative study. Mol. Med. **8**, 137–148 (2002)
86. Davydov, Y.I., Tonevitsky, A.G.: Prediction of linear B cell epitopes. Mol. Biol. **43**, 150–158 (2009)
87. Zhang, Q., et al.: Immune epitope database analysis resource (IEDB-AR). Nucleic Acids Res. **36**, W513–W518 (2008). doi:10.1093/nar/gkn254
88. Van Bergen, J., et al.: Get into the groove! Targeting antigens to MHC class II. Immunol. Rev. **172**, 87–96 (1999)
89. Tung, C.-W., Ziehm, M., Kamper, A., Kohlbacher, O., Ho, S.-Y.: POPISK: T cell reactivity prediction using support vector machines and string kernels. BMC Bioinf. **12**, 446 (2011). doi:10.1186/1471-2105-12-446
90. Stranzl, T., Larsen, M., Lundegaard, C., Nielsen, M.: NetCTLpan: pan-specific MHC class I pathway epitope predictions. Immunogenetics **62**, 357–368 (2010). doi:10.1007/s00251-010-0441-4
91. Kulkarni-Kale, U., Bhosle, S., Kolaskar, A.S.: CEP: a conformational epitope prediction server. Nucleic Acids Res. **33**, W168–W171 (2005). doi:10.1093/nar/gki460
92. Rubinstein, N.D., Mayrose, I., Pupko, T.: A machine-learning approach for predicting B cell epitopes. Mol. Immunol. **46**, 840–847 (2009)
93. Liang, S., Zheng, D., Zhang, C., Zacharias, M.: Prediction of antigenic epitopes on protein surfaces by consensus scoring. BMC Bioinf. **10**, 302 (2009). doi:10.1186/1471-2105-10-302
94. Liu, R., Hu, J.: Prediction of discontinuous B cell epitopes using logistic regression and structural information. J. Proteomics Bioinformatics **4**, 010–015 (2011)
95. Zhang, W., et al.: Prediction of conformational B cell epitopes from 3D structures by random forests with a distance-based feature. BMC Bioinf **12**, 341 (2011). doi:10.1186/1471-2105-12-341
96. Ryvkin, A., et al.: Deep Panning: steps towards probing the IgOme. PLoS One **7**, e41469 (2012). doi:10.1371/journal.pone.0041469
97. Doytchinova, I.A., Flower, D.R.: Identifying candidate subunit vaccines using an alignment-independent method based on principal amino acid properties. Vaccine **25**, 856–866 (2007)
98. Magnan, C.N., et al.: High-throughput prediction of protein antigenicity using protein microarray data. Bioinformatics **26**, 2936–2943 (2010). doi:10.1093/bioinformatics/btq551
99. Grandi, G.: Genomics and proteomics in reverse vaccines. Methods Biochem. Anal. **49**, 379–393 (2006)
100. Vivona, S., Bernante, F., Filippini, F.: NERVE: new enhanced reverse vaccinology environment. BMC Biotechnol. **6**, 35 (2006). doi:10.1186/1472-6750-6-35
101. Gardy, J.L., et al.: PSORT-B: improving protein subcellular localization prediction for Gram-negative bacteria. Nucleic Acids Res. **31**, 3613–3617 (2003). doi:10.1093/nar/gkg602
102. Sachdeva, G., Kumar, K., Jain, P., Ramachandran, S.: SPAAN: a software program for prediction of adhesins and adhesin-like proteins using neural networks. Bioinformatics **21**, 483–491 (2005). doi:10.1093/bioinformatics/bti028
103. Tusnády, G.E., Simon, I.: Principles governing amino acid composition of integral membrane proteins: application to topology prediction. J. Mol. Biol. **283**, 489–506 (1998)
104. Doytchinova, I.A., Flower, D.R.: VaxiJen: a server for prediction of protective antigens, tumour antigens and subunit vaccines. BMC Bioinf. **8**, 4 (2007). doi:10.1186/1471-2105-8-4
105. Flower, D.R., Macdonald, I.K., Ramakrishnan, K., Davies, M.N., Doytchinova, I.A.: Computer aided selection of candidate vaccine antigens. Immunome Res. **6**(Suppl 2), S1 (2010). doi:10.1186/1745-7580-6-s2-s1
106. Lawrence, E.: Henderson's dictionary of biology. Pearson Education Limited, Harlow (2005)

107. Lillehoj, H.S., Kim, C.H., Keeler, C.L., Zhang, S.: Immunogenomic approaches to study host immunity to enteric pathogens. Poult. Sci. **86**, 1491–1500 (2007)
108. Ohara, O.: From transcriptome analysis to immunogenomics: current status and future direction. FEBS Lett. **583**, 1662–1667 (2009)
109. Snoep, J.L., Bruggeman, F., Olivier, B.G., Westerhoff, H.V.: Towards building the silicon cell: a modular approach. Biosystems **83**, 207–216 (2006)
110. Tjalsma, H., Schaeps, R.M.J., Swinkels, D.W.: Immunoproteomics: from biomarker discovery to diagnostic applications. Peoteomics Clin. Appl. **2**, 167–180 (2008)
111. Poland, G.A., Ovsyannikova, I.G., Jacobson, R.M., Smith, D.I.: Heterogeneity in vaccine immune response: the role of immunogenetics and the emerging field of vaccinomics. Clin. Pharmacol. Ther. **82**, 653–664 (2007). doi:10.1038/sj.clpt.6100415
112. Bagnoli, F., et al.: In: Rappuoli, R., Bagnoli, F. (eds.) Vaccine design. Caister Academic Press, Norfolk (2011)
113. Sollner, J., et al.: Concept and application of a computational vaccinology workflow. Immunome Res. **6**(Suppl 2), S7 (2010). doi:10.1186/1745-7580-6-s2-s7
114. Petersen, T.N., Brunak, S., Von Heijne, G., Nielsen, H.: SignalP 4.0: discriminating signal peptides from transmembrane regions. Nat. Methods **8**, 784–786 (2011)
115. Bui, H.-H., Sidney, J., Li, W., Fusseder, N., Sette, A.: Development of an epitope conservancy analysis tool to facilitate the design of epitope-based diagnostics and vaccines. BMC Bioinf. **8**, 361 (2007). doi:10.1186/1471-2105-5-361
116. He, Y., Xiang, Z., Mobley, H.: Vaxign: the first web-based vaccine design program for reverse vaccinology and applications for vaccine development. J. Biomed. Biotechnol. (2010). doi:10.1155/2010/297505 (2010)
117. Sayers, S., Ulysse, G., Xiang, Z., He, Y.: Vaxjo: a web-based vaccine adjuvant database and its application for analysis of vaccine adjuvants and their uses in vaccine development. J. Biomed. Biotechnol. **13**, 2012 (2012). doi:10.1155/2012/831486

7 Adjuvants

Contents

7.1 Adjuvants: Immunology's Dirty Secret

The author of this book himself learnt the *dirty little secret* of vaccines the hard way:

> …So far all experiments with a therapeutical DNA vaccine against the equine arteritis virus (EAV) on the Clinic for Large Animals of the University of Leipzig/Germany, Faculty for Veterinary Medicine were successful. All horses developed a strong humoral and cellular response upon repeated subcutaneous immunization in a first clinical study. The great day came; we started to test our innovative vaccine at a national horse breeding farm near Hannover/Germany in a second study. Against all odds, the results of this important study were negative and the level of frustration in our team was tremendous…

This remembered the early days of commercial vaccine manufacture, when significant variations in the effectiveness of different batches of the same vaccine were observed. These variations were due to contamination of the manufacturing process. However, a stringent cleaning reduced the effectiveness of the vaccines. The dirty contaminants were responsible for driving the immune response (Deciphering Immunology's Dirty Secret by Kate Travis, 2007, The Scientist).

> ….Fortunately, we had stored reference samples of all horse vaccines and analyzed the two different manufactured vaccines. Much to our surprise we found that all vaccines of the first successful study were contaminated with endotoxin, LPS. Unbelievable. The purification process failed. The second study at a national horse-breeding farm used a vaccine manufactured by another biotech company - with a different purification protocol: the product was highly purified and without any efficacy. This was our dirty secret. The dirty contaminants were responsible for driving the immune response. Meanwhile, we routinely include bits of detoxified LPS (see No 6 in this chapter) as adjuvant of animal DNA vaccines. LPS induce Th1-type responses as described later.

7.2 Overview of Current Adjuvants

Adjuvants have been used for decades to improve the immune response to vaccine antigens. Strong vaccines such as attenuated live vaccines or vector-driven vaccines induce an effective

M. Giese, *Introduction to Molecular Vaccinology*, DOI 10.1007/978-3-319-25832-4_7

humoral and also a cellular immune response to the administered antigens with a long-term protection against the infection. Vaccines based on recombinant peptides, polysaccharides, nucleic acids, or killed vaccines share weak antigens and are generally insufficiently immunogenic. For those vaccines, adjuvants or combinations of various adjuvants are helpful to potentiate or modulate the immune response (e.g., increase, accelerate, prolong, and/or possibly target) or modulate to a different type (e.g., switch a Th1 immune response to a Th2 response or a humoral response to a cytotoxic T cell response).

Adjuvants can be classified according to their source (natural, synthetic, or endogenous), mechanism of action, or physical or chemical properties. The current most common described adjuvant classes are presented in Table 7.1.

The oldest and still used adjuvant is alum, already discovered by Alexander Glenny in 1926: toxoid precipitated with aluminum potassium sulfate induced a stronger antibody production when injected into guinea pigs than soluble toxoid alone [1, 14].

Table 7.1 Adjuvants, classified according to their source, based on EMEA/CHMP/VEG/134716/2004

1. Mineral salts	2. Oil emulsions and surfactant based formulations	3. Particulate adjuvants
• Alum salts (Al, aluminum hydroxide and aluminum phosphate)	• MF59 (microfluidised detergent stabilised oil-in-water emulsion • QS21 (purified saponin) • AS02 [SBAS2] (oil-in-water emulsion + MPL + QS-21) • ISA-51 and ISA-720 (stabilised water-in-oil emulsion)	• virosomes (unilamellar liposomal vehicles) • AS04 ([SBAS4] Al salt with MPL) • ISCOMS (structured complex of saponins and lipids) • PLG (polylactide co-glycolide)
4. Microbial derivatives (natural and synthetic)	**5. Endogenous human immunomodulators**	**6. Inert vehicles**
• MPL (monophosphoryl lipid A) • AGP [RC-529] (synthetic acylated monosaccharide) • OM-174 (lipid A derivative) • CpG (synthetic oligonucleotides) • LT and CT (modified bacterial toxins, heat-labile and cholera toxin)	• huGM-CSF, huIL-12 (human granulocyte macrophage colony-stimulating factor; interleukin)	• gold particles

7.3 Aluminum-Containing Formulas[1]

Today, alum is the most common adjuvant used in approved prophylactic vaccines because of its excellent safety profile and ability to enhance protective humoral immune responses. Currently, alum is still the only licensed vaccine adjuvant in the United States. In Europe, however, since the 1990s of the last century MF59, an oil-in-water emulsion, MPL (monophospholipid A, an LPS analog)+alum and AS03 are also approved for use [2, 3, 9]. In veterinary medicine, aluminum adjuvants have been used in a large number of vaccine formulations against viral and bacterial diseases [4].

7.3.1 Formulation of Aluminum-Containing Adjuvants

Numerous inaccuracies are found in literature when referred to the term “alum.” The most used term “alum” only applies to aluminum potassium sulfate [5, 6] (Table 7.2). Since problems have occurred during manufacturing, alum is not used anymore in vaccines. Instead, several other insoluble aluminum salts are used, such as aluminum hydroxide and aluminum phosphate, as they can be prepared in a more standardized manner and capture antigen by direct adsorption. Two different adsorption forces prevail adsorptive interaction between the antigen and the adjuvant [7, 8].

Electrostatic Interactions. They occur most strongly between negatively charged proteins and aluminum hydroxide and between positively charged proteins and aluminum phosphate. Anions present at time of preparation may co-precipitate and change the characteristics of “pure” aluminum hydroxide.

One very critical example of an anion having such influence is phosphate. Exposure of aluminum hydroxide adjuvant and phosphorylated antigens to phosphate ions in the formulation should be minimized to produce maximum adsorption of the antigen [10, 11].

Adsorption Force. Anionic ligand exchange is a covalent interaction that occurs when an antigen contains a phosphate group that can displace a hydroxyl group on the adjuvant surface. Ligand exchange is the strongest adsorption force and can occur even when an electrostatic repulsive force is present [12, 13]. Antigens that adsorb to aluminum-containing adjuvants by electrostatic attraction are more likely to elute upon intramuscular or subcutaneous administration than antigens that adsorb by ligand exchange. Antigen released from the adjuvant, antigen trapped in void spaces within the adjuvant, as well as antigen adsorbed to aluminum-containing adjuvants are all present for proper uptake of antigen by dendritic cells (DCs). Of note, absorbed antigen to either aluminum hydroxide or aluminum phosphate adjuvant can be completely eluted within 4 h or 15 min, respectively [7].

7.3.2 Working Mechanism

Three potential mechanisms are frequently cited to explain how adjuvants increase humoral immunity, although scarce experimental evidence is publicly available: firstly, the formation of a depot by which the antigen is slowly released to enhance the antibody production; secondly, the induction of inflammation, thus recruiting and activating antigen-presenting cells that capture the antigen [5, 6]; and thirdly, the conversion of soluble antigen into a particulate form so that it is phagocytosed by antigen-presenting cells such as macrophages, DCs, and B cells. The main theory has been that depot formation and the associated slow release of antigen [7, 15] are responsible for alum enhancement of antigen presentation and subsequent T and B cell responses. However, recently several papers show that the depot formation is dispensable for the adjuvanticity of alum [10, 11].

7.3.2.1 Cellular Pathways Activated by Aluminum-Containing Adjuvants

Injection of alum induces inflammation at the injection site, being it subcutaneous, intramuscular, or, in an experimental setting, intraperitoneal (Fig. 7.1). Within several hours after

[1] Mechanism of adjuvanticity of aluminum-containing formulas by *Bart N Lambrecht and Mirjam Kool* in Molecular Vaccines – From Prophylaxis to Therapy, Volume 2, Springer-Verlag Wien, 2013, Ed. Matthias Giese.

Table 7.2 Overview of different aluminum-containing adjuvant formulations

Commercial name	Chemical formulation	Chemical name	Used as adjuvant in
Alum	$AlK(SO_4)_2 \bullet 12H_2O$	Aluminum potassium sulfate	Not used anymore
Inject-alum	$Al(OH)_3+Mg(OH)_2$	Aluminum hydroxide and magnesium hydroxide	Experimental immunology
Alhydrogel	$Al(OH)_3$	Aluminum hydroxide	Human and veterinary vaccines
Adju-Phos	$Al(PO_4)_3$	Aluminum phosphate	Human and veterinary vaccines

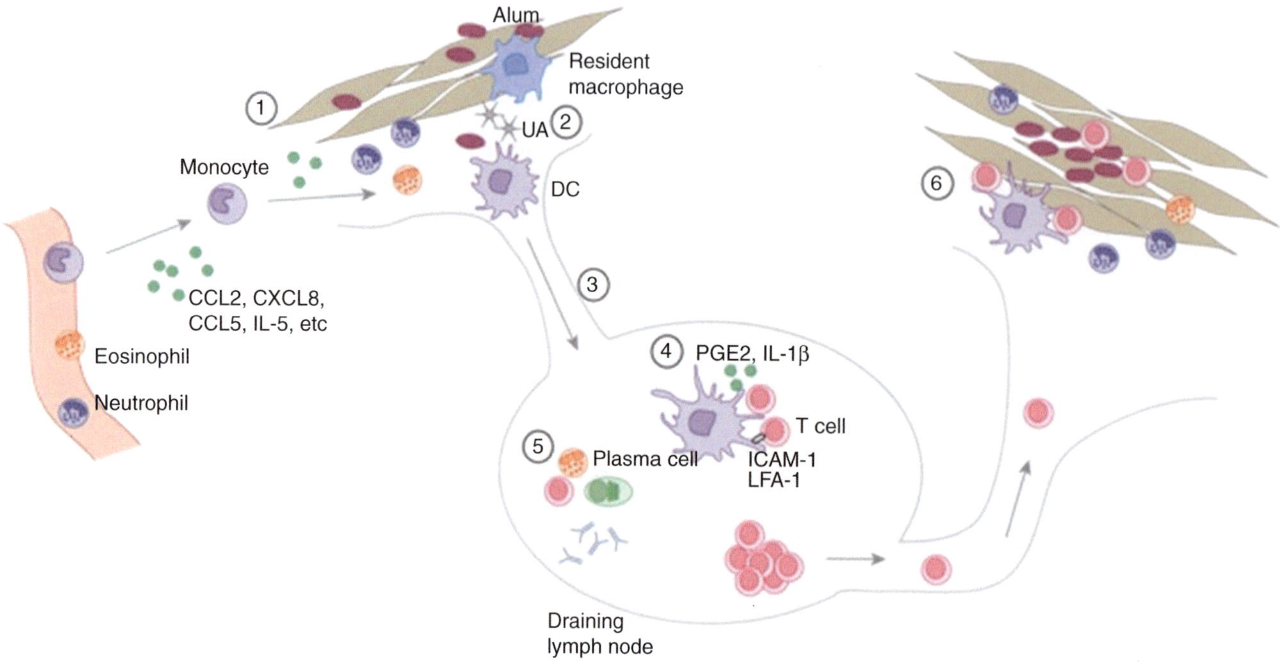

Fig. 7.1 Overview of cellular immune response induced by alum adjuvant. (*1*) After an alum-formulated antigen is injected intramuscularly, there is an immediate response of muscle cells to release chemokines and cytokines, like CCL2, CCL5, IL-5, and CXCL8, that attract cells of the innate immune system, like monocytes, eosinophils, and neutrophils to the site of injection. (*2*) In addition, there is the local release of uric acid (at least in some models) by local tissue damage or active production by macrophages. (*3*) Recruited monocytes differentiate into dendritic cells (DCs), take up antigen, and process it on MHCI and MHCII molecules on their way to the draining nodes. (*4*) In the nodes, mature DCs select antigen-specific T cells that differentiate into Th effector cells. Particularly in the mouse, this response is Th2 biased due to PGE2 and IL1β production and the expression of ICAM-1 and LFA-1. (*5*) In the spleen, and possibly in the draining nodes, there is also recruitment of $Gr1^+$, $IL-4^+$ eosinophils that stimulate B cell responses. Alum mainly induces long-lived B cell responses. (*6*) Effector T cells are recruited back to the site of injection and found around the depot of alum and antigen, where also DCs, neutrophils, and eosinophils reside. Possibly, depot formation could be involved in stimulating long-lasting memory. It is common knowledge that aluminum-containing adjuvants predominantly induce humoral immunity, while sparing cellular immunity

injection, there is a significant increase in the number of conventional and plasmacytoid DCs, neutrophils, NK cells, eosinophils, and inflammatory monocytes, and disappearance of mast cells and macrophages can be observed [16–19]. The recruitment of these innate cells was accompanied by the secretion of several necessary chemokines, such as monocyte chemotactic MCP1 (CCL2), MIP-1α (CCL2), MIP-1β (CCL4), the neutrophil chemotaxin KC/IL-8 (CXCL8), the eosinophil chemotaxin1 (CCL11), IL-5, and RANTES (CCL5) [16, 18].

It has been less clear if and how aluminum-containing adjuvants can induce DC mobilization and maturation. Most likely the mode of action of alum in vivo is upstream of the direct activation of DCs, as confirmed by in vitro data [20]. At least in vitro, alum did not enhance co-stimulatory molecule expression and DC maturation, leading to the proposal that they might induce activation of DCs only in vivo, upon release of endogenous danger signals by structural cells or inflammatory cells [21]. It has been demonstrated that both uric acid and dsDNA are released upon alum injection acting as danger signals [21].

In humans, it also appears that alum-formulated vaccines mainly act at the levels of the monocytes, inducing phenotypic and functional maturation [22]. These experiments demonstrate that monocyte-derived DCs are necessary and sufficient to mediate the adjuvant effects of alum. Alum also enhances the magnitude and duration of expression of peptide–MHC II complexes on the DC surface, with an accompanying increase in MHC II expression [23]. This together with increased ICAM-1 expression will lead to an enhance contact time with T cells, resulting in a strong $CD4^+$ T cell response [24].

Classical cell-mediated immunity measured by DTH responses and induction of $CD8^+$ CTL responses to a range of polypeptide and protein antigens is poorly induced by alum, because of a lack of cross-priming [25].

7.3.2.2 Molecular Pathways Activated in DCs by Aluminum-Containing Adjuvants

How exactly aluminum-containing adjuvants are recognized by antigen-presenting cells has been – and continues to be – a puzzle (Fig. 7.4). Several high-profile papers published over the last years have shown that Toll-like receptors (TLRs) and TLR signaling through the MyD88 or TRIF adaptor pathway, classical activators of innate immunity, and the DC network in vivo were not always necessary for alum to act as an adjuvant for humoral immunity [26].

Additionally, it has become clear that an alternative pathogen detection system exists, which relies on a family of intracellular receptors, called NOD-like receptors (NLRs) [27]. Whereas TLRs sense extracellular non-self-motifs of infectious organisms, NLRs sense stimuli of microbial origin as well as endogenous signals (DAMPs) rather than microbial patterns. They can recognize stress, abnormal self ,or danger signals such as DNA, RNA, and uric acid. NLRP3 (NALP3), a member of the NLR family, along with ASC and caspase-1 forms a molecular platform called the inflammasome. NLRP3 can be activated by several agonists, like endogenous ATP, uric acid, silica, and alum adjuvant, leading to the processing and release of IL-1β and IL-18.

The release of these pro-inflammatory cytokines requires two signals. The first signal is derived from TLR agonist such as lipopolysaccharide (LPS) and inflammatory cytokines, activating the NF-κB pathway, thereby initiating the transcription and accumulation of the precursor proteins. And secondly, cleavage and secretion of the cytokines is mediated by the inflammasome. IL-1β is a potent inflammatory cytokine, which is implicated in acute and chronic inflammatory disorders.

In contrast to the in vitro data showing that alum activates the NLRP3 inflammasome, there is considerable controversy if the inflammasome-IL-1β pathway is necessary for the humoral immune response induced by alum.

Recently it has been shown that alum can activate DCs through lipid raft formation due to its interaction with membrane lipids, such as sphingomyelin and cholesterol [24].

In contrast to uric acid crystals, which also induce the lipid raft formation and activation of Syk [28], alum is not phagocytosed by DCs. However, DCs that have been primed with alum interact stronger with $CD4^+$ T cells, which are antigen independent but were dependent on ICAM-1 and LFA-1 expression [24].

7.3.3 Inflammasome

Inflammasomes are large intracellular multimeric protein complexes that play a central role in innate immunity. Inflammasomes consist of specific PRRs such as NLRP1 and NLPR3 and the adaptor protein ASC (apoptosis-associated speck-like protein). This complex activates inflammatory via the caspase system and the production of cytokines of the IL-1 family. Caspase-1 is regarded as a key mediator of inflammatory processes and has an important role as cell death protease leading to apoptosis. A general scheme of activation of caspase-1 via NLRP3 by microbes is given in Fig. 7.2.

Alum adjuvant as salt is phagocytosed via lysosomes by the resident cells.After disruption of the lysosomes, cathepsin B, an enzymatic protein, is released. Cathepsin B may directly or indirectly induce K^+ efflux, which activates the NLR family, pyrin domain containing 3: NLRP3 inflammasome. The cytosolic K^+ concentration is the common step necessary for caspase-1 activation (Fig. 7.3 – see also Fig. 3.10 in Chap. 3).

7.3.3.1 The Involvement of Endogenous Danger Signals

Besides direct effects, alum adjuvant exerts some level of cytotoxicity [6]. In humans an increase in necrotic cells, a potential source of endogenous danger signals or damage-associated molecular patterns (DAMPs), can be found at the injection site. Dying cells release numerous molecules that act as DAMPs and which can alert the innate immune system through the activation of various PRR signaling pathways. Aluminum-containing adjuvants induce the endogenous release of uric acid (UA) and host dsDNA that will activate the immune system indirectly. UA is a danger signal produced during the catabolism of purines and is the end product in ureotelic mammals. Additionally, UA can be released from injured cells, after degradation of RNA and DNA and permutation of the liberated purines into UA (Fig. 7.4).

Host dsDNA is exposed to the immune system through the release from necrotic cells. Both DAMPs alert the immune system for cell death. After administration of alum in mice, both UA and dsDNA levels are rapidly increased at the site of injection [16]. Both UA and dsDNA are able to act as an adjuvant and boost Th2-associated humoral responses.

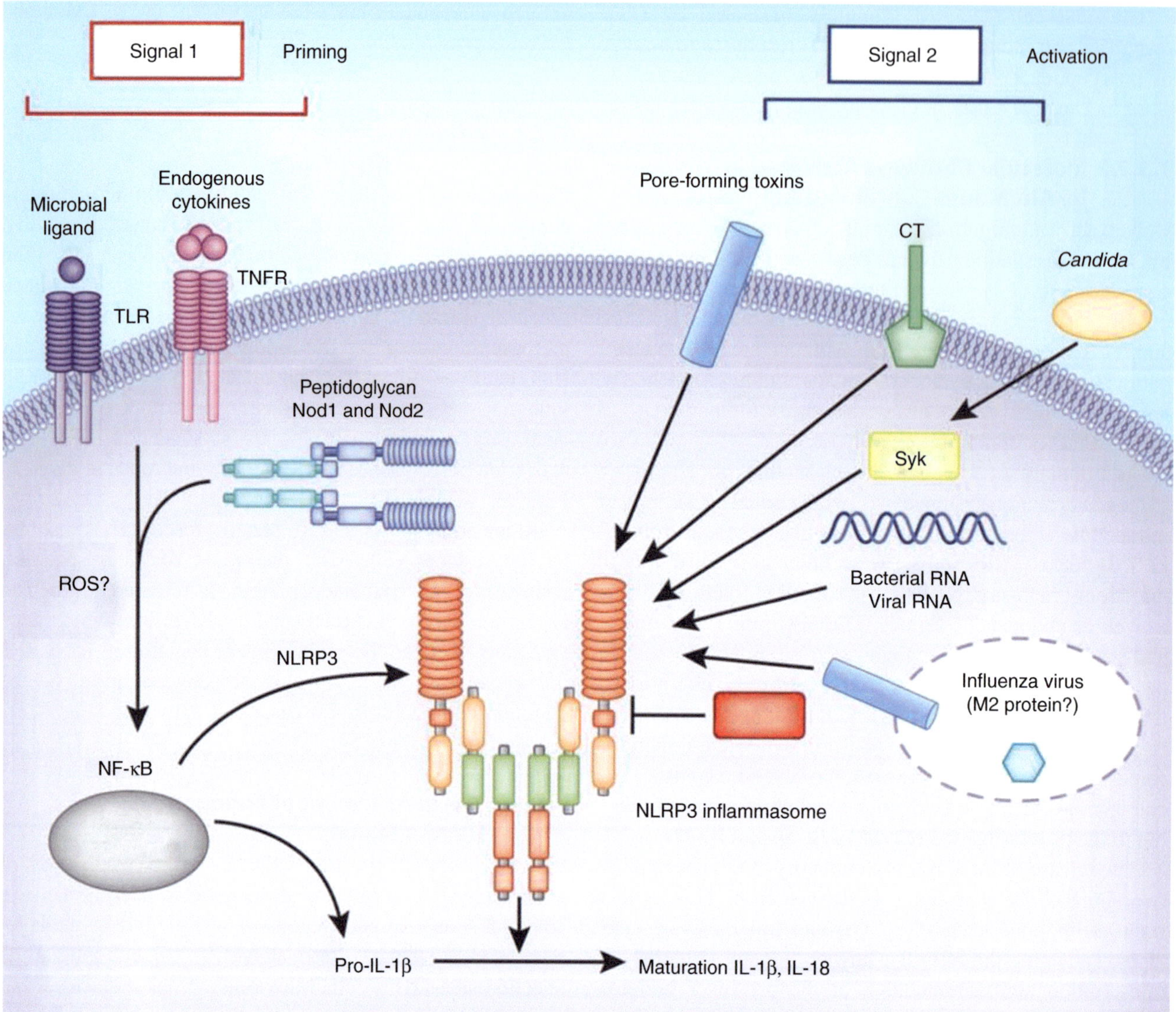

Fig. 7.2 Activation of caspase-1 via NLRP3 requires two signals. Signal 1 is represented by microbial molecules or endogenous cytokines and is required for the upregulation of NLRP3 and pro-IL-1β. Signal 2 activates the NLRP3 inflammasome. Activation by *S. aureus*, *S. pyogenes*, *S. pneumoniae*, and *V. cholerae* is mediated by pore-forming toxins. Other bacterial toxins can also induce the activation of the NLRP3 inflammasome, such as cholera toxin (*CT*) or *C. difficile* toxins TcdA and TcdB (not shown here); *C. albicans* induces activation of the NLRP3 inflammasome through the kinase Syk, although the mechanism involved is unclear. Influenza virus can induce the activation of the NLRP3 inflammasome, but it is controversial whether this is due to a pore-forming activity mediated by M protein or to sensing of viral RNA species in the cytosol. Cytosolic bacterial RNA induces activation of the NLRP3 inflammasome. TNFR, receptor for tumor-necrosis factor (Credit: L. Franchi et al., Sensing and reacting to microbes through the Inflammasomes, Nature Immunology, Mar 19, 2012, Nature Publishing Group)

Fig. 7.3 Alum salts are phagocytosed by the resident cells. After disruption of the lysosomes, cathepsin B, an enzymatic protein, is released. Cathepsin B may directly or indirectly induce potassium efflux, which activates the NLR family, pyrin domain containing 3: NLRP3 inflammasome (Figure by M. Giese Heidelberg/Germany)

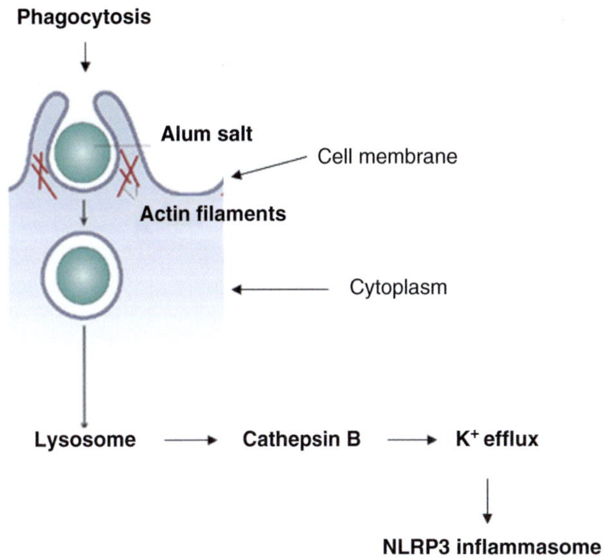

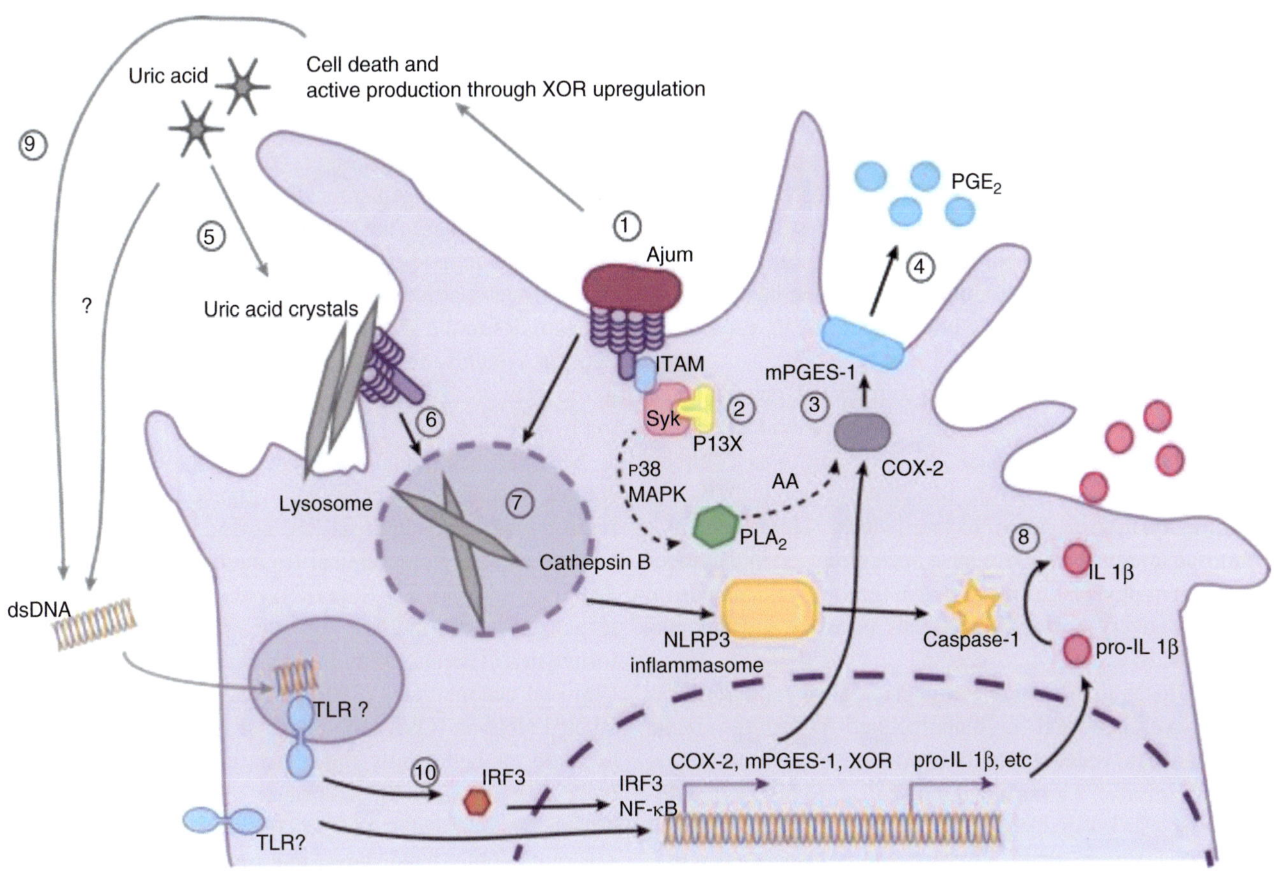

Fig. 7.4 The molecular pathways induced by alum in DCs and macrophages. (*1*) Alum binds to the cell membrane and thereby induces lipid raft formation. (*2*) In the lipid raft, ITAM-containing receptors cluster and activate the Syk-PI3Kδ pathway. (*3*) This pathway in turn activates cytosolic phospholipase A2 (cPLA2), probably via p38 MAP kinase, resulting in the release of arachidonic acid from membrane lipids. COX-2 and membrane-associated PGE synthase-1 (*mPGES-1*) converts arachidonic acid to prostaglandin E2 (*PGE2*). (*4*) PGE_2 is released from the cell and instructs the Th2 response. (*5*) Furthermore, alum induces the release of uric acid via the induction XOR. (*6*) Upon phagocytosis of alum or uric acid crystals, lysosomal damage is induced. (*7*) This activates the NLRP3 inflammasome resulting from the release of enzymes like cathepsin B into the cytoplasm. (*8*) Activated caspase-1 mediates the proteolytic cleavage of pro-IL1β in biologically active IL1β. (*9*) Besides the release of uric acid, alum also induces the release of dsDNA, probably through cell death. (*10*) dsDNA activates the immune system and more specifically monocytes through *Irf3* which is critical for the migration of inflammatory monocytes

7.4 Chitosan[2]

7.4.1 Formulation and Chemistry

Chitosan is commercially manufactured from the exoskeletons of crustaceans, recovered as a side product from the seafood industry. The manufacturing process involves strong alkaline treatment of chitin, a homopolymer consisting of 1–4-β-linked-N-acetyl-glucosamine units, to remove acetyl groups and form water-soluble chitosan. Chitosan is thus composed of N-acetyl-glucosamine and glucosamine (Fig. 7.5) at various ratios.

Degree of Deacetylation. The percentage of glucosamines in the chitosan is termed degree of deacetylation (DD). Standard manufacturing processes typically leads to a DD of 80–95 %, but the DD may vary considerably. The quality of chitosans applied in published studies is often inadequately defined, making it difficult to link physical and chemical composition of chitosans to stimulation of certain immune responses. Existing data mostly refer to chitosan in the 80–95 % DD range, since commercially available chitosans are generally highly deacetylated.

Due to its high content of glucosamines, chitosan is cationic [29] and muco-adherent [30, 31]. Moreover, chitosan possesses permeation-enhancing properties [32]. These characteristics are of importance for formulation of mucosal vaccines. However, one limitation for the medical application of chitosan is that it is only soluble in its protonated form, at pH below 6–6.5.

In order to keep chitosans in solutions at physiological conditions (neutral pH, salts, etc.), various chemical modifications have been attempted [30, 33]. The most common soluble chitosan derivatives for mucosal applications are N-trimethylated and carboxymethylated chitosans [34]. Chitosan and its derivatives have been produced in a number of different physical forms to match the various demands on vaccine delivery systems, e.g., as gels, powders, and nanoparticles [34, 35].

A chitosan that is soluble at physiological conditions has been developed and is manufactured under the name Viscosan. The water solubility is promoted by a random distribution of acetyl groups and a DD close to 50 %. In addition, Viscosan is rapidly degraded in a biological environment and it has a high purity. Viscosan can be processed into a viscoelastic hydrogel, ViscoGel. The gel is formed by cross-linking of chitosan chains to achieve a physically stable hydrogel consisting of 99 % water and 1 % Viscosan.

[2]Chitosan-based adjuvants *by Guro Gafvelin and Hans Grönlund* in Molecular Vaccines – From Prophylaxis to Therapy, Volume 2, Springer-Verlag Wien, 2013, Ed. Matthias Giese.

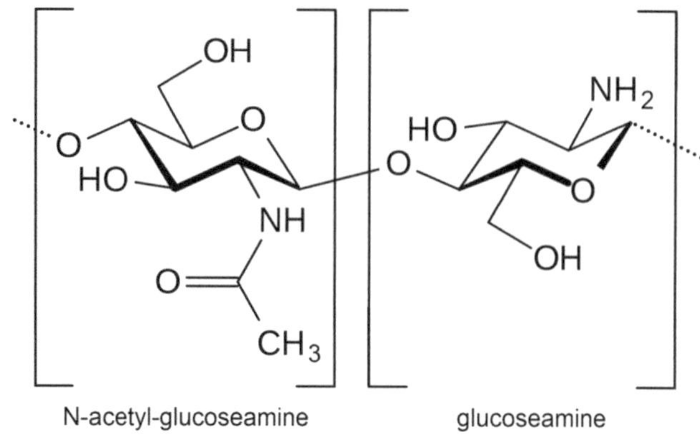

Fig. 7.5 Chitosan is a carbohydrate polymer composed of N-acetyl-glucosamine and glucosamine units. The polymer length, as well as the distribution and overall composition of N-acetyl-glucosamine and glucosamine units, varies between chitosans. The percentage of glucosamine units in the polymer denotes the degree of deacetylation (DD)

7.4.2 Microtechnology and Nanotechnology

The particulate form enables exposure of a large surface area and efficient display of antigen. Microparticles exhibit similar sizes as microorganisms, which the immune system has evolved to combat. Thus, they are efficiently phagocytosed and activate antigen-presenting cells (APCs). ViscoGel provides a microparticulate system and can be processed into gel particles in the size range from a few micrometers up to 200 μm. Notably, ViscoGel does not precipitate but remains in the form of clear transparent gel particles when subjected to physiological pH.

Nanoparticulate chitosan systems have especially been studied for mucosal vaccine applications. For example, chitosan nanospheres (approx. 350 nm) have been applied as vaccine carriers in preclinical testing of nasal delivery of a tetanus toxoid [36, 37]. Superior systemic and local immune responses were induced by the chitosan-nanoparticle-formulated tetanus toxoid compared to fluid vaccine. Chitosan nanoparticles (350 nm) loaded with fluorescently labeled albumin (OVA) have been shown to be internalized by nasal epithelial cells and transported to the submucosal layer after intranasal administration to rats [38]. In a mouse model for sublingual allergen-specific immunotherapy, it was on the other hand shown that treatment with the model allergen OVA formulated with chitosan microparticles (1–3 μm) was superior to a nanoparticle (300–800 nm) formulated vaccine. The uptake of OVA by sublingual APCs and the activation of OVA-specific T cell responses were increased for the microparticle formulated OVA, and furthermore, the airway hyperresponsiveness and inflammation in the lung was reduced after treatment with the microparticulate vaccine [39].

7.4.2.1 Working Mechanism

Immune activation by chitosan has been demonstrated after intranasal [36], oral [40], subcutaneous [41, 42], and intramuscular antigen administration [43]. The oral route is expected to induce tolerogenic immune responses. Chitosan given orally without any protein antigen stimulated a Th2/regulatory T cell-promoting milieu in the intestinal mucosa, characterized by secretion of IL-10 and expression of IL-4 and TGF-β [40]. When given by the subcutaneous or intramuscular route, chitosan stimulates both strong humoral and cellular responses to coadministered antigens. A mixed Th1/Th2 type of response as well as CTL activation has been demonstrated in mice [41, 43]. It has been proposed that chitin, the precursor to chitosan, activates innate immune responses through two main mechanisms: activation of pathogen pattern-recognition receptors (PRRs) and activation of chitinases [44]. The PRRs suggested to be activated by chitin include the mannose receptor, TLR-2 and dectin-1 [45, 46].

Depot Effect. There are few reports on how chitosan acts as an adjuvant. In an early study, chitosan was shown to activate macrophages [47]. Chitosan has later been demonstrated to provide an antigen depot effect, which has been suggested to enhance adjuvant activity [41]. It has also been reported that chitosan induces inflammasome activation in an NLRP3-dependent fashion, a mechanism that may be shared among particulate adjuvants, including alum. Interestingly, in an in vitro study performed on murine bone marrow-derived dendritic cells (DCs), it was shown that chitosan, in contrast to alum, did not inhibit stimulated production of the Th1-polarizing cytokine IL-12 from activated DCs, providing a possible explanation to why chitosan stimulates Th1 responses more readily than alum [48]. These and other studies suggest that chitosan activates innate immune signaling, but so far no candidate PRR specifically interacting with chitosan has been identified.

7.4.3 Preclinical Development, Safety, and Efficacy

A glycoconjugate vaccine to *Haemophilus influenzae* type b (Act-HIB) was used as model antigen. The model vaccine was chosen because it is approved for human use and the outcome of vaccination can be measured as antibody titers in standardized assays [49]. The vaccine was formulated as a mixture of Act-HIB with 200 μm ViscoGel particles. Groups of mice were immunized with the adjuvant-formulated vaccine and compared to non-adjuvanted Act-HIB [42]. Significantly enhanced IgG1 and IgG2a titers were found in sera from mice immunized with ViscoGel-formulated Act-HIB. In fact, the antigen dose could be reduced tenfold when ViscoGel was used as an adjuvant. Furthermore, the Act-HIB specific cellular response was significantly stronger and of a mixed type, based on the cytokine profile. Similar effects were seen when the adjuvant was administered either subcutaneously or intramuscularly.

The toxicity of ViscoGel, as well as for the formulated vaccine consisting of Act-HIB mixed with ViscoGel, was evaluated in mice and rabbits. No systemic toxic effects were recorded. The local reactions observed were mild and associated with the immunostimulating effect, which was confirmed by measurement of antibodies raised to Act-HIB by the vaccination. The possibility to develop an immune response to chitosan, and possibly an allergic, IgE-mediated response, has been addressed earlier [43]. In mice given intramuscular injections with chitosan alone or in combination either with an influenza vaccine or an added adjuvant (Freunds incomplete adjuvant), no significant anti-chitosan antibody responses were detected. Moreover, no increase of IgE to chitosan or to influenza antigen was recorded in sera from rats injected with chitosan or chitosan/vaccine [43]. The question if seafood-allergic individuals can react to chitosan has been raised [50]. This concern applies to the possible presence of trace amounts of allergenic proteins in chitosan preparations. Well-characterized chitosans of high purity, e.g., ViscoGel, are not associated with this risk.

7.4.4 Clinical Development

Even though several chitosan-based adjuvants have been developed and tested preclinically [34], few studies have evaluated chitosan as an adjuvant in man. So far, the clinical trials where the immunostimulatory effect has been studied involve mucosal vaccinations. Intranasal administration of a detoxified diphtheria toxin vaccine (CRM_{197}) formulated with chitosan glutamate generated significantly higher levels of neutralizing antitoxin serum antibodies compared to the non-adjuvanted intranasal vaccine and to intramuscular alum-formulated CRM_{197} [51]. Only the chitosan-formulated vaccine induced an antitoxin IgA response, and the nasal CRM_{197}/chitosan vaccine also generated a stronger Th2 type of cell response to diphtheria toxin than the vaccine given alone or by the intramuscular route with alum [52].

In another study, intranasal vaccination with a trivalent influenza vaccine formulated with chitosan glutamate was compared to vaccination by the conventional intramuscular route [53]. The intranasal immunization resulted in satisfactory protective responses that were not significantly different from those generated by the intramuscular vaccine. A third study investigated a *Neisseria meningitides* glycoconjugate vaccine administered intranasally with chitosan in comparison to the same vaccine formulated with alum and administered intramuscular [54]. The intranasal chitosan-formulated vaccine was well tolerated and generated protective antibody responses comparable to the parenteral vaccine. In addition, trials employing chitosan as adjuvant and vaccine vehicle, but without comparison to other administration routes or non-adjuvanted

Table 7.3 Advantages and restrains associated with the application of chitosan in vaccine development

Strengths	Weaknesses
Natural product; nontoxic, biodegradable	Natural product; formulation and characterization methods are not standardized
Controlled manufacturing process enables high purity without traces of allergenic components in high-quality chitosans	Chitosans of inferior qualities that contain impurities generate non-reliable results
May be manufactured in various forms, e.g., gel, powder, nano-/microparticles, chemical derivatives	Most non-modified chitosans are insoluble at physiological pH
Cationic and mucoadhesive; application as vehicle/adjuvant for mucosal vaccination, formulation for various administration routes possible	Few studies available on other administration routes than intranasal
Low cost of goods, "unlimited" access to raw material	Few medical grade, high-quality chitosans available
Different chemical (e.g., DD) and physical (e.g., particle size) characteristics determine immune response; versatility allows specific design of vaccines	Chemical and physical characteristics that determine immune responses are ill defined
Stimulates humoral and cellular immune responses	Mechanisms of action are poorly understood

vaccines, have been conducted with a Norwalk virus-like particle vaccine formulated with the adjuvant monophosphoryl lipid A (MPL) and chitosan for intranasal delivery.

This vaccine was evaluated in a safety and dose-finding study [55], followed by a randomized, double-blind, placebo-controlled, multicenter study [56]. It was concluded that the nasal vaccine was well tolerated and highly immunogenic and provided increased protection to experimentally induced Norwalk virus gastroenteritis. Chitosan has also been applied for intranasal vaccination in a Phase I trial (MUCOVAC2), evaluating an HIV viral coat vaccine administered via the intranasal, intramuscular, and vaginal routes [57]. Finally, chitosan has been employed as an immunoactivator in cancer immunotherapy. In a safety–efficacy study on late-stage metastatic breast cancer patients, glycated chitosan was applied in combination with laser immunotherapy [58]. The clinical outcome of this study was promising, exhibiting systemic antitumor responses with milder side effects than conventional treatments (Table 7.3).

7.5 Bacterial Toxins Used for Vaccination[3]

Many bacterial toxins are encoded by chromosome, plasmids, or phages and can be broadly divided in two groups referred to as endotoxins and exotoxins. Endotoxins are cell-associated structural components of bacteria cell envelope represented by peptidoglycan constituent muramyl dipeptide (MDP) and muropeptides or lipopolysaccharide (LPS) or lipooligosaccharide (LOS) which are located in the outer membrane of gram-negative bacteria.

Exotoxins are mostly protein toxins which belong to the most powerful human poisons known. They are actively transported from bacteria or released by cell lysis induced by host defense mechanisms or by the action of antibiotics. Some bacteria produce many toxins like staphylococci or streptococci, whereas other bacteria like *Corynebacterium diphtheriae* produce just one. Some toxins, e.g., pore-forming hemolysins or phospholipases exhibit broad cytotoxic activity toward various cell types, while others like clostridial neurotoxins act specifically only on neurons. Some bacterial toxins may serve as invasins; others damage the cellular integrity by means of enzymatic activity or pore formation causing cell death.

The cytotoxic activity of toxins has been utilized to treat various neurological disorders as well as to generate immunotoxins to kill malignant or virus-infected cells. Moreover, various bacterial toxins have been differentially modified either by single-point mutations, insertion of specific sequences, or deletion of parts of the toxin molecule to alter their binding abilities and/or abolish their enzymatic activity to be used for vaccination, antigen/drug delivery, or, most importantly, as adjuvants.

The specific immunotherapeutic use of bacterial toxins is listed in Table 7.4.

7.5.1 The Structure and Mode of Entry of Bacterial Toxins into Host Cells

The majority of toxins are referred as AB-toxins where the A moiety generally possesses an enzymatic activity and the monomeric or multimeric B moiety binds the toxin to cell-surface receptors. The B moiety can play a role in the translocation of the A moiety into the cytosol [59]. After receptor binding via B moiety, most protein toxins enter host cells predominantly via receptor-mediated endocytosis (Fig. 7.6).

A Moiety. Within the cell the translocated enzymatic A moiety interferes with components of the protein synthesis machinery, various cellular signaling pathways, actin polymerization, and intracellular trafficking of vesicles, causing, in most cases, the death of intoxicated cells. On contrary, *Bordetella pertussis* adenylate cyclase toxin (CyaA) after

[3]Bacterial toxins are successful immunotherapeutic adjuvants and immunotoxins by *Irena Adkins* in Molecular Vaccines – From Prophylaxis to Therapy, Volume 2, Springer-Verlag Wien, 2013, Ed. Matthias Giese.

Table 7.4 Experimental immunotherapeutic use of bacterial toxins

Toxin	Experimental immunotherapeutic use							
	Adjuvant	Antigen delivery[a]	Drug/DNA delivery	IT	Antiviral agent	Diagnostics/imaging	Cancer therapy	Therapy of neurological disorders/injury
Muramyl dipeptide/ Muropeptides	x		x		x		x	
Enterotoxins A,B,C	x						x	
Shiga toxin	x	x	x	x	x	x	x	
Shiga-like toxin	x	x		x	x	x	x	
Exotoxin A	x	x		x	x		x	
Diphtheria toxin	x	x		x	x		x	
Lethal toxin		x		x		x	x	
Tetanus toxin		x	x					x
Neurotoxins			x				x	x
Adenylate cyclase toxin	x	x					x	
Pertussis toxin	x	x			x			
Dermonecrotic toxin	x							
Edema toxin	x							
Cholera toxin	x							
Zonula occludens toxin	x	x	x				x	
C2 toxin			x				x	
C3 toxin								x
Toxin A							x	
CNF1	x							x
Heat-labile toxin	x							
Hemolysin		x						
Listeriolysin O	x	x	x				x	
Perfringolysin O	x	x	x					
Aerolysin				x		x	x	
Pneumolysin	x	x						
Intermedilysin			x		x			
Crystal proteins	x	x					x	

Abbreviations: *IT* immunotoxin

[a]Antigen genetically fused or chemically coupled to the toxin molecule

binding to its receptor CD11b translocates its enzymatic adenylate cyclase domain directly across the cellular membrane into the host cell cytosol where it generates nonphysiological levels of cAMP, thereby paralyzing innate immune functions of myeloid phagocytes and inducing cell death. After the receptor binding, pore-forming toxins act directly to form pores in the plasma membrane without the need of endocytosis, causing lysis of the target cells [60].

7.5.2 Bacterial Toxins Used as Adjuvants

Endotoxins as well as exotoxins have been exploited as adjuvants, mainly mutated toxins with ablated or reduced enzymatic activity or modified chemical structure to reduce their cytotoxic effects.

From bacterial exotoxins, *V. cholera* cholera toxin (CT) and *E. coli* heat-labile toxin (LT) represent the most potent oral–mucosal immunogens and adjuvants for a variety of coadministered antigens. Their inherent immunomodulatory properties depend on the ADP-ribosylating activity and structural properties of the A subunit together with the activity of the pentameric B subunit to bind to widely expressed GM1 gangliosides (Fig. 3.12).

Because of their toxicity, mainly the nontoxic B subunits have been extensively used as mucosal immunogens in humans, e.g., cholera vaccine. As the B subunits alone were poor mucosal adjuvant, CT and LT mutants were introduced where the enzymatically A subunit was mutated. These mutants behaved as strong mucosal adjuvants for all antigens tested when given orally, intranasally, or vaginally, inducing strong systemic and mucosal antigen-specific antibody response [61, 62]. Several of these mutants like LTK63 or LTR192G were tested as adjuvants in phase I clinical trials [63]. Some other modified adjuvant based on CT have been also described like CTA1-DD, where fully active CTA1 and

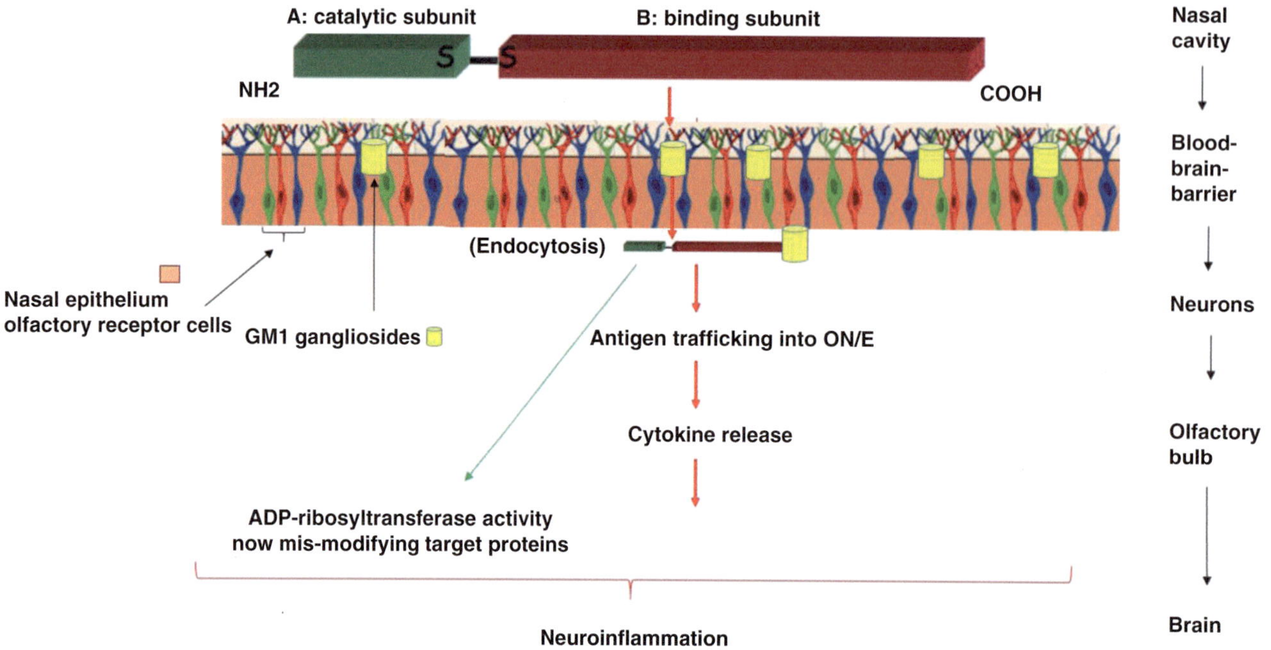

Fig. 7.6 A-B moiety of heat-labile enterotoxins crossing the blood–brain barrier. Inhaled substances, also particular vaccines, contact the main olfactory epithelium (OE) which contains various olfactory receptors. Olfactory neurons (ON) transduce receptor activation signals axonal to the olfactory bulbs (OBs). The process of antigen trafficking into the olfactory nerves/epithelium (*ON/E*) and subsequently the endocytosis into the nerve cell require ADP-ribosyltransferase activity of the A subunit of the enterotoxin-based adjuvant, as well as binding to GM1 gangliosides on neuroepithelial cells (monosialoganglioside) by the B subunit. A damaged blood–brain-barrier leads to the release of cytokines resulting in neuroinflammation (Figure by M. Giese Heidelberg/Germany)

an *S. aureus* protein A derivative named DD are genetically fused [64] or CTB coupled with CpG oligonucleotide [65].

On the other hand, CTB and LTB with conjugated antigens were shown to efficiently induce oral tolerance [66]. In experimental models, CTB–antigen conjugate was shown to suppress the development of several autoimmune diseases, type I allergies, and allograft rejection [60, 62]. An interesting alternative to CT and LT might be Cry proteins of entomopathogenic *B. thuringiensis* which exhibit similar potent mucosal and systemic immunogenicity and adjuvanticity to coadministered antigens [60, 67].

Superantigens. Another group of toxins, which were exploited as adjuvants, is represented by pyrogenic toxin superantigens like enterotoxins A, B, and C of *S. aureus* (SEA, SEB, and SEC). These toxins bind to distinct regions outside the peptide-binding cleft of the major histocompatibility class II (MHC II) molecules expressed on antigen-presenting cells and to specific Vβ elements on the T cell receptor which induces massive T cell proliferation and cytokine release (Fig. 7.7).

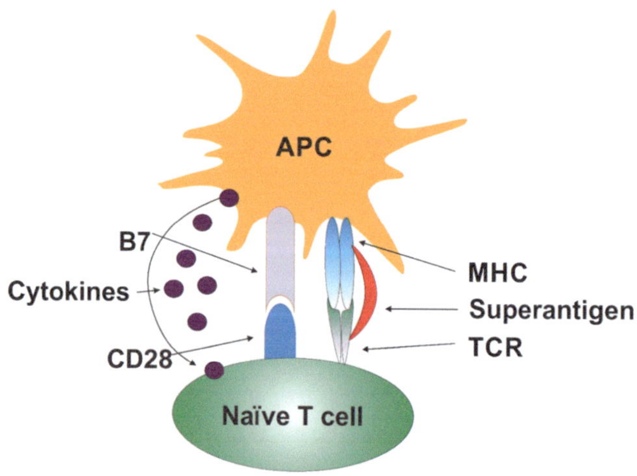

Fig. 7.7 A superantigen connects directly the MHC II of the antigen-presenting cell (*APC*) with the T cell receptor (*TCR*) outside of the normal antigen-binding groove. Cytokines are released in large amounts, causing the symptoms of toxic shock. Up to one in five T cells can be activated by superantigens (*B7* and *CD28*, accessory molecules) (Figure by M. Giese Heidelberg/Germany)

Many other bacterial toxins have been shown to enhance an antibody response to fused or coadministered antigens and/or to exert adjuvant activity toward the immune cells potentiating T cell adaptive responses [60]. However, their therapeutic potential as adjuvants has to be carefully evaluated, e.g., *B. pertussis* pertussis toxin exacerbated an experimental autoimmune encephalomyelitis in mouse model of multiple sclerosis [68].

7.5.3 Bacterial Toxins Commercially Used for Vaccination

Scientific advances in molecular engineering enabled the development of vaccines based on mutated bacterial toxins; however, only few are nowadays used for treatment and/or prevention of human diseases. Detoxified *C. diphtheriae* diphtheria toxoid or *C. tetani* tetanus toxoid is used for the universal vaccination against diphtheria or tetanus, respectively. The nontoxic B subunit of *V. cholerae* cholera toxin (CTB) used as a protective antigen together with killed vibrios in a widely licensed oral cholera vaccine. Similarly, *B. pertussis* pertussis toxoid (PT9K/129G) [69] has been approved for human use as a component of a vaccine against *B. pertussis* infection [70]. Although diphtheria toxoid is successfully used as a carrier in glycoconjugate vaccines against a variety of bacterial pathogens, four clinical trials failed to prove the benefit of *P. aeruginosa* exotoxin A in such vaccines.

7.6 Lipopolysaccharide[4]

The most studied bacterial endotoxins for their adjuvanticity are LPS, muramyl dipeptide (MDP), and muropeptides which are discussed in more detail here.

Lipopolysaccharide (LPS, endotoxin) is a component of the external leaflet of the outer membrane of gram-negative bacteria. It is a complex glycolipid formed by three domains, a fatty acid-rich domain (Lipid A), an oligosaccharide domain (core), and a repeating oligosaccharide domain (O antigen) [71]. Figure 7.8 represents the typical LPS organization.

[4]Bacterial lipopolysaccharide as adjuvants by *Jesús Arenas* in Molecular Vaccines – From Prophylaxis to Therapy, Volume 2, Springer-Verlag Wien, 2013, Ed. Matthias Giese.

The Lipid A domain is a β-1, 6-linked D-glucosamine disaccharide linked to variable number of ester- and amide-linked 3-hydroxy fatty acids and phosphate groups. Its architecture is highly conserved, but different microorganisms may present variations in the number and length of the fatty acid side chains, the presence of terminal phosphate residues, and associated modifications. The core domain is a branched oligosaccharide region formed by nine or ten sugars and its composition is more variable between species than the Lipid A. Finally, the O antigen, if present, is the most variable of the tree domains and consists of up to 50 repeating oligosaccharide units formed of 2–8 monosaccharide moieties. In addition, certain modifying enzymes can alter the composition of LPS, contributing to increase the LPS heterogeneity [72, 73].

7.6.1 Biological Activity

The Toll-like receptor 4 (TLR4), in complex with the glycoprotein MD-2, constitutes the LPS receptor [74]. Its stimulation requires the cooperation of associated molecules, like the LPS-binding protein and CD14 that facilitate LPS transfer to the receptor. TLR4 stimulation induces the formation of intracellular protein complexes that leads to the activation of intracellular signaling cascades. These reactions trigger the biosynthesis and secretion of diverse pro-inflammatory cytokines (IL-1, IL-8, IL-12, TNF-α, and IFN-γ) and the production of co-stimulatory molecules [75] that finally activates humoral and cellular responses including activation of the complement system [76], activation of macrophages [77], B and T cells, and enhancement of cellular cooperation. In contrast, high LPS dose, specially released to the blood system during sepsis, leads to large secretion of cytokines and inflammatory mediators with severe [78] and/or fatal consequences. Table 7.5 summarizes beneficial and harmful effects of LPS in humans. In summary, LPS is a strong activator of the immune system (adjuvant) but also a high toxic substance (endotoxin).

Table 7.5 Relevant effects of LPS in humans

Beneficial		Harmful	
Effect	**Mechanism**	**Effect**	**Mechanism**
Antimicrobial immunity	Activation of DC, priming B and T cells, opsonization, stimulation of natural killer cells, activation of macrophages	High fever	IL-1 release
Antiviral immunity	Stimulating CD8(+) T cell immunity	Strong inflammatory responses	Large secretion of various inflammatory mediators
Antitumor immunity	Stimulating CD8(+) T cell immunity	Disseminated intravascular coagulation	Reduction of elements involved in blood coagulation
Mitigation of Th2 response to Th1	Enhancing Th1 phenotype	Shock, hypotension, lymphopenia	Reduced blood flow

The Lipid A region is the major responsible of the TLR4 stimulation. Variations in its structure, mainly regarding the number and length of acyl acid chains and the charge, are crucial in this regard [79].

7.6.2 Lipid A Analogous Structures and Its Role as Adjuvants

Alum refers to several aluminum salts and is the most used adjuvant. It is safe and elicits predominantly a Th2-type antibody response that results effective in a large variety of vaccines. However, alum hardly promotes Th1-type antibody responses. Apart from that, alum poorly stimulates mucosal immunity. Mucosa tissues are the first line of defense against many pathogens and the ecological niche of commensal and opportunistic microorganisms, for example, *Neisseria meningitidis*.

7.6.2.1 MF59, AS03, and RC-529

Therefore, mucosal immunity is considered the gold therapy to evade pathogen colonization and confer herd immunity against certain particular pathogens. Vaccine adjuvants that target mucosal immunization must promote a large series of biological and complex activities as Th17 cell development, APC proliferation, and IgA production [80]. Alternatively to alum, three additional adjuvants were licensed: MF59, AS03, and RC-529. MF59 is an oil-in-water emulsion with low oil content and it is included in an approved influenza vaccine [81]. Although MF59 induces a more balanced Th1/Th2 response than alum, it shows partial efficacy, often requiring the coadministration of a Th1 enhancers. ASO3 and RC-529 contain LPS-based substances to be discussed later.

LPS has attracted large attention as adjuvant by its high capacity to induce Th1-type responses against coadministrated antigens. One of the most relevant factors involved in the development of this response is IL-12. Interestingly, TLR4 receptor are tactically present at mucosa surfaces; therefore it would be expected that TLR4 agonist can promote immune responses at local and distal mucosal sites. Variation of the LPS composition, in particular the Lipid A, by chemical treatments and chemical synthesis of Lipid A analogous are good examples (see detailed revision [82]). As a result, a diverse Lipid A species was generated although only few exhibited the desirable properties. Next, the most relevant substances and clinical applications are further discussed.

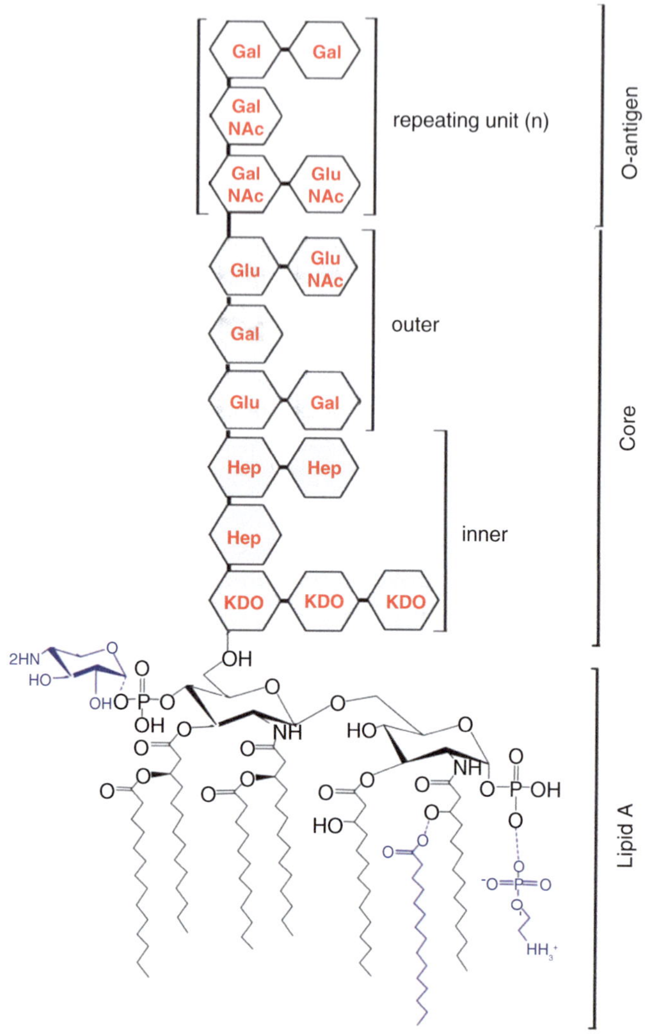

Fig. 7.8 General chemical structure of LPS of gram-negative bacteria. The LPS structure of *Escherichia coli* is depicted. LPS consists of three regions: lipid A, core, and O antigen. The chemical structure of the lipid A of *Escherichia coli* that display the maximal immunostimulatory or endotoxic activities in humans (the topic of this work) is further detailed (*black colored*). Additionally, those substituents that possess the lipid A of *Salmonella minnesota* used to obtain MPL are blue colored. Residues of core and O antigen region are schematized and abbreviated as KDO, 2-keto-3-deoxyoctonoic acid, Hep, D-glycero-D-mano-heptose, Glu, D-glucose, Gal, D-galactose, GluNAc, N-acetyl-glucosamine, GalNAc, N-acetyl-galactosamine. The length of the O antigen depends of the number of repeating units. Additional substituents or modifications can be found in nature but they are not shown for clarity

7.6.2.2 MPL

The chemical hydrolysis of the LPS of *Salmonella minnesota,* which contains a Lipid A with seven acyl chains and three phosphate groups as depicted in Fig. 7.8 (with blue-colored substituent), generated one of the most successful LPS-based adjuvants, the Monophosphoryl Lipid A (MPL). This derivate structure is a six acyl side chain Lipid A with one phosphoryl group [83] (Fig. 7.9). MPL demonstrated to be less toxic than the parent (0.1 % of toxicity) [84] with a toxic side effect profile comparable to alum [85, 86] while

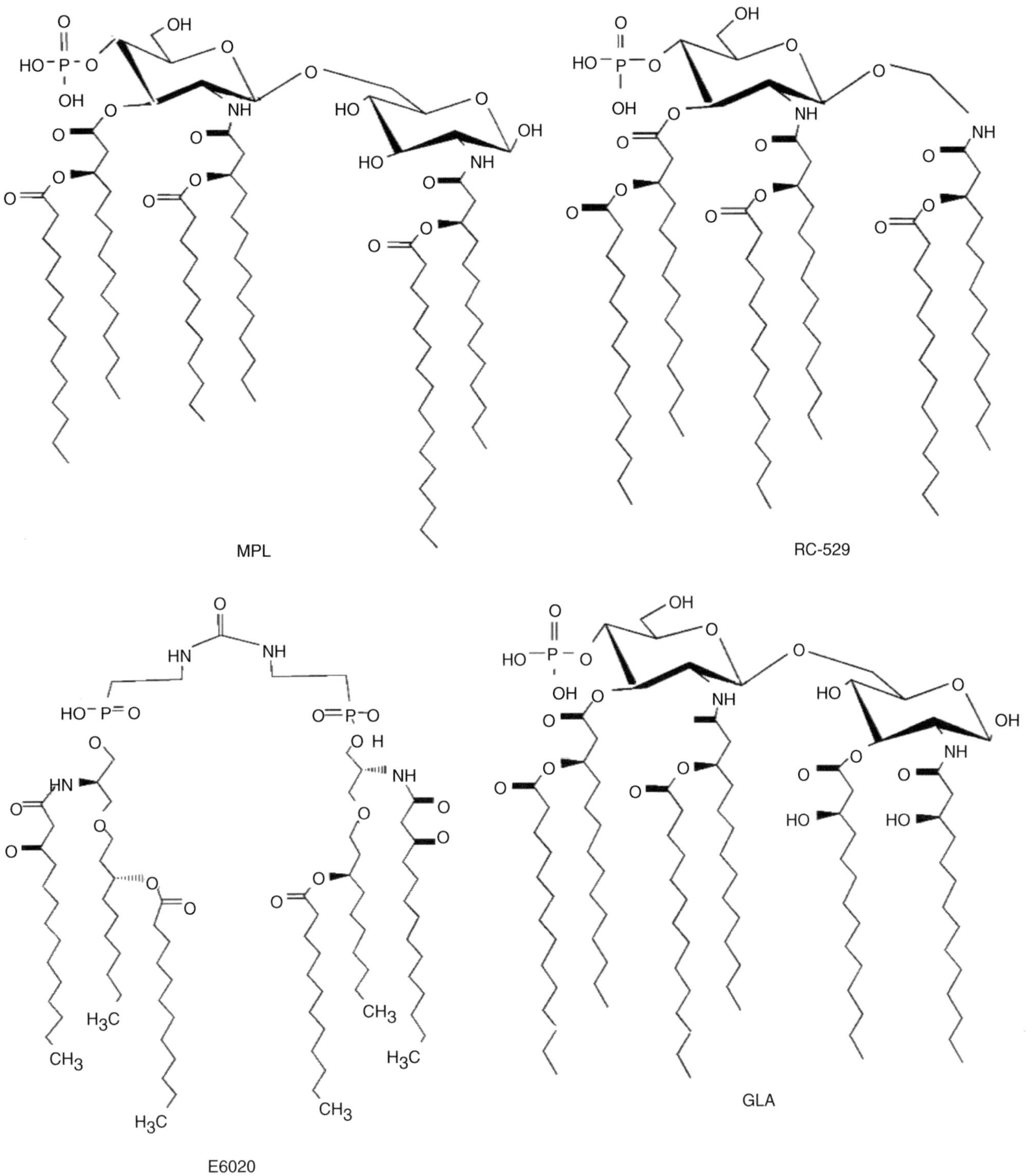

Fig. 7.9 Chemical structure of relevant LPS-based adjuvants

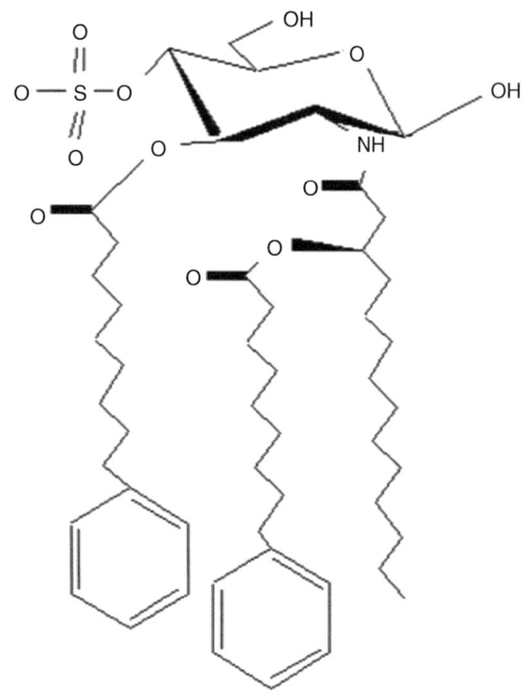

Fig. 7.9 (continued)

retaining stimulatory properties of LPS. At present, MPL is adjuvant of approved vaccine preparations for humans in Europe (human papilloma [Cervarix] [80] and pollen allergy [Pollinex Quatro] [87]) and Australia (hepatitis B virus [FENDrix] [88]), and it has been used extensively in human vaccine trials for several infectious disease like malaria [89], tuberculosis [90], or tumor growth [91].

Because MPL is highly hydrophobic and generates aggregates in aqueous solution that may considerably affect the TLR4 activation, it is often formulated in combination with alum or other delivery systems. These combinations, together with other factors (accompanying antigen or administration route), can alter its adjuvant action. For example, in aqueous formulations MPL promotes antibody production while in oil-in-water emulsions better stimulates T cell responses. In contrast, MPL combined with delivery systems is a strong stimulator of cytotoxic T-lymphocyte proliferation.

Delivery systems can also modify their biological properties. Incorporation of MPL into liposomes reduced the residual toxicity of MPL but retained intact its adjuvant potential; this effect was also observed with other detoxified LPS species [92]. Therefore, liposomal MPL formulations were extensively studied in human trials for different indications as malaria, pneumococcal disease [93], or genital herpes type 2 [94] and in experimental animals for *Streptococcus pyogenes* infections [95] or toxin neutralization of *E. coli* [96]. Finally, it is significant to notice that MPL has been successful in providing mucosal immunity after mucosal [97] and intramuscular administration. MPL formulations for mucosal vaccines have been extensively explored for the treatment of different diseases; genital herpes and mucosal leishmaniasis are good examples.

7.6.2.3 RC-529, E6020, GLA, ONO-4007

RC-529. is a synthetic analog of MPL composed by a monosaccharide backbone with six fatty acyl chains [84]. Like MPL, it is well tolerated and effective during clinical trials but with a lower production cost. In addition, several studies performed in experimental animals indicate that RC-529 has is an efficient mucosal adjuvant against pathogens that lack effective vaccine therapy. For example, it elicited bactericidal antibodies after intranasal immunization with the *Streptococcus pneumoniae* protein PppA and the meningococcal protein P2086, and it promoted high antibody titers in macaques at the nasal and genital mucosa against a HIV peptide immunogen [98]. Similarly, it reduced nasal colonization of non-typable *Haemophilus influenzae* and *Moraxella catarrhalis* in mice that were immunized nasally with recombinant proteins [99], and it conferred significant protection against lethal influenza challenge [100].

E6020. It is an hexa-acylated acyclic backbone [101] with higher biological activities than alum or MPL and with a reduced toxicity. Its simple structure allows the production of high pure material than other synthetic TLR4 agonists. Various works showed its high capacity to shift immune responses toward a Th1 profile when combined with conventional vaccines. Generation of this immune profile is especially relevant in cancer vaccines. Indeed, E6020 in combination with a monoclonal antibody (trastuzumab) enhanced significantly protection against tumor growth in animal models [102].

GLA. It is a hexa-acyl synthetic lipid A derivative composed of a disaccharide backbone with a single phosphate group. Results showed even more powerful adjuvant abilities than MPL while it exhibited a good safety profile in animals and in phase I trials [103]. GLA exhibits a strong ability to shift antigen-specific immune responses toward Th1 type being proposed as a better alternative than MPL to confer adequate protection against certain pathogens.

ONO-4007. It is a tri-acylated acyclic sulfonated backbone. This molecule induced tumor and metastases regression in animal models [104]. This property was due to its strong ability to stimulate secretion of tumor necrosis factor alpha (TNF-α) by macrophages. Studies in rodents showed remarkable but selective efficacy against TNF-α-sensitive tumors, which improved in combination with other antitumor therapies.

References

1. Glenny, A., Pope, C., Waddington, H., Wallace, V.: The antigenic value of toxoid precipitated by potassium-alum. J. Pathol. Bacteriol. **29**, 38–45 (1926)
2. Romero Méndez, I.Z., Shi, Y., HogenEsch, H., Hem, S.L.: Potentiation of the immune response to non-adsorbed antigens by aluminum-containing adjuvants. Vaccine **25**, 825–833 (2007)
3. Tritto, E., Mosca, F., De Gregorio, E.: Mechanism of action of licensed vaccine adjuvants. Vaccine **27**, 3331–3334 (2009)
4. Heegaard, P.M.H., et al.: Adjuvants and delivery systems in veterinary vaccinology: current state and future developments. Arch. Virol. **156**, 183–202 (2011)
5. Mannhalter, J.W., Neychev, H.O., Zlabinger, G.J., Ahmad, R., Eibl, M.M.: Modulation of the human immune response by the non-toxic and non-pyrogenic adjuvant aluminium hydroxide: effect on antigen uptake and antigen presentation. Clin. Exp. Immunol. **61**, 143–151 (1985)
6. Goto, N., et al.: Local tissue irritating effects and adjuvant activities of calcium phosphate and aluminium hydroxide with different physical properties. Vaccine **15**, 1364–1371 (1997)
7. Shi, Y., HogenEsch, H., Hem, S.L.: Change in the degree of adsorption of proteins by aluminum-containing adjuvants following exposure to interstitial fluid: freshly prepared and aged model vaccines. Vaccine **20**, 80–85 (2001)
8. Hem, S.L., HogenEsch, H., Middaugh, C.R., Volkin, D.B.: Preformulation studies – the next advance in aluminum adjuvant-containing vaccines. Vaccine **28**, 4868–4870 (2010)
9. Iyer, S., HogenEsch, H., Hem, S.L.: Effect of the degree of phosphate substitution in aluminum hydroxide adjuvant on the adsorption of phosphorylated proteins. Pharm. Dev. Technol. **8**, 81–86 (2003)
10. Hutchison, S., et al.: Antigen depot is not required for alum adjuvanticity. FASEB J. (2011). doi:10.1096/fj.11-184556
11. Noc, S.M., Green, M.A., HogenEsch, H., Hem, S.L.: Mechanism of immunopotentiation by aluminum-containing adjuvants elucidated by the relationship between antigen retention at the inoculation site and the immune response. Vaccine **28**, 3588–3594 (2010)
12. Munks, M.W., et al.: Aluminum adjuvants elicit fibrin-dependent extracellular traps in vivo. Blood **116**, 5191–5199 (2010)
13. Lambrecht, B.N., Kool, M., Willart, M.A.M., Hammad, H.: Mechanism of action of clinically approved adjuvants. Curr. Opin. Immunol. **21**, 23–29 (2009)
14. Jiang, D., Morefield, G.L., HogenEsch, H., Hem, S.L.: Relationship of adsorption mechanism of antigens by aluminum-containing adjuvants to in vitro elution in interstitial fluid. Vaccine **24**, 1665–1669 (2006)
15. Gupta, R.K., Chang, A.C., Griffin, P., Rivera, R., Siber, G.R.: In vivo distribution of radioactivity in mice after injection of biodegradable polymer microspheres containing 14C-labeled tetanus toxoid. Vaccine **14**, 1412–1416 (1996)
16. Kool, M., et al.: Alum adjuvant boosts adaptive immunity by inducing uric acid and activating inflammatory dendritic cells. J. Exp. Med. **205**, 869–882 (2008)
17. Seubert, A., et al.: Adjuvanticity of the oil-in-water emulsion MF59 is independent of Nlrp3 inflammasome but requires the adaptor protein MyD88. Proc. Natl. Acad. Sci. **108**, 11169–11174 (2011)
18. McKee, A.S., et al.: Alum induces innate immune responses through macrophage and mast cell sensors, but these sensors are not required for alum to act as an adjuvant for specific immunity. J. Immunol. **183**, 4403–4414 (2009)
19. Calabro, S., et al.: Vaccine adjuvants alum and MF59 induce rapid recruitment of neutrophils and monocytes that participate in antigen transport to draining lymph nodes. Vaccine **29**, 1812–1823 (2011)
20. Mosca, F., et al.: Molecular and cellular signatures of human vaccine adjuvants. Proc. Natl. Acad. Sci. **105**, 10501–10506 (2008)
21. Shi, Y., Evans, J.E., Rock, K.L.: Molecular identification of a danger signal that alerts the immune system to dying cells. Nature **425**, 516–521 (2003)
22. Ulanova, M., Tarkowski, A., Hahn-Zoric, M., Hanson, L.A.: The Common vaccine adjuvant aluminum hydroxide up-regulates accessory properties of human monocytes via an interleukin-4-dependent mechanism. Infect. Immun. **69**, 1151–1159 (2001)
23. Ghimire, T.R., Benson, R.A., Garside, P., Brewer, J.M.: Alum increases antigen uptake, reduces antigen degradation and sustains antigen presentation by DCs in vitro. Immunol. Lett. **147**(1–2), 55–62 (2012). doi:10.1016/j.imlet.2012.06.002
24. Flach, T.L., et al.: Alum interaction with dendritic cell membrane lipids is essential for its adjuvanticity. Nat. Med. **1–10**, 479–487. doi:10.1038/nm.2306 (2011)
25. Wijburg, O.L., et al.: The role of macrophages in the induction and regulation of immunity elicited by exogenous antigens. Eur. J. Immunol. **28**, 479–487 (1998)
26. Gavin, A.L., et al.: Adjuvant-enhanced antibody responses in the absence of toll-like receptor signaling. Science **314**, 1936–1938 (2006)
27. Martinon, F., Tschopp, J.: Inflammatory caspases and inflammasomes: master switches of inflammation. Cell Death Differ. **14**, 10–22 (2007)
28. Ng, G., et al.: Receptor-independent, direct membrane binding leads to cell-surface lipid sorting and Syk kinase activation in dendritic cells. Immunity **29**, 807–818 (2008)
29. Sorlier, P., Denuziere, A., Viton, C., Domard, A.: Relation between the degree of acetylation and the electrostatic properties of chitin and chitosan. Biomacromolecules **2**, 765–772 (2001)
30. Bonferoni, M.C., Sandri, G., Rossi, S., Ferrari, F., Caramella, C.: Chitosan and its salts for mucosal and transmucosal delivery. Expert Opin. Drug Deliv. **6**, 923–939 (2009). doi:10.1517/17425240903114142
31. Kumar, M.N., Muzzarelli, R.A., Muzzarelli, C., Sashiwa, H., Domb, A.J.: Chitosan chemistry and pharmaceutical perspectives. Chem. Rev. **104**, 6017–6084 (2004). doi:10.1021/cr030441b
32. Illum, L., Farraj, N.F., Davis, S.S.: Chitosan as a novel nasal delivery system for peptide drugs. Pharm. Res. **11**, 1186–1189 (1994)
33. Alves, N.M., Mano, J.F.: Chitosan derivatives obtained by chemical modifications for biomedical and environmental applications. Int. J. Biol. Macromol. **43**, 401–414 (2008), S0141-8130(08)00208-0 [pii]. doi:10.1016/j.ijbiomac.2008.09.007
34. Jabbal-Gill, I., Watts, P., Smith, A.: Chitosan-based delivery systems for mucosal vaccines. Expert Opin. Drug Deliv. **9**, 1051–1067 (2012). doi:10.1517/17425247.2012.697455
35. Luppi, B., Bigucci, F., Cerchiara, T., Zecchi, V.: Chitosan-based hydrogels for nasal drug delivery: from inserts to nanoparticles. Expert Opin. Drug Deliv. **7**, 811–828 (2010). doi:10.1517/17425247.2010.495981
36. Vila, A., Sanchez, A., Tobio, M., Calvo, P., Alonso, M.J.: Design of biodegradable particles for protein delivery. J. Control. Release **78**, 15–24 (2002), S0168365901004862 [pii]
37. Vila, A., et al.: Low molecular weight chitosan nanoparticles as new carriers for nasal vaccine delivery in mice. Eur. J. Pharm. Biopharm. **57**, 123–131 (2004), S0939641103001620 [pii]
38. Amidi, M., et al.: Preparation and characterization of protein-loaded N-trimethyl chitosan nanoparticles as nasal delivery system. J. Control. Release **111**, 107–116 (2006), S0168-3659(05)00652-8 [pii]. doi:10.1016/j.jconrel.2005.11.014
39. Saint-Lu, N., et al.: Targeting the allergen to oral dendritic cells with mucoadhesive chitosan particles enhances tolerance induction. Allergy **64**, 1003–1013 (2009), ALL1945 [pii]. doi:10.1111/j.1398-9995.2009.01945.x

40. Porporatto, C., Bianco, I.D., Correa, S.G.: Local and systemic activity of the polysaccharide chitosan at lymphoid tissues after oral administration. J. Leukoc. Biol. **78**, 62–69 (2005), jlb.0904541 [pii]. doi:10.1189/jlb.0904541
41. Zaharoff, D.A., Rogers, C.J., Hance, K.W., Schlom, J., Greiner, J.W.: Chitosan solution enhances both humoral and cell-mediated immune responses to subcutaneous vaccination. Vaccine **25**, 2085–2094 (2007), S0264-410X(06)01225-4 [pii]. doi:10.1016/j.vaccine.2006.11.034
42. Neimert-Andersson, T., et al.: Improved immune responses in mice using the novel chitosan adjuvant ViscoGel, with a Haemophilus influenzae type b glycoconjugate vaccine. Vaccine **29**, 8965–8973 (2011), S0264-410X(11)01447-2 [pii]. doi:10.1016/j.vaccine.2011.09.041
43. Ghendon, Y., et al.: Evaluation of properties of chitosan as an adjuvant for inactivated influenza vaccines administered parenterally. J. Med. Virol. **81**, 494–506 (2009). doi:10.1002/jmv.21415
44. Lee, C.G., Da Silva, C.A., Lee, J.Y., Hartl, D., Elias, J.A.: Chitin regulation of immune responses: an old molecule with new roles. Curr. Opin. Immunol. **20**, 684–689 (2008), S0952-7915(08)00185-4 [pii]. doi:10.1016/j.coi.2008.10.002
45. Shibata, Y., Metzger, W.J., Myrvik, Q.N.: Chitin particle-induced cell-mediated immunity is inhibited by soluble mannan: mannose receptor-mediated phagocytosis initiates IL-12 production. J. Immunol. **159**, 2462–2467 (1997)
46. Da Silva, C.A., Hartl, D., Liu, W., Lee, C.G., Elias, J.A.: TLR-2 and IL-17A in chitin-induced macrophage activation and acute inflammation. J. Immunol. **181**, 4279–4286 (2008), 181/6/4279 [pii]
47. Peluso, G., et al.: Chitosan-mediated stimulation of macrophage function. Biomaterials **15**, 1215–1220 (1994)
48. Mori, A., et al.: The vaccine adjuvant alum inhibits IL-12 by promoting PI3 kinase signaling while chitosan does not inhibit IL-12 and enhances Th1 and Th17 responses. Eur. J. Immunol. (2012). doi:10.1002/eji.201242372
49. Hallander, H.O., Lepp, T., Ljungman, M., Netterlid, E., Andersson, M.: Do we need a booster of Hib vaccine after primary vaccination? A study on anti-Hib seroprevalence in Sweden 5 and 15 years after the introduction of universal Hib vaccination related to notifications of invasive disease. APMIS **118**, 878–887 (2010). doi:10.1111/j.1600-0463.2010.02674.x
50. Muzzarelli, R.A.: Chitins and chitosans as immunoadjuvants and non-allergenic drug carriers. Mar. Drugs **8**, 292–312 (2010). doi:10.3390/md8020292
51. Mills, K.H., et al.: Protective levels of diphtheria-neutralizing antibody induced in healthy volunteers by unilateral priming-boosting intranasal immunization associated with restricted ipsilateral mucosal secretory immunoglobulin a. Infect. Immun. **71**, 726–732 (2003)
52. McNeela, E.A., et al.: Intranasal immunization with genetically detoxified diphtheria toxin induces T cell responses in humans: enhancement of Th2 responses and toxin-neutralizing antibodies by formulation with chitosan. Vaccine **22**, 909–914 (2004), doi:10.1016/j.vaccine.2003.09.012S0264410X03006728
53. Read, R.C., et al.: Effective nasal influenza vaccine delivery using chitosan. Vaccine **23**, 4367–4374 (2005), S0264-410X(05)00463-9 [pii]. doi:10.1016/j.vaccine.2005.04.021
54. Huo, Z., et al.: Induction of protective serum meningococcal bactericidal and diphtheria-neutralizing antibodies and mucosal immunoglobulin A in volunteers by nasal insufflations of the Neisseria meningitidis serogroup C polysaccharide-CRM197 conjugate vaccine mixed with chitosan. Infect. Immun. **73**, 8256–8265 (2005), 73/12/8256 [pii]. doi:10.1128/IAI.73.12.8256-8265.2005
55. El-Kamary, S.S., et al.: Adjuvanted intranasal Norwalk virus-like particle vaccine elicits antibodies and antibody-secreting cells that express homing receptors for mucosal and peripheral lymphoid tissues. J. Infect. Dis. **202**, 1649–1658 (2010). doi:10.1086/657087
56. Atmar, R.L., et al.: Norovirus vaccine against experimental human Norwalk Virus illness. N. Engl. J. Med. **365**, 2178–2187 (2011). doi:10.1056/NEJMoa1101245
57. Mucovac2. http://public.ukcrn.org.uk/Search/StudyDetail.aspx?StudyID=11679. (2012)
58. Li, X., et al.: Preliminary safety and efficacy results of laser immunotherapy for the treatment of metastatic breast cancer patients. Photochem. Photobiol. Sci. **10**, 817–821 (2011). doi:10.1039/c0pp00306a
59. Sandvig, K., van Deurs, B.: Delivery into cells: lessons learned from plant and bacterial toxins. Gene Ther. **12**, 865–872 (2005). doi:10.1038/sj.gt.3302525
60. Adkins, I., Holubova, J., Kosova, M., Sadilkova, L.: Bacteria and their toxins tamed for immunotherapy. Curr. Pharm. Biotechnol. **13**, 1446–1473 (2012)
61. Pizza, M., et al.: Mucosal vaccines: non toxic derivatives of LT and CT as mucosal adjuvants. Vaccine **19**, 2534–2541 (2001)
62. Sanchez, J., Holmgren, J.: Cholera toxin – a foe & a friend. Indian J. Med. Res. **133**, 153–163 (2011)
63. Lapa, J.A., et al.: Randomized clinical trial assessing the safety and immunogenicity of oral microencapsulated enterotoxigenic Escherichia coli surface antigen 6 with or without heat-labile enterotoxin with mutation R192G. Clin. Vaccine Immunol. **15**, 1222–1228 (2008)
64. Lycke, N.: Targeted vaccine adjuvants based on modified cholera toxin. Curr. Mol. Med. **5**, 591–597 (2005)
65. Adamsson, J., et al.: Novel immunostimulatory agent based on CpG oligodeoxynucleotide linked to the nontoxic B subunit of cholera toxin. J. Immunol. **176**, 4902–4913 (2006)
66. Sun, J.B., Holmgren, J., Czerkinsky, C.: Cholera toxin B subunit: an efficient transmucosal carrier-delivery system for induction of peripheral immunological tolerance. Proc. Natl. Acad. Sci. U. S. A. **91**, 10795–10799 (1994)
67. Vazquez, R.I., Moreno-Fierros, L., Neri-Bazan, L., De La Riva, G.A., Lopez-Revilla, R.: Bacillus thuringiensis Cry1Ac protoxin is a potent systemic and mucosal adjuvant. Scand. J. Immunol. **49**, 578–584 (1999)
68. Munoz, J.J., Bernard, C.C., Mackay, I.R.: Elicitation of experimental allergic encephalomyelitis (EAE) in mice with the aid of pertussigen. Cell. Immunol. **83**, 92–100 (1984)
69. Pizza, M., et al.: Mutants of pertussis toxin suitable for vaccine development. Science **246**, 497–500 (1989)
70. Podda, A., et al.: Metabolic, humoral, and cellular responses in adult volunteers immunized with the genetically inactivated pertussis toxin mutant PT-9K/129G. J. Exp. Med. **172**, 861–868 (1990)
71. Rietschel, E.T., et al.: Bacterial endotoxins: chemical structure, biological activity and role in septicaemia. Scand. J. Infect. Dis. Suppl. **31**, 8–21 (1982)
72. Guo, L., et al.: Lipid A acylation and bacterial resistance against vertebrate antimicrobial peptides. Cell **95**, 189–198 (1998)
73. Reynolds, C.M., et al.: An outer membrane enzyme encoded by *Salmonella typhimurium lpxR* that removes the 3′-acyloxyacyl moiety of lipid A. J. Biol. Chem. **281**, 21974–21987 (2006)
74. Palsson-McDermott, E.M., O'Neill, L.A.: Signal transduction by the lipopolysaccharide receptor, Toll-like receptor-4. Immunology **113**, 153–162 (2004)
75. Alexander, C., Rietschel, E.T.: Bacterial lipopolysaccharides and innate immunity. J. Endotoxin Res. **7**, 167–202 (2001)
76. Morrison, D.C., Kline, L.F.: Activation of the classical and properdin pathways of complement by bacterial lipopolysaccharides (LPS). J. Immunol. **118**, 362–368 (1977)
77. Conti, P., et al.: Activation of human natural killer cells by lipopolysaccharide and generation of interleukin-1 alpha, beta, tumour necrosis factor and interleukin-6. Effect of IL-1 receptor antagonist. Immunology **73**, 450–456 (1991)

78. Annane, D., Bellissant, E., Cavaillon, J.M.: Septic shock. Lancet **365**, 63–78 (2005)
79. Miller, S.I., Ernst, R.K., Bader, M.W.: LPS, TLR4 and infectious disease diversity. Nat. Rev. Microbiol. **3**, 36–46 (2005)
80. Chen, K., Cerutti, A.: Vaccination strategies to promote mucosal antibody responses. Immunity **33**, 479–491 (2010)
81. O'Hagan, D.T.: MF59 is a safe and potent vaccine adjuvant that enhances protection against influenza virus infection. Expert Rev. Vaccines **6**, 699–710 (2007)
82. Arenas, J.: The role of bacterial lipopolysaccharides as immune modulator in vaccine and drug development. Endocr Metab Immune Disord Drug Targets **12(3)**, 221–235 (2012)
83. Baldridge, J.R., Crane, R.T.: Monophosphoryl lipid A (MPL) formulations for the next generation of vaccines. Methods **19**, 103–107 (1999)
84. Evans, J.T., et al.: Enhancement of antigen-specific immunity via the TLR4 ligands MPL adjuvant and Ribi.529. Expert Rev. Vaccines **2**, 219–229 (2003)
85. Ulrich, J.T., Myers, K.R.: Monophosphoryl lipid A as an adjuvant. Past experiences and new directions. Pharm. Biotechnol. **6**, 495–524 (1995)
86. Vajdy, M., Singh, M.: The role of adjuvants in the development of mucosal vaccines. Expert Opin. Biol. Ther. **5**, 953–965 (2005)
87. Drachenberg, K.J., Wheeler, A.W., Stuebner, P., Horak, F.: A well-tolerated grass pollen-specific allergy vaccine containing a novel adjuvant, monophosphoryl lipid A, reduces allergic symptoms after only four preseasonal injections. Allergy **56**, 498–505 (2001)
88. Kundi, M.: New hepatitis B vaccine formulated with an improved adjuvant system. Expert Rev. Vaccines **6**, 133–140 (2007)
89. Aide, P., et al.: Four year immunogenicity of the RTS, S/AS02(A) malaria vaccine in Mozambican children during a phase IIb trial. Vaccine **29**, 6059–6067 (2011)
90. Polhemus, M.E., et al.: Evaluation of RTS, S/AS02A and RTS, S/AS01B in adults in a high malaria transmission area. PLoS One **4**, e6465 (2009)
91. Brichard, V.G., Lejeune, D.: Cancer immunotherapy targeting tumour-specific antigens: towards a new therapy for minimal residual disease. Expert Opin. Biol. Ther. **8**, 951–968 (2008)
92. Arenas, J., et al.: Coincorporation of LpxL1 and PagL mutant lipopolysaccharides into liposomes with *Neisseria meningitidis* opacity protein: influence on endotoxic and adjuvant activity. Clin. Vaccine Immunol. **17**, 487–495 (2010)
93. Vernacchio, L., et al.: Effect of monophosphoryl lipid A (MPL) on T-helper cells when administered as an adjuvant with pneumocococcal-CRM197 conjugate vaccine in healthy toddlers. Vaccine **20**, 3658–3667 (2002)
94. Olson, K., et al.: Liposomal gD ectodomain (gD1-306) vaccine protects against HSV2 genital or rectal infection of female and male mice. Vaccine **28**, 548–560 (2009)
95. Hall, M.A., et al.: Intranasal immunization with multivalent group A streptococcal vaccines protects mice against intranasal challenge infections. Infect. Immun. **72**, 2507–2512 (2004)
96. Tana, Watarai, S., Isogai, E., Oguma, K.: Induction of intestinal IgA and IgG antibodies preventing adhesion of verotoxin-producing *Escherichia coli* to Caco-2 cells by oral immunization with liposomes. Lett. Appl. Microbiol. **36**, 135–139 (2003)
97. Baldridge, J.R., Yorgensen, Y., Ward, J.R., Ulrich, J.T.: Monophosphoryl lipid A enhances mucosal and systemic immunity to vaccine antigens following intranasal administration. Vaccine **18**, 2416–2425 (2000)
98. Egan, M.A., et al.: A comparative evaluation of nasal and parenteral vaccine adjuvants to elicit systemic and mucosal HIV-1 peptide-specific humoral immune responses in cynomolgus macaques. Vaccine **22**, 3774–3788 (2004)
99. Mason, K.W., et al.: Reduction of nasal colonization of nontypeable *Haemophilus influenzae* following intranasal immunization with rLP4/rLP6/UspA2 proteins combined with aqueous formulation of RC529. Vaccine **22**, 3449–3456 (2004)
100. Baldridge, J.R., et al.: Immunostimulatory activity of aminoalkyl glucosaminide 4-phosphates (AGPs): induction of protective innate immune responses by RC-524 and RC-529. J. Endotoxin Res. **8**, 453–458 (2002)
101. Ishizaka, S.T., Hawkins, L.D.: E6020: a synthetic Toll-like receptor 4 agonist as a vaccine adjuvant. Expert Rev. Vaccines **6**, 773–784 (2007)
102. Wang, S., et al.: Effective antibody therapy induces host-protective antitumor immunity that is augmented by TLR4 agonist treatment. Cancer Immunol. Immunother. **61**, 49–61 (2012)
103. Coler, R.N., et al.: A synthetic adjuvant to enhance and expand immune responses to influenza vaccines. PLoS One **5**, e13677 (2010)
104. Ueda, H., Yamazaki, M.: Induction of tumor necrosis factor in a murine tumor by systemic administration of a novel synthetic lipid A analogue, ONO-4007. J. Immunother. **20**, 65–69 (1997)

Micro- and Nanotechnology

8

Contents

8.1 Nanostructures and Nanopharmaceuticals

> Nano-technology mainly consists of the processing of separation, consolidation, and deformation of materials by one atom or one molecule. (Richard Feynman: There's Plenty of Room at the Bottom, 1959)

By definition, *nanopharmaceuticals are based on the manipulation of matter with at least one dimension sized from 1 to 100 nm, where unique phenomena enable novel applications not feasible when working with bulk materials or even with single atoms or molecules.* (National Nanotechnology Initiative, USA).

1 nanometer (nm) is one billionth, or 10^{-9}, of a meter.

Thereby, nanotechnology is defined by size. By comparison: a DNA double helix has a diameter around 2 nm. On the other hand, the smallest cellular life forms, *Mycoplasma*, are around 200 nm in length. Poxviruses are exceptionally large viruses, their size is around 200 nm in diameter and 300 nm in length, and *picornaviruses* are around 27–30 nm in diameter.

Colloid Chemistry. The term "nano" partly masks the good, old colloid chemistry: a colloid is prepared by reducing large particles to colloidal size (between 1 and 1000 nm) or increasing small particles (single molecules) to the size of colloidal particles. In so doing, e.g., colloidal gold particles *mutated* to nano gold particles. Fortunately, liposomes still refer as liposomes and not as nanoliposomes. In the case of liposomes, these particles can range between 25 and 1000 nm. The most commonly used liposomes display a size between 50 and 200 nm.

Microparticles. The limits for nano is clearly defined and sized from 1 to 100 nm. All tendencies to stretch the upper limits are a creeping maceration of the definition. Particles of more than 100 nm are microparticles and nothing else (Fig. 8.1).

The synthesis of nanoparticles is still demanding, but novel tools enable the control of particle properties and may

M. Giese, *Introduction to Molecular Vaccinology*, DOI 10.1007/978-3-319-25832-4_8

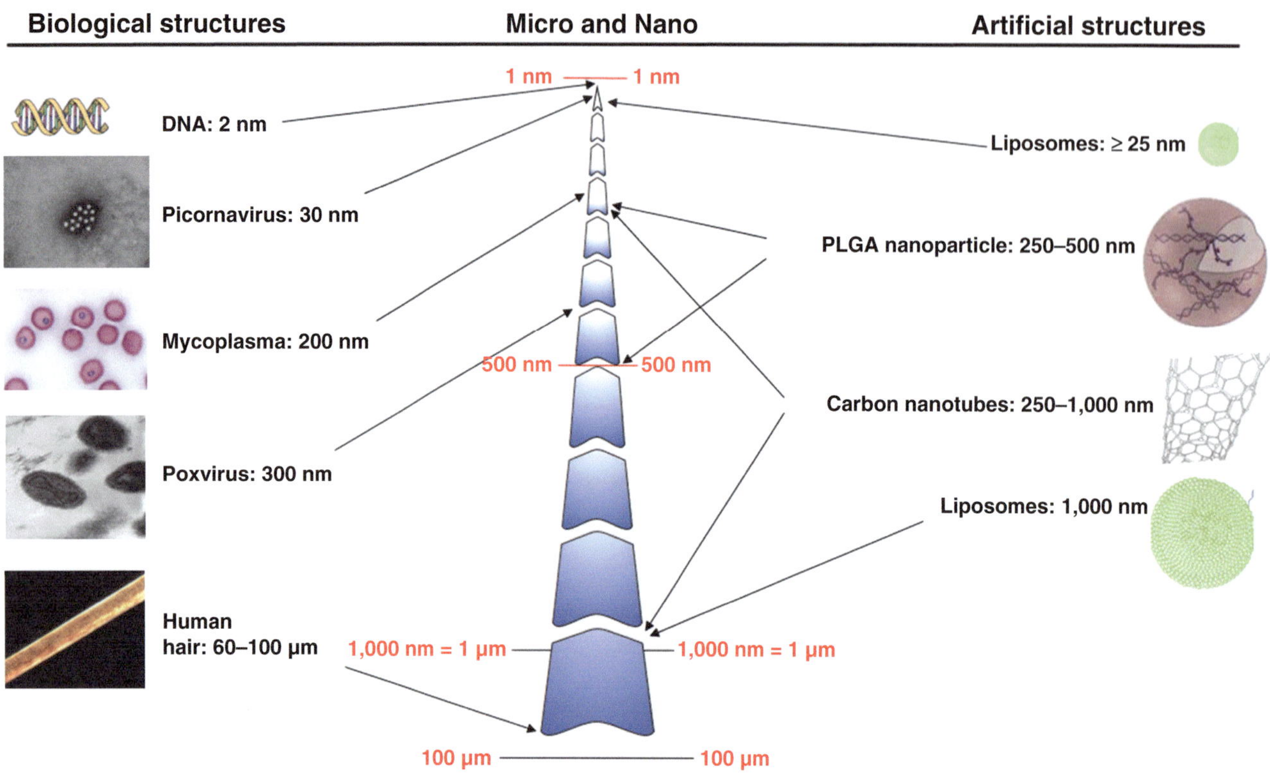

Fig. 8.1 Nanotechnology is defined by size. Biological structures: a DNA double helix has a diameter around 2 nm. The smallest cellular life forms, *Mycoplasma*, are around 200 nm in length. *Poxviruses* are exceptionally large viruses, and their size is around 200 nm in diameter and 300 nm in length, and picornaviruses are around 27–30 nm in diameter. Artificial structures: Liposomes can range between 25 and 1000 nm. The most commonly used liposomes display a size between 50 and 200 nm. Particles of more than 100 nm are microparticles (Figure prepared for this book by S. Giese, Institute of Virology, University of Freiburg/Germany)

allow the optimized synthesis of immunomodulating nanomedicine for effective vaccination approaches.

8.2 Basics in Nanotechnology[1]

Nanoparticles can be made up of a variety of materials and, because of their large surface to volume ratio, often possess different properties from the bulk material they are made of. Nanoparticles can be synthesized by bottom-up or top-down approaches. In general, these nano-sized systems can be inorganic colloids, organic colloids (synthesized by emulsion polymerization or mini-/nanoemulsion techniques), polymeric aggregates (micelles or polymersomes), core cross-linked aggregates (nanohydrogels, cross-linked micelles, or polyplexes), multifunctional polymer coils, dendritic polymers, or perfect dendrimers.

For example, a paramagnetic iron oxide core can be used for magnetic resonance imaging (MRI) or a biodegradable core to release a bioactive by diffusion while degrading. Due to their size, they can be used to combine different functionalities among one object leading to multifunctionality or multivalency. Additionally, those systems can be able to encapsulate bioactive compounds. Shielding the cargo requires core–shell structures, while the core encapsulates the cargo, the shell provides solubility and suppresseses protein absorption or aggregation.

Nanomedicine. When these nano-sized objects are applied to diagnose or treat diseases, they become so-called nanomedicines, an umbrella term encompassing nanopharmaceuticals, nanoimaging agents, and theranostics.

The interaction of a nanoparticle with its environment takes place at the interface of particle and surrounding media – the particle surface. Thus, the molecules stabilizing the particle surface toward its surroundings determine the interaction with biological matter and the in vivo fate. In many cases, the characterization of nanoparticles is difficult as described later. In respect to this fact, it is necessary to carefully consider, understand, and design nanoparticles – in particular when they are utilized for complex in vivo applications.

[1] From polymers to nanomedicines: New materials for future vaccines by *Philipp Heller, David Huesmann, Martin Scherer, and Matthias Barz* in Molecular Vaccines – From Prophylaxis to Therapy, Volume 2, Springer-Verlag Wien, 2013, Ed. Matthias Giese.

Terminology in Nanoparticle Synthesis

Polymers

Polymers are chemical compounds consisting of basic structural repeating units called monomers. A polymer may be formed from one or multiple kinds of monomers during a process called polymerization. The material properties are not only determined by the chemical composition of the monomer(s) but also by the number of monomer molecules connected to each other to form the macromolecule (degree of polymerization) and the structural alignment.

Dispersity

Apart from a few examples (proteins, DNA, or perfect dendrimers), polymers often consist of a mixture of macromolecules differing in molecular weight/degree of polymerization due to a variance in the number of monomers the individual polymer molecule consists of. The dispersity $Đ$ is defined as

$$Đ = \frac{M_w}{M_n}$$

where M_w is the mass-average molar mass

$$M_w = \frac{\sum M_i^2 \cdot N_i}{\sum M_i \cdot N_i}$$

and M_n is the number-average molar mass

$$M_n = \frac{\sum M_i \cdot N_i}{\sum N_i}.$$

A low dispersity (near 1) means that a large fraction of molecules have similar degrees of polymerization.

Block Copolymers

Block copolymers are an important type of copolymers (polymers consisting of more than one monomeric species). This term is applied when a sequence of a single type of monomer (homopolymer) is followed by a sequence formed from another species. Block copolymers may consist of two (diblock copolymer), three (triblock copolymer), or more blocks (multiblock copolymer). The chemical nature of the different blocks in a covalent macromolecule can lead to unique properties (such as tenside-like amphiphilicity in the case of hydrophilic/hydrophobic block copolymers) or can enable the block-specific functionalization (e.g., with dyes, receptor molecules, etc.).

Colloids

Colloids are particles ranging from 1 to 1000 nm which are microscopically dispersed in a continuous medium. Colloidal solutions are an interstage between true solutions and suspensions and exhibit no colligative properties. Colloidal systems can be made of organic as well as inorganic particles. To prevent colloids from coagulation – which is thermodynamically favored – particles must be kept separate from each other by electrostatic or steric repulsion.

Amphiphiles

Amphiphiles are molecules having both hydrophilic (polar) and hydrophobic (nonpolar) properties. When in contact with water, amphiphiles will self-assemble into different superstructures in order to minimize the interphase energy. In this way, various aggregates such as micelles, polymersomes (polymer-based liposome-like structures), or double-layer membranes can be formed. The precise structure depends on the ratio of hydrophilic versus hydrophobic domains as well as environmental conditions during preparation and storage.

Dendrimers/Dendrons

Dendrimers are polymeric molecules which are repetitively branched and exhibit a highly symmetrical and well-defined structure. They are synthesized in repeated cycles where new generations of monomers are added to a core exhibiting two or more reactive sites. The reactive groups (again, more than one per unit) of the newly added outer sphere then act as basis for the addition of the next generation. Alternatively, in a convergent approach, dendrons (branched molecules with a single reactive group, the so-called focal point) are synthesized which are then coupled to the multifunctional core in a final step. In both cases, monodisperse dendrimers are formed which exhibit a large number of functional peripheral groups.

Micelles

Micelles are an important type of colloidal aggregate formed from amphiphilic molecules such as low molecular weight surfactants or amphiphilic polymers. Above the *critical micelle concentration* (CMC), the surfactant molecules will spontaneously arrange in an order where the polar head groups are directed toward the water phase (or other polar solvent) and the tails form the hydrophobic inner core which can be employed to encapsulate hydrophobic cargo.

Surfactants

Surfactants *(surface-active agents)* are molecules lowering the surface tension of a liquid or the interfacial tension between two immiscible phases. They are amphiphilic compounds which will adsorb at the interface between hydrophilic and hydrophobic phase with the polar head group arranged in the hydrophilic environment and the nonpolar part extending into the hydrophobic phase, respectively. Surfactants are widely applied in interphase science and technology, serving as detergents or dispersants, wetting agents, and as stabilizers for emulsification.

Apart from both natural and synthetic small-molecule surfactants, polymer-based surfactants have attracted huge interest. Due to the variability of block materials and the possibility for postpolymerization modification, such amphiphiles can be specifically tailored for the intended application. Their high molecular weights result in stronger adsorption and superior stabilization properties since – in contrast to small-molecule amphiphiles – steric stabilization becomes an important aspect.

Emulsions

Emulsions are disperse systems which consist of droplets of one liquid phase (dispersed phase) which are dispersed in a second liquid phase (continuous phase) it is not miscible with. Typically, a stable emulsion requires the addition of surfactants and a co-stabilizer which is dissolved in the dispersed phase. Via different methods, droplet sizes on the order of around 30 to a few hundred nanometers can be achieved. This so-called *miniemulsion* fabrication has become an interesting tool in nanoparticle synthesis. Such particles can either be obtained by *miniemulsion polymerization* or by (polymer) coating and stabilization of preformed droplets (*miniemulsion technique*).

8.2.1 Favorable Properties of Nanoparticles

During the last decades, nanoparticles have shown great potential for the application in drug delivery and vaccination, and they are expected to provide solutions to various current issues in this field. The first one is the fundamental problem of solubility: according to Torchilin [1], about half of potentially valuable drug candidates identified by high-throughput screening technologies including those with the highest activities demonstrate poor solubility in water and – for this reason – never enter further development. By encapsulation or binding to a nanoparticulate carrier, this problem can be overcome.

Additionally, encapsulation of sensitive agents such as DNA, RNA, or peptides protects them against premature enzymatic or proteolytic degradation.

In combination with a "stealth" surface of the carrier, which prevents opsonization through steric repulsion, a prolonged circulation can be achieved. Moreover, through chemical modification, defined recognition and site-specific release are possible.

One main objective in using nanocarriers is to increase the specificity toward certain cells or tissues. This can either be achieved by passive targeting as in the accumulation in well-vascularized tumors driven by the EPR (enhanced permeability and retention) effect [2] or actively by binding of the particles to specific receptors presented by certain cells. Such targeted localization is enabled by functionalizing the particle surface with ligand molecules binding to those receptors, as has been carried out using antibodies, sugar moieties, transferrin, or folates, for instance.

In combination, encapsulation and targeting improve the bioavailability of the respective therapeutic agent. Furthermore, the toxic side effects associated with many drugs are minimized if the active component is shielded from the environment and only released at the designated site of action. As an example, by employing doxorubicin as HPMA-copolymer conjugates PK1/PK2, the maximum tolerated dose (MTD) of the drug was increased threefold [3]. Controlled release can be triggered by factors such as pH, redox potential, enzyme activity, temperature, or magnetic, electric, and ultrasonic signals (Table 8.1).

Table 8.1 Controlled-release strategies

Trigger	Linkage (examples)	Site of release
pH	Cleavage of covalent bonds in acetals, hydrazones, esters	Acidic environment (e.g., endosomal/lysosomal compartment)
Reduction potential	Cleavage of disulfides or benzoquinones	Reductive environment (cytosol)
Enzyme activity	Cleavage of peptide bonds	Specific cells/tissues/diseases
Temperature	Phase transition or change in solubility	Hyperthermic tissue/where hyperthermia is applied
Magnetic signal	Pore formation through movement of magnets	Where signal is applied
Electric signal	Pore formation through electrically stimulated polymer swelling or piezoelectric elements	Where signal is applied
Ultrasonic signal	Polymer degradation	Where signal is applied

As pointed out by Little, another promising aspect of nanoparticles in vaccine development is the multiple presentation of subunit antigens [4]. Such synthetic particles can be designed to exhibit a repetitive orientation of the antigen on the surface, giving the potential of generating B cell receptor cross-linking and enhanced activation [5].

8.2.2 Stabilization of Nanoparticles

Employing nanoparticles as carriers in drug delivery, several aspects need to be taken into consideration: not only must the carrier itself remain in a colloidal form, but nonspecific aggregation in the body has to be avoided or at least controlled.

The two main mechanisms concerning the stabilization of dispersed or emulsified systems are electrostatic and steric stabilization. The electrostatic interaction is described by the *DLVO theory* named after Derjaguin, Landau, Verwey, and Overbeek. Steric stabilization results from polymers adsorbed or covalently linked to the particle surface. This is mostly due to entropic effects concerning the polymer chains, but there is also an enthalpic contribution via solvation energies [6].

For in vivo applications, electrostatic stabilization is difficult to achieve, since serum proteins include polycationic as well as anionic macromolecules, which will adsorb onto oppositely charged colloids. The human body has developed a series of protective mechanisms against foreign material far beyond the scope of this article. One of them is the removal of unprotected foreign particles larger than the renal threshold from the bloodstream. However, this includes the removal of nano-sized drug carriers, a process initiated by opsonization by the mononuclear phagocyte system (MPS). Monocytes of the MPS can remove unprotected particles within seconds of intravenous administration which impedes their application as drug carriers due to premature clearance.

Opsonization. Even though the exact mechanism of this complicated process is not fully understood yet, it is widely accepted that opsonization is started by a series of proteins including immunoglobulins and components of the complement system and other serum proteins. The (incomplete) list of relevant proteins identified so far contains C3, C4, C5, laminin, fibronectin, C-reactive protein, type I collagen, and many more [7]. Those proteins approach the nanocarrier by random Brownian motion and, once close enough to the surface, may bind to the particle via different forces: van der Waals or ionic forces, just to name two of them. The step of opsonin binding is followed by the attachment of phagocytes to the nanoparticle. Phagocytes cannot recognize the carrier themselves but will dock to the particle via surface-bound opsonins. Two alternative mechanisms are the stimulation of phagocytosis by nonspecific adherence to the opsonins and complement activation, which results in binding of the foreign particle by mononuclear phagocytes.

In a final step, the particle is taken up by phagocytes, typically by endocytosis or phagocytosis. Once the particle is endocytosed, it is degraded by various enzymes and chemical substances or – in case of a nondegradable material – stored and enriched in the body.

As of today, there is no universal solution to completely prevent the opsonization of particles. However, a general trend is observed that hydrophilic but neutral ligands hamper the adsorption of proteins and therefore slow down the clearance from the bloodstream.

Thus, steric stabilization appears to be the method of choice for in vivo applications. Steric stabilization can be achieved by the use of commercial polymeric surfactants (e.g., Tween 20/40/60/80, Pluronics, Cremophor) or synthetic polymers. Block copolymers form more stable layers at the interface of particle and aqueous solution as reported by Scheibe et al. [8] and Kelsch et al. [9] and can suppress aggregation in blood serum. In addition, the polymer can be modified with functional groups, which can later on be addressed for further functionalization.

8.2.3 Types of Nanoparticulate Carriers and Fabrication Methods

As stated above, the precise location of the bioactive compound does have an influence on its action. For example, in vaccination, the immune response can be modulated by the location of the antigen. Depending on the specific aim and the nature of the agent, it can be advantageous to encapsulate the antigen to prevent it from premature degradation, while in other cases the presentation in a repetitive orientation on the outside of the carrier for optimized immune response may be preferred. Consequently, a variety of different colloidal carriers can be employed.

Among the most frequently used systems are liposomes, solid lipid nanoparticles (SLNs), immunostimulating complexes (ISCOMs), micelles, hydrogels, polymer colloids prepared by miniemulsions, and polymer nanoparticles such as those fabricated by particle replication in non-wetting templates (PRINT) (Fig. 8.2).

Polymeric micelles [10], core cross-linked micelles [11], nanohydrogels [12], and polyplexes [13] are mostly based on the assembly of block copolymers into superstructures, which is mainly driven by four forces [14]. Often, hydrophobic (micelles and core cross-linked micelles) and electrostatic (polyplexes) interactions are involved, while metal complexation and the formation of H bonds are only applicable in specific cases. For *hydrophobic interactions*, a different

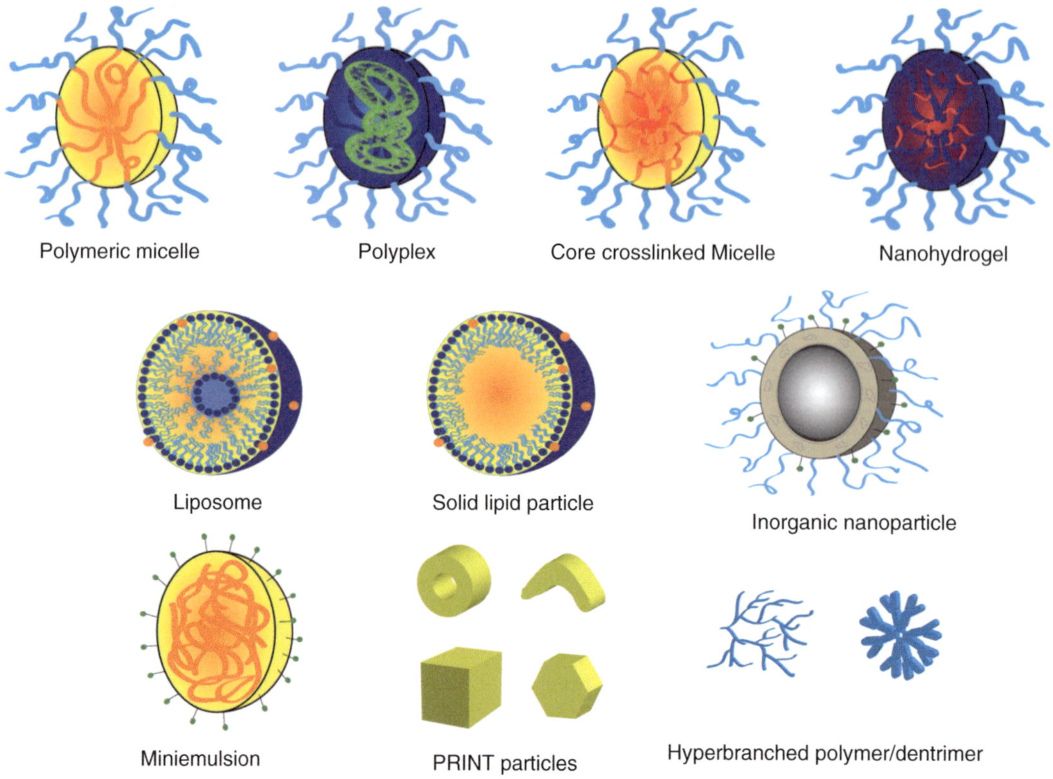

Fig. 8.2 Nanoparticulate carriers

polarity of the blocks leads to a phase separation, resulting in the formation of polymeric micelles where the hydrophobic part aggregates to avoid contact to water. In core–shell structures, the hydrophobic core can then be used for the transport of a hydrophobic payload. In this case, the release of the encapsulated compound is based on passive diffusion or disintegration of the micelle. *Electrostatic interactions* on the other hand relay on the interaction of oppositely charged molecules to form superstructures. A typical example for the formation of so-called polyplexes is the interaction of a positively charged polymer (e.g., polylysine) and negatively charged nucleic acids (DNA or RNA).

Polymeric Micelles. Polymeric micelles form above their critical micelle concentration (CMC), but are always in equilibrium with free unimer. The CMC is also the maximum concentration of free unimer in solution underlining the dynamics of these systems. Upon injection into the blood, the micellar solution is rapidly diluted, potentially leading to disassembly of the micelles. Although the CMC of polymeric micelles is much lower than that of surfactant micelles, this might still pose a problem.

Cross-linked Micelles. Therefore, micelles that are further stabilized are of interest. The easiest way to further stabilize micelles is to cross-link the core chemically [15]. These *core-cross-linked micelles* find themselves in the dilemma of both stably encapsulating the cargo but also needing to be capable of releasing it, once the vesicle has reached its destination. To achieve this, the cross-linking has to be reversible and a stimulus at the destination has to break the stabilizing bonds. This has been realized with various stimuli-responsive cross-linkers. The stimuli used most often are pH or redox potential, but also temperature, enzymes, light, and others have been realized (see Table 8.1). pH-labile bonds are cleaved during endocytosis in the endosome, while redox-labile bonds are cleaved in the reducing environment of the cytoplasm, thus leading to a release of the cargo after uptake by the cell.

Liposomes. Liposomes are spherical structures composed of one or more phospholipid bilayers surrounding an aqueous core, mimicking the basic structure of cell membranes. Depending on the number of bilayers, their size ranges from around 20 nm to several micrometers. Their structural composition gives liposomes great versatility with respect to the way of loading pharmaceutically active agents and the agent's properties. Antigens or immunopotentiators can be encapsulated within the core, embedded in the lipid bilayer, or linked to the outer surface [16]. Liposomes are commonly produced by thin-film hydration, solvent injection, or reverse-phase evaporation.

In order to produce smaller vesicles and narrow the size distribution, sonication and extrusion techniques are used. Liposomes are often modified with polymers to shield the liposome and reduce protein adsorption (e.g., PEGylation) [17] or to integrate pH-responsive elements [18] and molecules for the specific targeting of cells of the immune system like mannose derivatives [19]. Being inherently non-immunogenic, liposomes can be designed not only to carry antigens but also adjuvants to stimulate the innate immune response. Liposomal formulations currently in clinical use include virosomal influenza and hepatitis A vaccines.

Limitations. Despite the aforementioned benefits, employment of liposomes is still limited by several issues. These include long-term physical instability and the low entrapment rate of molecules but also the difficult large-scale production resulting in high costs. Some of these issues can be tackled by *polymersomes* [20]. Vesicular carriers built up analog to liposomes but from block copolymer amphiphiles instead of lipids. Due to their molecular weight, which exceeds the molecular weight of lipids by up to two orders of magnitude, polymersomes have superior material properties and storage capacities. *In contrast to lipids, most polymers, however, do not have GRAS (generally regarded as safe) status by the FDA.*

ISCOMs. Another type of lipid-based nanoparticles are *immunostimulating complexes (ISCOMs).* They have a spherical open lattice structure which, additional to the antigen, is formed from phospholipids, cholesterol, and Quil-A saponin, a strong adjuvant (Fig. 8.16). Such ISCOMs can carry a variety of antigens and have been reported to be about ten times more immunogenic than similar colloidal particles because of the saponin [21]. It also has to be mentioned that there are concerns regarding the toxicity of Quil-A due to its hemolytical activity [22].

Solid Lipid Nanoparticles (SLNs). SLNs are also lipid based, but exhibit a structure different from liposomes. They consist of a core formed from lipids, which are in a solid state under physiological conditions, surrounded by an emulsifier shell. The approach here is to combine the advantages of conventional lipid-based carriers (good biocompatibility, ease of production/scaling up) with those of polymeric nanoparticles (solid matrix for physical and chemical stabilization) [23]. SLNs are mainly produced via high-pressure homogenization and miniemulsion methods. For processing the solid lipids, elevated temperatures are required, but the use of organic solvents can be avoided. A major issue of SLNs is polymorphic transitions due to alteration of the lipid packing (e.g., crystallization), affecting the particle shape which has an influence on the interaction with the physiological environment [24].

Emulsion Techniques. Emulsion techniques are versatile methods for particle formation, giving rise to different classes of colloid carriers in vaccination and drug delivery. This includes nano- and microemulsion particles directly administered as well as polymer or inorganic nanoparticles produced by emulsion polymerization or processing of previously formed emulsion droplets [22].

(Mini)Emulsions. (Mini)Emulsions are composed of droplets of one liquid (dispersed phase) in another, immiscible liquid (continuous phase). Depending on their composition and way of fabrication, miniemulsions occupy a size range of about 30–500 nm [25] (Fig. 8.3).

By the use of surfactants, resulting in electrostatic or steric repulsion, the droplets are stabilized against coalescence. A second additive mixed into the dispersed phase can prevent the destabilization of dispersed droplets by net mass flux of molecules due to the different Laplace pressure of differently sized particles. Such additives are of a highly

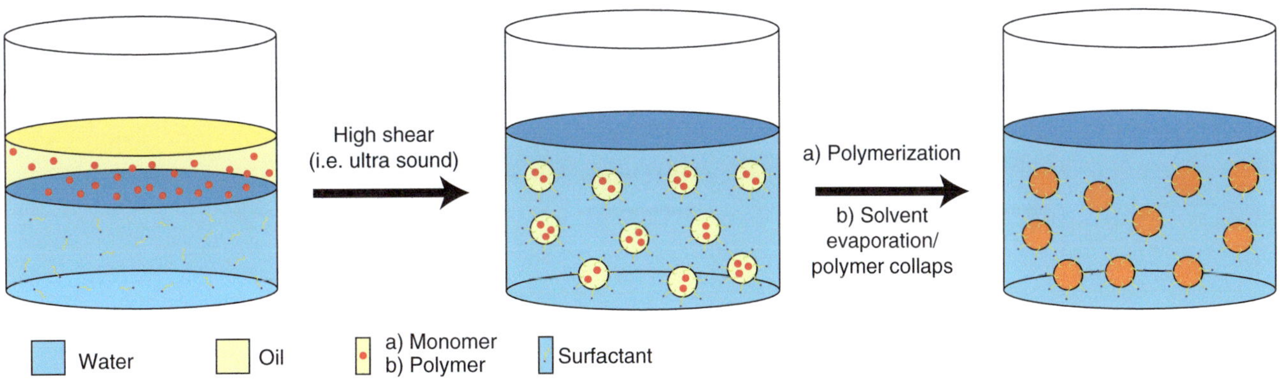

Fig. 8.3 Miniemulsion polymerization (**a**) and miniemulsion technique (**b**)

hydrophobic nature, keeping them from diffusing from one droplet to another and therefore establishing an osmotic pressure counteracting the Laplace pressure. The effectiveness of this process is governed by the hydrophobicity of the additive. Many different types of molecules have been employed as such hydrophobes in the past, including alkanes, dyes, and hydrophobic initiators for polymerization. Given the aforementioned mechanisms and their nanometer size providing kinetic stability against sedimentation, miniemulsions are considered as thermodynamically stable, and time scales for the stability of such emulsions are reported to be in the order of months.

Nano- or miniemulsion – as well as dispersion – of one species in another is a process comprising two major aspects: the disruption of the to-be-emulsified phase resulting in droplets of high specific surface areas and the stabilization of these interfaces by a surfactant. In the emulsification process, the oil phase consisting of the molecules to be emulsified and the hydrophobe is dispersed in the water phase by means of an adequate surfactant and then homogenized. The required high-shear forces are provided by ultrasonication, rotor-stator dispersers, microfluidizers, or high-pressure homogenizers. After homogenization, a second charge of surfactant is added to poststabilize the system effectively [26].

Apart from the facts already mentioned, an important advantage of emulsion techniques is the relatively easy scale-up. While this is a critical point with any kind of highly ordered, self-assembled structures, the bulk production of emulsion formulations affords homogenous and highly stable results in short periods of time.

Evaporation. Among the most common emulsification methods for antigen encapsulation are solvent evaporation and coacervation. Both methods include the formation of a double emulsion (water phase 1/oil phase/water phase 2, see Fig. 8.4) and share the first step, where an aqueous solution of the respective agent is emulsified in an organic polymer solution. In solvent evaporation, this first W/O emulsion is then further dispersed in an aqueous solution containing an appropriate emulsifier – poly(vinyl alcohol) that is frequently employed for this purpose. Finally, the organic solvent is evaporated under reduced pressure, leading to hardening of the polymer and formation of the desired particle.

Coacervation. Coacervation is a phase separation process in which a nonsolvent for the polymer (and antigen) is added to the previously formed W/O emulsion. This results in a phase separation to form a coacervate phase encapsulating the antigen.

Nanoprecipitation. Another possibility for the formation of nanocarriers is nanoprecipitation, also known as solvent displacement method. Here, stabilized nanoparticles are formed by the interfacial deposition of a preformed polymer onto emulsion droplets. An inverse emulsion is formed in a mixed solvent/nonsolvent medium containing a surfactant and the polymer for shell formation. Adding nonsolvent leads to the precipitation of the polymer and deposition on the large surface droplets. After precipitation, the particles can be transferred into water.

However, the formation of nano-sized carriers requires more harsh conditions compared to their micrometer-sized analogs [27]. Consequently, sensitive molecules such as DNA might be structurally damaged, and utmost care needs to be taken when engineering the conditions for forming such particles. Such measures may include the complexation of the agent with cationic amphiphilic molecules (hydrophobic ion pairing, HIP), the judicious choice of solvents, and the adsorption of antigens on the surface of preformed particles [28].

PLA and PLGA. A class of polymeric materials widely used to form drug carriers are polyesters such as poly (D,L-lactide) (PLA) and poly (D,L-lactic-co-glycolic acid) (PLGA). They are biodegradable through hydrolysis and exhibit excellent biocompatibility and sustained-release properties. To stabilize such polymers during mini- or nano-emulsion processes, PEG-b-PLA copolymers appear advantageous since the PLA block mixes well with the polyester core and collapses during solvent evaporation, while the

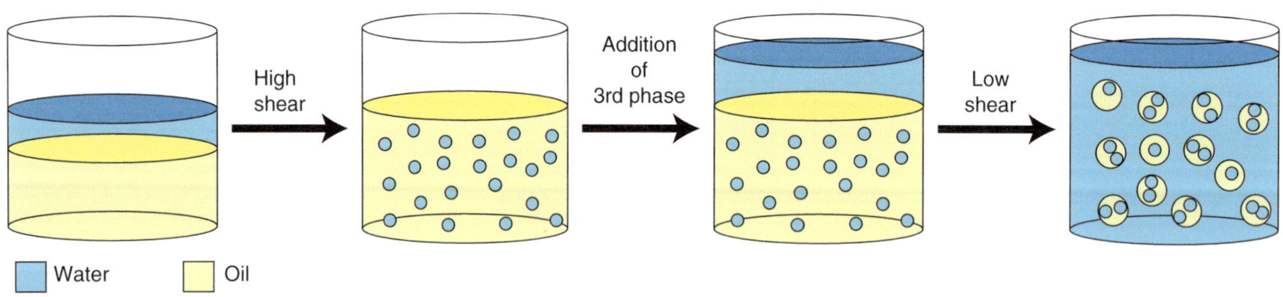

Fig. 8.4 Preparation of a double emulsion

PEG block forms a hydrophilic, protein-resistant corona. Whenever a corona with higher functionality is required, multifunctional PHPMA-b-PLA copolymers as developed by Barz and coworkers can be applied [29].

However, natural or semisynthetic polymers are also widely employed. Such polymers are usually polysaccharide- or protein-based, and to review them all is beyond the scope of this chapter. Therefore, only dextrans and chitosan shall be mentioned here as two important examples.

Dextrans. Dextrans are polymers mainly consisting of α-1,6-glycosides and a small percentage of 1,3-linkages leading to branching [30]. They are well soluble in water and relatively stable due to the glycosidic bonds, being hydrolyzed only under extremely acidic or alkaline conditions. The hydroxyl groups allow for derivatization, for example, a partial hydrophobization to obtain amphiphilic molecules. Chitosan is not water soluble at physiological pH and is therefore chemically modified at the amine or hydroxyl group to obtain soluble derivatives. Chitosans have shown great potential for mucosal delivery due to their mucoadhesive properties (see Chap. 7).

PRINT. An interesting approach to forming quasi-monodisperse and shape-specific polymeric nanoparticles is a method of preparation called PRINT (particle replication in non-wetting templates), developed by the group of J. DeSimone [31] (see Fig. 8.2). In this "top-down" approach, particles are formed in a mold made from perfluoropolyethers. The molecules the particle is made from – such as poly(ethylene glycol) trisacrylate or *p*-hydroxystyrene – are filled into the mold as a solution or melt and then cured by UV radiation or chemical means. This is enabled by the low surface energy of perfluoropolyethers which allows for filling the cavities trough capillary action, but prevents the deposition of material between the cavities [32]. Loading of the particles with therapeutic agents can be achieved either by inclusion into the particle matrix or by post-fabrication functionalization. As an example, siRNA for gene silencing was recently incorporated into PRINT particles [33].

Metal Nanoparticles. Apart from particles made from organic materials, colloidal particles from inorganic matter have also been explored. Here, research has mainly focused on particles consisting of gold and magnetite (Fe_3O_4). A broad variety of routes for particle synthesis has been described in the literature [34]. Metal nanoparticles are typically prepared by reduction of metal salts using suitable reducing agents while metal oxide nanoparticles are usually prepared through base hydrolysis of molecular precursors. Stabilization of the colloids is achieved by adequate ligands, e.g., chelating polymers, which are either added directly during the initial synthesis, or post-synthesis by modification of the ligand sphere by exchange or polymer coating.

Gold Nanoparticles. Gold nanoparticles have so far essentially been studied for passive immunotherapy of tumors. Absorbing near-infrared (NIR) light, gold nanoparticles can locally increase the temperature when targeted to tumors via tumor-specific antibodies and thus have a perspective use in photothermal cancer therapy [35]. Recently, gold nanoparticle-epitope-Fc conjugates were also successfully employed as antigen carriers, exhibiting better activities and immunological responses compared to liposomes [36].

Magnetite Nanoparticles. Magnetite nanoparticles too have been investigated for hyperthermia therapy with a focus on heat shock protein expression for antitumor T-lymphocyte-mediated immunity [37]. Furthermore, they have been investigated as MRI contrast agents [38]. In all the abovementioned cases, it has to be kept in mind that a stabilizing and solubilizing agent is required to make inorganic nanoparticles applicable to in vivo applications. For the same reasons stated for organic colloids, polymers are preferable over tensides or other low molecular weight components to fulfill this task.

Basic Requirements. In summary, there are many kinds of nanoparticles and not all of them are useful as carriers in the body. To be considered for transporting cargo in humans, the particles have to fulfill some basic requirements. Obviously, they need to be biocompatible or, better yet, biodegradable to avoid acute toxicity or storage diseases as reported for PEG. They need to be water soluble and they need to show little or no interaction with proteins in order to ensure smooth circulation in the blood. Materials that do not interact with proteins need to be hydrophilic, electrically neutral, and have hydrogen bond acceptors but no hydrogen bond donors. This concerns the outer material of the particle that is in contact with the body and therefore determines how the body reacts to it (or not), for example, through uptake by the MPS. While in many cases the particles are shielded by PEG, there are some interesting alternatives available, which we would like to introduce in the following sections.

Polymer Structures. Since many nanoparticles are made up of polymers or use them to form a shell around the particle, a brief description of polymer structures available appears reasonable (Fig. 8.5). Macromolecules, consisting of multiple repeating units, can have different levels of complexity. The simplest structure is a linear homopolymer that has only one type of repeating unit. Block copolymers and random copolymers consist of two or more repeating units. But while the

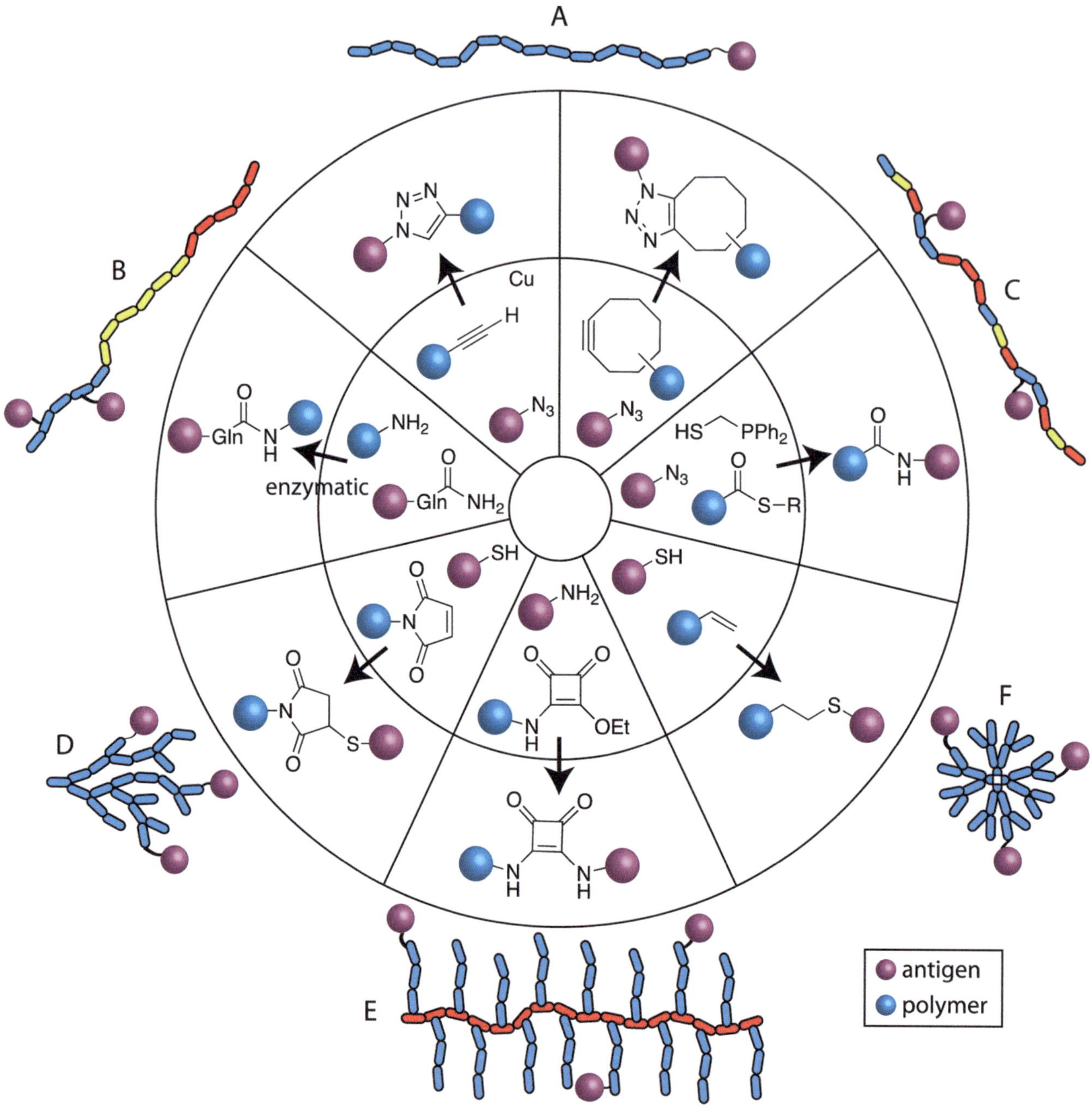

Fig. 8.5 Polymer architectures and possible antigen conjugation. *A* homopolymer, *B* block copolymer, *C* random copolymer, *D* hyperbranched polymer, *E* polymer brush, *F* dendrimer. Antigens can be attached using (clockwise from top left): copper-catalyzed azide-alkyne-cycloaddition [40], copper-free azide-alkyne-cycloaddition [40], traceless Staudinger ligation [41], thiol-ene chemistry [42], squaric acid [43], maleimide [40], enzymatic conjugation [43], and other chemical methods [44])

repeating units are ordered in distinct blocks in the first case, they are randomly distributed along the chain in the second.

When multifunctional monomers are used, branched structures and brushes are also available. A special case is the perfect dendrimer, a branched structure where every generation of branches is synthesized in a different step. In contrast to classical polymers, which have a more or less broad distribution in the number of repeating units per molecule, these dendrimers are exactly defined. The high density and defined arrangement of functional groups on their surface allow them to engage in multivalent interactions. Glycopeptide dendrimers, for example, have been employed in immunotherapy [39].

Besides variations in polymer architecture, the material of which the polymers consist of can be varied as well. Within the next paragraph we would like to introduce polymers, which are of interest as materials building a hydrophilic corona around nanoparticles and thus making them applicable to the development of systems for in vivo applications, e.g., drug delivery, imaging, or vaccination.

8.2.4 Polymeric Materials

8.2.4.1 Poly(Meth)Acrylates and Acrylamides

The development of controlled radical polymerization (CRP) techniques has had a tremendous impact on synthetic polymer chemistry, since it has enabled the controlled polymerization of (meth)acrylates and acrylamides. The CRP techniques were developed to reduce termination as well as uncontrolled transfer of radicals and can be divided into three subgroups:

1. Stable free radical polymerization (e.g., NMP)
2. Degenerative transfer polymerization (e.g., RAFT, MADIX)
3. Transition metal-mediated controlled radical polymerization (e.g., ATRP)

Among these, atom transfer radical polymerization (ATRP) and RAFT (reversible addition-fragmentation chain transfer) polymerization are arguably the most commonly used and most versatile processes. There have been various reviews describing mechanism as well as recent developments of either RAFT [45] or ATRP [46] (Table 8.2).

The CRP techniques can be used in the synthesis of complex polymer architectures, e.g., (multi)block copolymers, branched polymers, or hybrid systems [47].

A group of (meth)acrylates bearing great potential are systems with oligoethylene glycol side chains (OEGMA) – e.g., diethylene glycol methacrylate (DEGMA) or polyethylene glycol methacrylate (PEGMA). The interest in these systems has grown recently. Polymers based on these monomers possess beneficial properties, such as a high solubility in water, non-immunogenicity and low toxicity, a lower critical solution temperature (LCST), and enhanced blood circulation times [48]. The LCST can be nicely tuned by copolymerization of both monomers. It was reported by Lutz and Hoth that the LCST can be adjusted from 26 to 90 °C by changing the ratio of OEGMA to DEGMA units in the copolymer [49].

Cytotoxicity was investigated in various cell lines, such as Caco-2, HT29-MTX-E12, or HepG2, ensuring nontoxic behavior up to a concentration of 5 mg mL^{-1} and 72 h exposure.

PMPC Polymersomes. Another interesting polymer is poly(2-(meth)acryloyloxyethyl phosphorylcholine) (PMPC). The monomer structure is highly bio-inspired since the side chain contains the head group of natural PC phospholipids, ensuring high biocompatibility.

PMPC-based polymersomes have been synthesized and applied to study diffusion across oral epithelium. Additionally, PMPC-based block copolymers have been used for transfection by Lomas et al. [50]. PMPC polymersomes showed pronounced cellular uptake as well as nontoxic behavior up to 3 mg mL^{-1}. Furthermore, PMPC polymers were used for protein conjugation by Lewis and coworkers [51]. A reduced tissue migration compared to PEG–protein conjugates of the same hydrodynamic volume was observed. Thus, an improved depot effect in the tissue as well as subsequent longer elimination half-life may lead to improved pharmacokinetics. These findings underline the potential of PMPC-based polymeric systems.

HPMA Polymers. Finally, also well-established polymers such as 2-(hydroxypropyl) methacrylamide (HPMA) can be prepared in a controlled manner by the CRP methods. HPMA was the first polymer entering clinical trials as polymer drug conjugate in the 1990s [52] and HPMA-based copolymers can be synthesized directly or using postpolymerization modifications.

Those three types of monomers may be the material future nanomedicines are made of. However, it has to be kept in mind that neither the polymer backbone of poly(meth)acrylates nor acrylamides can be degraded in vivo. Thus, polymers need to be excreted, limiting the molecular weight of the single polymer as well as the potential application.

Table 8.2 Comparison of free radical polymerization (FRP) to controlled radical polymerization (CRP)

	FRP	CRP
Advantages	Compatible with a broad variety of monomers	Low dispersity/narrow molecular weight distribution
	Insensitive to impurities	Good control over polymer architecture (chain topology, end-group functionality)
	Employed in industry for decades	
Disadvantages	Lack of control over chain topology (no block architecture, no defined end groups!)	Inferior reaction rate due to limited number of active species
	Little control over dispersity/broad molecular weight distribution	Higher sensitivity to impurities

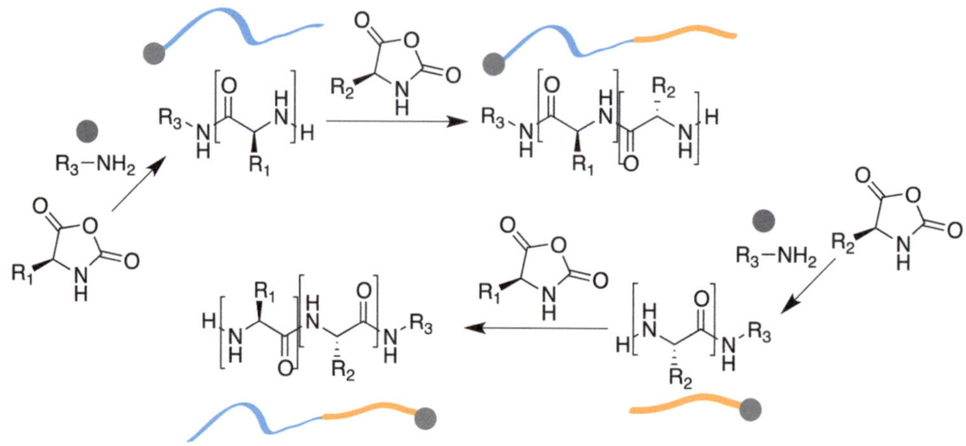

Fig. 8.6 Synthesis of block copolypeptides

8.2.4.2 Polypeptides

Polypeptides are one of the major building blocks in nature and a very versatile class of materials. They naturally have multiple functionalities, which allow them to respond to stimuli like change in pH or oxidation potential.

There are various methods of synthesizing polypeptides. The use of biotechnological methods that allow production of peptides in cells or the solid-phase peptide synthesis leads to sequence-defined polypeptides, but are limited in amino acids, are expensive, and can only be performed on a relatively small scale and therefore will not be discussed here. Where large quantities of homo or block copolypeptides are required, the polymerization of α-amino acid-*N*-carboxyanhydrides (NCAs) is a suitable production method (Fig. 8.6). The polymerization of NCAs is known since the beginning of the last century, and the work since then has been summarized in excellent books and reviews. Only in recent years different ways of controlling this type of polymerization have been developed [53].

Since synthetic polypeptides, just like natural proteins, are made up of amino acids, they can be nontoxic, biocompatible, and degradable in the body while they remain stable in aqueous solution. Because of their similarity to natural proteins, immunogenicity is a concern that has to be addressed. Although immunogenicity has not been observed for homo and block copolypeptides, new polypeptides have to be studied in this respect especially when various amino acids are incorporated.

The multitude of different side chains enable the design of peptidic superstructures like polyion complexes, polymer micelles, polymer vesicles, nanofibers or nanotubes, and hydrogels.

All these different structures give rise to a wide range of biomedical applications. In the field of DNA and RNA transport, peptidic polyplexes have evolved from simple polylysine to highly complex structures that contain a removable hydrophilic shell [54] and respond to stimuli like change in pH, oxidation potential, or ATP concentration.

PEG. Polypeptides are also used to encapsulate hydrophobic drugs. Probably, the most prominent example is PEG-block-poly(aspartate) where the Asp is modified with 4-phenyl-1-butanol to make it more hydrophobic. Loaded with paclitaxel, this micellar formulation is currently in a phase III clinical trial for breast cancer under the name NK105.

Polypeptides have also found their way into the field of diagnostics. For example, PEGylated polylysine with an NIR dye was used as an in vivo imaging probe to visualize tumor-associated proteases in nude mice [55].

Copaxone. Polypeptides can also work as bioactive agents themselves. The immunomodulator drug Copaxone is a random copolymer of alanine, lysine, glutamic acid, and tyrosine and is approved for the treatment of multiple sclerosis [56]. The exact mode of action of Copaxone is still under discussion, but it is believed that due to the similarity of Copaxone and the myelin basic protein (MBP), the drug can divert the autoimmune response away from the myelin sheath of neurons.

Opaxio. Also the covalent attachment of drugs to polypeptides is very promising. In Opaxio (formerly known as Xyotax or CT-2103), paclitaxel is conjugated to polyglutamic acid (PGA) via an ester bond and the conjugate is currently in phase III clinical trials for ovarian and non-small cell lung cancer. Here paclitaxel is only released when the polymer is degraded by tumor-associated proteases leading to a selective release of the chemotherapeutic agent [57].

Lysine-block-leucine copolypeptides were used by Deming for the preparation of the first stable double emulsions below 100 nm [58]. These double emulsions consist of water droplets and oil droplets in a water phase and have the capacity to carry hydrophobic as well as hydrophilic drugs, which makes them attractive for delivery applications.

Table 8.3 Polypeptides in clinical trials

Name	Polypeptide	Drug	Indication	Phase
NK105	PEG-b-Asp(buPh)	Paclitaxel	Stomach cancer	III
			Breast cancer	II
NK012	PEG-b-Glu	SN-38	Small-cell lung cancer	II
			Breast cancer	II
NC-6004	PEG-b-Glu	Cisplatin	Pancreatic cancer	II
			Solid cancer	I
NC-4016	PEG-b-Glu	DACH-platin	Solid cancer	I
Opaxio	p(Glu)	Paclitaxel	Ovarian cancer	III
			Non-small cell lung cancer	III
CT-2106	p(Glu)	Camptothecin	Ovarian cancer	II
			Solid cancer	I
Copaxone	Ala-Lys-Glu-Tyr copolymer	Peptide itself	Multiple sclerosis	FDA/EMA/PMDA approved
VivaGel	Modified p(Lys) dendrimer	Peptide itself	Bacterial vaginosis	III

Polypeptides in clinical trials, as carriers or as active agents, are summarized in Table 8.3 [59–61].

Although most of the polypeptides in the clinics are for the treatment of cancer, they underline the potential of polypeptides as carriers. Their multifunctionality, biocompatibility, and biodegradability make them ideal materials for the transport of bioactive substances in the body.

8.2.4.3 Polyglycerols

An important class of biocompatible branched polymers are polyglycerols (PGs), which can be synthesized as dendrons, dendrimers, or with hyperbranched architectures [62].

When compared to linear polymers of similar molecular weight, dendrimers and hyperbranched polymers have interesting properties like globular structure and low intrinsic viscosities. The chemical structure of PG is similar to that of PEG with which PGs share their low affinity to proteins. But while PEG only offers two sites for modification, PG has many free OH groups which might be used to attach bioactive molecules or targeting moieties.

Dendrons and Dedrimers. While dendrons and dendrimers are synthesized in multistep processes, highly defined hyperbranched polyglycerols can be prepared via anionic polymerization of glycidol. The polymers can be modified in the core [63] or in the shell by chemically addressing the alcohol groups in the corona.

For linear and hyperbranched PG (molecular weight 6.4 kg mol^{-1}) complement activation, red blood cell aggregation and coagulation were not observed to a significant extent. Cytotoxicity of the PGs was comparable to the controls PEG and hetastarch (80 % cell viability at a concentration of 10 mg ml^{-1}; L-929 fibroblasts). Hyperbranched polyglycerols were found to be well tolerated by mice even when injected in doses of up to 62.5 mg kg^{-1} [64].

Hyperbranched PGs. The biocompatibility of larger hyperbranched PGs (160 and 540 kg mol^{-1}) was investigated in vitro [65] and in vivo [66]. The in vitro tests were similar to the ones performed with low molecular weight PG and came to a similar conclusion, i.e., that PGs are highly biocompatible. These polymers were tested in vivo in mice for their pharmacokinetic behavior. The plasma half-lives were 32 h and 57 h, respectively. No toxicity was observed with a dose of 1 g kg^{-1}. However, due to the high molecular weight of the PGs, urinary excretion was very low, and significant accumulation by the mononuclear phagocyte system was observed. PGs were detectable in the liver and spleen for at least 30 days. This again highlights the need for biodegradable materials.

Due to their good biocompatibility, there are plenty of biomedical applications of PGs. Bioactive compounds can be transported by PG either through covalent attachment or encapsulation.

For covalent attachment, there has been great interest to add functionality to the alcohol-terminated PG. The introduction of amine groups, for example, allows the attachment of acids via an amide, while thiols on the PG surface have been used to attach drugs via a biodegradable peptide linker. Doxorubicin has been attached to PG via an acid cleavable linker. The conjugate was tested in vitro and in an ovarian carcinoma A2780 xenograft model, showing a distinct increase in tolerability and antitumor efficacy with tumor remissions for up to 30 days [67]. Also, triple bonds have been introduced for facile *click chemistry*, which has been employed to synthesize sugar-terminated PGs with high binding affinities to selectins. Equal results have been found for negatively charged PG sulfates. Such systems use their multivalency to achieve high binding affinities.

The nondegradability of PG was partially addressed by synthesizing PG in an inverse miniemulsion process via an acid-catalyzed ring-opening polyaddition of disulfide containing polyols and polyepoxides [68]. These nanoparticles can be cleaved in a reductive environment yielding smaller fragments that can be excreted from the body.

The application of PGs also includes hydrogel scaffolds for tissue engineering, which will not be discussed here.

Since dendrimers are quite small (1–5 nm) and hyperbranched architectures are not much bigger (2–20 nm), assembly into superstructures is desirable to get into a size range of 20–100 nm.

Microgels. Microgels were prepared using the inverse miniemulsion technique [69]. The particles were between 23 and 80 nm in diameter and seemed to accumulate in the perinuclear region of human lung cancer cells. An MTT essay showed no influence of the microgel on human hematopoietic U-937 cell metabolic activity below 0.5 mg ml^{-1}.

So-called megamers were prepared by cross-linking hyperbranched PG, modified with azides and alkynes, using the miniemulsion technique [70]. Hydrophilic as well as hydrophobic megamers were prepared with diameters of 25–90 nm.

With their low protein adsorption and their good biocompatibility, polyglycerols are a promising class of materials, which have already proven their benefits in a wide range of biomedical applications. In the future, they promise to lead to more advanced, highly functionalizable transport systems of bioactive molecules.

8.2.4.4 Polyoxazolines

Poly(2-oxazoline)s (POx) can be expected to be one of the upcoming polymer platforms for nanomedicines [71]. POx meet the specific requirements needed for the development of next-generation nanomedicines such as biocompatibility, high modulation of solubility, variation of size, architecture, as well as chemical functionality. POx are synthesized by cationic ring-opening polymerization of 2-oxazolines (Fig. 8.7). This methodology offers precise control over molecular weight and chain-end functionality ($Đ \leq 1.2$) [72] and therefore allows chemists to adjust the polymers to meet the necessary requirements.

POx have a lower critical solution temperature (LCST), a temperature below which the polymers are fully soluble in aqueous solution. Above this temperature, they become insoluble, leading to polymer precipitation. The LCST of POx depends on the polymer composition and structure and can be adjusted by copolymerization of the monomers nPrOx with iPrOx from about 26–38.7 °C and with the even more hydrophilic EtOx from 35 to 75.1 °C.

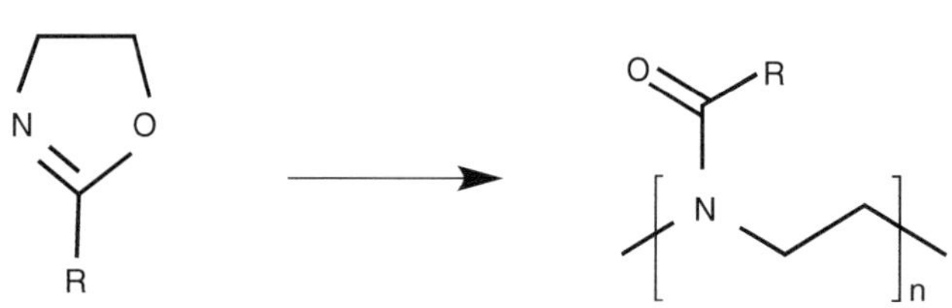

Fig. 8.7 Synthesis of polyoxazolines

Those properties may enable the specific accumulation by precipitation of polymers in parts of the body with higher temperature induced externally (hyperthermia). Furthermore, POx fulfill several important aspects of polymers used for in vivo applications. Considering in vitro cytotoxicity, different POx-based polymers were found to be nonhazardous in general [73]. In addition to that, PEtOx exhibited no hemolytic effects at 20 g L^{-1} [74]. Results for hybrid systems with a POx part are variable. The triblock copolymers poly(L-lactide)-*b*-PEtOx-*b*-poly(L-lactide) and PEtOx-*b*-PCL-*b*-PEtOx were found to be non-cytotoxic at concentrations of up to 50 g L^{-1} and 10 g L^{-1}, respectively. Contrary to that, PEtOx-*b*-poly(ε-caprolactone) copolymers showed explicit cytotoxicity at concentration of below 1 g L^{-1}, although in another experiment of the same study, no hemolytic effects of PEtOx-b-PCL were observed at 10 g L^{-1}.

Previous studies on in vivo toxicity of poly(2-oxazoline)s focused mainly on PEtOx and PMeOx. Viegas et al. intravenously injected repeated doses of 10 kg mol^{-1} PEtOx (2 g kg^{-1}) and 50 kg mol^{-1} (50 mg kg^{-1}) into rats. No adverse effects were observed and histology of the kidney, liver, and spleen showed no abnormalities.

Similar to other polymer systems, the susceptibility of poly(2-oxazoline)s to interaction with proteins depends on their hydrophilicity or hydrophobicity, respectively. Overall, hydrophilic poly(2-oxazoline)s like PMeOx and PEtOx show low affinity to protein adsorption [75]. Consequently, they exhibit stealth properties and may be used to mediate them, for example, as coating moiety for liposomes. The biodistribution profile of PMeOx and PEtOx is consistent with their stealth properties, i.e., low organ uptake and rapid or slow elimination through the kidneys depending on the molecular weight [76].

With regard to potential immunogenicity, different block copolymers of PMeOx, PEtOx, PBuOx, and PPheOx were screened for their capability to activate the complement system. Compared to negative controls, levels of complement proteins were elevated significantly [77]. Although much has been done, further clinical data is necessary to underline the potential of POx, making it a substitute for PEG in general.

8.2.5 Characterization of Nanoparticles

Besides developing different kinds of nanoparticles based on novel materials, another focus needs to be set on the characterization of nanomedicines, especially when those systems are applied in targeted delivery or vaccination.

The synthesized particles can be characterized in solution by (cryo-) transmission electron microscopy (TEM), scanning electron microscopy (SEM), or atomic force microscopy (AFM). Furthermore, light scattering techniques as well as fluorescence correlation spectroscopy can be used to determine hydrodynamic diameters of particles. All these tools, however, are somehow limited to artificial conditions and thus often cannot provide information regarding protein adsorption or protein-induced aggregation.

Especially in vaccination, when a nanoparticle should deliver an antigen and/or adjuvant to an antigen presenting cell, a protein corona may cause an immune reaction against the undesirably absorbed serum proteins causing autoimmune diseases. To tackle those important questions, novel methodologies are required and some of them will be briefly described.

As stated above, the absorption of proteins might not be hindered by charge-stabilized nanoparticles, since proteins can be regarded as polyelectrolytes containing anionic or cationic groups. In salt-containing solution, charges are compensated by counter ions. Those ions are set free whenever a multivalent binding partner is present since the systems entropy is increased by the freely diffusing ions. Though enthalpy contributions to the system's energy also play a role, for macromolecules, usually entropic contributions are the major factor. Thus, steric stabilization of nanoparticles appears reasonable, but in all cases, protein adsorption needs to be investigated carefully.

Zeta (ζ) Potential. Often particles are characterized in aqueous solution at low ionic strength and in absence of proteins by measuring and interpreting electrokinetic phenomena. In many cases, zeta (ζ) potential measurements are carried out using commercial systems. The ζ-potential itself cannot be measured but has to be derived from electrokinetic signals using sophisticated models considering surface properties such as nature of the surface, roughness, charge, electrolyte concentration, and the nature of the electrolyte and of the solvent used in the measurements. Since those parameters differ easily from one particle to the other, an IUPAC technical report highly recommends to use this methodology carefully and not to over-interpret the results obtained [78]. However, the ζ-potential can be a helpful tool in quality control of the particles synthesized.

Dynamic Light Scattering. More suitable methodologies may be dynamic light scattering in serum to determine changes in hydrodynamic radius as reported by Rausch and coworkers [9, 79]. This method allows studying the aggregation behavior of nanoparticles in serum. Even small traces of aggregated particles can be identified. The drawback of this methodology is that the adsorption of a single or few proteins cannot be detected since the changes in hydrodynamic radius are below the accuracy of measurements.

Isothermal Titration Calorimetry. In a more artificial setup, isothermal titration calorimetry (ITC) can be used to measure the heat flow and therefore quantify an average adsorption energy over all particles. In combination with quantitative label-free liquid chromatography and mass spectrometry (MS), adsorbed proteins can be identified and quantified [80].

Imaging of Biodistribution. In addition, in vivo imaging of the biodistribution of nanoparticles is necessary to monitor local accumulation at the target side or to ensure excretion from the organism. This requires nanoparticles to be labeled by near-infrared dyes or radioactive isotopes for single photon emission computed tomography (SPECT) or positron emission tomography (PET). During the last decade, various methodologies have been developed to label nanoparticles. Labeling methods for polymers using prosthetic groups for ^{18}F as well as $^{72/74}Ar$ have been established [81].

8.2.6 Nanoparticulate Vaccine Formulations

8.2.6.1 Advantages of Particle-Based Vaccines

The next years will see an increasing use of synthetic subunit antigen vaccines because they provide many advantages over traditional vaccines derived from live attenuated or killed pathogens However, it is a well-known fact that (synthetic) peptides often lack the immunogenicity to induce a strong immune response. Therefore, efficient vaccination requires the use of adjuvants. In the field of tumor immunotherapy, adjuvants are especially important to reverse tumor immunosuppression mediated, for example, by regulatory T cells or myeloid-derived suppressor cells.

Adjuvants among other things promote the maturation of antigen-presenting cells by interaction with receptors of the innate immune system, e.g., dendritic cells. Only mature dendritic cells are able to generate co-stimulatory signals, which, together with the presented antigen, lead to the desired effector T cell responses. Thus, it is important that antigen and adjuvant act on dendritic cells concomitantly. Most of today's human vaccine formulations use aluminum-based compounds as adjuvants. However, as recent years have seen intense research for more potent and specific alternatives, new means of co-delivery are required.

Another problem of subunit antigen vaccines is their susceptibility to enzymatic degradation. To increase their lifetime and biological activity, protective carrier molecules are needed. Nanoparticles have become of great interest as an instrument to protect antigens and adjuvants against blood serum proteins and to ensure their safe and simultaneous delivery to dendritic cells.

Alongside their capability for protection and co-delivery of antigen and adjuvant, nanoparticles show several other advantages:

- They can deliver an antigen together with combinations of adjuvants overcoming immune suppression by regulatory T cells [82].
- They trap their cargo, thus preventing systemic distribution and toxicity [83].
- They can be used as a platform to present multiple copies of an antigen on their surface which especially improves B cell activation [84].
- They can promote the cytosolic accumulation of antigens in dendritic cells. This is important for cross-presentation, the key mechanism for $CD8^+$ T cell activation.
- Modification of nanoparticles with inert substances like poly(ethylene glycol) that mediate stealth properties [85] can minimize protein absorption and lower their immunogenicity. This increases their blood circulation time [86].
- Surface functionalization of nanoparticles with receptor ligands or antibodies enables specific tissue or cellular targeting [86]. Thereby, antigen and adjuvant are retained at the site of action so that unspecific distribution is reduced, lower doses are needed, and adverse reactions to vaccination are minimized.
- Nanoparticles provide a sustained release of adjuvants and thus a prolonged exposure to the immune system which is essential for a proper activation of dendritic cells [87].

8.2.7 Approaches

Big potential for nanoparticulate vaccine formulations most likely lies in cancer immunotherapy. In addition to this, applications for vaccination against various infectious diseases are investigated. These include, for example, nanoparticle-based vaccines against influenza [88], West Nile encephalitis [89], and malaria [90].

The components of a typical nanoparticulate vaccine formulation combine an antigen (T cell and/or B cell epitopes), adjuvant, and targeting moiety on one particle. A wide variety of antigens such as peptides/proteins, lipoproteins, glycopeptides, tumor-associated carbohydrate antigens (TACAs), and carbohydrate mimetic peptides are tested in combination with nanoparticulate carriers.

Two basic concepts can be distinguished for targeting dendritic cells with antigens: ex vivo pulsing and subsequent administration of matured dendritic cells or direct in vivo targeting of immature dendritic cells. Nanoparticles are especially evaluated for in vivo strategies [91].

TLRs and Nanoparticles. The group of adjuvants mainly studied in the context of nanoparticulate vaccines are several Toll-like receptor ligands. LPS, the major component of the outer membrane of gram-negative bacteria, is a pathogen-derived TLR4 ligand. While being far too toxic for systemic application as an immunopotentiator for classic vaccines, LPS shows promising results in vitro and in mouse models, when administered within PLGA nanoparticles [92].

7-acyl lipid A, a component of LPS, is also investigated in mice as an additive for PLGA-based vaccines [93]. In addition to pathogen-derived TLR ligands, synthetic molecules mimicking pathogen-associated molecular patterns (PAMPs) are evaluated. Representatives of this group are CpG oligodeoxynucleotides (CpG ODN), binding to TLR9, and polyribosinic:polyribocytidic acid (Poly I:C), a TLR3 ligand [82]. Alongside the general activation of dendritic cells, the application of certain TLR ligands like CpG oligodeoxynucleotides and LPS together with nanoparticulate carriers might be of special interest as they, contrary to alum, elicit a Th1-biased immune response [94].

Demento et al. developed PLGA nanoparticles loaded with a recombinant envelope protein antigen from the West Nile virus and surface functionalized with CpG ODN. In several experiments, they compared this system with unmodified nanoparticles and an aluminum hydroxide vaccine formulation. In mice, CpG ODN-modified nanoparticles produced a Th1 immune response-biased antibody profile in contrast to a Th2 profile elicited by aluminum hydroxide. Moreover, immunization of mice with modified nanoparticles induced a higher number of circulating effector T cells and an enhanced antigen-specific IL-2 and IFN-γ production compared to control groups. In a mouse model of West Nile encephalitis, modified nanoparticles showed a superior protection in comparison to aluminum hydroxide.

Studies suggest that some nanoparticles, probably by binding to Toll-like receptors, can act as adjuvants themselves [95]. This has been shown for high molecular weight γ-PGA particles, PLGA nano- and microparticles, poly(anhydride) nanoparticles, liposomes, polystyrene nano- and microparticles, and acid-degradable cationic polyacrylamide nanoparticles. However, particle size and concentration seem to be critical for activation of dendritic cells as in other experiments PLGA particles failed to induce dendritic cell maturation [96].

In one experiment, mucosal immunization of mice against highly pathogenic influenza A H5N1 virus was carried out. The vaccine consisted of recombinant influenza hemagglutinin (rHA) antigen and γ-PGA/chitosan nanoparticles. This system was compared to two other formulations: inactivated virus with γ-PGA/chitosan nanoparticles and cholera toxin with recombinant influenza hemagglutinin antigen. The γ-PGA/chitosan nanoparticles in combination with rHA antigen led to potent virus-specific humoral and cellular immune responses. Compared to cholera toxin, the adjuvant properties of the γ-PGA/chitosan nanoparticles were equally good. Immunized mice were protected against challenge with a lethal dose of highly pathogenic influenza A H5N1 virus [97].

Nanoparticle-Based Vaccines. A different concept for nanoparticle-based vaccines investigated in multiple studies involves the delivery of nucleic acids (RNA or DNA) encoding a defined antigen into dendritic cells. In contrast to peptide antigens, RNA and DNA have to remain intact and functional all along the endocytic route until they have reached the cytosol or the nucleus, respectively. After being endocytosed, nanoparticles functionalized with buffering groups or cell-penetrating peptides can protect nucleic acids against hydrolytic enzymes and foster endosomal escape [98]. Once nucleic acids have reached their destination inside the cell, expression of the encoded peptide antigen can start.

One advantage of DNA is that it can encode for various peptide antigens. Thus, one nanoparticulate system that is able to transport DNA can be used for a broad range of vaccinations. Further DNA can function as an immunostimulant because it contains CpG sequences recognized by TLR9 [99].

Sudowe et al. investigated the potential of in vivo DNA vaccination to generate an immune response against βGal as model antigen. Plasmids encoding βGal under the control of DC-specific, keratinocyte-specific, or unspecific promoters were adsorbed on gold nanoparticles and applied to the skin of mice via gene gun. As a result, Th1-biased immune responses were observed. Moreover, with regard to $CD8^+$ T cell priming, it was shown that the presentation of endogenous antigen produced by transfected skin dendritic cells is equally effective as the cross-presentation of exogenous antigen [100].

As mentioned above, the surface of nanocarriers can be functionalized with a multitude of different ligands, including proteins, peptides, antibodies, antibody fragments, aptamers, and small molecules [86]. By targeting defined cell surface structures with receptor ligands or antibodies attached to nanoparticles, an increased and/or more specific cellular uptake might be achieved. Considering vaccine formulations in particular, the configuration of the carrier system with ligands for pattern recognition receptors, e.g., Toll-like receptors or C-type lectin receptors, might augment its immunogenicity and contribute to dendritic cell activation.

Different targeting concepts have been realized with various particulate carriers and have shown stronger immune responses compared to nontargeted carriers [101]. Mannose is a ligand for a C-type lectin receptor expressed on dendritic cells. Multiple research projects have examined its performance for targeting dendritic cells and macrophages [102]. In experiments comparing mannose-decorated PLGA particles with plain PLGA particles, it was shown that mannose only causes a slight increase in cellular uptake. Presumably, because depending on the experimental conditions, nonspecific uptake usually predominates specific uptake. However, in another study, it was demonstrated that mannan, a natural polymannose derived from the cell wall of *Saccharomyces cerevisiae,* when conjugated to PLGA particles leads to increased antigen-specific $CD4^+$ and $CD8^+$ T cell responses [103].

Other methods for addressing dendritic cells reported in literature are the deployment of Fc receptor ligands or anti-DEC-205 antibodies. Raghuwanshi et al. evaluated a two-component vaccine formulation, one element being biotinylated PLGA nanoparticles loaded with ovalbumin as model antigen, the other a bifunctional fusion protein consistent of truncated core-streptavidin and an anti-DEC-205 single-chain antibody. They observed a twofold increase in receptor-mediated uptake of functionalized nanoparticles compared to nontargeted nanoparticles. OVA-specific IgG responses of mice immunized with anti-DEC-205-modified nanoparticles in connection with αCD40 as adjuvant were considerably higher than those of control groups [104].

To trigger an antibody response, an antigen has to be recognized and processed not only by dendritic cells but also by B cells. Consequently, alongside T cell epitopes, the inclusion of B cell epitopes into a vaccine formulation is a central approach. As mentioned before, nanoparticles can be used to present multiple copies of epitopes on their surface [84]. This enables the induction of T cell-independent type I antibody responses as has been shown for virus-like particles. T cell-independent type II antibody responses can be realized through co-delivery of adjuvants suited for B cell activation [105].

Especially in tumor immunotherapy, the delivery of B cell epitopes derived from glycopeptides, TACA, or carbohydrate mimetic peptides is of great interest. In several studies, Kunz et al. investigated the B cell activating potential of different synthetic tumor-associated MUC1 glycopeptides which contain the Thomsen-Friedenreich antigen, its precursor or its sialylated derivatives. They chemically linked the glycopeptides to bovine serum albumin (BSA) or tetanus toxoid as carrier molecules. These vaccine systems were applied to Balb/c mice. In the case of the BSA formulations, complete Freud's adjuvant was coadministered. For all vaccines, strong specific antibody responses against the MUC1 antigens were observed.

Brinãs et al. used gold nanoparticles to co-deliver MUC4 glycopeptides containing the Thomsen-Friedenreich antigen together with a peptide derived from the complement protein C3d as B cell-activating adjuvant. Mice immunized with these nanoparticles showed statistically significant immune responses.

8.3 Engineered Liposomes[2]

Liposomes (phospholipid bilayer vesicles) represent an almost ideal carrier system for the preparation of synthetic vaccines due to their biodegradability and capacity to protect and transport molecules of different physicochemical properties (including size, hydrophilicity, hydrophobicity, and charge).

Liposomal carriers can be applied by invasive (e.g., *i.m.*, *s.c.*, *i.d.*) as well as noninvasive (transdermal and mucosal) routes. In the last 15 years, liposome vaccine technology has matured and several vaccines containing liposome-based adjuvants have been approved for human and veterinary use or have reached late stages of clinical evaluation.

Given the intensifying interest in liposome-based vaccines, it is important to understand precisely how liposomes interact with the immune system and how they stimulate immunity. It has become clear that the physicochemical properties of liposomal vaccines – method of antigen attachment, lipid composition, bilayer fluidity, particle charge, and other properties – exert strong effects on the resulting immune response.

Lyme disease is discussed as example for a liposome-based vaccine development.

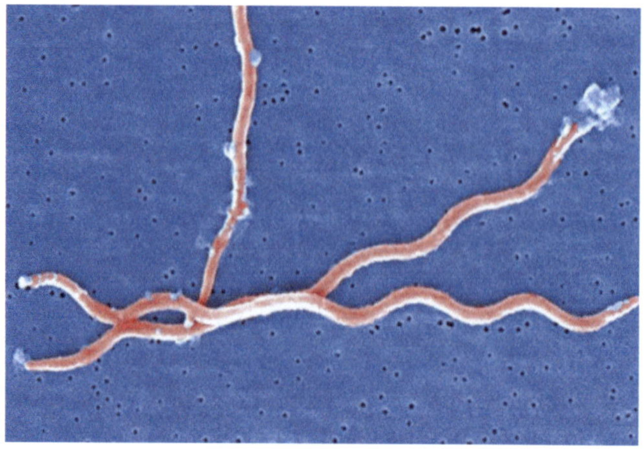

Fig. 8.8 Scanning electron micrograph image of *Borrelia burgdorferi. Borreliae* are typical for their spiral-shaped cells, 10–30 μm in length and 0.2–0.3 μm in diameter. *Borrelia* lacks the rigid cell wall and the surface is composed mainly of lipoproteins. *Borrelia* is a spirochete. Spirochetes are a group of phylogenetically distinct bacteria that have a unique mode of motility by means of axial filaments (endoflagella). The spirochetes are not classified as either gram positive or gram negative (Photo credit: Janice Haney Carr, CDC/USA)

8.3.1 Lyme Diseases

Lyme disease is the most frequent zoonosis both in Europe and the United States. Disease may progress into a chronic form and cause damage of the nervous or cardiovascular system, joints, skin, or eyes. Infected patients can be affected by prolong work disability or even permanent invalidity. Prevention and treatment of disease thus becomes a long-term priority for medical research.

8.3.1.1 History

Some symptoms typical for Lyme disease have been known since the beginning of the twentieth century – acrodermatitis chronica atrophicans, erythema migrans, lymphocytoma, and meningo-polyradiculoneuritis [106]. Nevertheless, the etiological agent *Borrelia burgdorferi* was described quite recently on the basis of endemic juvenile arthritis accompanied with erythema migrans [107, 108] (Fig. 8.8).

Later, it was shown that *B. burgdorferi sensu lato* is a complex of several sibling species. Currently, 12 species are distinguished and new variants are identified continuously, so the number of *Borrelia* species is probably not final. Three of species are known to be pathogenic for human – *B. burgdorferi sensu stricto, B. afzelii*, and *B. garinii*. The number of annually reported Lyme disease cases continually increases in many geographical areas. This may be due to the actual spread of the disease or alternatively, to improved diagnostic methods [109].

8.3.1.2 Etiological Agents

The genus *Borrelia* Swellengrebel 1907 is a member of the family Spirochaetaceae together with genera *Leptospira* and *Treponema*. In the USA, the only one causative agent – *B. burgdorferi s.s.* was described. In Europe, two species – *B. afzelii* and *B. garinii* – are the most common.

Borreliae are typical for their spiral shaped cells, 10–30 μm in length and 0.2–0.3 μm in diameter. This shape is caused by periplasmatic flagella responsible for the high motility in viscous environment like connective tissue. *Borrelia* lacks the rigid cell wall and the surface is composed mainly of lipoproteins with strictly controlled expression pattern, essential for adaptation for external conditions [110].

8.3.1.3 Epidemiology, Clinical Disease, and Treatment

The disease has a vector character. Most of the time, it is transmitted to humans by infected ticks of the genus *Ixodes*, but *Borrelia* has also been found in the midgut of the mosquitoes and other blood-sucking insect. Role of hematophagous insect in disease transmission is still unclear [111, 112]. Reservoir competence has been described in the broad

[2]Functionalised nanoliposomes for construction of recombinant vaccines: Lyme disease as an example by *Jaroslav Turánek, Josef Mašek, Michal Křupka and Milan Raška* in Molecular Vaccines – From Prophylaxis to Therapy, Volume 2, Springer-Verlag Wien, 2013, Ed. Matthias Giese.

spectrum of wildlife animals, e.g., rodents (genera *Apodemus, Clethrionomys, Microtus, Rattus, etc.*), squirrels (*Sciurus* sp.*)*, hares (*Lepus* sp.), and birds (genera *Turdus, Phasianus, Fratercula, etc.*). Human is a terminal host, incapable of further spreading of infection [113].

Lyme Disease. Lyme disease can have three stages – early localized infection, early disseminated infection, and late persistent infection, but not all stages develop in every infected individual. It appears that a significant portion of infections has asymptomatic course without clinical symptoms, but with elevated levels of anti-*Borrelia*-specific antibodies. The first stage is characteristic by nonspecific symptoms including fever, chills, headache, lethargy, and/or muscle and joint pain, in about 70 % accompanied by erythema migrans at the site of bacterial entry. If the infection is not eliminated by the host immune system or antibiotics treatment, it may disseminate and affect the central nervous system (meningitis, radiculopathy, seventh cranial nerve palsy) or cardiovascular system (atrioventricular heart block, myopericarditis). The late persistent infection may develop months to years after the transmission and commonly affects the nervous system, skin, joints, or less frequently heart, eyes, or other organs.

Treatment of Lyme Disease. Treatment is based on the application of antibiotics. For adults, administration of doxycycline is recommended. For children, mainly beta-lactam antibiotics are prescribed. For the treatment of advanced forms, cephalosporins or G-penicillin are recommended. Long-term usage of antibiotics in persistent forms of Lyme disease has only limited effect [114].

First effort to design vaccine against the Lyme disease followed shortly after the discovery of *Borrelia* as the etiological agent causing this disease. First experiments demonstrated the immunogenicity of bacterial whole cell lysates. Later, specific proteins were identified to be recognized by the host immune system [115].

8.3.1.4 Antigens and Immune Response

Expression of surface antigens by *Borrelia* is highly variable. In the tick host, *Borrelia* expresses outer surface proteins A (OspA) and B (OspB). Genes coding both proteins are located within one operon and expression of these proteins is dependent on housekeeping sigma factor RpoD (σ^{70}). Presumed function of OspA and OspB is the adhesion to tick gut epithelium. When tick starts blood feeding on the vertebrate host, both proteins are downregulated.

At the same time the expression of proteins dependent on alternative sigma factor RpoS (σ^{38}) is induced, e.g., (OspC) and OspF, decorin-binding proteins DbpA and DbpB, and some others. These proteins are required for *Borrelia* transmission to vertebrate and for initial stages of vertebrate infection. In later stages, OspC is downregulated and the expression of VlsE protein (Vmp-like sequence, expressed) is induced. It enables *Borrelia* escape from specific humoral response due to high VlsE variability.

Early humoral response to *Borrelia* is characterized by production of IgM antibodies specific to OspC, flagellins (p39 and p41), and BmpA (p39). Later IgG antibodies against p39, p41, p83/100, DbpA, and VlsE arise. In some cases, antibodies against OspA and OspB can be detected in later stages of the disease.

Subunit Vaccines of First Generation. These were based on OspA antigen, which is highly expressed during cultivation of Lyme disease spirochetes in vitro. Preclinical trials with vaccines based on OspA antigen demonstrated protection in animal models. OspA antigen was produced either as a recombinant protein or lipoprotein, or it was expressed on the surface of *E. coli*, *Salmonella typhimurium*, or *Mycobacterium bovis*.

ImuLyme and LYMErix Vaccines. Two OspA-based vaccine candidates were developed and tested. The ImuLyme vaccine (Pasteur Merieux Connaught) was based on purified recombinant OspA antigen expressed in *E. coli* and LYMErix (GlaxoSmithKline) containing purified recombinant OspA from *B. burgdorferi s.s.* [116]. In both vaccines, protein was adsorbed on aluminum hydroxide. In clinical trials involving more than 10,000 people, LYMErix vaccine was found to confer protective immunity to *Borrelia* in 76 % of adults and 100 % of children with only mild or moderate and transient adverse effect. Based on these results, LYMErix was approved by the Food and Drug Administration (FDA) on December 21, 1998.

Autoimmune Side Effects. Subsequently, hundreds of vaccinees reported the development of autoimmune side effects. Supported by some patient advocacy groups, a number of class-action lawsuits were filed against GlaxoSmithKline, alleging the vaccine had caused these health problems. These claims were investigated by the FDA and the US Centers for Disease Control (CDC), who found no connection between the vaccine and the autoimmune complaints [117, 118]. Despite the lack of evidence, sales plummeted and LYMErix was withdrawn from the US market by GlaxoSmithKline in February 2002 in the setting of negative media coverage and fears of vaccine side effects.

There are a number of reasons for the slow development of a Lyme disease vaccine, including reluctance by pharmaceutical companies to get burned in a similar way to LYMErix manufacturers. Others argue that it is simply more profitable for drug manufacturers to "treat" the symptoms of Lyme palliatively, giving anti-inflammatory medications, pain relievers, and other medications where antibiotics fail to address a patient's ailments.

The continued availability of a Lyme disease vaccine for dogs has made many people question the motives of drug companies and the psychological component of many symptoms often blamed on Lyme disease.

8.3.2 Licensed Veterinary Lyme Disease Vaccines

Unlike humane medicine, several licensed veterinary Lyme disease vaccines are available for companion pets. Three are formulations of *B. burgdorferi* bacterin (Merilym, Merial, Germany; Galaxy Lyme, Schering Plough, USA; LymeVax, Fort Dodge, USA). A European vaccine based on combination of bacterins from *B. garinii* and *B. afzelii* is produced for dogs (Biocan, Bioveta, Czech Republic) [119]. There are also available veterinary subunit vaccines based on recombinant OspC antigen (ProLyme, Intervet, USA; Recombitek Lyme, Merial, USA). All of the veterinary vaccines are applied in two-dose immunization scheme with boosters recommended yearly. Safety data are limited and minor cross-reactivity between heterologous *Borrelia* species has been reported [120]. Thus, the poor cross-protective coverage is a problem of currently available vaccines.

Second Generation of OspA Subunit Vaccines. This is based on recombinant OspA with genetically removed potentially cross-reactive T cell epitopes, formerly suspected for the induction of autoimmunity [121]. Development of broadly cross-protective rOspA vaccine must address issues pertaining to sequence variation, because at least seven serotypes of OspA do exist. Multivalent-chimeric OspA proteins have been developed by molecular cloning incorporating the protective epitopes from several OspA serotypes [122]. Nevertheless, OspA antigen-based vaccines require repeated vaccination to keep high titer of specific antibodies in vaccinee serum to prevent transfer of bacteria from tick into human host.

8.3.2.1 Ferritin

New interesting antigen for vaccine development is tick ferritin 2, which is responsible for maintaining iron homeostasis. Iron is an essential but potentially toxic element; therefore, during feeding, ticks must deal with the challenge of an enormous iron supply in the blood meal. Ferritins, the iron-storage proteins, play a pivotal role in this process.

It was shown that vaccination with recombinant FER2 significantly reduces tick infestations in vaccinated rabbits infected with *I. ricinus* and in cattle infected with *R. microplus* and *R. annulatus*. These results support the inclusion of FER2 as a promising candidate antigen for development of new anti-tick vaccines [123]. In spite of the fact that ferritin 2 is not the antigen derived from *Borrelia*, the vaccination with this antigen prevents long-term feeding of tick and transmission of *Borrelia* as well as other tick-transmitted pathogens into host. In this aspect ferritin 2 could be superior to OspA and is of interest to include it in development of combined multiantigen vaccine.

8.3.2.2 OspC Antigen

As mentioned above, several new antigens were discovered and studied as possible targets for new vaccines. We focus on OspC antigen, which received considerable attention in the effort to develop a broadly protective Lyme disease vaccine. OspC is an essential virulence factor that is critical for the establishment of early infection in mammals [124], and the sequence of the protein is not undergoing mutation during infection [125]. OspC is a 22 kDa immunodominant lipoprotein that is anchored in the spirochete outer membrane by an *N*-terminal tripalmitoyl-S-glyceryl-cysteine [126].

The factor complicating the exploitation of OspC as a vaccine candidate is the existence of OspC variation. Molecular phylogenetic analyses have revealed that OspC sequences form at least 38 distinct OspC types. This OspC variation arises primarily through genetic exchange and recombination and not by hypermutation with concomitant immune selection [127]. Owing to this sequence variation, the protective range of single OspC-based vaccine is narrow. A potential approach to solve the high variability of the OspC is to prepare (a) polyvalent vaccine containing several OspC variants [128], (b) generation of recombinant chimeric protein that consists of protective epitopes from those OspC types associated with disease [129], and (c) combination of two or more different recombinant immunogens like OspC, DbpA, and fibronectin-binding protein (BBK32) [130].

From the biotechnological point of view, the full-length OspC is difficult to express in a high yield and purity as a recombinant protein [131]. The removal of the lipidization signal substantially increases both the yield (28 mg per 1 L of the bacterial culture) and purity (93 %) of the recombinant OspC protein [132]. On the other side, delipidized rOspC exerted very low immunogenicity [133, 134], and strong adjuvanticity of vaccine formulation is necessary to induce specific antibody response especially in IgG2 subclass (in experimental mice) important for effective complement activation and opsonization.

In effort to adhere to all above requirement for OspC vaccine, we developed experimental vaccine based on functionalized metallochelating nanoliposomes and synthetic non-pyrogenic adjuvants derived from muramyl dipeptide. This formulation induced strong immune response in experimental mice, which was superior to aluminum hydroxide formulation. Owing to the versatility and safety as an adjuvant, liposomes thus represent promising platform for developing the clinically acceptable vaccine against Lyme disease.

8.3.3 Liposomes as Carriers for Recombinant Vaccines

Of the numerous particulate delivery systems that have been developed until now, phospholipid bilayer vesicles (liposomes) are among the most promising. Gregoriadis and Allison first reported the use of liposomes as immunological adjuvants in 1974 [135, 136]. Since that time, liposomes and related vesicular carriers have been established as robust systems for induction of humoral and cell-mediated immunity to a broad spectrum of infectious diseases and cancers [137].

Liposomes represent the oldest nanoparticle systems described for applications in biological studies as model membranes and in medicine (Fig. 8.9). Over 44 years, liposomes have been shown to be suitable drug delivery systems for applications ranging from cosmetics and dermatology to medical applications such as therapy of infections, anticancer therapy, and veterinary vaccination [138].

Liposome-based vaccines have been around for approximately 30 years, and numerous liposome variants have been developed, some with evident immunostimulatory properties and attractive safety profiles, resulting in registration of several products on the market and progressing of others to advanced stage of clinical testing. Epaxal® (Crucell, Hepatitis A, Formalin-inactivated Hepatitis A virus adsorbed to virosomes) and Inflexal® V, (Crucell, Influenza, Virosomes – reconstituted influenza viral membranes) are two examples of marketed liposome-based vaccines in man. Inflexal® V is licensed in 43 countries with over 60 million doses applied [139, 140].

Furthermore, at least eight liposome-based adjuvant systems are currently approved for human use or undergoing clinical evaluation [141].

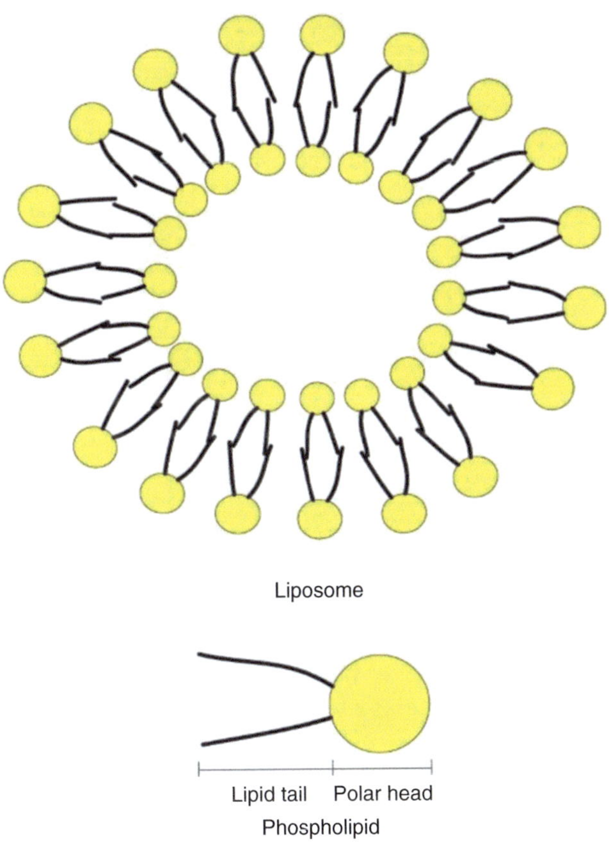

Fig. 8.9 Liposomes are made of phospholipid molecules but can also include other lipids, such as egg phosphatidylethanolamine or phosphatidylglycerol (PG). The lipid molecules spontaneously self-assemble into spherically closed bilayer membranes. The polar heads are hydrated, and the hydrophobic lipid tails interact with each other. The lipid composition defines membrane surface properties. The thickness of the lipid bilayer is typically about 5 nm (Figure by M. Giese Heidelberg/Germany)

8.3.4 Physicochemical Properties of Liposome-Based Vaccines

Liposomes represent almost ideal carrier/delivery systems for the components of synthetic vaccines due to their biodegradability and their ability to retain/incorporate a variety of essential vaccine components simultaneously, even components possessing quite different physicochemical properties (different size, hydrophobicity, charge, etc.).

Different synthetic vaccine components can be encapsulated within the aqueous cavities of liposomes (if hydrophilic) or associated with liposome bilayers (if at least partially hydrophobic in character). Furthermore, essential components can be attached to either internal or external outer leaflet membrane by electrostatic, covalent, or metallochelation interactions.

Biochemically, the most diverse vaccine components are adjuvants required for efficacious activation of innate immunity cells including antigen-presenting cells (APCs) (e.g., monophosphoryl lipid A, CpG oligonucleotides, muramyl dipeptide, and analogs). In addition, adjuvants can be combined with antigens such as soluble or membrane proteins to provoke strong specific immune response. Finally, the liposomes may present carrier for targeting of antigens and adjuvants to antigen-presenting cells [142]. The laboratory and industrial procedures for the liposome preparation have been established, and liposomes have been approved by the US Food and Drug Administration for biomedical applications. The potential for the participation of liposome-based recombinant vaccines in the human and veterinary vaccine market is very promising [143].

The beneficial effect of liposomal carriers consists in their ability to ensure:

1. Protection and stabilization of the antigen, including reconstitution of its native conformation
2. Enhanced uptake by APC by passive or active targeting
3. Enhanced or controlled antigen processing after uptake

Interaction of liposomal vaccine and liposomal immunomodulators with immune cells and cooperation between innate and adaptive branches of immune system is schematically represented in Fig. 8.10.

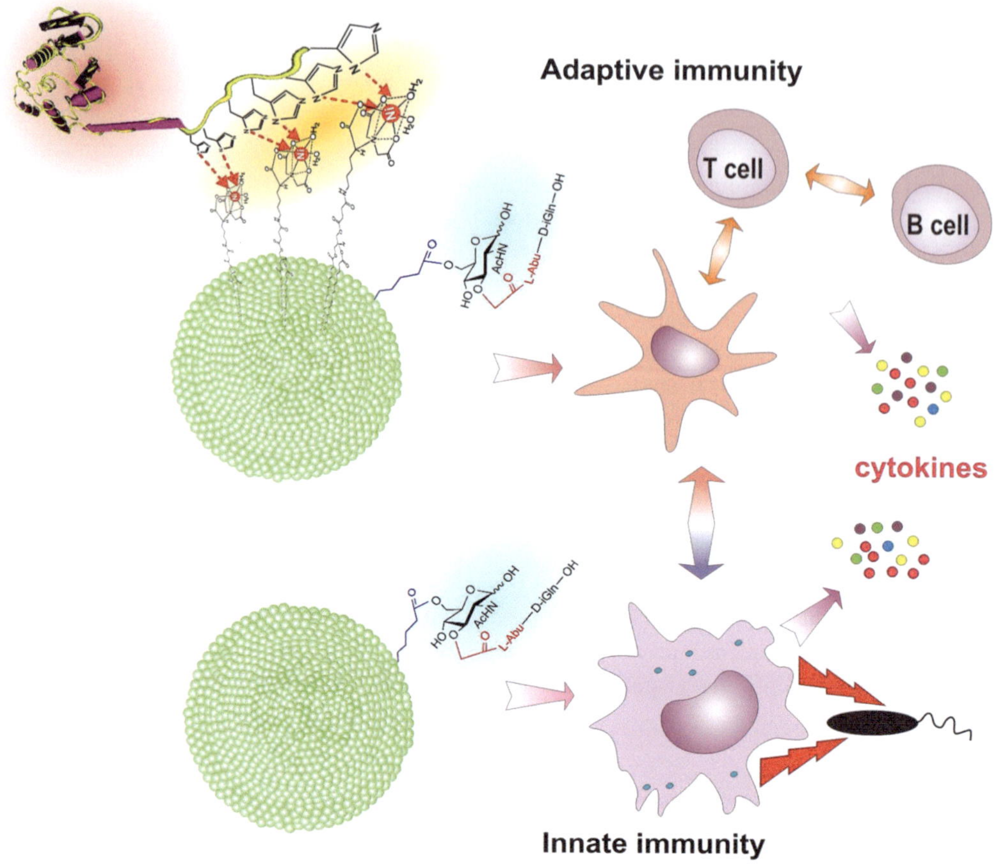

Fig. 8.10 Interaction of liposome-based immunomodulators and proteoliposomal vaccines with immune cells. Functionalized nanoliposomes facilitate co-delivery of antigen to immune cells (dendritic cells, macrophages, and B cells). Highly oriented protein antigen on the liposomal surface is able to interact with membrane-bound immunoglobulins on B cells followed by internalization of whole complex liposomal antigen. Synthetic lipophilic derivative of muramyl dipeptide (norAbuMDP) provides the danger signal via intracellular receptors like NOD2 and NALP-3 to induce innate and adaptive immune responses. Moreover, glycopeptide part of the molecule exposed on the liposomal surface forms molecular pattern recognized by immune cells and enhancing internalization of liposomes (liposomes and immune cells are not in scale)

Liposome-based nanoparticle formulations used for vaccination can be broadly grouped into several classes:

A. *Conventional* (*classical*) *liposomes* composed of neutral lipids and cholesterol and have been the most widely studied due to the greatest versatility – desired formulation parameters can be achieved through modification of the lipid composition or vesicle preparation method. These liposomes were used for steric entrapment of protein antigens in early stage of liposome-based vaccine research.

These classical liposomes are relatively ineffective at enhancing the immunogenicity of antigens because the phospholipids do not act as adjuvants. Adjuvant effect of these liposomes is based on multimeric presentation of antigen, and their adjuvant effect can be optimized by variation of lipid composition, co-incorporation of various adjuvant molecules (e.g. MLP-A, MDP, CpG oligonucleotides, trehalose dibehenate, etc.), and attachment of antigen.

B. *Transferosomes* are ultradeformable liposomes with enhanced skin-penetration properties. They are composed of phosphatidylcholine and cholate (9:2 molar ratio). Presence of cholate endowed these vesicles with high elasticity that enables them to squeeze through pores in the stratum corneum. As a result of high elasticity of bilayer, vesicles of the size of 200–300 nm can pass the highly compact stratum corneum and deliver their content into deep part of skin. Transferosomes are utilized as carrier system for topical application of vaccines [144]. Cationic transferosomes were also tested for noninvasive topical vaccination with pDNA vaccine against hepatitis B [145].

A general process of membrane-mediated incorporation of liposome into cell is illustrated in Fig. 8.11.

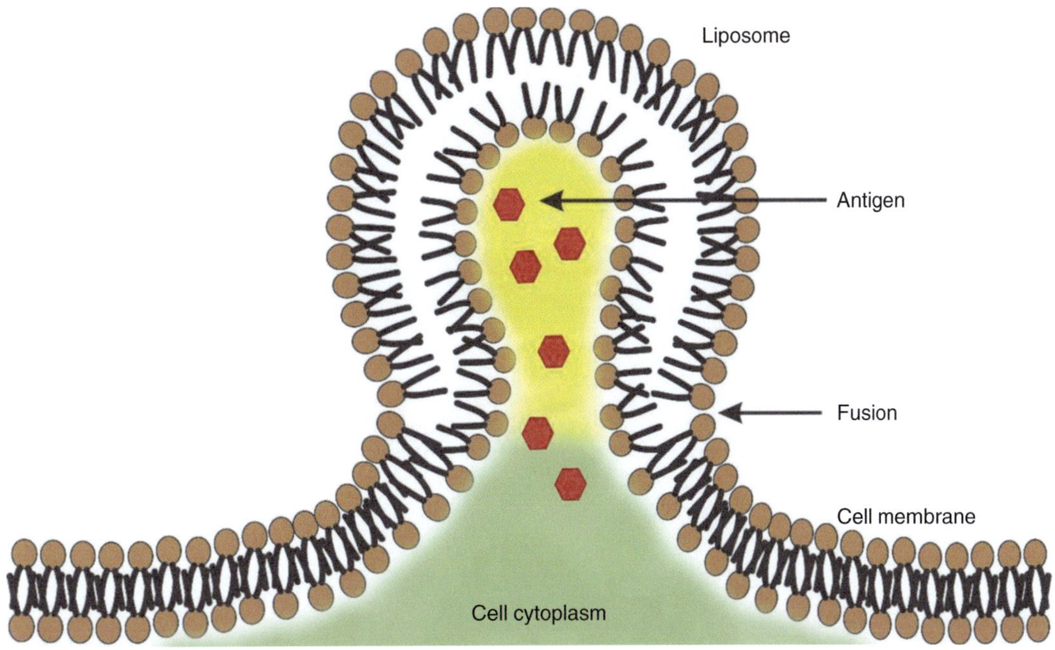

Fig. 8.11 Membrane fusion. The lipid composition defines membrane surface properties. Liposomes deliver antigens or drugs into a cell either by fusion with its membrane, or by endocytosis (see also Fig. 3.10) (Figure by M. Giese Heidelberg/Germany)

8.3.4.1 Cationic Liposomes

Surface adsorption on the cationic liposomes, via electrostatic interactions, is another useful method for attachment of antigens (primarily proteins) on liposomes. The recent work of Christensen, Perrie, and others with protein antigens adsorbed to cationic DDA/TDB (dimethyldioctadecylammonium/trehalose-6,6-dibehenate) liposomes has demonstrated that formulations with surface-adsorbed antigens can be highly stable and elicit robust antibody- and cell-mediated immune responses in mice and ferrets [146–148].

Incorporation of synthetic immunostimulatory molecules like lipophilic TDB into cationic liposomes is able to potentiate significantly their adjuvant effect. It was also observed that certain cationic lipids, originally synthesized as transfection reagents, induce robust IFN-γ and TNF-α response in serum and anti-tumor immunity in murine models of pulmonary metastasis and fibrosarcoma [149]. DOTAP is an example of such a cationic lipid used for many years as component of liposomal gene delivery system exerted an enantiospecific adjuvant effect in dendritic cells [150].

A. *Virosomes* are a special class of proteoliposomes prepared from reconstituted influenza virus membranes supplemented with PC [151]. The physicochemical features of virosomes are constrained by their well-defined composition and method of preparation, but these vesicles benefit greatly from the inherent delivery properties (efficient cell binding, internalization, and cytosolic release) and immunogenicity of the influenza virus (Fig. 8.12).
B. *Archaeosomes* are liposomes prepared from special lipids isolated from Archaebacteria, which are extremophiles and their cell membranes contain lipids and proteins resistant to extreme temperatures, pH, and salt concentration. These lipids are less sensitive to oxidation and the membrane of archeosomes is resistant to action of bile acid salts. Therefore, they are suitable for enteral application. Immune responses induced by archeosomes are comparable to those induced by complete Freund's adjuvants [152].

Functionalized Liposomes in General. These represent various liposomal structures having their surface modified by various ligands (biotin, oligosaccharides, peptides), lipids with reactive head groups, pH- or temperature-sensitive polymers, monoclonal antibodies or their fragments, lectins, etc., to tailor their functions with respect to selective interaction with targeted extra- or intracellular structures (e.g., pathogenic microorganisms, tumor cells, immune cells, blood clothes, etc.). Targeting of antigen to antigen-presenting cells is of great importance for enhancement of efficacy of subunit recombinant vaccines. In this chapter, we will introduce a new system for construction of liposomal based vaccines. This system employs metallochelating lipids for binding of HIS-tagged recombinant antigens onto the surface of liposomes.

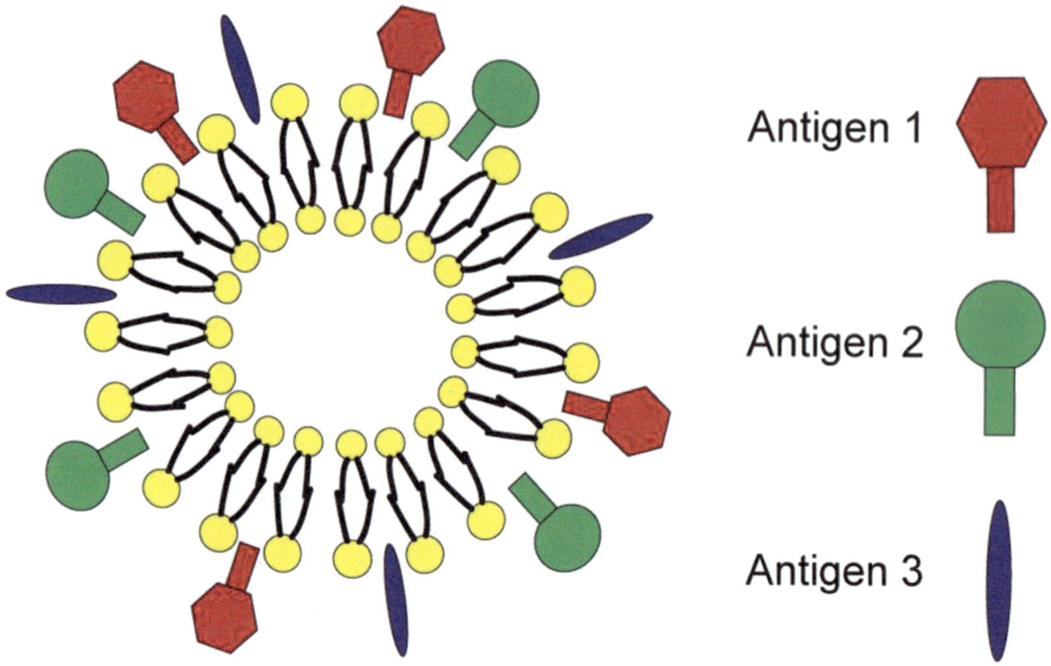

Fig. 8.12 Virosomes are a special class of proteoliposomes prepared from reconstituted influenza virus membranes. The surface of a virosome–liposome carries viral protein antigens, here marked as antigen 1–3 (Figure by M. Giese Heidelberg/Germany)

8.3.5 Binding of Antigen to Liposomes

One of the most critical parameters influencing the immunogenicity of liposomal vaccines is the method by which the antigen is physically or chemically associated with the formulation. The most common modes of association include covalent lipid conjugation (either pre- or post-vesicle formation), non-covalent surface attachment (via biotin, NTA-Ni-HIS, or antibody–epitope interactions), encapsulation, and surface adsorption (Fig. 8.13). Many of the early studies of liposomal peptide and protein antigenicity in mice compared encapsulated antigens to those conjugated to the surface of preformed liposomes. Early studies by Alving, Gregoriadis, Therien, and others confirmed that both methods are generally effective for inducing antibody and T cell responses to associated protein antigens such as albumin and tetanus toxoid [153–155].

In some cases, covalent antigen conjugation results in superior antibody induction, which is not surprising because B cell receptors can recognize intact antigen on the liposome surface [156]. As the size and complexity of the antigen decreases, the benefit of their surface conjugation for antibody induction becomes more pronounced, as found for the synthetic peptides for which surface conjugation provides immune responses superior to encapsulation [156, 157].

8.3.6 Metallochelating Bond and Metallochelating Liposomes

With respect to potential application of metallochelating liposomes for the construction of vaccines, the question of in vitro and especially in vivo stability is of great importance. This problem could be divided into two fields. First, the stability of the liposomes themselves and second, the effect of the components presented in biological fluids (e.g., proteins and ions) on the stability of the metallochelating bond.

In the example of OspC proteoliposomes, the gel-permeation chromatography data indicated a good in vitro stability of the OspC proteoliposomes during the chromatographic process, within which they experience a shear stress and dilution. Also after incubating OspC proteoliposomes in serum at 37 °C, we demonstrated the stability of the metallochelating bond linking the protein to the liposomal surface [132]. In fact, in vivo fate of liposomes after the intradermal application is different from the situation after intravenous injection. First, dilution of proteoliposomes after intramuscular application is not so rapid, and second, the ratio of tissue fluid proteins to proteoliposomes is more favorable to proteoliposomes owing to their relatively high concentration at the site of application. In the case of another route of application – intradermal – the flow rate of tissue fluid within intradermal extracellular matrix is even lower in comparison with muscle tissue or blood vessels.

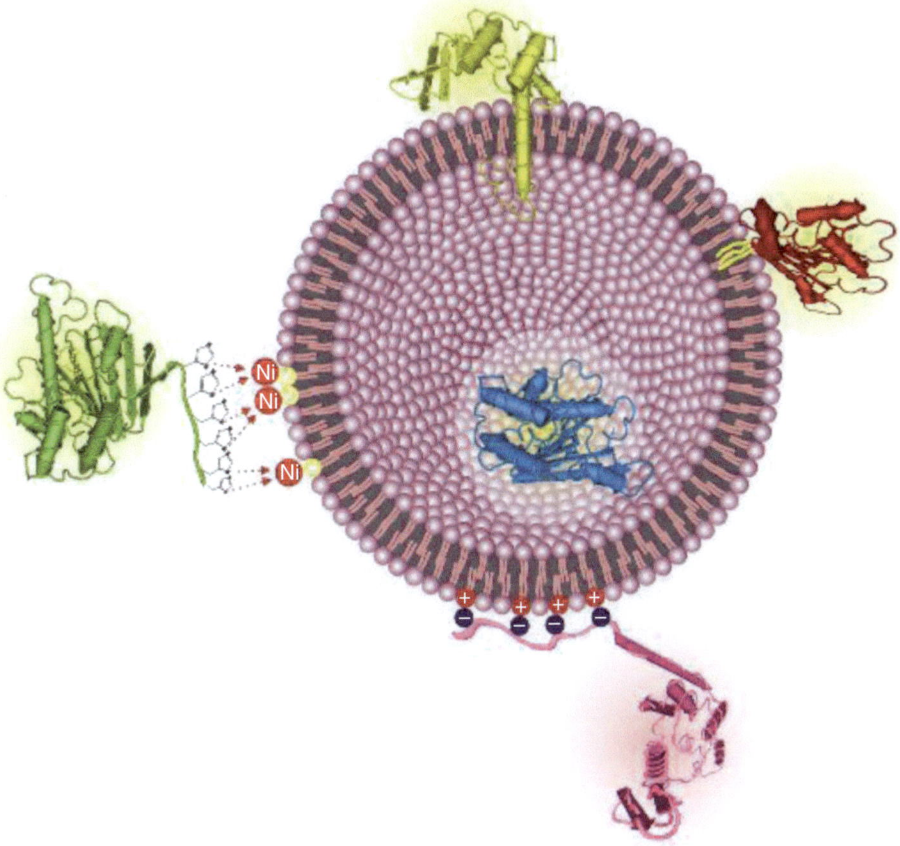

Fig. 8.13 Association of protein antigen with liposome. Protein antigen can be associated with liposome by various ways. Membrane protein can be reconstituted in their natural conformation in liposome membrane (*yellow*), lipophilized protein (e.g., palmitoyled protein) can be anchored in lipid membrane by lipidic residue (*red*). Functionalized liposomes can be prepared to facilitate covalent or non-covalent binding of protein onto the surface of liposomes

Stability of Metallochelating. This fact is often overlooked. The stability of metallochelating bond probably depends also on the character of particular protein. It was shown that Ni-NTA3–DTDA liposomes (containing three-functional chelating lipid) with single-chain Fv fragments (anti-CD11c) bound onto the liposomal surface were able to target dendritic cells in vitro as well as in vivo. The application of Ni-NTA3–DTDA probably endows the metallochelating bond with a higher in vivo stability [158], but this improved stability did not influence higher immunogenicity [159].

Generally, metal ions, physical-chemical character of the metallochelating lipids, and their surface density belong to the factors that could be optimized to get a required in vivo stability and therefore strong immune response.

Binding of recombinant OspC (rOspC) onto metallochelating liposomes was confirmed by TEM, GPC, SDS PAGE, and dynamic light-scattering methods. Stability of the metallochelating bond in model biological fluids was studied by the incubation of rOspC liposomes with human serum. This study showed that after 1 h incubation at 37 °C, more than 60 % of rOspC was still associated with liposomes. Based on this data, therefore, the half-life of rOspC proteoliposomes in serum was estimated to be at least 1 h. Increase in stability of surface-exposed antigens on the liposomes can be achieved by chemical binding onto the outer liposomal surface that is appropriately functionalized. With respect to a potential application for the construction of vaccines, the question of in vitro and especially in vivo stability is of great importance.

There are only few references reporting the metallochelating bond implemented in the construction of supramolecular structures as vaccine carriers [159–164]. Various ways for association of protein antigen with liposome are depicted in Fig. 8.13. Real structures revealed by various microscopy methods are presented in Fig. 8.15.

Selective metallochelating bond is applicable for His-tagged recombinant proteins (green), and this non-covalent bond can be transformed to covalent one via carbodiimide conjugation (see Fig. 8.14b). All abovementioned examples represent highly oriented binding of protein onto liposomal surface.

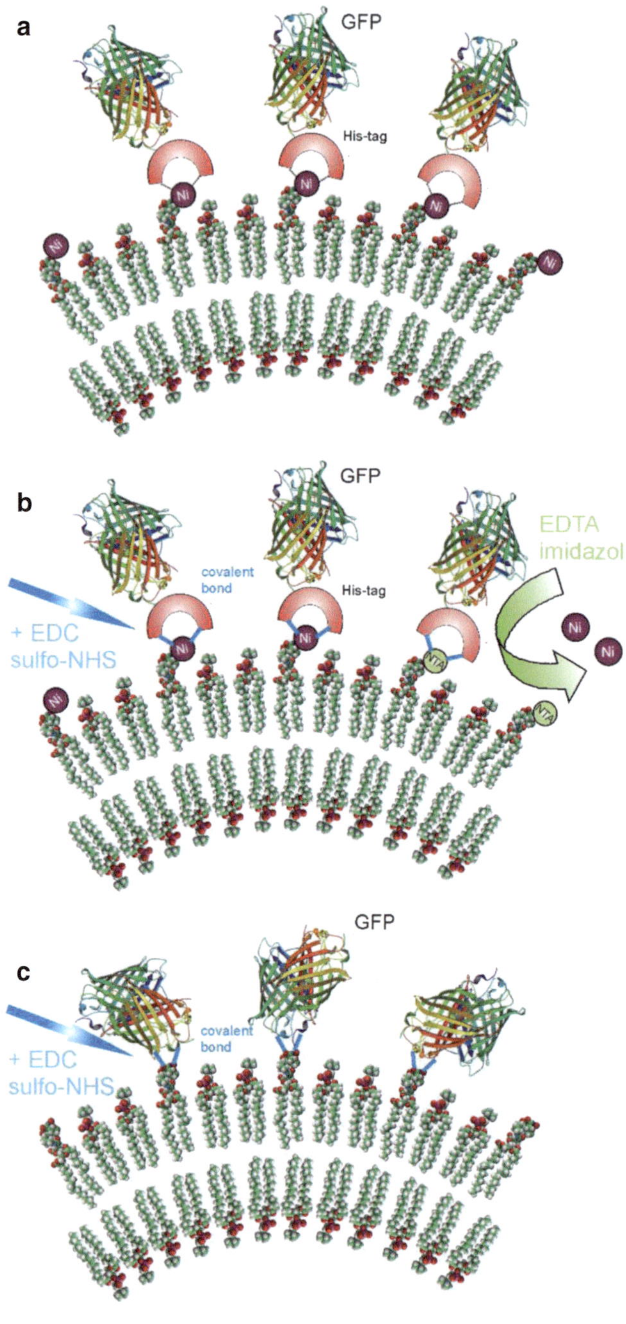

Fig. 8.14 Binding of protein onto liposomal surface. (**a**) Oriented non-covalent binding of HIS-tagged GFP (green fluorescent protein) onto liposomal surface. (**b**) Transformation of metallochelating bond into covalent amide bond via carbodiimide chemistry preserving oriented binding of GFP. Ni+2 ions are removed by EDTA as a metallochelation agent. (**c**) Example of random orientation of GFP bound onto liposomal surface by application of carbodiimide chemistry without pre-orientation via metallochelating bond

Covalent coupling of protein onto liposomal surface functionalized by, e.g., reactive maleimide phospholipid head group leads to random orientation of bound protein (Fig. 8.14b).

Electrostatic interaction represents another way for association of proteins with liposomes. This association is non-specific and relatively labile in biological milieu (*pink*). Molecule of soluble protein can be also sterically entrapped in water compartment of liposome (blue). This is of importance especially for peptide antigens and protein antigens intended for direct delivery into cytoplasm of immune cells to mimic virus-like pathways for antigen processing. The structure of metallochelating liposomes is illustrated in Fig. 8.15.

8.4 Adjuvants for Liposomal Based Vaccines

The interaction between the innate and the adaptive immune responses is paramount in generating an antigen-specific immune response. The initiation of innate immune responses begins with the interaction of pathogen-associated molecular patterns (PAMPs) on the pathogen side with pattern-recognizing receptors (PRR) such as Toll-like receptors (TLRs) on the host cells involved in the innate immunity (e.g., dendritic cells). A major functional criterion commonly used for the evaluation of various new adjuvants involves their ability to stimulate the innate immunity cells. This would include engaging other PRRs and the co-receptors and intracellular adaptor signaling proteins with which they are associated. PAMPs and their derivatives are utilized by adjuvant developers to harness the power of innate immunity to channel the immune response in a desired direction.

Based on the identification of several TLRs and PAMPs recognized by them, various PAMP agonists were tested as adjuvants. Examples of TLR–PAMP-specific interaction include bacterial or viral unmethylated immunostimulating CpG oligonucleotides interacting with TLR9, liposaccharide, and its component monophosphoryl lipid A (MPL-A) interacting with TRL4. These two types of adjuvants are in advanced stage of testing in clinical trials and some already licensed vaccines contain MPLA in liposomal form [165, 166].

New lipophilic adjuvant suitable for construction of liposome-based vaccines is the mycobacterial cord factor trehalose-6,6-dimycolate (TDM), and its synthetic analog trehalose-6,6-dibehenate (TDB) is potent adjuvant for Th1/Th17 vaccination that activates Syk-Card9 signaling in APCs [167].

The last group of potent synthetic or semisynthetic adjuvants is derived from muramyl dipeptide (MDP) and discussed in Chap. 7.

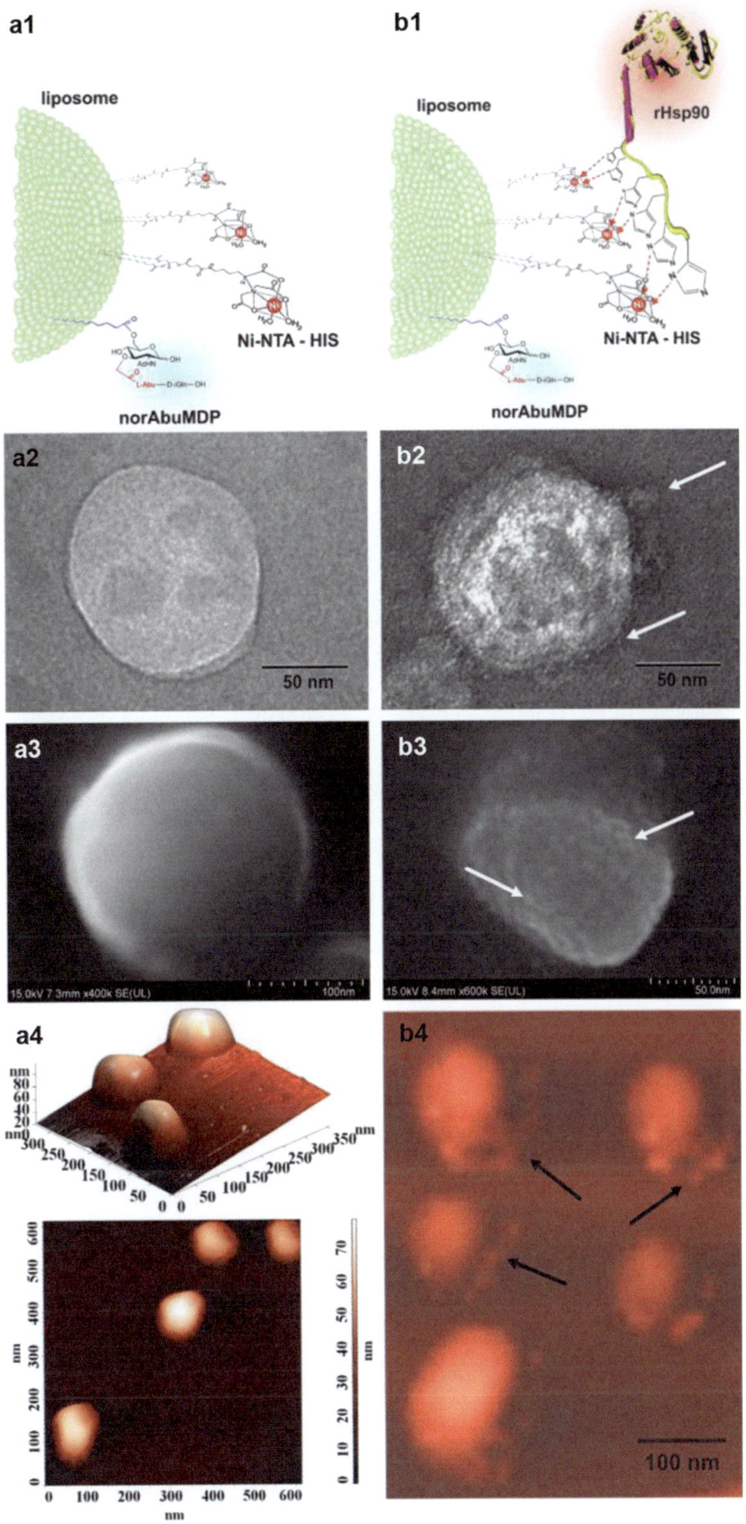

Fig. 8.15 Structure of metallochelating liposomes and proteoliposomes revealed by TEM, SEM, and AFM. Recombinant heat shock protein derived from *Candida albicans* was used as illustrative example. (**a1**) Schematic presentation of a metallochelating liposome with metallochelating lipids and incorporated lipidized norAbuMDP molecules. (**a2**) TEM photograph of a metallochelating liposome with metallochelating lipids and incorporated lipidized norAbuMDP molecules. (**a3**) SEM photograph of a metallochelating liposome with metallochelating lipids and incorporated lipidized norAbuMDP molecules. (**a4**) AFM photograph of a metallochelating liposome with metallochelating lipids and incorporated lipidized norAbuMDP molecules. (**b1**) Schematic presentation of a metallochelating liposome (**a1**) with rHsp90 bound via metallochelating bond. (**b2**) TEM photograph of a metallochelating liposome with rHsp90 bound via metallochelating bond. (**b3**) SEM photograph of a metallochelating liposome with rHsp90 bound via metallochelating bond. (**b4**) AFM photograph of a metallochelating liposome with rHsp90 bound via metallochelating bond. *White arrows* indicate the metallochelating bond linking the protein rHsp90 to the liposomal surface. *Black arrows* indicate the metallochelating bond linking the protein rHsp90 to the liposomal surface

8.5 Selected Applied Micro- and Nanostructures

8.5.1 Immunostimulatory Complexes (ISCOMs)

Typically, ISCOMs are spherical, hollow, rigid, cagelike structures with particle size approximately 40 nm with a strong negative charge [168, 169]. ISCOMs are composed of phospholipid, cholesterol, saponin, and immunogen (antigen) usually a protein. These systems are actually designed for effective vaccine delivery. They mimic the virus particles in various aspects such as their size, orientation of surface proteins associated with a powerful immunostimulatory activity due to saponins [170] (as shown in Fig. 8.17c).

These characteristics of ISCOMs furnish them with an ability to induce strong immune responses to a variety of antigens in a number of species. In contrast to many other carrier systems, ISCOMs promote a broad immune response by simultaneous induction of both high levels of antibody titer and strong T cell response, including enhanced cytokine secretion and activation of cytotoxic T-lymphocyte (CTL) responses [171].

ISCOM-Based Vaccine. The ability to stimulate CTL may be important in generating effective immune responses to virus-infected cells where strong T cell response is desired. A further attraction of ISCOMs is their reduced toxicity and reactogenicity compared with other saponin-based formulations. Presently, ISCOM-based vaccine for veterinary use is available in the market against equine influenza.

A critical question concerning the use of ISCOMs as a general vaccine adjuvant is whether the results in animal models such as the efficient induction of CTL responses can be reproduced in humans. The potential for ISCOMs to induce significant and sustained levels of CTL activity in humans may be of particular importance to viral vaccines [172]. Hopefully, the ongoing clinical trials of ISCOM-based vaccines will provide superior results in forthcoming years.

Saponins. Saponins are natural bioactive glycosides consisting of a triterpene or steroid aglycone with a range of pharmacological properties, found in wild or cultivated plants, lower marine animals, and some bacteria. Saponins induce a strong adjuvant effect to T-dependent as well as T-independent antigens and provoke a strong cytotoxic CD8+ lymphocyte response. Saponins are suitable to act as mucosal adjuvants.

However, saponins are surface-active agents and cause hemolysis of red blood cells. The LD50 for intravenously administered Quil-A is 0.67 mg/kg in rats, and doses of greater than 25 µg of Quil-A given intraperitoneally can be toxic in the B6D2F1 strain of mice. Figure 8.16 illustrates the chemical structure of quillaia saponin.

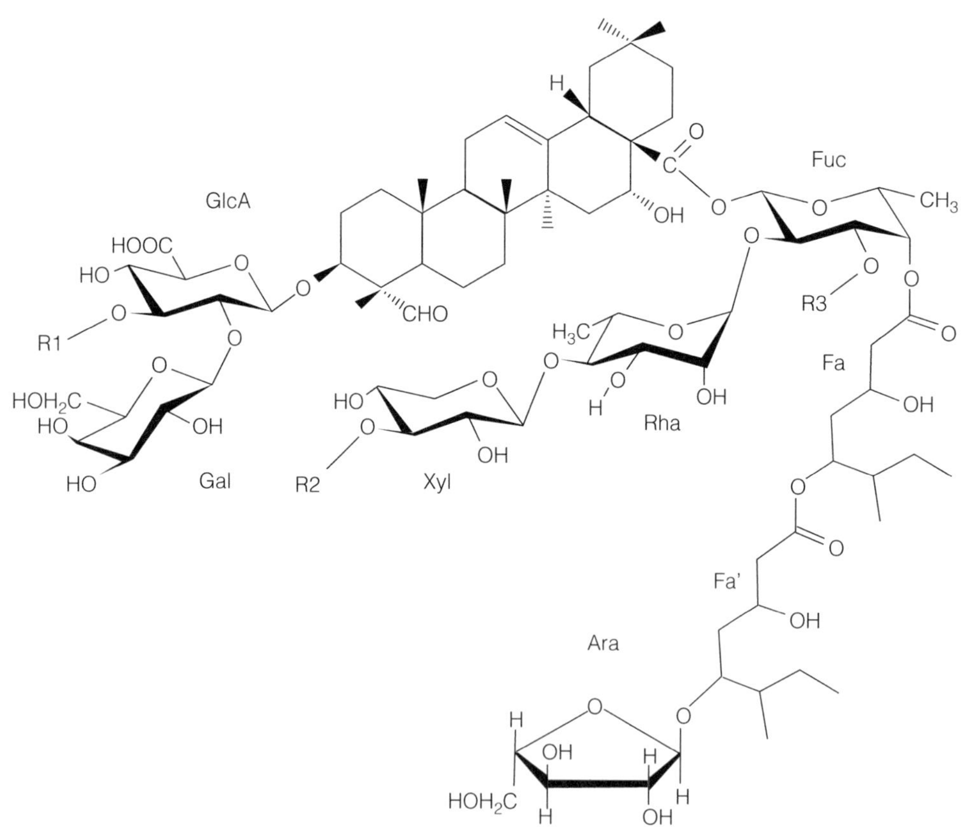

Fig. 8.16 Structure of quillaia saponin

Several ISCOM™ and ISCOMATRIX™ vaccines have shown to induce humoral and cellular response in animal models. These systems can access both the MHC I and MHC II pathways and act as a potent immunomodulator of both the innate and adaptive immune systems. Intranasal delivery of influenza ISCOMATRIX™ vaccine in humans has shown to induce systemic and mucosal responses, and therefore the ISCOMATRIX™ adjuvant can be used as a mucosal adjuvant [173].

Antigen-specific CTL, T helper cells, and antibodies can be induced by ISCOMs and ISCOMATRIX™ vaccines for cancer and infectious diseases [174]. Another modification of ISCOM with regard to charge resulted in cationic ISCOM derivatives (PLUSCOMs), which offered high anionic antigen loading and therefore enhanced T cell response in comparison to classic anionic ISCOMs against a model protein antigen (ovalbumin) [175]. Moreover, these complexes can reduce the dose of antigen required to induce immune response [176].

8.5.2 Polymeric Micelles

Polymeric micelles (as shown in Fig. 8.17e) are a well-organized nano-sized assembly of synthetic polymers. These fall in the category of association colloids that are formed spontaneously when the ampihiliic molecules or hydrophilic regions are maintained at an appropriate concentration and temperature [177, 178]. They are not held together by covalent bonds and hence can be dissociated easily. This property of micelles can be exploited as per their applications [179].

They have shown high stability in vitro as well as in vivo. Physical and chemical properties of polymeric micelles can be manipulated by selection of suitable hydrophilic and hydrophobic polymers. In a study by Morein et al., a 30S protein subunit micellar vaccine induced a detectable antibody titer as well as protective immunity in a challenge study against pneumonia caused by the PI-3 virus [180]. Prabakaran et al. performed similar studies where they used soya phosphatidylcholine micelles against H5N1 infection. Higher levels of serum IgG, mucosal IgA, and HI titers were observed when compared to the free antigen. Hence micelles can serve as a promising carrier for vaccine antigens.

8.5.3 Dendrimers

Dendrimers (as shown in Fig. 8.17f) are highly branched, monodispersed polymeric nanoparticles. Dendrimers are composed of three different components, an initiator core,

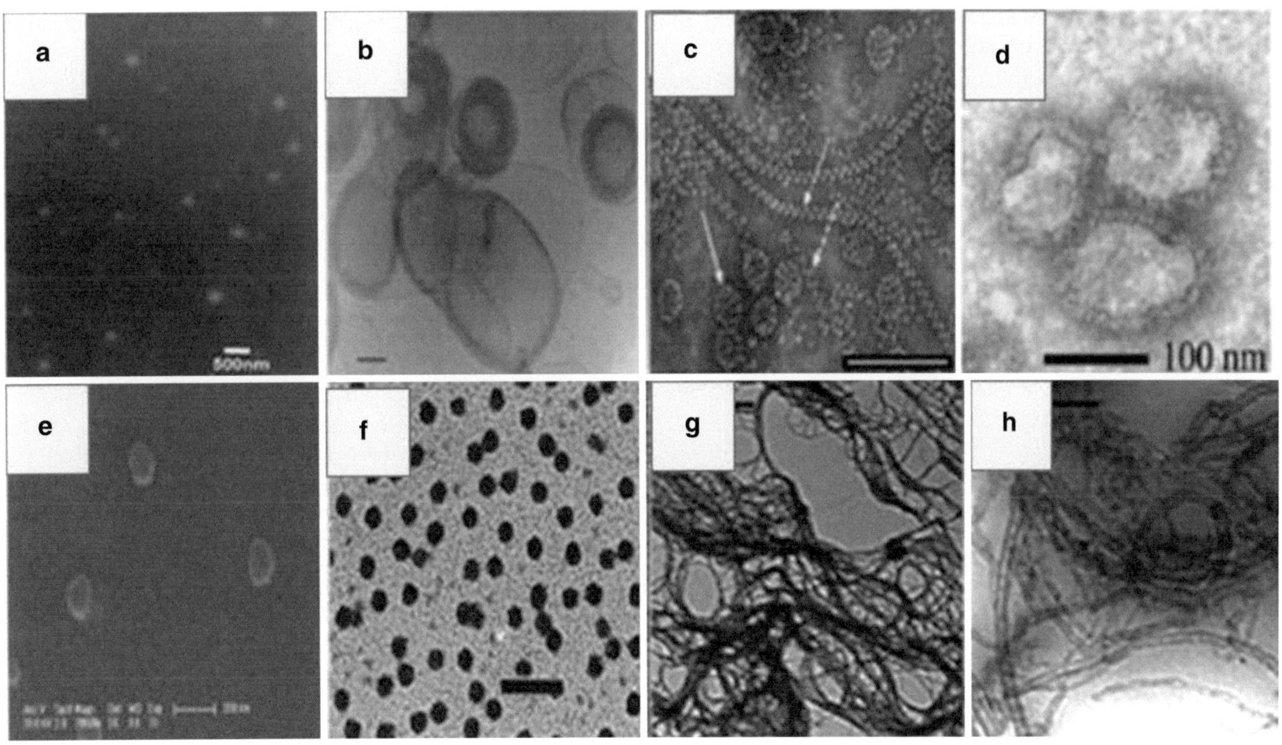

Fig. 8.17 Different nanocarriers for vaccine delivery: (**a**) TEM image of PEG-PLGA nanoparticle (scale bar corresponds to 500 nm), (**b**) Cryo-EM image of cationic liposomes entrapping DNA (*scale bar* corresponds to 200 nm), (**c**) TEM image of ISCOMs of different types such as typical cagelike (*solid arrow*), helices (*dashed arrow*) and double helices (*dotted arrows*), (*scale bar* corresponds to 200 nm), (**d**) EM image of influenza H1N1 virus-like particles (scale corresponds to 100 nm), (**e**) SEM image of PEG-PEI-PBLG copolymeric micelles (scale corresponds to 200 nm), (**f**) TEM image of PAMAM dendrimer, (**g**, **h**) TEM images of single-walled (**g**) and multi-walled (**h**) carbon nanotubes (*scale bar* corresponds to 1 μm and 250 nm, respectively)

branches, and terminal functional groups. The initiator core is the main component of dendrimers and the branches extend in the outer directions. The terminal groups can be modified based on charge/hydrophilic/lipophilic properties. They are similar to polymeric micelles but are linked covalently unlike micelles and thus have more stronger bonds and do not tend to dissociate easily [181]. The external surface can be easily modified and alterations of the internal cavity make dendrimers a promising carrier for various biomedical and industrial applications.

Recent work by Baker et al. involves coupling of various functional molecules including sensing units, MRI contrast agents, triggering devices, and targeting molecules to the surface of a generation 5 dendritic polymer (MW 25,000 daltons, diameter 5 nm) [182]. A specific class of dendrimers called as multiple antigenic peptide (MAP) systems has been used widely for the vaccine purposes. MAP-based malaria vaccine has been tested in phase I clinical trials [183]. Having the potential to enter the clinical trials, these delivery systems are expected to be available on market shortly.

8.5.4 Carbon Nanotubes

Recently, inorganic nanomaterials such as nanocrystals, nanowires, and nanotubes have been receiving an increasing amount of attention for vaccine delivery. Carbon nanotubes (as shown in Fig. 8.17g, h) are explored as a vehicle for vaccines because of their capacity to link to an antigen while maintaining their conformation and thus inducing antigen-specific antibody response.

They can also be modified in a non-immunogenic material. Functionalized carbon nanotubes can be used as nanovectors for the delivery of antigen/s by forming covalent bonds or supramolecular assemblies based on non-covalent interactions [184]. However, carbon nanotubes remain an area of interest for current researchers; still extensive work is required before they can enter the clinical trials.

References

1. Torchilin, V.P.: Micellar nanocarriers: pharmaceutical perspectives. Pharm. Res. **24**, 1–16 (2007)
2. Hobbs, S.K., et al.: Regulation of transport pathways in tumor vessels: role of tumor type and microenvironment. Proc. Natl. Acad. Sci. U. S. A. **95**, 4607–4612 (1998)
3. Hopewell, J.W., Duncan, R., Wilding, D., Chakrabarti, K.: Preclinical evaluation of the cardiotoxicity of PK2: a novel HPMA copolymer–doxorubicin–galactosamine conjugate antitumour agent. Hum. Exp. Toxicol. **20**, 461–470 (2001)
4. Little, S.R.: Reorienting our view of particle-based adjuvants for subunit vaccines. Proc. Natl. Acad. Sci. **109**, 999–1000 (2012)
5. Moon, J.J., et al.: Enhancing humoral responses to a malaria antigen with nanoparticle vaccines that expand T fh cells and promote germinal center induction. Proc. Natl. Acad. Sci. U. S. A. **109**, 1080–1085 (2012)
6. Prokop, A., Davidson, J.M.: Nanovehicular intracellular delivery systems. J. Pharm. Sci. **97**, 3518–3590 (2008)
7. Johnson, R J.: The complement system. Biomaterials Science: An Introduction to Materials in Medicine 318–328 (2004)
8. Scheibe, P., Barz, M., Hemmelmann, M., Zentel, R.: Langmuir-Blodgett films of biocompatible poly(HPMA)-block-poly(lauryl methacrylate) and poly(HPMA)-random-poly(lauryl methacrylate): influence of polymer structure on membrane formation and stability. Langmuir **26**, 5661–5669 (2010)
9. Kelsch, A., et al.: HPMA copolymers as surfactants in the preparation of biocompatible nanoparticles for biomedical application. Biomacromolecules **13**, 4179–4187 (2012)
10. Riess, G.: Micellization of block copolymers. Prog. Polym. Sci. **28**, 1107–1170 (2003)
11. O'Reilly, R.K., Hawker, C.J., Wooley, K.L.: Cross-linked block copolymer micelles: functional nanostructures of great potential and versatility. Chem. Soc. Rev. **35**, 1068–1083 (2006)
12. Kabanov, A.V., Vinogradov, S.V.: Nanogels as pharmaceutical carriers: finite networks of infinite capabilities. Angew. Chem. Int. Ed. **48**, 5418–5429 (2009)
13. Miyata, K., Nishiyama, N., Kataoka, K.: Rational design of smart supramolecular assemblies for gene delivery: chemical challenges in the creation of artificial viruses. Chem. Soc. Rev. **41**, 2562–2574 (2012)
14. Kataoka, K., Harada, A., Nagasaki, Y.: Block copolymer micelles for drug delivery: design, characterization and biological significance. Adv. Drug Deliv. Rev. **47**, 113–131 (2001)
15. Nuhn, L., et al.: Cationic nanohydrogel particles as potential siRNA carriers for cellular delivery. ACS Nano **6**, 2198–2214 (2012)
16. Torchilin, V.P.: Recent advances with liposomes as pharmaceutical carriers. Nat. Rev. Drug Discov. **4**, 145–160 (2005)
17. Lasic, D.D.: Sterically stabilized vesicles. Angew. Chem. Int. Ed. **33**, 1685–1698 (1994)
18. Allen, T.M., Cullis, P.R.: Drug delivery systems: entering the mainstream. Science **303**, 1818–1822 (2004)
19. White, K.L., Rades, T., Furneaux, R.H., Tyler, P.C., Hook, S.: Mannosylated liposomes as antigen delivery vehicles for targeting to dendritic cells. J. Pharm. Pharmacol. **58**, 729–737 (2006)
20. Levine, D.H., et al.: Polymersomes: a new multi-functional tool for cancer diagnosis and therapy. Methods **46**, 25–32 (2008)
21. Osterhaus, A., Rimmelzwaan, G.F.: Induction of virus-specific immunity by ISCOMs. Modulat. Immune Response Vaccine Antigens 49–58 (1998)
22. Saupe, A., McBurney, W., Rades, T., Hook, S.: Immunostimulatory colloidal delivery systems for cancer vaccines. Expert Opin. Drug Deliv. **3**, 345–354 (2006)
23. Bunjes, H.: Lipid nanoparticles for the delivery of poorly water-soluble drugs. J. Pharm. Pharmacol. **62**, 1637–1645 (2010)
24. Petersen, S., Steiniger, F., Fischer, D., Fahr, A., Bunjes, H.: The physical state of lipid nanoparticles affects their in vitro cell viability. Eur. J. Pharm. Biopharm. **79**, 150–161 (2011)
25. Landfester, K.: Synthesis of colloidal particles in miniemulsions. Annu. Rev. Mater. Res. **36**, 231–279 (2006)
26. Landfester, K.: Recent developments in miniemulsions – formation and stability mechanisms. Macromol. Symp. **150**, 171–178 (2000)
27. Mok, H., Park, T.G.: Direct plasmid DNA encapsulation within PLGA nanospheres by single oil-in-water emulsion method. Eur. J. Pharm. Biopharm. **68**, 105–111 (2008)
28. Kazzaz, J., Neidleman, J., Singh, M., Ott, G., O'Hagan, D.T.: Novel anionic microparticles are a potent adjuvant for the induction of cytotoxic T lymphocytes against recombinant p55 gag from HIV-1. J. Control. Release **67**, 347–356 (2000)
29. Barz, M., et al.: P(HPMA)-block-P(LA) copolymers in paclitaxel formulations: polylactide stereochemistry controls micellization, cellular uptake kinetics, intracellular localization and drug efficiency. J. Control. Release **163**, 63–74 (2012)

30. Aspinall, G.O.: The Polysaccharides 35. Academic, New York (1982)
31. Rolland, J.P., et al.: Direct fabrication and harvesting of monodisperse, shape-specific nanobiomaterials. J. Am. Chem. Soc. **127**, 10096–10100 (2005)
32. Gratton, S.E., et al.: Nanofabricated particles for engineered drug therapies: a preliminary biodistribution study of PRINT nanoparticles. J Control. Release **121**, 10–18 (2007)
33. Dunn, S.S., et al.: Reductively responsive siRNA-conjugated hydrogel nanoparticles for gene silencing. J. Am. Chem. Soc. **134**, 7423–7430 (2012)
34. Laurent, S., et al.: Magnetic iron oxide nanoparticles: synthesis, stabilization, vectorization, physicochemical characterizations, and biological applications. Chem. Rev. **108**, 2064–2110 (2008)
35. Bernardi, R.J., Lowery, A.R., Thompson, P.A., Blaney, S.M., West, J.L.: Immunonanoshells for targeted photothermal ablation in medulloblastoma and glioma: an in vitro evaluation using human cell lines. J. Neuro. Oncol. **86**, 165–172 (2008)
36. Cruz, L.J., et al.: Targeting nanosystems to human DCs via Fc receptor as an effective strategy to deliver antigen for immunotherapy. Mol. Pharm. **8**, 104–116 (2011)
37. Ito, A., Honda, H., Kobayashi, T.: Cancer immunotherapy based on intracellular hyperthermia using magnetite nanoparticles: a novel concept of "heat-controlled necrosis" with heat shock protein expression. Cancer Immunol. Immunother. **CII 55**, 320–328 (2006)
38. Masoudi, A., Madaah Hosseini, H.R., Shokrgozar, M.A., Ahmadi, R., Oghabian, M.A.: The effect of poly(ethylene glycol) coating on colloidal stability of superparamagnetic iron oxide nanoparticles as potential MRI contrast agent. Int. J. Pharm. **433**, 129–141 (2012)
39. Niederhafner, P., Reinis, M., Sebestík, J., Jezek, J.: Glycopeptide dendrimers, part III: a review. Use of glycopeptide dendrimers in immunotherapy and diagnosis of cancer and viral diseases. J. Pept. Sci. **14**, 556–587 (2008)
40. Günay, K.A., Theato, P., Klok, H.-A.: Standing on the shoulders of Hermann Staudinger: post-polymerization modification from past to present. J. Polym. Sci. A: Polym. Chem. **51**, 1–28 (2013)
41. Grandjean, C., Boutonnier, A., Guerreiro, C., Fournier, J.-M., Mulard, L.A.: On the preparation of carbohydrate-protein conjugates using the traceless Staudinger ligation. J. Org. Chem. **70**, 7123–7132 (2005)
42. Xu, P., et al.: Simple, direct conjugation of bacterial O-SP-core antigens to proteins: development of cholera conjugate vaccines. Bioconjug. Chem. **22**, 2179–2185 (2011)
43. Scaramuzza, S., et al.: A new site-specific monoPEGylated filgrastim derivative prepared by enzymatic conjugation: production and physicochemical characterization. J. Control. Release **164**, 355–363 (2012)
44. Jung, B., Theato, P.: Chemical strategies for the synthesis of protein – polymer conjugates. Bio-synthet. Poly. Conjugates 37–70 (2013)
45. Moad, G., Rizzardo, E., Thang, S.H.: Living radical polymerization by the RAFT process. Aust. J. Chem. **58**, 379 (2005)
46. Braunecker, W.A., Matyjaszewski, K.: Controlled/living radical polymerization: features, developments, and perspectives. Prog. Polym. Sci. **32**, 93–146 (2007)
47. Marsden, H.R., Kros, A.: Polymer-peptide block copolymers – an overview and assessment of synthesis methods. Macromol. Biosci. **9**, 939–951 (2009)
48. Lutz, J.-F.: Polymerization of oligo(ethylene glycol) (meth)acrylates: toward new generations of smart biocompatible materials. J. Polym. Sci. A Polym. Chem. **46**, 3459–3470 (2008)
49. Lutz, J.-F., Hoth, A.: Preparation of ideal PEG analogues with a tunable thermosensitivity by controlled radical copolymerization of 2-(2-Methoxyethoxy)ethyl Methacrylate and Oligo(ethylene glycol) Methacrylate. Macromolecules **39**, 893–896 (2006)
50. Lomas, H., et al.: Non-cytotoxic polymer vesicles for rapid and efficient intracellular delivery. Faraday Discuss. **139**, 143–159 (2008)
51. Lewis, A., Tang, Y., Brocchini, S., Choi, J.-W., Godwin, A.: Poly(2-methacryloyloxyethyl phosphorylcholine) for protein conjugation. Bioconjug. Chem. **19**, 2144–2155 (2008)
52. Kopecek, J., Kopecková, P.: HPMA copolymers: origins, early developments, present, and future. Adv. Drug Deliv. Rev. **62**, 122–149 (2010)
53. Hadjichristidis, N., Iatrou, H., Pitsikalis, M., Sakellariou, G.: Synthesis of well-defined polypeptide-based materials via the ring-opening polymerization of alpha-amino acid N-carboxyanhydrides. Chem. Rev. **109**, 5528–5578 (2009)
54. Takae, S., et al.: PEG-detachable polyplex micelles based on disulfide-linked block catiomers as bioresponsive nonviral gene vectors. J. Am. Chem. Soc. **130**, 6001–6009 (2008)
55. Weissleder, R., Tung, C.H., Mahmood, U., Bogdanov, A.: In vivo imaging of tumors with protease-activated near-infrared fluorescent probes. Nat. Biotechnol. **17**, 375–378 (1999)
56. Arnon, R.: The development of Cop 1 (Copaxone), an innovative drug for the treatment of multiple sclerosis: personal reflections. Immunol. Lett. **50**, 1–15 (1996)
57. Shaffer, S.A., et al.: In vitro and in vivo metabolism of paclitaxel poliglumex: identification of metabolites and active proteases. Cancer Chemother. Pharmacol. **59**, 537–548 (2007)
58. Hanson, J.A., et al.: Nanoscale double emulsions stabilized by single-component block copolypeptides. Nature **455**, 85–88 (2008)
59. Matsumura, Y.: Poly (amino acid) micelle nanocarriers in preclinical and clinical studies. Adv. Drug Deliv. Rev. **60**, 899–914 (2008)
60. http://www.clinicaltrials.gov. At: http://clinicaltrials.gov
61. Li, C., Wallace, S.: Polymer-drug conjugates: recent development in clinical oncology. Adv. Drug Deliv. Rev. **60**, 886–898 (2008)
62. Khandare, J., Calderón, M., Dagia, N.M., Haag, R.: Multifunctional dendritic polymers in nanomedicine: opportunities and challenges. Chem. Soc. Rev. **41**, 2824–2848 (2012)
63. Barriau, E., et al.: Systematic investigation of functional core variation within hyperbranched polyglycerols. J. Polym. Sci. A: Polym. Chem. **46**, 2049–2061 (2008)
64. Kainthan, R.K., Janzen, J., Levin, E., Devine, D.V., Brooks, D.E.: Biocompatibility testing of branched and linear polyglycidol. Biomacromolecules **7**, 703–709 (2006)
65. Kainthan, R.K., Hester, S.R., Levin, E., Devine, D.V., Brooks, D.E.: In vitro biological evaluation of high molecular weight hyperbranched polyglycerols. Biomaterials **28**, 4581–4590 (2007)
66. Kainthan, R.K., Brooks, D.E.: In vivo biological evaluation of high molecular weight hyperbranched polyglycerols. Biomaterials **28**, 4779–4787 (2007)
67. Calderón, M., et al.: Development of efficient acid cleavable multifunctional prodrugs derived from dendritic polyglycerol with a poly(ethylene glycol) shell. J. Control. Release **151**, 295–301 (2011)
68. Steinhilber, D., et al.: Synthesis, reductive cleavage, and cellular interaction studies of biodegradable, polyglycerol nanogels. Adv. Funct. Mater. **20**, 4133–4138 (2010)
69. Sisson, A.L., et al.: Biocompatible functionalized polyglycerol microgels with cell penetrating properties. Angew. Chem. Int. Ed. **48**, 7540–7545 (2009)
70. Sisson, A.L., Papp, I., Landfester, K., Haag, R.: Functional nanoparticles from dendritic precursors: hierarchical assembly in miniemulsion. Macromolecules **42**, 556–559 (2009)
71. Luxenhofer, R., et al.: Poly(2-oxazoline)s as polymer therapeutics. Macromol. Rapid Commun. **33**, 1613–1631 (2012)
72. Knop, K., Hoogenboom, R., Fischer, D., Schubert, U.S.: Poly(ethylene glycol) in drug delivery: pros and cons as well as potential alternatives. Angew. Chem. Int. Ed. **49**, 6288–6308 (2010)

73. Luxenhofer, R., et al.: Structure–property relationship in cytotoxicity and cell uptake of poly(2-oxazoline) amphiphiles. J. Control. Release **153**, 73–82 (2011)
74. Viegas, T.X., et al.: Polyoxazoline: chemistry, properties, and applications in drug delivery. Bioconjug. Chem. **22**, 976–986 (2011)
75. Zhang, N., et al.: Tailored poly(2-oxazoline) polymer brushes to control protein adsorption and cell adhesion. Macromol. Biosci. **12**, 926–936 (2012)
76. Gaertner, F.C., Luxenhofer, R., Blechert, B., Jordan, R., Essler, M.: Synthesis, biodistribution and excretion of radiolabeled poly(2-alkyl-2-oxazoline)s. J. Control. Release **119**, 291–300 (2007)
77. Luxenhofer, R., et al.: Doubly amphiphilic poly(2-oxazoline)s as high-capacity delivery systems for hydrophobic drugs. Biomaterials **31**, 4972–4979 (2010)
78. Delgado, A.V., González-Caballero, F., Hunter, R.J., Koopal, L.K., Lyklema, J.: Measurement and interpretation of electrokinetic phenomena. J. Colloid Interface Sci. **309**, 194–224 (2007)
79. Rausch, K., Reuter, A., Fischer, K., Schmidt, M.: Evaluation of nanoparticle aggregation in human blood serum. Biomacromolecules **11**, 2836–2839 (2010)
80. Tenzer, S., et al.: Nanoparticle size is a critical physicochemical determinant of the human blood plasma corona: a comprehensive quantitative proteomic analysis. ACS Nano **5**, 7155–7167 (2011)
81. Herth, M.M., Barz, M., Jahn, M., Zentel, R., Rösch, F.: 72/74As-labeling of HPMA based polymers for long-term in vivo PET imaging. Bioorg. Med. Chem. Lett. **20**, 5454–5458 (2010)
82. Lee, Y.-R.Y.-H., et al.: Biodegradable nanoparticles containing TLR3 or TLR9 agonists together with antigen enhance MHC-restricted presentation of the antigen. Arch. Pharm. Res. **33**, 1859–1866 (2010)
83. Malyala, P., O'Hagan, D.T., Singh, M.: Enhancing the therapeutic efficacy of CpG oligonucleotides using biodegradable microparticles. Adv. Drug Deliv. Rev. **61**, 218–225 (2009)
84. O'Hagan, D.T., Singh, M., Ulmer, J.B.: Microparticle-based technologies for vaccines. Methods **40**, 10–19 (2006)
85. Sherman, M.R., et al.: Conjugation of high-molecular weight poly(ethylene glycol) to cytokines: granulocyte-macrophage colony-stimulating factors as model substrates. ACS Symp. Ser **680**, 155–169 (1997). At: http://scholar.google.com/scholar?hl=en&btnG=Search&q=intitle:Poly(ethylene+glycol):+Chemistry+and+Biological+Applications#5
86. Alexis, F., Pridgen, E., Molnar, L.K., Farokhzad, O.C.: Factors affecting the clearance and biodistribution of polymeric nanoparticles. Mol. Pharm. **5**, 505–515 (2008)
87. Yang, Y., Huang, C.-T., Huang, X., Pardoll, D.M.: Persistent Toll-like receptor signals are required for reversal of regulatory T cell-mediated CD8 tolerance. Nat. Immunol. **5**, 508–515 (2004)
88. Galloway, A.L., et al.: Development of a nanoparticle-based influenza vaccine using the PRINT® technology. Nanomed. Nanotechnol. **9(4)**, 523–31 (2013)
89. Demento, S.L., et al.: TLR9-targeted biodegradable nanoparticles as immunization vectors protect against West Nile encephalitis. J. Immunol. **185**, 2989–2997 (2010)
90. Tyagi, R.K., Garg, N.K., Sahu, T.: Vaccination Strategies against Malaria: novel carrier(s) more than a tour de force. J. Control. Release **162**, 242–254 (2012)
91. Reddy, S., Swartz, M., Hubbell, J.: Targeting dendritic cells with biomaterials: developing the next generation of vaccines. Trends Immunol. **27**, 573–579 (2006)
92. Demento, S.L., et al.: Inflammasome-activating nanoparticles as modular systems for optimizing vaccine efficacy. Vaccine **27**, 3013–3021 (2009)
93. Hamdy, S., et al.: Co-delivery of cancer-associated antigen and Toll-like receptor 4 ligand in PLGA nanoparticles induces potent CD8+ T cell-mediated anti-tumor immunity. Vaccine **26**, 5046–5057 (2008)
94. Barton, G.M., Medzhitov, R.: Control of adaptive immune responses by Toll-like receptors. Curr. Opin. Immunol. **14**, 380–383 (2002)
95. Akagi, T., Baba, M., Akashi, M.: Biodegradable nanoparticles as vaccine adjuvants and delivery systems: regulation of immune responses by nanoparticle-based vaccine. Adv. Polym. Sci. **247**, 31–64 (2011). doi:10.1007/12
96. Sun, H., Pollock, K.G.J., Brewer, J.M.: Analysis of the role of vaccine adjuvants in modulating dendritic cell activation and antigen presentation in vitro. Vaccine **21**, 849–855 (2003)
97. Moon, H.-J., et al.: Mucosal immunization with recombinant influenza hemagglutinin protein and poly gamma-glutamate/chitosan nanoparticles induces protection against highly pathogenic influenza A virus. Vet. Microbiol. **160**, 277–289 (2012)
98. Varkouhi, A.K., Scholte, M., Storm, G., Haisma, H.J.: Endosomal escape pathways for delivery of biologicals. J. Control. Release **151**, 220–228 (2011)
99. Krieg, A.M.: CpG motifs in bacterial DNA and their immune effects. Annu. Rev. Immunol. **20**, 709–760 (2002)
100. Sudowe, S., et al.: Uptake and presentation of exogenous antigen and presentation of endogenously produced antigen by skin dendritic cells represent equivalent pathways for the priming of cellular immune responses following biolistic DNA immunization. Immunology **128**, e193–e205 (2009)
101. Joshi, M.D., Unger, W.J., Storm, G., Van Kooyk, Y., Mastrobattista, E.: Targeting tumor antigens to dendritic cells using particulate carriers. J. Control. Release **161**, 25–37 (2012)
102. Saraogi, G.K., et al.: Mannosylated gelatin nanoparticles bearing isoniazid for effective management of tuberculosis. J. Drug Target. **19**, 219–227 (2011)
103. Hamdy, S., Haddadi, A., Shayeganpour, A., Samuel, J., Lavasanifar, A.: Activation of antigen-specific T cell-responses by mannan-decorated PLGA nanoparticles. Pharm. Res. **28**, 2288–2301 (2011)
104. Raghuwanshi, D., Mishra, V., Suresh, M.R., Kaur, K.: A simple approach for enhanced immune response using engineered dendritic cell targeted nanoparticles. Vaccine **30**, 7292–7299 (2012)
105. Brinãs, R.P., et al.: Design and synthesis of multifunctional gold nanoparticles bearing tumor-associated glycopeptide antigens as potential cancer vaccines. Bioconjug. Chem. **23**, 1513–1523 (2012)
106. Stanek, G., Strle, F., Gray, J., Wormser, G.P.: In Gray, J.S., Kahl, O., Lane, R.S., Stanek G. History and characteristics of Lyme borreliosis. Lyme borreliosis – biology, epidemiology and control, Vol 1, Chap 1, pp. 1–28. CABI Publishing (2002)
107. Steere, A.C., et al.: Erythema chronicum migrans and Lyme arthritis. The enlarging clinical spectrum. Ann Intern Med **86**, 685–698 (1977)
108. Burgdorfer, W., et al.: Lyme disease-a tick-borne spirochetosis? Science **216**, 1317–1319 (1982)
109. Krupka, M., et al.: Biological aspects of Lyme disease spirochetes: unique bacteria of the Borrelia burgdorferi species group. Biomed. Pap. Med. Fac. Univ. Palacky Olomouc Czech Repub. **151**, 175–186 (2007)
110. Krupka, M., Zachova, K., Weigl, E., Raska, M.: Prevention of lyme disease: promising research or sisyphean task? Arch. Immunol. Ther. Exp. (Warsz.) **59**, 261–275 (2011)
111. Zakovska, A., Nejedla, P., Holikova, A., Dendis, M.: Positive findings of Borrelia burgdorferi in Culex (Culex) pipiens pipiens larvae in the surrounding of Brno city determined by the PCR method. Ann. Agric. Environ. Med. **9**, 257–259 (2002)
112. Nejedla, P., Norek, A., Vostal, K., Zakovska, A.: What is the percentage of pathogenic borreliae in spirochaetal findings of mosquito larvae? Ann. Agric. Environ. Med. **16**, 273–276 (2009)
113. Gern, L., Humair, P.F.: In Gray, J.S., Kahl, O., Lane, R.S., Stanek G. History and characteristics of Lyme borreliosis. Lyme

borreliosis – biology, epidemiology and control, Vol 1, Chap 1, pp. 149–174. CABI Publishing (2002)
114. Klempner, M.S., et al.: Two controlled trials of antibiotic treatment in patients with persistent symptoms and a history of Lyme disease. N. Engl. J. Med. **345**, 85–92 (2001)
115. Poland, G.A., Jacobson, R.M.: The prevention of Lyme disease with vaccine. Vaccine **19**, 2303–2308 (2001)
116. Sigal, L.H., et al.: A vaccine consisting of recombinant Borrelia burgdorferi outer-surface protein A to prevent Lyme disease. Recombinant Outer-Surface Protein A Lyme Disease Vaccine Study Consortium. N. Engl. J. Med. **339**, 216–222 (1998)
117. Abbott, A.: Lyme disease: uphill struggle. Nature **439**, 524–525 (2006)
118. Nigrovic, L.E., Thompson, K.M.: The Lyme vaccine: a cautionary tale. Epidemiol. Infect. **135**, 1–8 (2007)
119. Tuhackova, J., et al.: Testing of the Biocan B inj. ad us. vet. vaccine and development of the new recombinant vaccine against canine borreliosis. Biomed. Pap. Med. Fac. Univ. Palacky Olomouc Czech Repub. **149**, 297–302 (2005)
120. Topfer, K.H., Straubinger, R.K.: Characterization of the humoral immune response in dogs after vaccination against the Lyme borreliosis agent A study with five commercial vaccines using two different vaccination schedules. Vaccine **25**, 314–326 (2007)
121. Trollmo, C., Meyer, A.L., Steere, A.C., Hafler, D.A., Huber, B.T.: Molecular mimicry in Lyme arthritis demonstrated at the single cell level: LFA-1 alpha L is a partial agonist for outer surface protein A-reactive T cells. J. Immunol. **166**, 5286–5291 (2001)
122. Gern, L., Hu, C.M., Voet, P., Hauser, P., Lobet, Y.: Immunization with a polyvalent OspA vaccine protects mice against Ixodes ricinus tick bites infected by Borrelia burgdorferi ss, Borrelia garinii and Borrelia afzelii. Vaccine **15**, 1551–1557 (1997)
123. Hajdusek, O., et al.: Characterization of ferritin 2 for the control of tick infestations. Vaccine **28**, 2993–2998 (2010)
124. Stewart, P.E., et al.: Delineating the requirement for the Borrelia burgdorferi virulence factor OspC in the mammalian host. Infect. Immun. **74**, 3547–3553 (2006)
125. Hodzic, E., Feng, S., Barthold, S.W.: Stability of Borrelia burgdorferi outer surface protein C under immune selection pressure. J. Infect. Dis. **181**, 750–753 (2000)
126. Brooks, C.S., Vuppala, S.R., Jett, A.M., Akins, D.R.: Identification of Borrelia burgdorferi outer surface proteins. Infect. Immun. **74**, 296–304 (2006)
127. Earnhart, C.G., Marconi, R.T.: OspC phylogenetic analyses support the feasibility of a broadly protective polyvalent chimeric Lyme disease vaccine. Clin. Vaccine Immunol. **14**, 628–634 (2007)
128. Earnhart, C.G., Marconi, R.T.: An octavalent lyme disease vaccine induces antibodies that recognize all incorporated OspC type-specific sequences. Hum. Vaccin. **3**, 281–289 (2007)
129. Buckles, E.L., Earnhart, C.G., Marconi, R.T.: Analysis of antibody response in humans to the type A OspC loop 5 domain and assessment of the potential utility of the loop 5 epitope in Lyme disease vaccine development. Clin. Vaccine Immunol. **13**, 1162–1165 (2006)
130. Brown, E.L., Kim, J.H., Reisenbichler, E.S., Hook, M.: Multicomponent Lyme vaccine: three is not a crowd. Vaccine **23**, 3687–3696 (2005)
131. Krupka, M., et al.: Isolation and purification of recombinant outer surface protein C (rOspC) of Borrelia burgdorferi sensu lato. Biomed. Pap. Med. Fac. Univ. Palacky Olomouc Czech Repub. **149**, 261–264 (2005)
132. Krupka, M., et al.: Enhancement of immune response towards non-lipidized Borrelia burgdorferi recombinant OspC antigen by binding onto the surface of metallochelating nanoliposomes with entrapped lipophilic derivatives of norAbuMDP. J. Control. Release **160**, 374–381 (2012)
133. Weis, J.J., Ma, Y., Erdile, L.F.: Biological activities of native and recombinant Borrelia burgdorferi outer surface protein A: dependence on lipid modification. Infect. Immun. **62**, 4632–4636 (1994)
134. Gilmore Jr., R.D., et al.: Inability of outer-surface protein C (OspC)-primed mice to elicit a protective anamnestic immune response to a tick-transmitted challenge of Borrelia burgdorferi. J. Med. Microbiol. **52**, 551–556 (2003)
135. Allison, A.G., Gregoriadis, G.: Liposomes as immunological adjuvants. Nature **252**, 252 (1974)
136. Gregoriadis, G., Allison, A.C.: Entrapment of proteins in liposomes prevents allergic reactions in pre-immunised mice. FEBS Lett. **45**, 71–74 (1974)
137. Henriksen-Lacey, M., Korsholm, K.S., Andersen, P., Perrie, Y., Christensen, D.: Liposomal vaccine delivery systems. Expert Opin. Drug Deliv. **8**, 505–519 (2011)
138. Gregoriadis, G.: Engineering liposomes for drug delivery: progress and problems. Trends Biotechnol. **13**, 527–537 (1995)
139. Bovier, P.A.: Epaxal: a virosomal vaccine to prevent hepatitis A infection. Expert Rev. Vaccines **7**, 1141–1150 (2008)
140. Herzog, C., et al.: Eleven years of Inflexal V-a virosomal adjuvanted influenza vaccine. Vaccine **27**, 4381–4387 (2009)
141. Watson, D.S., Endsley, A.N., Huang, L.: Design considerations for liposomal vaccines: influence of formulation parameters on antibody and cell-mediated immune responses to liposome associated antigens. Vaccine **30**, 2256–2272 (2012)
142. Altin, J.G., Parish, C.R.: Liposomal vaccines – targeting the delivery of antigen. Methods **40**, 39–52 (2006)
143. Adu-Bobie, J., Capecchi, B., Serruto, D., Rappuoli, R., Pizza, M.: Two years into reverse vaccinology. Vaccine **21**, 605–610 (2003)
144. Gupta, P.N., et al.: Non-invasive vaccine delivery in transfersomes, niosomes and liposomes: a comparative study. Int. J. Pharm. **293**, 73–82 (2005)
145. Mahor, S., et al.: Cationic transfersomes based topical genetic vaccine against hepatitis B. Int. J. Pharm. **340**, 13–19 (2007)
146. Henriksen-Lacey, M., et al.: Comparison of the depot effect and immunogenicity of liposomes based on dimethyldioctadecylammonium (DDA), 3beta-[N-(N', N'-Dimethylaminoethane)carbomyl] cholesterol (DC-Chol), and 1,2-Dioleoyl-3-trimethylammonium propane (DOTAP): prolonged liposome retention mediates stronger Th1 responses. Mol. Pharm. **8**, 153–161 (2011)
147. Henriksen-Lacey, M., Devitt, A., Perrie, Y.: The vesicle size of DDA:TDB liposomal adjuvants plays a role in the cell-mediated immune response but has no significant effect on antibody production. J. Control. Release **154**, 131–137 (2011)
148. Henriksen-Lacey, M., et al.: Liposomal cationic charge and antigen adsorption are important properties for the efficient deposition of antigen at the injection site and ability of the vaccine to induce a CMI response. J. Control. Release **145**, 102–108 (2010)
149. Whitmore, M., Li, S., Huang, L.: LPD lipopolyplex initiates a potent cytokine response and inhibits tumor growth. Gene Ther. **6**, 1867–1875 (1999)
150. Vasievich, E.A., Chen, W., Huang, L.: Enantiospecific adjuvant activity of cationic lipid DOTAP in cancer vaccine. Cancer Immunol. Immunother. **60**, 629–638 (2011)
151. Daemen, T., et al.: Virosomes for antigen and DNA delivery. Adv. Drug Deliv. Rev. **57**, 451–463 (2005)
152. Conlan, J.W., Krishnan, L., Willick, G.E., Patel, G.B., Sprott, G.D.: Immunization of mice with lipopeptide antigens encapsulated in novel liposomes prepared from the polar lipids of various Archaeobacteria elicits rapid and prolonged specific protective immunity against infection with the facultative intracellular pathogen, Listeria monocytogenes. Vaccine **19**, 3509–3517 (2001)
153. Davis, D., Gregoriadis, G.: Liposomes as adjuvants with immunopurified tetanus toxoid: influence of liposomal characteristics. Immunology **61**, 229–234 (1987)

154. Shahum, E., Therien, H.M.: Liposomal adjuvanticity: effect of encapsulation and surface-linkage on antibody production and proliferative response. Int. J. Immunopharmacol. **17**, 9–20 (1995)
155. Shahum, E., Therien, H.M.: Immunopotentiation of the humoral response by liposomes: encapsulation versus covalent linkage. Immunology **65**, 315–317 (1988)
156. White, W.I., et al.: Antibody and cytotoxic T-lymphocyte responses to a single liposome-associated peptide antigen. Vaccine **13**, 1111–1122 (1995)
157. Frisch, B., Muller, S., Briand, J.P., Van Regenmortel, M.H., Schuber, F.: Parameters affecting the immunogenicity of a liposome-associated synthetic hexapeptide antigen. Eur. J. Immunol. **21**, 185–193 (1991)
158. van Broekhoven, C.L., Parish, C.R., Demangel, C., Britton, W.J., Altin, J.G.: Targeting dendritic cells with antigen-containing liposomes: a highly effective procedure for induction of antitumor immunity and for tumor immunotherapy. Cancer Res. **64**, 4357–4365 (2004)
159. Watson, D.S., Platt, V.M., Cao, L., Venditto, V.J., Szoka Jr., F.C.: Antibody response to polyhistidine-tagged peptide and protein antigens attached to liposomes via lipid-linked nitrilotriacetic acid in mice. Clin. Vaccine Immunol. **18**, 289–297 (2011)
160. Masek, J., et al.: Metallochelating liposomes with associated lipophilised norAbuMDP as biocompatible platform for construction of vaccines with recombinant His-tagged antigens: preparation, structural study and immune response towards rHsp90. J. Control. Release **151**, 193–201 (2011)
161. Masek, J., et al.: Immobilization of histidine-tagged proteins on monodisperse metallochelation liposomes: preparation and study of their structure. Anal. Biochem. **408**, 95–104 (2011)
162. Chikh, G.G., Li, W.M., Schutze-Redelmeier, M.P., Meunier, J.C., Bally, M.B.: Attaching histidine-tagged peptides and proteins to lipid-based carriers through use of metal-ion-chelating lipids. Biochim. Biophys. Acta **1567**, 204–212 (2002)
163. Malliaros, J., et al.: Association of antigens to ISCOMATRIX adjuvant using metal chelation leads to improved CTL responses. Vaccine **22**, 3968–3975 (2004)
164. Patel, J.D., O'Carra, R., Jones, J., Woodward, J.G., Mumper, R.J.: Preparation and characterization of nickel nanoparticles for binding to his-tag proteins and antigens. Pharm. Res. **24**, 343–352 (2007)
165. Alving, C.R., Rao, M., Steers, N.J., Matyas, G.R., Mayorov, A.V.: Liposomes containing lipid A: an effective, safe, generic adjuvant system for synthetic vaccines. Expert Rev. Vaccines **11**, 733–744 (2012)
166. Kim, D., Kwon, H.J., Lee, Y.: Activation of Toll-like receptor 9 and production of epitope specific antibody by liposome-encapsulated CpG-DNA. BMB Rep. **44**, 607–612 (2011)
167. Schoenen, H., et al.: Cutting edge: Mincle is essential for recognition and adjuvanticity of the mycobacterial cord factor and its synthetic analog trehalose-dibehenate. J. Immunol. **184**, 2756–2760 (2010)
168. Rimmelzwaan, G.F., Osterhaus, A.D.: A novel generation of viral vaccines based on the ISCOM matrix. Pharm. Biotechnol. **6**, 543–558 (1995)
169. Morein, B.: Iscom – an immunostimulating complex. Arzneimittelforschung **37**, 1418 (1987)
170. Morein, B., Sundquist, B., Hoglund, S., Dalsgaard, K., Osterhaus, A.: Iscom, a novel structure for antigenic presentation of membrane proteins from enveloped viruses. Nature **308**, 457–460 (1984)
171. Barr, I.G., Mitchell, G.F.: ISCOMs (immunostimulating complexes): the first decade. Immunol. Cell Biol. **74**, 8–25 (1996). doi:10.1038/icb.1996.2
172. Sjolander, A., Cox, J.C., Barr, I.G.: ISCOMs: an adjuvant with multiple functions. J. Leukoc. Biol. **64**, 713–723 (1998)
173. Drane, D., et al.: Immunopotentiators in modern vaccines, pp. 191–215. Academic, Boston (2006)
174. Sun, H.X., Xie, Y., Ye, Y.P.: ISCOMs and ISCOMATRIX. Vaccine **27**, 4388–4401 (2009)
175. McBurney, W.T., et al.: In vivo activity of cationic immune stimulating complexes (PLUSCOMs). Vaccine **26**, 4549–4556 (2008)
176. Boyle, J., et al.: The utility of ISCOMATRIX adjuvant for dose reduction of antigen for vaccines requiring antibody responses. Vaccine **25**, 2541–2544 (2007)
177. Torchilin, V.P.: Structure and design of polymeric surfactant-based drug delivery systems. J. Control. Release **73**, 137–172 (2001)
178. Tian, H.Y., et al.: Biodegradable cationic PEG-PEI-PBLG hyperbranched block copolymer: synthesis and micelle characterization. Biomaterials **26**, 4209–4217 (2005)
179. Chadwick, S., Kriegel, C., Amiji, M.: Nanotechnology solutions for mucosal immunization. Adv. Drug. Deliv. Rev. **62**, 394–407 (2010)
180. Morein, B., Sharp, M., Sundquist, B., Simons, K.: Protein subunit vaccines of parainfluenza type 3 virus: immunogenic effect in lambs and mice. J. Gen. Virol. **64**(Pt 7), 1557–1569 (1983)
181. Patri, A.K., Majoros, I.J., Baker, J.R.: Dendritic polymer macromolecular carriers for drug delivery. Curr. Opin. Chem. Biol. **6**, 466–471 (2002)
182. Baker, J.R. Jr.: Dendrimer-based nanoparticles for cancer therapy. Hematol. Educ. Prog. Am. Soc. Hematol. 708–719 (2009)
183. Nardin, E.H., et al.: A totally synthetic polyoxime malaria vaccine containing Plasmodium falciparum B cell and universal T cell epitopes elicits immune responses in volunteers of diverse HLA types. J. Immunol. **166**, 481–489 (2001)
184. Klumpp, C., Kostarelos, K., Prato, M., Bianco, A.: Functionalized carbon nanotubes as emerging nanovectors for the delivery of therapeutics. Biochim. Biophys. Acta **1758**, 404–412 (2006)

9 Types of Recombinant Vaccines

Contents

9.1 Live and Non-live Vaccines

The original scientific strategy behind vaccinology has historically been to "isolate, inactivate, and inject," first invoked by Louis Pasteur.

The recombinant DNA and nanotechnology did much enlarge the repertoire on vaccines, which is today based on three adjusted principles, attenuation, inactivation, and recombination, as shown in Fig. 9.1. The three principles are regarded as equal, and all experimental possibilities for a new vaccine development against a pathogen should be studied in detail. The recombinant DNA and nanotechnology did not change the basic scientific strategy: live and non-live vaccines. Live vaccines are non-adjuvanted, and non-live vaccines are generally adjuvanted.

New developments against tuberculosis (TB) highlight this broad experimental approach:

Today, it estimated that about one-third of the world population is infected with the TB bacillus. Approximately 54 million people are infected every year, 9.4 million develop the disease, and 1.7 million die from this curable disease. The TB bacillus kills more people than any other infectious agent alone.

1921 and BCG. Currently, BCG (Bacillus Calmette–Guérin) is the only vaccine recommended by the WHO, with more than three billion doses administered since its introduction in 1921. BCG is prepared from a strain of the attenuated live bovine tuberculosis bacillus, *Mycobacterium bovis*, which lost its virulence in humans by being specially subcultured in an artificial medium. However, although it protects newborns and children from severe forms of TB, its efficacy against pulmonary TB in adolescents and adults is far from optimal, with protection rates varying between 0 and 80 % according to the geographical area.

M. Giese, *Introduction to Molecular Vaccinology*, DOI 10.1007/978-3-319-25832-4_9

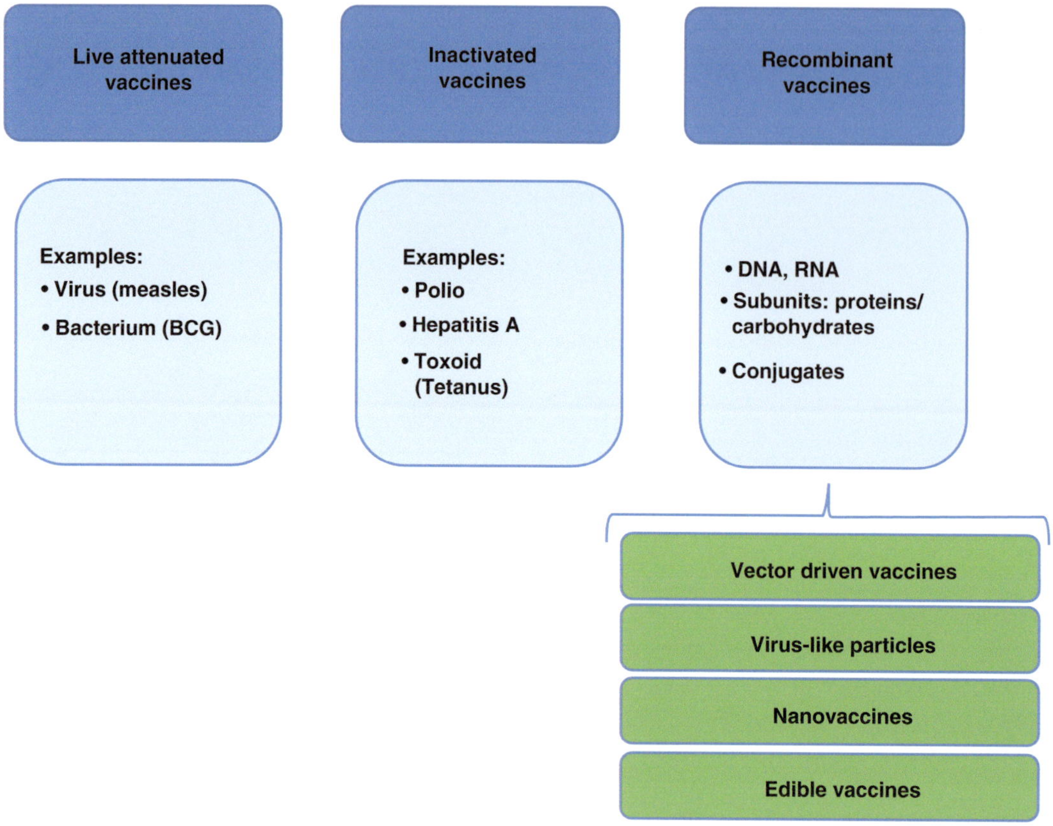

Fig. 9.1 The three basic principles of all vaccines are attenuation, inactivation, or recombination and are regarded as equal. The recombinant DNA and nanotechnology did not change the basic scientific strategy behind vaccinology: live and non-live vaccines

New vaccines and vaccination strategies are being developed including the use of attenuated live mycobacteria, recombinant microorganisms, and subunits, prime-boost strategies based on the successive administration of a certain mycobacterial antigen under two different vaccine vectors, and DNA vaccines [1].

9.2 Efficacy and Safety Aspects

The various types of vaccines differ in eliciting an immune response. Live attenuated vaccines (LAVs) mimic a natural infection without being virulent and trigger the activation of the innate immune system through PAMPs. Following injections, LAVs rapidly disseminate throughout the vascular network to the draining lymph nodes. Therefore, the route of application of LAVs does not specifically influence the immune response. LAVs also don't need an adjuvant; they possess a natural intrinsic adjuvancy. Safety concerns exist because of the replication competence and the possibility of recombination with a wild type.

Non-live vaccines, inactivated and most recombinant vaccines, whether containing proteins or carbohydrates (−conjugates), are less effective. In the absence of replication, vaccine-induced immune reactions remain more limited, and therefore the route of vaccination influences the efficacy and the duration of the immune reaction. Non-live vaccines induce a lower antibody response and generally no cytotoxic T lymphocyte activation. Compared to LAV, all non-live vaccines are regarded as biologically safe (Fig. 9.2).

9.3 DNA Vaccines

DNA vaccines entail the direct, in situ inoculation of DNA-based eukaryotic expression vectors that encode the sequence of a pathogenic protein antigen. The constructed plasmids are then subsequently grown in bacteria like *E. coli* and highly purified via chromatographic methods. LPS contamination of plasmids has to be prevented because of the immunotoxic properties of natural LPS.

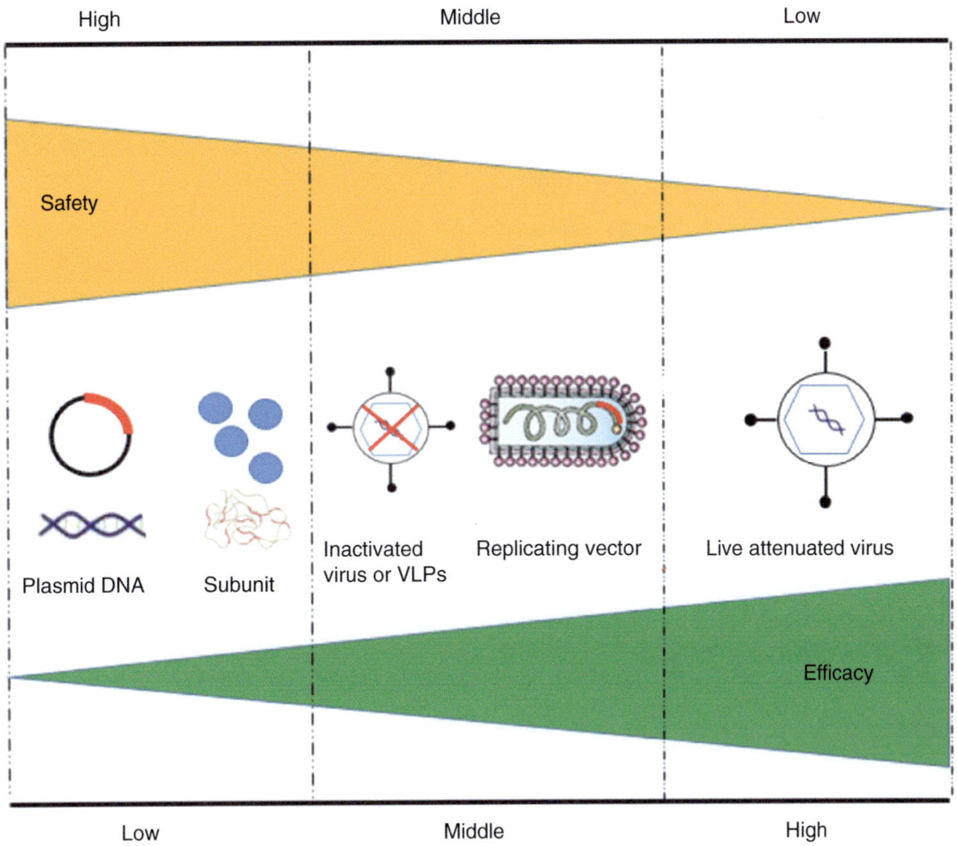

Fig. 9.2 Safety and efficacy of various vaccine types. The various types of vaccines differ in eliciting an immune response and in safety aspects. Some of the most efficacious vaccines in use today are based on live attenuated viruses, such as the measles, mumps, and rubella vaccines. However, these vaccines, also vector-based vaccines, are replication competent and are potentially of higher risk as nonreplicating inactivated viruses, virus like particles (*VLPs*) or subunit or plasmid DNA-based vaccines. These types of vaccines are perceived to be safer but need strong adjuvants to enhance their weak immunogenicity

After purification the circular double-stranded DNA plasmids are ready for vaccination. The de novo production of the encoded antigens in the host results in the elicitation of both the antibody and the cellular response by activating cytotoxic T lymphocytes (CTLs). Vaccine proteins made by the host are natural proteins and contain important posttranslational modifications such as the correct glycosylation. But like subunit vaccines, DNA vaccines must be adjuvanted. Naked DNA does not work.

The unique advantage of DNA vaccines is their ability to mimic the effects of live attenuated vaccines without the risk associated with the administration of infectious albeit attenuated material. DNA vaccines are able to stimulate a complete, humoral and cellular immune response. Peptide fragments are processed via the endogenous pathway, resulting in the presentation of antigen on the cell surface by MHC class I molecules.

Plasmid DNA is very stable also beyond a cold chain. Therefore, the storage, transportation, and distribution of DNA vaccines are more practical and also cheaper [2].

Mostly all plasmid DNA constructs (Fig. 9.3) used for vaccination share five main characteristics:

- Strong promoter/enhancer sequence for driving the incorporated foreign gene
- Convenient cloning site for insertion of foreign genes
- Origin of replication for initiation of plasmid replication
- Polyadenylation/termination sequence for production of mature mRNA
- Resistance/antibiotic marker for selection
- Immunomodulators, e.g., CpGs, interleukins, ubiquitin, etc.
- (on the same plasmid or on extra plasmids)

Uptake of Plasmid DNA. Some biological barriers have to be overcome by DNA vaccines on the way to the cell nucleus where the plasmid DNA is translated into cellular mRNA. After delivery of plasmid DNA to the target tissue, e.g., skeletal muscle or skin, lots of tissue nucleases attack

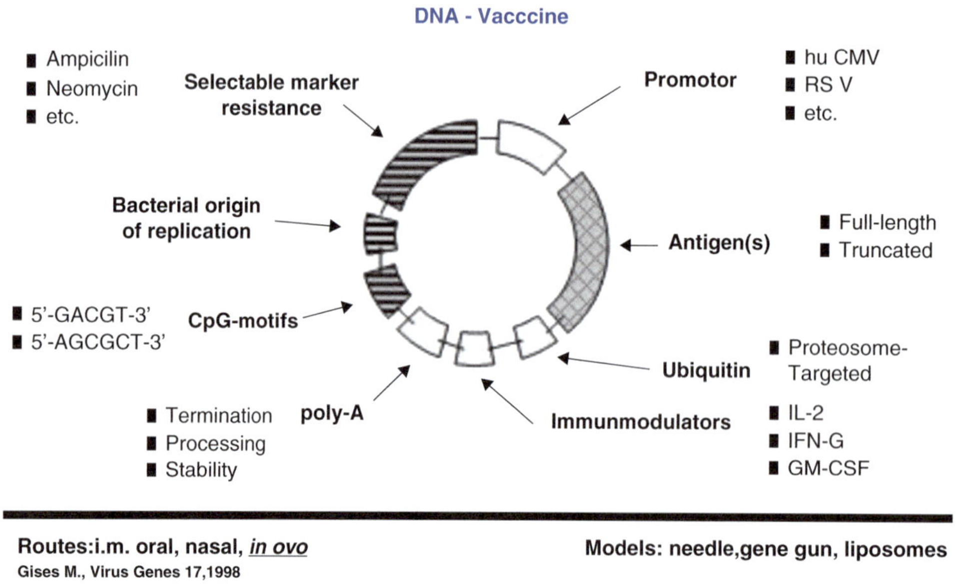

Fig. 9.3 Model of an expression plasmid used for DNA vaccination. Individual elements comprising functional expression cassettes. The encoded antigen, as full-length or truncated cDNA, is under control of strong promoter/enhancer and polyadenylation sequences. Co-expression of cytokines will specifically enhance the immune response. Unspecific activation of the immune system can be initiated by CpGs. Vaccines focusing on a strong cellular response can be enhanced by co-expression of ubiquitin targeting the proteasome pathway. Various application routes and modes of administrations are possible

and degrade a large amount of the applicated DNA. Also the extracellular matrix with collagen and hyaluronic acid influences the passage from the application site to the cell membrane.

Only a small portion (1 % estimated) of the still intact plasmid DNA will cross the cell membrane by phagocytosis or pinocytosis. Inside the cell the route toward the nucleus is also spiked with exo- and endonucleases so that probably only 0.1 % (estimated) is successfully and actively transported through the nucleus pore membrane (NPC). Small particles (<~40 kDa) are able to pass through the nuclear pore complex (NPC) by passive diffusion; larger particles need the support of carrier proteins for efficient passage through the complex.

Because of this enormous loss of plasmid DNA (up to 99.9 %), various tools were developed to protect the plasmid DNA and thus increase the efficacy such as encapsulation into liposomes or binding of DNA to dendrimers. Figure 9.4 illustrates the passage of plasmid DNA from the extracellular matrix (ECM) to the nucleus.

Whereas in human medicine clinical trials with DNA vaccines are still ongoing without any registered product on the market, the first approved DNA vaccines for the veterinarian medicine are available since 2005 and are discussed now.

Approved DNA Vaccines in Veterinary Medicine

The first veterinarian DNA vaccines were developed for horses (Davis B.S., 2001 for WNV [3]; Giese M., 2002 for EAV [4]). Today the number of current clinical trials worldwide with veterinary DNA vaccines is unmanageable and probably all species are hit.

9.3.1 Dogs: Canine Malignant Melanoma

Canine malignant melanoma (CMM) typically begins in the mouth or around the toes and can spread within the body to the heart, lungs, intestines, and other organs. Canine malignant melanoma is known for being one of the most aggressive cancers in dogs and deadly. CMM is most commonly seen in golden retrievers, Scottish terriers, dachshunds, labradors, and poodles (Fig. 9.5).

Metastases of the tumors will be found very often in distant parts of the body. The overall biology of CMM is similar to the biology of human melanoma. However the melanomas in dogs have diverse biologic behaviors due to the race and a variety of factors. Standardized treatments such as surgery, radiation, and chemotherapy are the common tools to fight canine malignant melanoma. These traditional tools have afforded minimal to modest stage-dependent clinical benefits.

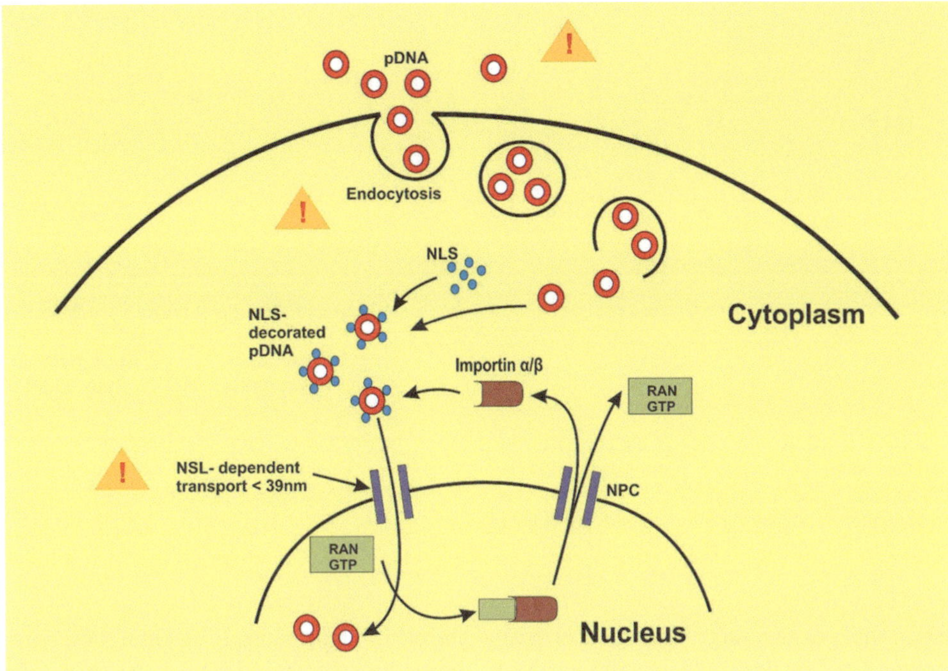

Fig. 9.4 Some biological barriers have to be overcome by DNA vaccines on the way to the cell nucleus where the plasmid DNA is translated into cellular mRNA. After delivery of pDNA, nucleases attack and degrade a large amount of pDNA. Also the extracellular matrix (ECM) with collagen and hyaluronic acid influences the passage from the application site to the cell membrane. Only a small portion of pDNA will cross the cell membrane and faces exo- and endonuclease. But a small portion is tagged with NLS (nuclear localization sequence). This NLS decoration is recognized by importin that transport the DNA cargo from the cytoplasm through the nuclear pore complex (NPC) into the nucleus. Only molecules smaller than 39 nm can pass. Once inside the nucleus, interaction with Ran-GTP causes a conformational change in the importin, resulting in the dissociation from its cargo. The resulting complex of importin and Ran-GTP translocates to the cytoplasm, where Ran-GTP will be separated from importin, a process called the Ran-GTP nuclear transport cycle (biological barriers ⚠)

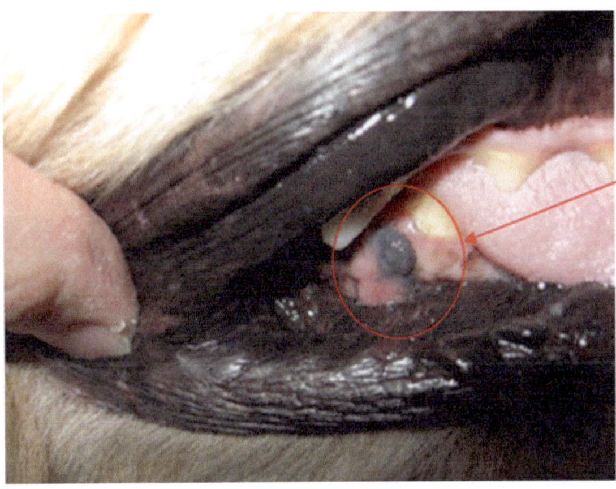

Fig. 9.5 Dog with oral melanoma which typically begins in the mouth or around the toes. A golden retriever, named Olympus, diagnosed with malignant melanoma at the age of 9 years. This dog was involved in a melanoma vaccine study at the University of Florida, USA (Photo kindly provided by the dog-owner Jessica Tan, Florida, USA – *in memoriam Olympus*)

Xenogeneic DNA Vaccine. The plasmid DNA contains a cDNA for the human tyrosinase, huTyr, a tumor antigen (TA). This is a non-mutated differentiation antigen and specific to melanoma. Tyrosinase is a glycoprotein and essential in the process of melanin synthesis (Fig. 9.6). Like other TAs tyrosinase is overexpressed in tumor cells and therefore an ideal target in cancer therapy. Normally there is no strong immune reaction against the body's own protein. But immunization of dogs with xenogeneic huTyr cDNA can break the immune tolerance against this self tumor differentiation antigen and induce antibody and cytotoxic T cell response against melanoma cells [5]. Tyrosinase is highly conserved from dog to mouse to man.

Immunization Regime. In a recent clinical trial with 58 dogs diagnosed with stage II and III canine oral melanoma, the safety and efficacy of the xenogeneic DNA vaccine was investigated. Dogs received a 4-vaccination treatment series following surgical removal of the primary tumor and

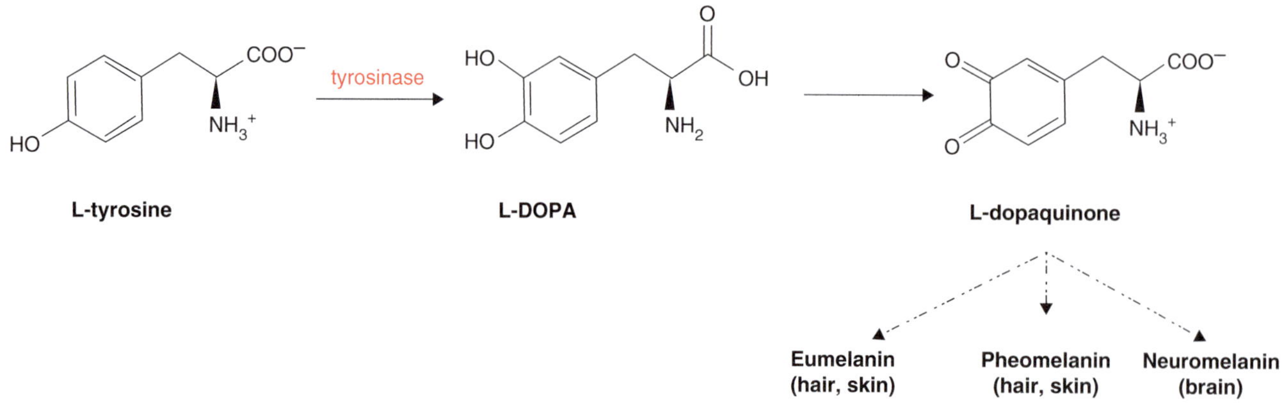

Fig. 9.6 Melanin synthesis. There are three types of melanin: eumelanin, pheomelanin, and neuromelanin. The most common type of melanin is eumelanin. The melanin in the skin is produced by melanocytes. The first step of the biosynthetic pathway for all melanin types is catalyzed by tyrosinase. Tyrosinase is essential in the process of melanin synthesis. Like other TAs tyrosinase is overexpressed in tumor cells and therefore an ideal target in cancer therapy

radiotherapy in cases with positive surgical margins or positive regional lymph nodes. One dose contains 102 μg DNA given in a volume of 0.4 ml by the transdermal route via a needle-free vaccination device. Booster immunizations were given at 6-month intervals.

In March 2007 the drug manufacturer received a conditional license for ONCEPT from the USDA and a full license in 2010.

The results of the xenogeneic immunization of dogs with huTyr cDNA as an adjunct therapy for CMM demonstrate a significant increase of survival time compared to the control group. None of the dogs developed systemic adverse reactions; no toxicity was seen. The overall safety of this DNA vaccine is confirmed. This vaccine development represents a tremendous milestone in DNA science and technology.

9.3.2 Horses: West Nile Virus, A Severe Zoonotic Infection

Virus. West Nile virus (WNV) is a mosquito-borne member of the family *Flaviviridae*, genus *Flavivirus*, and was first identified in 1937 in Uganda, Africa. It is a positive-sense, single-strand RNA virus, (+)ssRNA, of about 11 kb that encodes a single polyprotein with seven nonstructural proteins and three structural proteins. The RNA strand is held within a nucleocapsid. WNV replicates in the cytoplasm of infected cells.

WNV is a zoonotic virus. The primary reservoir is birds with a significant impact to spread the infection across countries and continents. More than 170 different species are described as carrier of this virus. WNV is spread from bird to bird by mosquitoes when they bite, or take a blood meal, from birds that are infected with the virus. Birds from some species get ill and die; others have no clinical signs and survive. Mosquitoes are also capable of spreading the virus to horses, dogs, cats, mice, alligators, and lots of other mammals but also to humans.

Disease. One-third of all horses bitten by carrier mosquitoes develop the disease and die or are so affected that euthanasia is required. The incubation period ranges from 3 to 14 days. Horses that do become ill vary in symptoms: muscle trembling, skin twitching, ataxia, sleepiness, dullness, and listlessness. WNV may cross the placenta from mother to gestating foal. Horses cannot spread the disease to humans.

WNV produces different outcomes in humans like in horses: fever, headache, chills, diaphoresis, weakness, swollen lymph nodes, drowsiness, and pain in the joints comparable to symptoms of influenza. More severe neuroinvasive infection includes meningitis and encephalitis.

WNV-DNA Vaccine. The surface envelope protein E is the main target for the antibody response. There are more than 180 copies of the E protein in a mature WNV virion. The E function is the interaction between the cell surface and the fusion between virus and cellular membrane. The premembrane protein prM is cleaved during viral maturation into a smaller membrane M peptide. The expression of prM and E protein in cells results in the formation of virus-like particles, VLP. These VLP share many of the antigenic and structural properties of fully mature viruses and are of special interest for a vaccine development (Fig. 9.7).

The final expression plasmid for immunization of horses contains the human cytomegalovirus early gene promoter, signal sequences from Japanese virus, and a fusion gene of

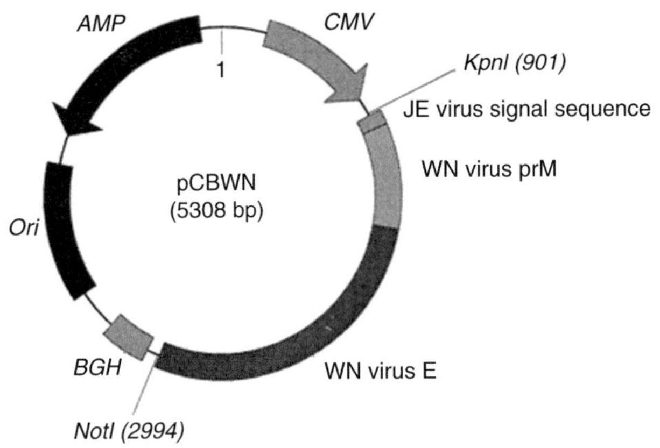

Fig. 9.7 Map of the recombinant WN virus plasmid pCBWN. The transcription unit contains the human cytomegalovirus early gene promoter (CMV), JE virus signal sequence, WN virus prM and E gene region, and bovine growth hormone poly(A) signal (BGH) (Credit: Gwong-Jen J. Chang, Division of Vector-Borne Infectious Diseases NCEID, CDC Fort Collins, CO 80521)

prM and E. The WNV DNA vaccines induce a stable and long-lasting complete immune response (12 months) and are safe in horses.

This vaccine was approved for veterinary use by USDA in July 2005 and released to public in December 2008.

9.3.3 Fish: Salmon and the First Commercial DNA Vaccine

Part of the fishing industry is aquaculture, also known as aqua farming, but it can be contrasted with commercial fishing, which is the harvesting of wild fish. Aquaculture involves cultivating freshwater and saltwater fish and other populations (shrimp, oyster) under controlled conditions. Salmon is one of the main food-producing fish in the world. A DNA vaccine for fish must be not only safe for the animal but especially safe for the fish consumer.

Salmon is the major economic contributor to the world production of farmed fish, representing over U$1 billion annually in the United States. Salmon farming is also very big in Norway, Scotland, Canada, and Chile and is the source for most salmon consumed in the United States and Europe. Like all other animals also fish is threatened by viruses, bacteria, and parasites. One major problem for salmons is the infectious hematopoietic necrosis (IHN) virus [6].

Virus. Infectious hematopoietic necrosis (IHN) virus is a common viral pathogen of both wild and farmed salmonids, in particular Pacific salmonids, rainbow trout, and Atlantic salmon. IHN virus is enzootic to the Pacific Northwest; however it has varying effects on different Pacific salmonids. It is a negative-sense single-stranded, (−)ssRNA virus that is a member of the *Rhabdoviridae* family, genus *Novirhabdovirus*. The RNA genome is 11,133 nucleotides long and contains a leader (L) and trailer (T) sequences at its 3′-end and 5′-end, respectively. The coding regions are N, P, M, G, NV, and L genes. G encodes the surface glycoprotein, so-called spikes, main target for the immune response.

Transmission. IHNV is transmitted following shedding of the virus in the feces, urine, sexual fluids, and external mucus and by direct contact or close contact with surrounding contaminated water. The virus gains entry into fish at the base of the fins. Salmons are carnivorous and are currently fed a meal produced from catching other wild fish and other marine organisms – a permanent origin of possible infections with IHNV.

Disease. Clinical signs of infection with IHNV include anemia, skin darkening, bulging of the eyes, fading of the gills, and abdominal distension. Infected fish commonly hemorrhage in several areas, like the mouth, the pectoral fins, muscles near the anus, and the yolk sac of fry. Diseased fish weaken, eventually floating on the surface of the water. Necrosis is common in the kidney and spleen and sometimes in the liver. Mortality rates in older fish (2–3 kg) tend to range from 10 to 20 %; in smolts the mortality rate often exceeds 85 %. The average cumulative mortality following an outbreak is estimated at 47 %.

IHNV-DNA Vaccine. The antigen is the viral surface glycoprotein (G) capable of eliciting neutralizing antibody and the production of a protective immune response. The G gene was cloned into a eukaryotic expression vector by insertion of an intermediate-early promoter and a polyadenylation signal. But the speciality of this vaccine is to be prepared as a two-component vaccine in a single vaccine, one plasmid or more.

The second component is a portion of the nucleic acid sequence encoding a second peptide, derived from a fish pathogen other than the said rhabdovirus resulting in a fusion. This second pathogen can be any fish pathogen, e.g., ISAV, IPNV, iridovirus, NNV, SPDV, SVCV, VHSV, koi herpes virus, and more. The rationale behind this is that the presence of the IHNV G protein boosts the immune response to the second protein, resulting in a protective effect against infection by this fish pathogen. The vaccine is given intramuscularly with a dosage of only 10 μg in 50 μl on the left dorsal flank, in the area just below the dorsal fin [7, 8].

This first DNA fish vaccine was licensed in 2005 in Canada by the Veterinary Biologics Section (VBS), Animal Health and Production Division, Canadian Food Inspection Agency (CFIA) and is also used now in studies in Norway.

9.3.4 Honey Bees: *Varroa Destructor*[1]

There are many environmental stressors and diseases which influence and seriously threat the life of European honey bees, *Apis mellifera.* The European honey bee is professionally managed worldwide for honey production and pollination. The bee was imported to the United States 400 years ago with the first European settlers and called "white man's fly" by the native Americans, the Indians.

CCD. First reported in the United States, a mysterious so-called colony collapse disorder (CCD) decimated the bee colonies there between 50 and 90 %, first observed during the winters of 1995–1996 and then 2000–2001 and without interruptions up to now. A similar situation is also given in Europe. About 20,000–60,000 bees live in a colony.

The first description originated from the 1950s. In the early nineteenth century, the colony losses were known in England as "Isle of Wight disease," and the Americans called this phenomenon "disappearing disease" in the 1960s, whereas these colony losses in France in the late 1990s were called "mysterious bee losses." Where have all the bees gone?

Economic Value. The huge loss of honey bees as pollinators has a dramatic impact on agricultural pollination. About 130 crops, nuts, fruits, and vegetables are pollinated by *A. mellifera*, with an overall value of more than $ 15 billion in the United States and more than € 14 billion for the EU in 2005. A bee colony produces some 1 kg/2205 lb honey per day. In return, these bees have to pollinate 10–15 million flowers.

One should keep in mind that besides European honey bees, wild insects, among them 30,000 species of wild bees, have also a very great impact on pollination and seem to be more efficient in pollination as managed honey bees [9]. The industrial farming threatens also the natural biotope of wild insect pollinators.

Ecologic Value. The total global economic value of honey bee pollination was calculated in 2005 to more than € 150 billion or $ 202 billion. The Food and Agriculture Organization (FAO) of the United Nations estimates that there are 65 million managed honey bee colonies worldwide. Beside this professional agriculture, honey bees are irreplaceable for the biodiversity. This organism appeared during evolution with the first flower plants and exists since 100 million years as described in Chap. 2, Fig. 2.10. After swine and cattle, bees are in Europe and North America the third important farm animal and since 2007 formally listed as farm animal in Switzerland. Therefore, CCD is not only an economical but also an essential global ecological problem which urgently must be solved in the future. "The bee is more than honey."

What Is Causing CCD? The colony collapse disorder of the last years seems to differ from past outbreaks: The worker bees disappear instead of dying in place, leaving behind the queen and young bees. High levels of bacteria, viruses, and fungi are measured in the gut of the remaining bees. Collapses can occur within 2 days.

A Complex Problem. Different theories are discussed about what is causing CCD. Pesticide contamination, hotly debated to interfere with the nerve system affecting foraging behavior of bees, lead them to abandon their hives. Fungal diseases such as *Nosema* spp. is known for big bee losses in Spain. Monocultures or gene-manipulated crops. Electro smoke (radio waves) caused by cell phones destroys the bee's compass. The rigors of travelling in trucks from crop to crop in the USA. Down from February professional US beekeepers travel with their colonies through the country until December. Thereby the bees must relocate up to 15 times. In Europe the bee colonies begin the winter sleep around September. Also the climate change, the temperature sensitivity is discussed to have an impact on crop pollination. CCD is likely caused by a combination of factors [10, 11].

Varroa destructor**.** But in all CCD cases, an overload of bloodsucking varroa mites is detectable and varroa is currently considered the major threat for apiculture. The infection and disease is called varroosis. *Varroa destructor* is an ectoparasite, has a reddish-brown flat shape, and is 1–1.8 mm long and 1.5–2 mm wide, with eight legs. *V. destructor* infest worker bees and drones and its brood. The mite develops inside the brood cells. *Varroa* is a real colossus compared to the size of bees as can be seen in Fig. 9.1. Varroa mites belong to the scientific class of Arachnida, subclass Acari. There are 50,000 species described alone from mites. Some mites prefer carbohydrates as food such as meal or crops. The house dust mites feed flakes of shed human skin. Varroa mites prefer fresh "blood" and the hemolymph of bees and can feed 0.1 mg/0.0000002205 lb within 2 h.

Varroa is transported into the hives via piggyback by worker bees. The female mite enters broad cells, preferentially drone cells. Once the cell is capped, varroa lays eggs on the larvae. The development from egg to insect takes 7 days. Bee larvae and mites hatch in about the same time and the newborn varroa mites spread to other bees [12, 13]. The lifetime of summer mites are 3–6 weeks, whereas fall mites

[1] Oral vaccination of honey bees against Varroa destructor by *Sebastian Giese and Matthias Giese* in Molecular Vaccines – From Prophylaxis to Therapy, Volume 2, Springer-Verlag Wien, 2013, Ed. Matthias Giese.

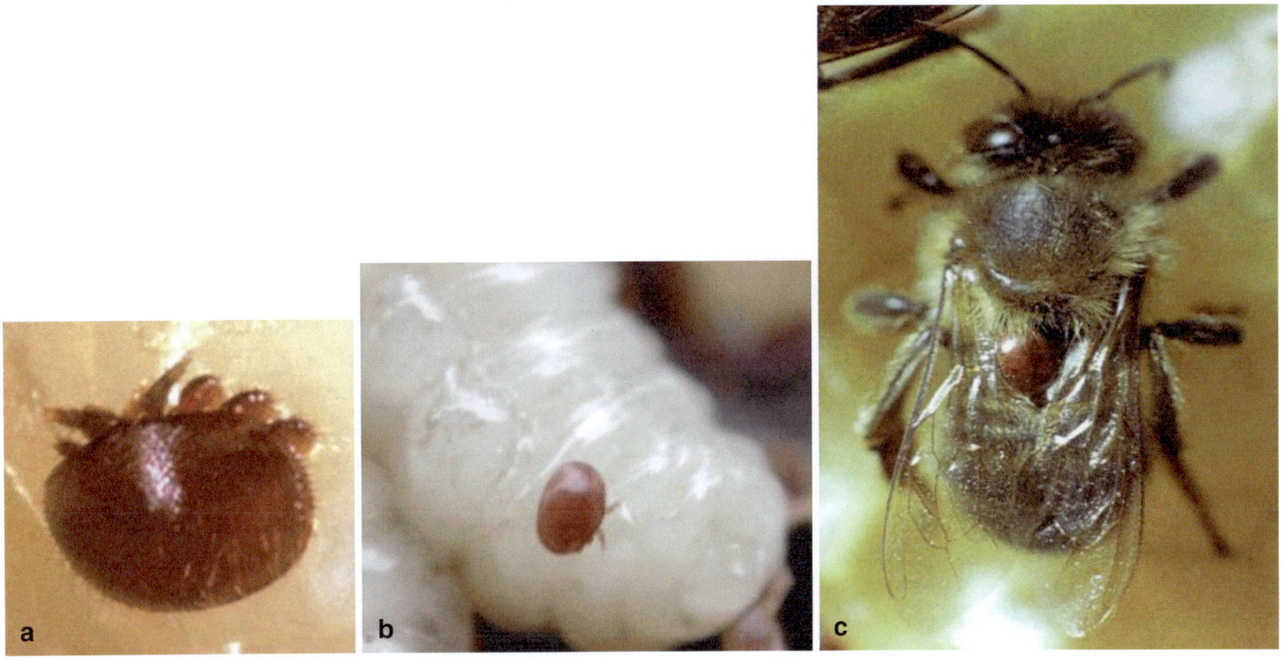

Fig. 9.8 (**a**) Varroa mite, reddish-brown, flat-shaped, 1–1.8 mm long and 1.5–2 mm wide, with eight legs. (**b**) *V. destructor* mite on a bee larva. (**c**) *V. destructor* infests worker bees and drones. Varroa mites are important vectors for viruses and spread these viruses throughout the hive (Credit: Dr. J. Mueller, Magdeburg, Germany)

can live for several months. Varroa can only reproduce in honey bees and thus are considered harmless to other insects. Varroa is more than a disease. It is a global pest having devastating effects on bees (Fig. 9.8).

***Varroa* as Vector.** *Varroa* may be not considered as isolated agent for the disease. The mortality of adult bees and its brood must be considered in the context with secondary viral infections. At least 18 various viruses are able to infect honey bees, mostly ssRNA viruses. Eight viruses are known to be associated with varroa mites: acute bee paralysis virus (ABPV), black queen cell virus (BQCV), chronic bee paralysis virus (CBPV), deformed wing virus (DWV), Kashmir bee virus (KBV), sacbrood bee virus (SBV), cloudy wing virus (CWV), and slow bee paralysis virus (SBPV) [14–17].

Varroa Control. A number of natural and synthetic chemicals are commercially available for the control of varroa infestations. The first compounds were bromopropylate, fluvalinate, or other pyrethroid insecticides. And to make a long story short, varroa mites became resistant not only against one product of a given chemical class; the resistance was against the entire class with several related synthetic products. Also the use of natural products, such as formic acid, mineral oil, or thymol, is only partially and temporally effective and show adverse effects [18]. There is no successful chemical treatment. Mites will quickly develop resistance to all chemicals.

The Immune System of Insects. The basic difference between insect and vertebrate immunity is the missing highly specific antigen response of the acquired immune system in insects. Nevertheless, in the 400 million years of evolution, insects developed a powerful defense strategy against bacteria, fungi, viruses, and parasites. Only protected by this "primitive" immune system insects were so successful that they colonized all terrestrial ecosystems.

The insect innate immunity shows many similarities to the vertebrate and to the human innate immunity, is multifaceted, and involves both humoral and cellular components [19]. Most insights on insect immunity are provided by *Drosophila melanogaster* research. The key mechanism is also observed in honey bees.

The humoral and systemic response to bacterial and fungal infections is controlled by antimicrobial peptides (AMPs). There are circulating receptors sensing a danger signal and activating the Toll pathway, whereas membrane-bound receptors activate the Imd pathway. Both pathways lead to the translocation of NF-kB-like transcription factors and the production of AMPs. NF-kB response elements can be detected in the promoter region of the diptericin gene.

The cellular immune response is mediated by specialized blood cells, the hemocytes, plasmatocytes, crystal cells, and lamellocytes [20]. Plasmatocytes represent 95 % of the majority of hemocytes. They express phagocytic receptors and patrol through the body, clear microorganism and cell debris, and signal infections to the fat bodies. The bee genome was completely sequenced in 2006 [21].

The Bee DNA Vaccine. An expression plasmid was constructed with a CMV promoter. Surprisingly, no bee or other insect specific promoter was essential to drive the expression of the protein. The enhanced green fluorescent protein (EGFP) was chosen as reporter gene and inserted into the multiple cloning site, together with an SV40 enhancer element. The plasmid construct was produced in *E. coli* and highly purified by standard techniques.

European honey bees (*Apis mellifera*) were obtained from local beekeepers and cultivated under lab conditions. Varroa mites were collected from infested bees.

The oral vaccination of the EGFP plasmid was operated by feeding the bees with a mixed solution of sugar and plasmid DNA (vaccine sugar). Standard sugar solutions made by the beekeeper are the normal food for winter bees.

Results. Over 10 days after onset of feeding, we measured the expression of EGFP by immunofluorescence and Western blot analysis with EGFP antibodies. Between day 3 and 10, a clear EGFP signal was detected in the thorax and especially in the Malpighian tubules. Control bees fed with DNA lacking the reporter did not show any signal. In parallel, control experiments with transformed *E. coli* were done to study the possibility of EGFP expression in gut bacteria instead of bee cells. No EGFP signal was detected in transformed bacteria.

Most surprisingly, we found the EGFP signal after 5 days in varroa mites sucking hemolymph of bees which were fed by the vaccine sugar solution and no signals in control mites of infested control bees. Feeding of plasmid DNA results in expression of a reporter gene in different bee tissues over a period of several days, and finally varroa absorbs this protein via bloodsucking. The bee blood is not carried by arteries and veins but flows loosely around the body. No EGFP signals were detected either in the honey stomach or in the feces. Figure 9.9 illustrates the EGFP passage through the bee body and toward the varroa mite.

We started with the simple idea that the biochemistry in eukaryotic cells remains the same, irrespective of the organism. A difference is given in the configuration of the immune system. That means, an insect can successfully fight against parasites and infections but with different weapons. No T cells, no B cells, and consequently no antibodies and no memory. We are able to stimulate targeted immune genes of bees and measure an insect typical immune response. A standard plasmid DNA vaccine, first developed for horses, bridges the evolution from fish to insects to mammals. No other vaccine type is able to do this job. How fascinating biology is!

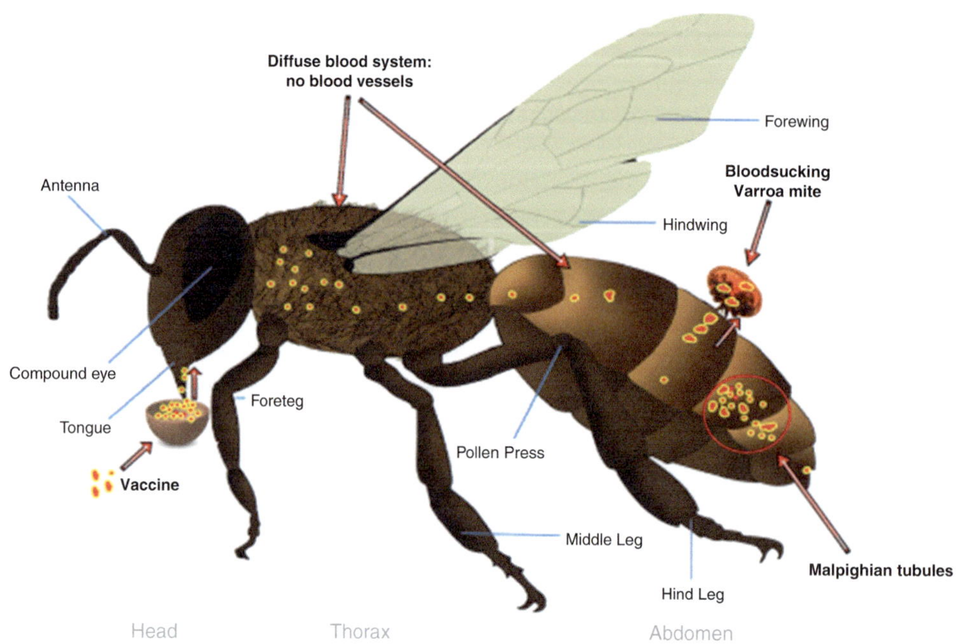

Fig. 9.9 Oral vaccination. Plasmid DNA-encoding EGFP as placeholder for a vaccine antigen is mixed to a standard sugar solution dissolved in water. Such sugar solutions are the nutrition for winter bees and are normally handmade by the beekeeper. The experimental DNA concentration was 500 μg DNA/ml sugar solution. DNA feeding was for 24 h. No booster feeding

9.4 Protein and Carbohydrate (Subunit) Vaccines

A protein subunit is based on a single protein molecule and able to stimulate a humoral immune response, but usually not a cellular response. After phagocytosis proteins are degraded by acid-dependent proteases in endosomes (endosomal or exogenous pathway), resulting in an MHC II presentation of the antigenic peptides. A peptide is one form of a subunit.

Carbohydrates are also used as subunits with a poor and age-dependent immunogenicity. Carbohydrate antigens induce a T cell-independent B cell response as discussed in Chap. 6. Therefore carbohydrates are mainly linked to a protein (conjugation) to enhance toe immune reaction as discussed here with the Hib conjugate vaccine.

Conjugate Vaccines. The polyribosylribitol phosphate (PRP) capsule of *Haemophilus influenzae* type b (Hib) is a major virulence factor for the organism. PRP is a T cell-independent antigen characterized by, e.g., induction of a poor antibody response in less than 18-month-old infants and children and the inability to induce a booster response. Polysaccharide vaccines based on PRP alone were developed in the 1970s.

By covalent linkage of PRP with T cell dependent protein antigens, a conjugated vaccine was created to overcome the T cell independent characteristics of PRP. At present three different licensed protein carriers are linked to PRP:

- HbOC: Diphtheria CRM protein 197, mutant *Corynebacterium* – linkage: no spacer
- HbOMP: Outer membrane protein, OMP, *Neisseria meningitidis* – linkage: spacer
- PRP-D: Diphtheria toxoid, D – linkage: spacer

These Hib conjugate vaccines differ by protein carrier, polysaccharide size, and method of chemical conjugation, including use of a spacer between the PRP and protein carrier.

A standard chemical conjugation between a polysaccharide and a protein is illustrated in Fig. 9.10.

Subunit vaccines, while offering greater safety, are intrinsically poorly immunogenic and strong adjuvants are essential to boost the activation of immune responses.

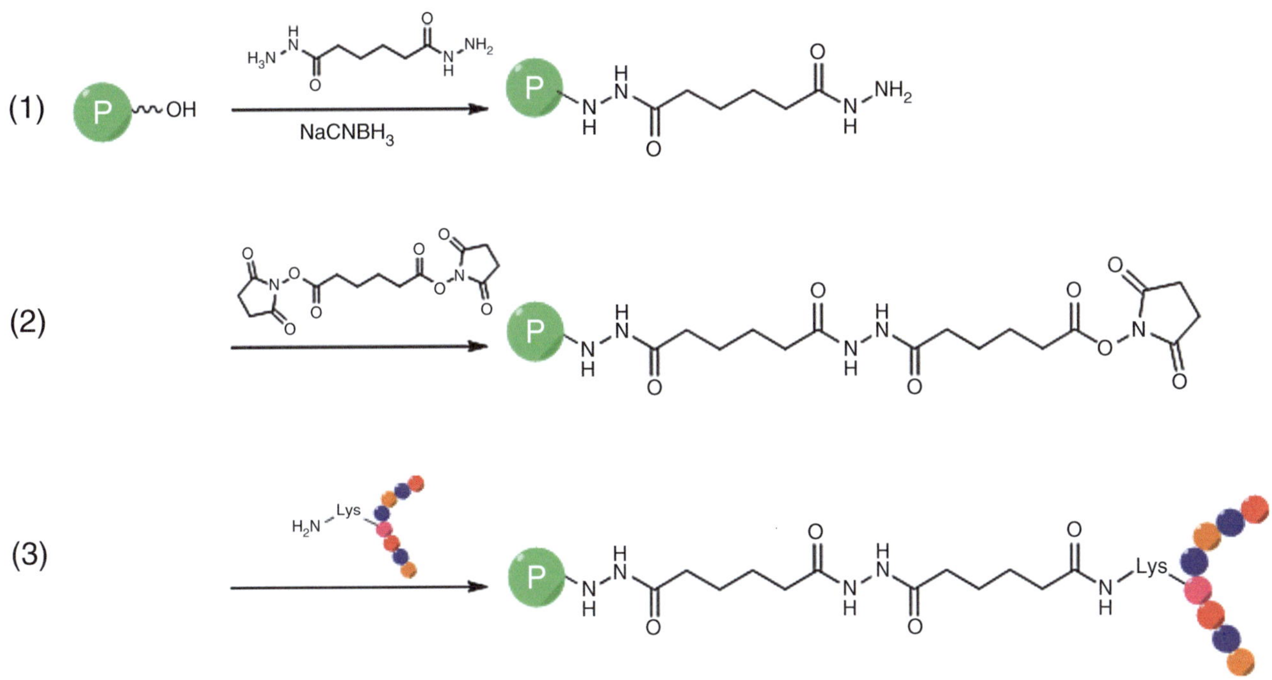

Fig. 9.10 Linkage sugar and protein. For the conjugation of carbohydrates to proteins, activated ester techniques are frequently used. This figure depicts the use of *N*-hydroxysuccinimide (NHS) esters as a prominent example. In this example, an unprotected hydroxyl group of the polysaccharide (*P*) is reacted with adipic acid dihydrazide in a mildly reductive amination (*1*). The residual hydrazide moiety is then converted with adipic acid bis(*N*-hydroxysuccinimide) (*2*). In a final step, the second NHS ester is aminolysed to link the polysaccharide and the protein via a long and flexible spacer (*3*) (Figure prepared for this book by M. Scherer, Institute of Organic Chemistry, University of Mainz, Germany)

9.4.1 Protein Subunit: Shigellosis[2]

Shigellosis remains an important cause of morbidity and mortality, with about 90 million episodes occurring each year and about 100,000 deaths per year. About 60 % of deaths occur in infants under 5 years of age living in third world countries. Four different species (*S. flexneri, S. sonnei, S. boydii, and S. dysenteriae*) have been described so far, along with more than 50 O-antigen serotype variations.

Serotype variability is dictated by modifications of the O-antigen portion of LPS. O antigens vary in the number of oligosaccharide unit repeats, the types and distribution of carbohydrates, and the intra- and intermolecular linkages [22]. In *S. flexneri*, these genes are encoded in the bacterial chromosome. In contrast, *S. sonnei*, which shows no serotype variability, expresses plasmid-encoded O-antigen modification enzymes. The O antigen is one of the major immunogenic components of *Shigella* and is a virulence factor, in part, due to masking the exposure of type three secretion apparatus [23].

The inclusion of conserved proteins in vaccine compounds potentially solves the issue of serotype specificity, thus allowing the generation of a highly desirable pan-*Shigella* vaccine. In addition, recombinant proteins usually have increased safety profiles.

Another important impact in *Shigella* epidemiology that prompts vaccine development is the increasing frequency of antibiotic-resistant strains. Antibiotic resistance is continually rising for this pathogen [24].

***Shigella* spp. as Causative Agent of Shigellosis.** First defined as a causative agent of bacillary dysentery by Shiga in Japan, *Shigella* is a gram-negative bacillus that is noncapsulated and nonmotile. Diagnosis is generally based on symptoms [25] since bloody, mucoid stools are indicative of *Shigella* infections. However, because several diarrheal infections caused by other microorganisms share these symptoms (enteroinvasive *E. coli* and *Campylobacter*, among others), the sole analysis of symptoms is insufficient for an accurate diagnosis. Therefore, clinical diagnosis must be complemented with microbiological isolation from culture.

***Shigella* Invasion and Pathogenesis.** *Shigella* is transmitted through the fecal–oral route by consumption of contaminated food and water. Following ingestion, the acid-tolerant *Shigella* passes through the stomach and small intestine into the large intestine [26] (Fig. 9.11). Here, they are taken up by M cells, transcytosed to the basolateral face of the colonic epithelium, and presented to resident macrophages wherein IpaB of the type three secretion system (T3SS) induces apoptosis by caspase 1 activation, thereby escaping killing by the macrophage [27]. *Shigella* then invades epithelial cells using its T3SS to create a translocation pore in the host cell membrane to initiate an orchestrated flow of effectors into the host cell cytoplasm to induce actin rearrangements that ultimately result in uptake of bacteria. Once inside, *Shigella* quickly escapes its vacuole, replicates, and moves about the cytoplasm via actin-based motility. In a T3SS-dependent manner, the *Shigella* then forms a protrusion into a neighboring uninfected cell with the resulting vacuole being quickly lysed to complete the process of intercellular spread.

The genes associated with the T3SS are encoded on a 220-kB plasmid which is highly conserved among the *Shigella* species. At the heart of the T3SS is the type three secretion apparatus (T3SA) which is composed of a basal body similar to that of flagellar systems and an extracellular needle [28]. Invasion plasmid antigen D (IpaD) is a 37 kDa protein that forms a pentameric ring at the tip of the needle. It controls secretion of effector proteins and is the environmental sensor for mobilization of IpaB to the T3SA tip complex. IpaB is a 64 kDa translocator that forms a ring atop the IpaD ring and is responsible for host cell contact. This contact is required for mobilization of IpaC to the needle tip and formation of a complete unidirectional conduit from the bacterial cytoplasm to the host cell cytoplasm. The initiation of inflammation and invasion processes occurs exclusively at the basolateral side of host cells, highlighting the importance of the previous steps of macrophage subversion in *Shigella* colonization of the gut.

Animal Models. Shigellosis is strictly a human disease. While the basis of this restriction is unknown, it complicates the ability to investigate the pathogenesis of *Shigella*. However, several animal models have been developed to study the pathogenesis of *Shigella*, the resulting immune response against *Shigella* antigens, and the protection efficacy of candidate vaccines against shigellosis:

Mouse lethal pulmonary challenge: Many of the recent vaccine development efforts have been tested in the mouse lethal pulmonary model. In this model, a high dose of virulent *Shigella* is administered to mice intranasally.

Mouse colonic infection: Another mouse model more recently developed involves the use of streptomycin to clear the intestinal commensal bacteria. After such treatment, *Shigella* is able to colonize the colon with viable *Shigella* being isolated from fecal samples for up to 30 days [29].

[2]Development of subunit vaccines against shigellosis: An update by *Francisco J. Martinez-Becerra, Olivia Arizmendi, Jamie C. Greenwood II and Wendy L. Picking* in Molecular Vaccines – From Prophylaxis to Therapy, Volume 2, Springer-Verlag Wien, 2013, Ed. Matthias Giese.

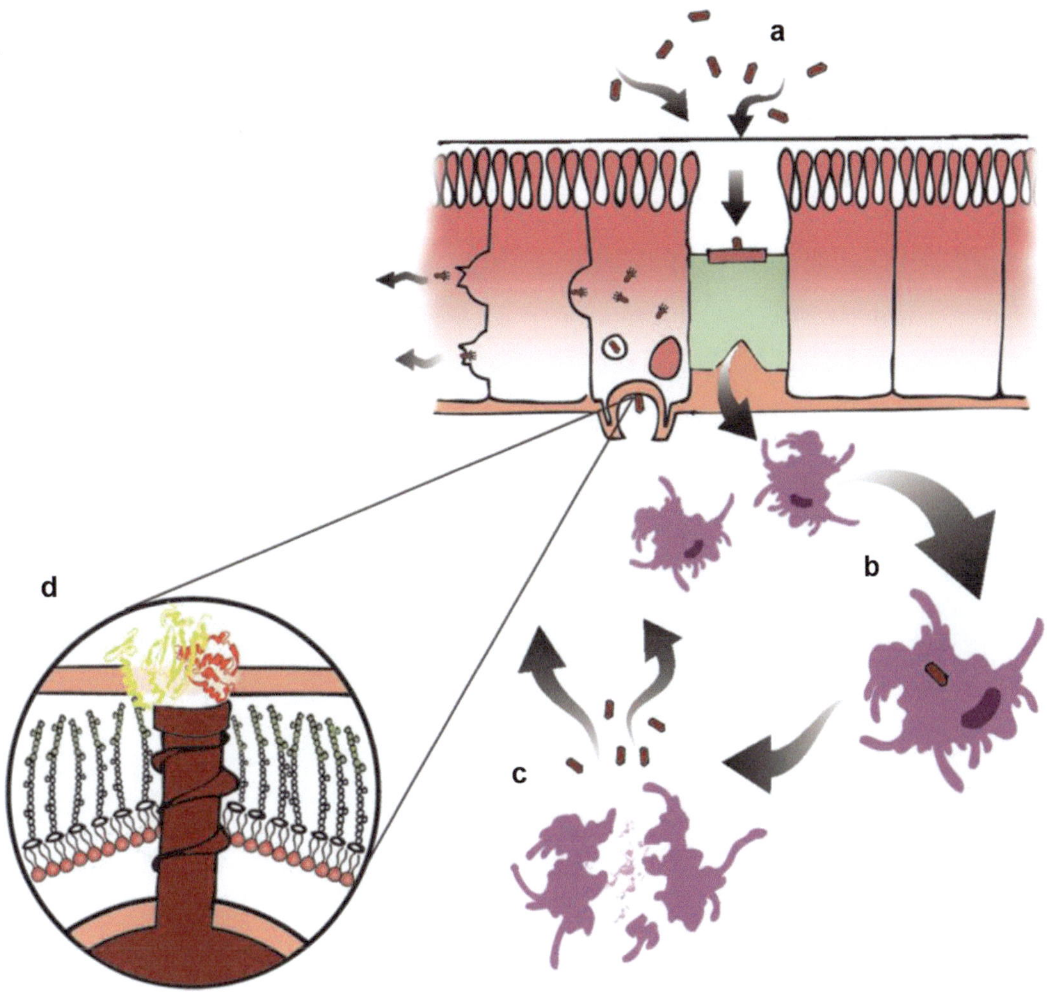

Fig. 9.11 Current model for invasion of epithelial cells by *Shigella*. *Shigella* reaches the lumen of the intestine and is taken up by M cells (**a**) and released to the basal side. Subsequently, *Shigella* is phagocytosed by macrophages residing under the M cells (**b**). After escaping by inducing apoptosis (**c**), *Shigella* invades epithelial cells using its type three secretion system (**d**)

Sereny test: The Sereny test model [30] has long been used to test the invasive capabilities of *Shigella*. In this model, guinea pigs are inoculated in the eye with *Shigella,* which induces a keratoconjunctivitis. This model allows examination of *Shigella* invasion and the protective efficacy of candidate vaccines.

Rabbit cecal ligation model: In this model, diarrhea is used as an indicator of infection and disease. Although this model can be used to characterize the interactions of *Shigella* and the intestinal mucosa at the natural site of infection, it has the difficulty that is introduced by surgery in laboratory animals [31].

Nonhuman primate (NHP) models: NHP models have been used to define the ability of vaccines to elicit immune responses and protection (rhesus and cynomolgus monkeys) [32]. The main advantage of this model is that *Shigella* is able to colonize the large intestine and generate symptoms that these bacteria generate in human infection.

Various Subunits Development

O antigen/proteosome: O antigen represents the variable portion of *Shigella* LPS (Fig. 9.12). Administration of LPS or O antigen alone in animal models is not enough to elicit immune responses, making them ineffective immunogens. To solve this limitation, these molecules have been used in conjunction with different proteins as carriers. Several variants of LPS/O-antigen mixtures have been developed and characterized. One of these protein combination approaches uses *S. flexneri* and *S. sonnei* LPS complexed with *Neisseria meningitidis* outer membrane protein proteosomes [33, 34]. LPS is extracted from *S. flexneri* or *S. sonnei* by hot phenol extraction and mixed with detergent-extracted outer membrane proteins from *N. meningitidis*. The complex was then separated from free LPS present in the mixture by gel filtration chromatography. The concept behind this vaccine is that the proteins present in the *N. meningitidis* proteosome are able to act as carriers for T cell stimulation, thus allowing the recognition of LPS.

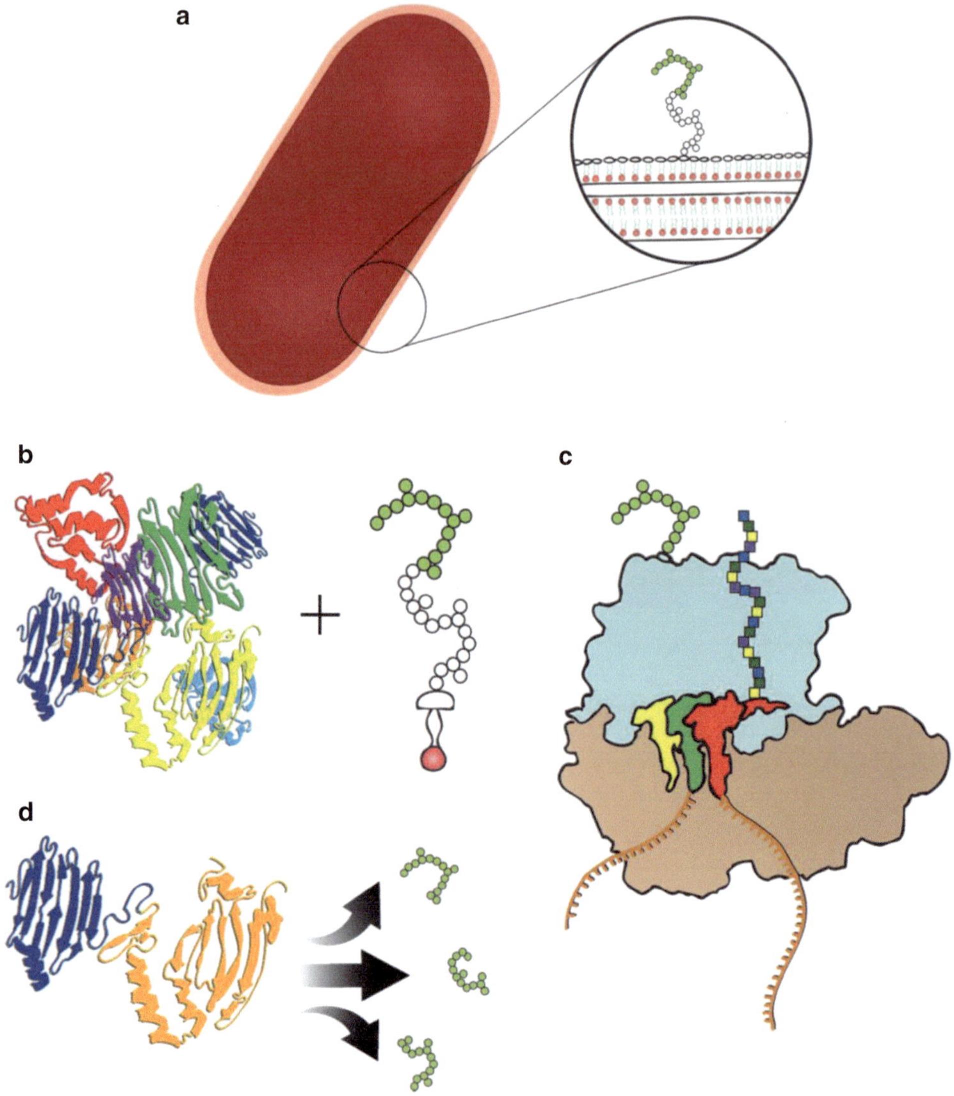

Fig. 9.12 Depiction of LPS/O-antigen-based vaccines. LPS (**a**) extracted from *Shigella flexneri* or *sonnei* is admixed with protein preparations from *N. meningitides* and used as a carrier. When this complex is administered orally and intranasally to mice and guinea pigs [33], serum IgG and mucosal IgA in intestines and lungs are vaccine compound (**b**). O antigen purified from LPS is delivered in combination with exoprotein A from *P. aeruginosa* (**c**). Finally, O antigen from different *Shigella* serogroups is combined with ribosomes from *Shigella* and is depicted in (**d**)

***Shigella* Outer Membrane Vesicles.** Outer membrane vesicles (OMVs) are particles composed of LPS, proteins, and nucleic acids. In a proposed vaccine formulation, these particles were purified from liquid cultures of *S. boydii* by centrifugation with subsequent filtering (Fig. 9.13). The precise identity and amount of the proteins included in this preparation is not currently known, although the presence of proteins having the same mass as IpaB, IpaC, and IpaD suggests its composition includes these proteins. When these OMVs are administered orally to mice, antibodies are generated against OMV lysates.

This vaccine has the advantage of heterologous protection (as shown by challenge against strains from each *Shigella* serogroup) and the absence of adjuvant dependency. In addition, immunity can be passively transferred to offspring, suggesting that the protective mechanism involves antibodies and raising the possibility that this vaccine can be used in infants, which is the main target population for a *Shigella* vaccine. The use of live, fully virulent *Shigella* during its formulation process, the presence of LPS, and lot-to-lot consistency are possible downsides of this preparation.

Invaplex. Another vaccine candidate that uses T3SS proteins and LPS as part of the formulation is the Invaplex [35]. These complexes are obtained by aqueous extraction followed by ion exchange chromatography (Fig. 9.13). The precise composition of these extracts has not been completely characterized but includes LPS, IpaB, and IpaC [36]. These complexes are able

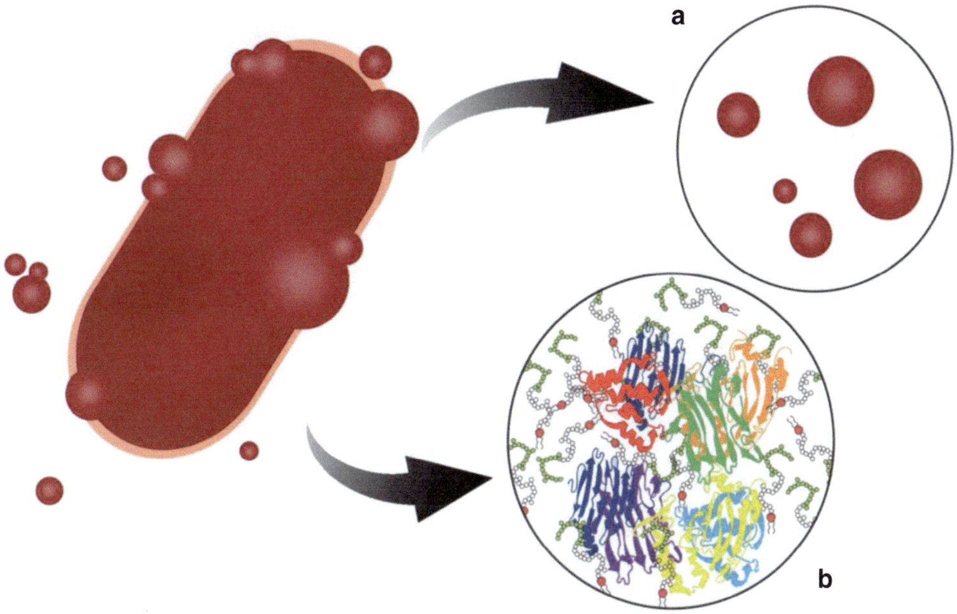

Fig. 9.13 Depiction of vesicle-based vaccines. A vaccine preparation consists of outer membrane vesicles purified from *S. boydii*. (**a**) These vesicles are naturally generated by all *Shigella* spp. (**b**). Another conjugate known as Invaplex consists of water extracts from *Shigella flexneri* or *sonnei*. This is composed primarily of LPS and proteins, in particular IpaB and IpaD

to elicit IgG and IgA responses against Ipa proteins as well as LPS in both mice and guinea pigs. In addition, they are protective against the *Shigella* species/serotype used for extract generation [37] in the mouse and guinea pig challenge models.

Two phase one studies have been performed using the Invaplex vaccine on adult volunteers [38] and showed no major side effects to delivery of intranasal doses of up to 690 μg. The highest dose employed in these studies generated an ASC response to LPS in 58 % of the volunteers. An advantage of this approach is that, other than the Invaplex itself, no additional adjuvants need to be administered. A drawback of this vaccine consists in a challenging production process that includes cultures of virulent *Shigella* as well as the presence of bacterial LPS products in the intermediate steps and final formulation. Another possible caveat is the uniformity of protein composition in these complexes through manufacturing lots.

Finally, this vaccine was not designed to protect against multiple serotypes. A solution for this possible drawback, however, is the generation of formulations that include Invaplex complexes generated from more than one particular serotype, which increases an already difficult manufacturing process. This would allow the generation of vaccine formulations specific for the serotypes prevalent in a particular region.

Recombinant T3SS Proteins. A vaccine candidate that targets conserved *Shigella* virulence proteins includes some of the T3SS Ipa proteins (Fig. 9.14). Recombinant IpaB and IpaD can be expressed in *E. coli* at high levels. IpaD is then easily purified from the *E. coli* cytosol while IpaB must be purified as a complex with its cognate chaperone IpgC. The chaperone is needed to maintain the hydrophobic IpaB in a soluble state and to provide stability for IpaB from proteolytic degradation. IpaB can then be further purified after separation from IpgC in low concentrations of detergent. Analyses have indicated that IpaB is greater than 90 % pure following this scheme. In its final formulation, this Ipa-based vaccine also contains a double mutant of heat-labile enterotoxin from *E. coli* (dmLT) [39] as an adjuvant. The mechanism of protection for this vaccine has not yet been worked out. Nevertheless, it was tested in the mouse lethal pulmonary model [40] where it exhibited over 90 % homologous protection (against *S. flexneri*) and greater than 60 % heterologous protection (using *S. sonnei* during the challenge experiments). IgG and mucosal IgA were generated after intranasal administration along with antigen-specific IFN-γ-secreting cells.

OmpA. A 34-kDa outer membrane protein (OMP) was purified from *S. flexneri* 2a using ion exchange chromatography. Incubation of macrophages with this 34-kDa protein induced the production of nitric oxide and increased production of IL-12 and TNF-α. This protein was delivered parenterally five times in rabbits, giving protection against challenge by *S. flexneri* in the rabbit cecal ligation model [41]. Subsequent work using a recombinant protein purified by affinity chromatography identified this 34-kDa OMP as OmpA, part of a family of immunomodulating proteins present in numerous gram-negative bacteria. This protein showed

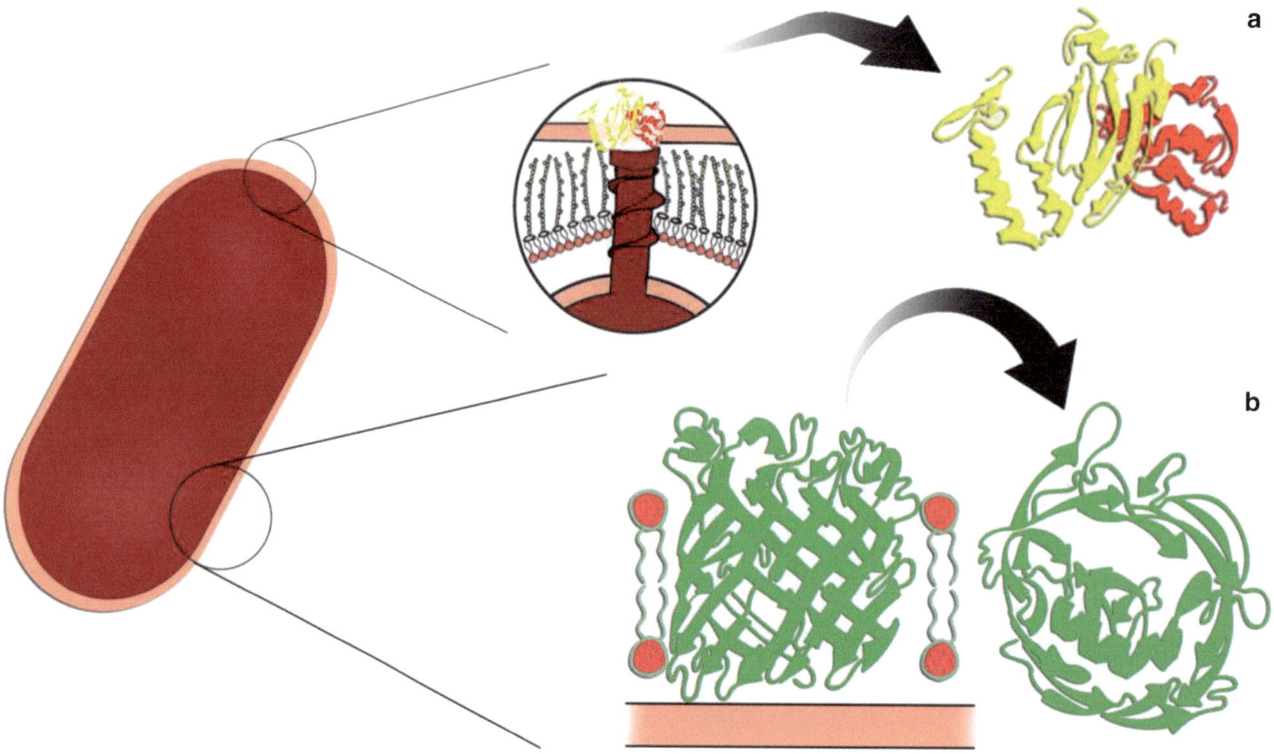

Fig. 9.14 Depiction of *Shigella* recombinant protein vaccines. IpaB and IpaD, key components of the T3SS of *Shigella* spp., are expressed in *E. coli* and administered with the adjuvant dmLT (**a**). The outer membrane protein OmpA is expressed in *E. coli* and delivered without additional adjuvants (**b**)

high protective efficacy in the mouse lethal pulmonary model [42] where it elicited serum IgG and mucosal IgA.

9.4.2 Protein Subunit: Ticks[3]

Ticks are widely distributed throughout the world, affecting 80 % of the world's cattle population [43]. The economic importance of ticks and tick-borne diseases (TBDs) has been estimated by a number of studies; however they most likely represent an underestimation of the real impact of these arthropod vectors and their transmitted diseases.

Tick feeding has devastating effects including disease transmission, paralysis, toxicosis, and secondary infections of the tick-feeding site [44]. The effect of ticks and tick-borne diseases is particularly pronounced in the livestock sector where it is repeatedly rated highly for its impact on the livelihood of farmers, particularly in countries of the South which are heavily dependent on agricultural production.

There are six genera of ixodid ticks of importance, namely, *Amblyomma*, *Dermacentor*, *Haemaphysalis*, *Hyalomma*, *Rhipicephalus*, and *Ixodes*.

Historically, tick and tick-borne disease control has focused on the control of ticks at tolerable levels through acaricide use and treatment of disease with appropriate drugs. In some cases acaricide-based tick control is often the only method of reducing tick populations without sacrificing productivity [45].

Acaricides are commercially available in a number of formulations that are applied either directly onto livestock or in dipping vats where multiple animals can be passed through at regular time intervals. Acaricide application relies heavily on correct formulation and administration to be effective. A large number of chemical compounds have been found to be effective against ticks including arsenic (introduced ~1983), DDT (~1946), cyclodienes and toxaphene (~1947), organophosphates-carbamate group (~1955), formamides (~1975), and macrocyclic lactones (~1981). The potency and usefulness of many of the abovementioned compounds is gradually eroding with resistance developing in many tick species of *Rhipicephalus*, *Amblyomma*, and *Hyalomma*.

Multiple acaricide-resistant tick stocks have been identified, limiting or entirely excluding the use of many acaricides [46]. In addition to resistance, chemical control through

[3]Anti-tick vaccines for the control of ticks affecting livestock by Cassandra Olds, Richard Bishop and Claudia Daubenberger in Molecular Vaccines – From Prophylaxis to Therapy, Volume 2, Springer-Verlag Wien, 2013, Ed. Matthias Giese.

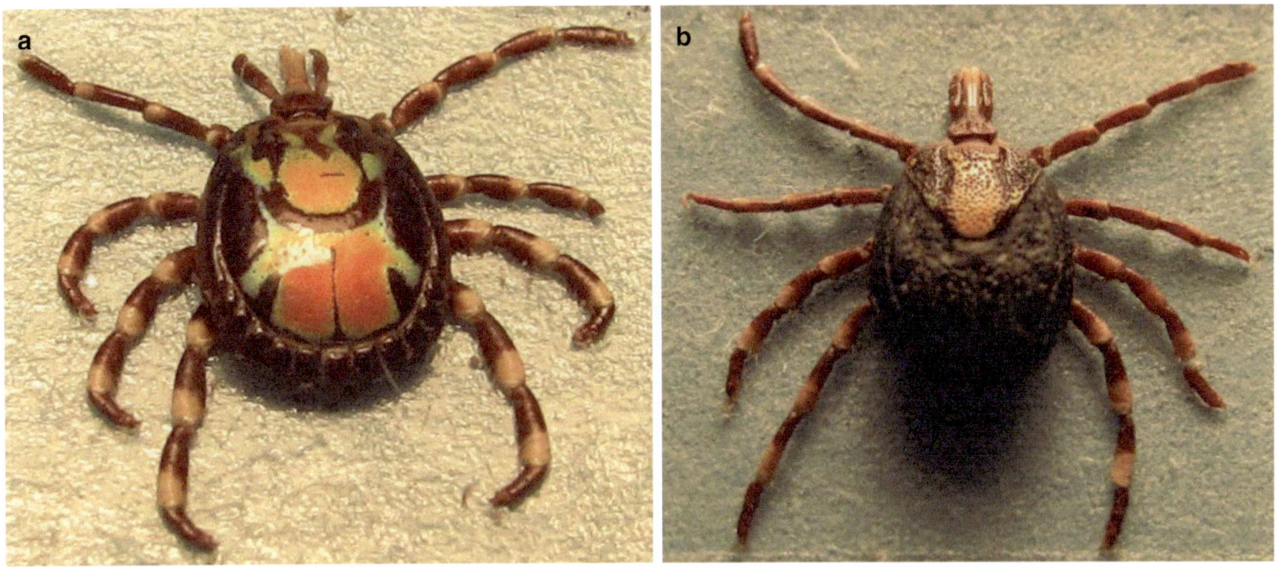

Fig. 9.15 Due to their large mouthparts, feeding by Amblyomma ticks may result in severe secondary infections of the tick feeding site. (**a**) *Amblyomma variegatum* adult male tick, (**b**) *Amblyomma variegatum* adult female tick

acaricide application results in environmental pollution and residue tainting of meat and milk products.

Figures 9.15, 9.16, 9.17, and 9.18 give an overview on ticks are found in Africa only.

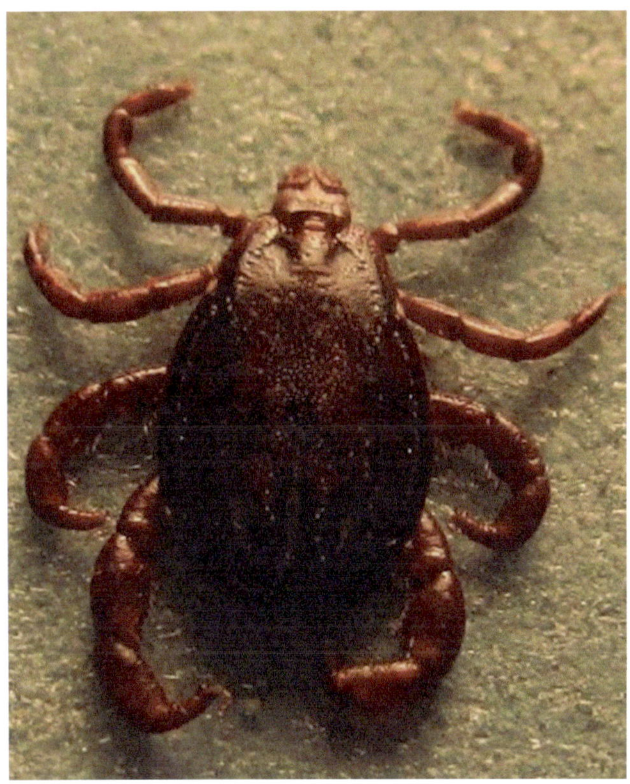

Fig. 9.16 Adult *Rhipicephalus appendiculatus* tick. Most known for the transmission of *Theileria parva* to cattle (East Coast fever), the tick species also transmits *Theileria taurotragi* (benign bovine theileriosis), *Anaplasma bovis* (bovine ehrlichiosis), *Rickettsia conorii* (tick typhus), and Nairobi sheep disease virus

Vaccination Against Ticks

The guiding principle for anti-tick vaccination stems from early studies conducted on acquired host resistance to tick infestations. Repeated exposure of hosts to ticks or tick organ homogenates induced resistance to tick re-infestation. While the degree of resistance may vary between different tick and host species, evidence strongly suggests that natural resistance against tick infestation develops based on adaptive immune response mechanisms [47]. Ticks feeding from hosts vaccinated with tick components take up effector molecules during feeding that mediate deleterious effects on the ticks. This effect manifests as reduction of feeding time, tick mortality (during or after feeding), reduced engorgement weights, and reduced reproductive capacity of adult females. Eggs laid from ticks fed on vaccinated hosts may also show reduced hatching rates. The overall result culminates in reduction of tick populations and tick-borne diseases.

Anti-tick Vaccine Candidates. Many of the anti-tick vaccine targets have been identified using conventional immune-screening techniques. Immunization of vertebrate hosts with tick homogenates or purified tick extracts generates immune sera. These sera are used to screen for tick antigens detected by the host.

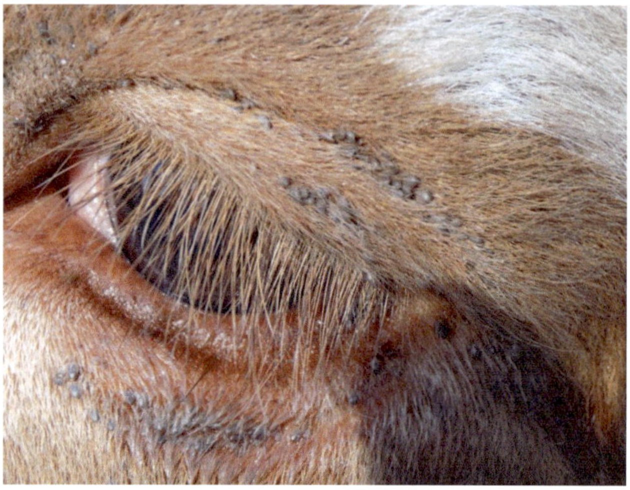

Fig. 9.17 Immature *Rhipicephalus* ticks feeding around the eye of cattle (Courtesy of S. Mwaura)

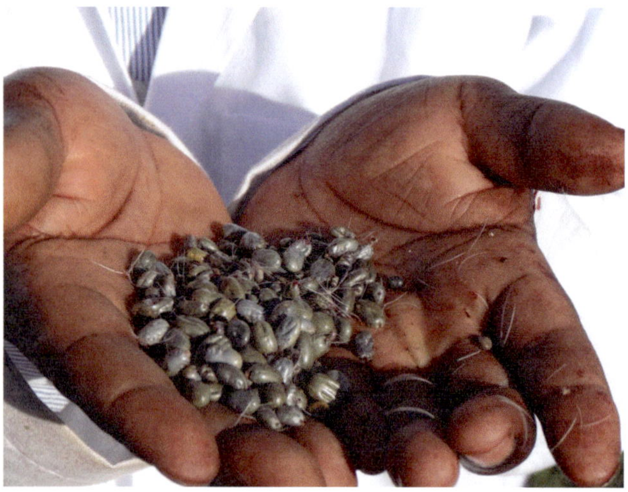

Fig. 9.18 Collection of acaricide resistant adult *Rhipicephalus* ticks in Kenya (Courtesy of S. Mwaura)

The identification of tick proteins essential for tick survival is a useful method for more targeted antigen discovery, which is made increasingly possible as information is gathered on tick biology. With the availability of genome sequences for a number of tick species, the number of candidates for discovery is expanding through reverse vaccinology. The use of other techniques such as RNA interference (RNAi) has been useful in confirming the importance of anti-tick vaccine candidates and is likely to play a role in future anti-tick vaccine antigen discovery [48].

Exposed or Concealed Antigens. Anti-tick vaccine candidates have been classified into two categories: exposed or concealed antigens. Exposed antigens are secreted in tick saliva during attachment and feeding on a host while concealed antigens are normally hidden from the host immune response. Molecular mimicry by ticks of host components has been observed, and vaccination may induce host sensitivity and autoimmune reactions when exposed antigens are used [49].

One advantage of using exposed antigens is that natural boosting occurs through tick feeding. Mechanistically, vaccination with exposed antigens is thought to induce a focal hostile environment unsupportive for tick attachment and feeding. Concealed antigens do not come into contact with the host immune response during natural tick feeding. Although often contained within the thoracic cavity of the tick, some salivary gland proteins can be characterized as concealed if they are not secreted into the tick-feeding site.

One difficulty in the development of concealed anti-tick vaccines is that the antigen must be accessible to the induced humoral vaccine response. This often limits the number of candidates to those coming into prolonged and direct contact with the blood meal or where the humoral response can be transported over the gut barrier into the hemolymph [50–52]. The second limitation of concealed antigens relates to natural boosting of the immune response. As the antigens do not come into contact with the immune response within the host, sufficiently high antibody levels must be induced through repeated vaccination.

As the blood meal acts as the carrier for the effector immune responses, the anti-tick effect can take place over a longer period of time compared to exposed antigens. This effect may even extend beyond the mere feeding period into the inactive stages where digestion and molting/egg laying takes place.

Bm86 Anti-tick Vaccine. The Bm86-based anti-tick vaccine remains the only anti-tick vaccine commercially produced and has become the benchmark for future anti-tick vaccine development and evaluation. The gut-associated Bm86 glycoprotein was first identified in *R. microplus* although homologues in other tick species have since been identified [53–55]. The biological function of Bm86 remains unknown although it is thought to play a role in the digestion of the blood meal [56]. In *R. microplus*, expression of Bm86 is increased during embryogenesis, reaching the highest level in unfed larvae. Expression decreases during feeding and molting with lowest levels of expression detected during the resting stages of the tick.

Bm86 has a translated coding sequence of 650 amino acids and a size of 71.7 kDa. The protein contains four potential N-linked glycosylation sites and a leader peptide suggesting transport to the cell surface. Localization studies have shown the molecule is located predominantly on the microvilli of gut epithelial cells. A single C-terminal transmembrane sequence is present in the unprocessed protein which is replaced by a glycosylphosphatidylinositol anchor in the mature protein. The protein also contains multiple predicted EGF repeats rich in cysteine residues.

Vaccination has been performed mostly with the whole molecule, and protective epitopes for Bm86 have not been well determined. The site of a protective B cell epitope was defined and additional epitopes are likely to exist. Overlapping cross-reactive immune-reactive epitopes have been found between Bm86 and the *R. decoloratus* homologue, Bd86. Vaccine efficacy is directly related to anti-Bm86 antibody titer and the ability to control tick populations is directly related to achieving a strong antibody response.

Substantial animal-to-animal variation has been observed in the ability to generate anti-Bm86 antibody titers which is likely related to the MHC class II haplotypes expressed. Antibodies to Bm86 and cattle complement system are taken up during the blood meal. Antibody binding results in lysis of the gut epithelial cells culminating in impaired blood meal digestion. Strong antibody responses may induce tick mortality due to blood leakage from the gut into the hemolymph and ticks may turn reddish instead of gray.

The development of the antibody response in cattle [57] after immunization with rBm86 is demonstrated in Fig. 9.19.

Recombinant expression of Bm86 has been attempted in several expression systems including *Escherichia coli*, *Aspergillus nidulans*, *Aspergillus niger*, and *Pichia pastoris*. Vaccine trials showed that Bm86 vaccination targeted mainly the adult stage of *R. microplus*, particularly the number of adult females fully engorging and post-engorgement mortality. Reproductive capacity of adult *R. microplus* females was affected in terms of egg-laying capacity and hatching of eggs [58].

Under field situations, vaccination of cattle reduced tick numbers by 56 % within a single generation and reduced the reproductive capacity by 72 %. Reversal of negative effects of tick feeding on live weight of vaccinated animals by an average increase in live weight of 18.6 kg over a 6-month period was observed. Extensive field trials in Cuba, Brazil, Argentina, and Mexico showed between 55 and 100 % control of *R. microplus* ticks within a 36-week period [59].

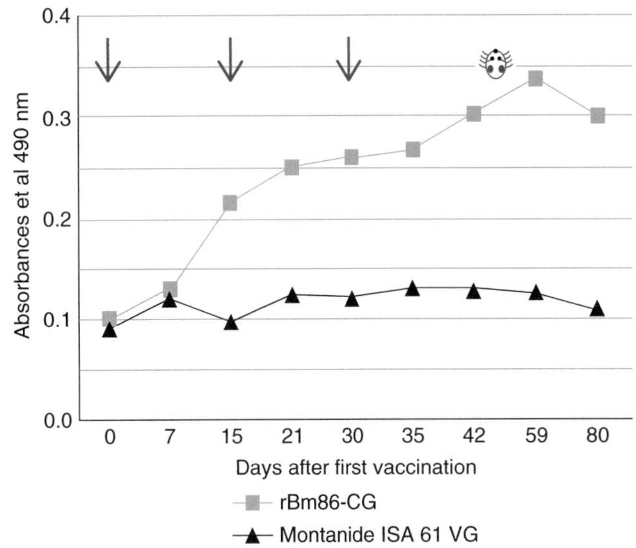

Fig. 9.19 Antibody response of cattle vaccinated with rBm86-CG antigen. Control animals were injected adjuvant Montanide ISA 61 VG alone. Antibody titers of immunized cattle are depicted as the OD480 nm value of the 1:100 dilution of serum samples that were pooled for each day of testing. Arrows indicate the day cattle were vaccinated. Tick icon indicates day 51 after the first vaccination, which is when cattle were infested (Credit: R. Andreotti, Embrapa Beef Cattle, Brazilian Agricultural Research Corporation, Brazil)

Importantly, complete control of acaricide-resistant ticks could be accomplished by integrating Bm86 vaccination with acaricide use [52], showing that integrated control systems are effective in controlling tick populations. Vaccination also decreased the amount of acaricides required to control tick populations and prolonged the time interval between cattle dipping. Bm86 vaccination has been extensively evaluated for its ability to control other tick species. Almost complete cross-protection against *Rhipicephalus annulatus* has been reported [60]. Significant protection against *Hyalomma anatolicum*, *H. dromedarii*, and *R. decoloratus* has been observed; however no cross-protection was seen against *R. appendiculatus* or *Amblyomma variegatum*.

9.5 Vector Vaccines

Genetically attenuated microorganisms, viruses and bacteria, can be engineered to deliver recombinant heterologous antigens to stimulate the host immune system. Some experimental vector systems are summarized in Table 9.1.

Table 9.1 Genetic attenuated microorganisms as vaccine delivery systems

Viral vector systems	Biosafety level	Bacterial vector systems	Biosafety level
Adenovirus (e.g., AdV5)	BSL-2	*Lactococcus lactis* and *Lactobacillus plantarum*	BSL-1 BSL-1
Adeno-associated virus (AAV)[a]	BSL-1	*Salmonella typhimurium*	BSL-1/2
Modified vaccinia virus (MVV) strain Ankara	BSL-2	*Salmonella typhi*[b]	BSL-2
Alphaviral vector (e.g., Semliki forest virus (SFV)	BSL-2	Bacillus Calmette–Guérin	BSL-2
Avipoxvirus (NYVAC and ALVAC)	BSL-2	*Shigella flexneri*	BSL-2
Baculovirus	BSL-1	*Listeria monocytogenes*[b]	BSL-1

[a]In 2012, the European Medicines Agency (EMA) recommends AAV as vector in the first gene therapy for approval
[b]Phase I clinical trials

Biosafety. The first *Laboratory Biosafety Manual* was published in 1983 and is now available with the third edition. The manual covers risk assessment and safe use of recombinant DNA technology and provides guidelines for certification of laboratories. The primary factors to consider in risk assessment fall into the main two categories, agent hazards and laboratory procedure hazards. The four biosafety levels, BSLs, consist of combinations of laboratory practices and techniques, safety equipment, and laboratory facilities and are measured as BSL 1, 2, 3, and 4 in rising order of danger.

Work with vectors classified as BSL-1 does not require biosafety program approval. Work with vectors classified as BSL-2 or higher requires approval by the local Biosafety Committee.

Safety Concerns. As demonstrated for adenovirus 5 (Ad5), following i.m. injection, the vector persisted mainly near the injection site and in draining lymph nodes for up to 6 months. Low levels of integration into chromosomal DNA were observed, with a calculated mutation rate of 2×10^{-7} mutations per cell. The spontaneous mutation rate of a cell is 2×10^{-6} and therefore tenfold higher. Ad5 is classified as biosafety level 2 (BSL-2).

Live vectors are able to stimulate the mucosal as well as a systemic humoral and cellular immunity. A severe drawback of the vector technology is that, once used, the vector cannot be effectively used in the patient again because it will be recognized by antibodies. Repeated booster immunization will fail. Also preexisting immunity in the patient against the vector could render the vaccination ineffective. A heterologous prime-boost and vector priming as described in Chap. 2 could circumvent this barrier.

9.5.1 Lactic Acid Bacteria Vector and Plague Disease[4]

9.5.1.1 *Lactobacillus plantarum* Platform

Lactic acid bacteria have *generally recognized as safe* (GRAS) status and have been developed in the past decade as potent adjuvants for mucosal delivery of vaccine. A platform technology based on *Lactobacillus plantarum* (Fig. 9.21) was developed to deliver antigens against plague disease caused by *Yersinia pestis*, an aerobic, nonmotile, gram-negative bacillus belonging to the family *Enterobacteriaceae*, which is transmitted to humans via fleabite or via aerosol droplet, causing bubonic or pneumonic plague, respectively [61].

Most human plague cases present as one of three primary forms – bubonic, septicemic, or pneumonic. Secondary plague septicemia, pneumonia, and meningitis are the most common complications. The pathogenicity of *Y. pestis* results from its impressive ability to overcome the defenses of the mammalian host and to overwhelm it with massive growth.

9.5.1.2 The Enzootic Cycle and Transmission

Plague is enzootic in rodents in Africa, Asia, South America, and North America. *Y. pestis* is transmitted from host to host by fleas via blood feeding, through consumption or handling of infectious host tissues, or through inhalation of infectious materials. *Y. pestis* infects an astonishingly broad range of mammals and uses rats, squirrels, mice, prairie dogs, marmots, or gerbils as reservoirs and several arthropod vectors for transmission [62] (Fig. 9.20).

[4]Lactic acid bacteria vector vaccines by *Maria Gomes-Solecki* in Molecular Vaccines – From Prophylaxis to Therapy, Volume 2, Springer-Verlag Wien, 2013, Ed. Matthias Giese.

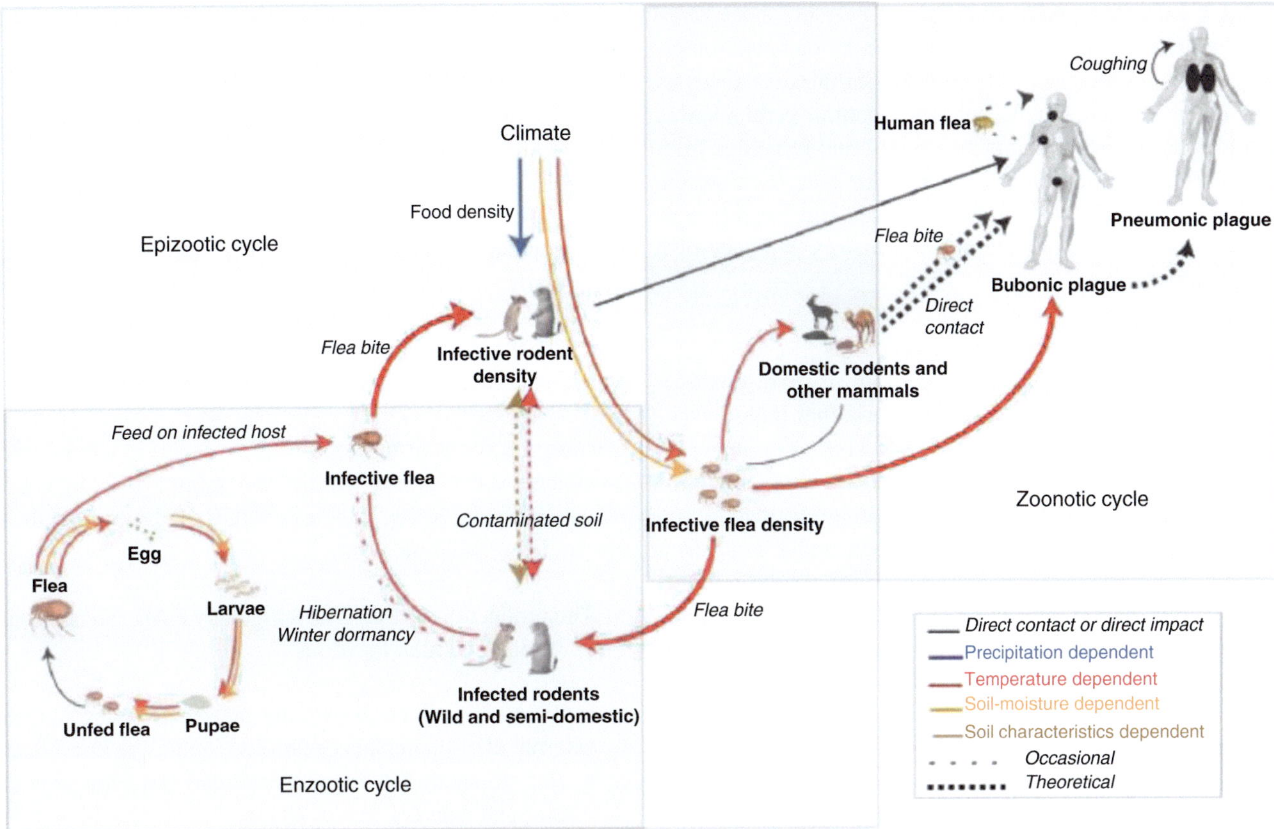

Fig. 9.20 Schematic of the plague cycle with small mammals as hosts and fleas as vectors. *Arrows* represent connections affected by climate with a color coding depending on the most influential climate variable on this link (i.e., precipitation, temperatures, and other variables indirectly depending on them such as soil characteristics and soil moisture). *Grey rectangles* somewhat arbitrarily delimit epizootic, enzootic, and zoonotic cycles. Note that despite their location at the far end of the cycle, humans often provide the only available information on plague dynamics

Humans acquire this zoonotic infection via an atypical bite from animal fleas, sometimes prompted by an animal's death from plague, after which the flea seeks a new source of blood. Most infected fleas come from the domestic black rat *Rattus rattus* or the brown sewer rat *Rattus norvegicus*.

Y. pestis cells spread from the site of the infected fleabite to the regional lymph nodes, grow to high numbers causing the formation of a bubo, and spill into the bloodstream where bacteria are removed in the liver and spleen. Growth continues in these organs, spreads to others, and causes septicemia. Fleas feeding on septicemic animals complete the infection cycle. In humans, bubonic plague can develop into an infection of the lung (secondary pneumonic plague) that can lead to aerosol transmission (primary pneumonic plague) [63]. Multiple antibiotic-resistant strains of *Y. pestis* occur naturally and they can be easily bioengineered. Thus, plague is a category A bioterrorism agent in need for novel strategies for its prevention.

9.5.1.3 Clinical Disease

Bubonic plague is the classic form of the disease. Patients usually develop symptoms of fever, headache, chills, and swollen, extremely tender lymph nodes (buboes) within 2–6 days of contact with the organism either by fleabite or by exposure of open wounds to infected materials. Primary septicemic plague is generally defined as occurring in a patient with positive blood cultures but no palpable lymphadenopathy. Patients are febrile, and most have chills, headache, malaise, and gastrointestinal disturbances. Primary pneumonic plague is a rare but deadly form of the disease that is spread via respiratory droplets through close contact (2–5 ft) with an infected individual. It progresses rapidly from a febrile flu-like illness to an overwhelming pneumonia with coughing and the production of bloody sputum. The incubation period for primary pneumonic plague is between 1 and 3 days. In general, patients who develop secondary plague pneumonia have a high fatality rate.

9.5.1.4 Laboratory Diagnosis

The laboratory diagnosis of plague is based on bacteriological and/or serological evidence [64]. Samples for analysis can include blood, bubo aspirates, sputum, cerebrospinal fluid in patients with plague meningitis, and scrapings from skin lesions, if present. Staining techniques such as the Gram, Giemsa, Wright, or Wayson stain can provide supportive but not presumptive or confirmatory evidence of a plague infection.

9.5.1.5 LAB-Based Vector Vaccines

Lactic acid bacteria (LAB) are a group of gram-positive, nonpathogenic, non-sporulating bacteria that include species of *Lactobacillus* (Fig. 9.21), *Lactococcus*, *Leuconostoc*, *Pediococcus*, and *Streptococcus*. They have limited biosynthetic abilities and require preformed amino acids, B vitamins, purines, pyrimidines, and a sugar as a carbon and energy source. These nutritional requirements restrict their habitats to those in which the required compounds are abundant. Thus, these highly specialized bacteria occupy a range of niches including milk, plant surfaces, the oral cavity, the gastrointestinal tract, and the vagina of vertebrates [65].

LAB have been consumed for centuries by humans in fermented foods and have an extraordinary safety profile. These intrinsic advantages turn LAB into excellent delivery vectors of novel preventive and therapeutic molecules for humans. A number of studies of oral vaccines generated from genetically engineered pathogenic or commensal bacteria have been reported [66, 67].

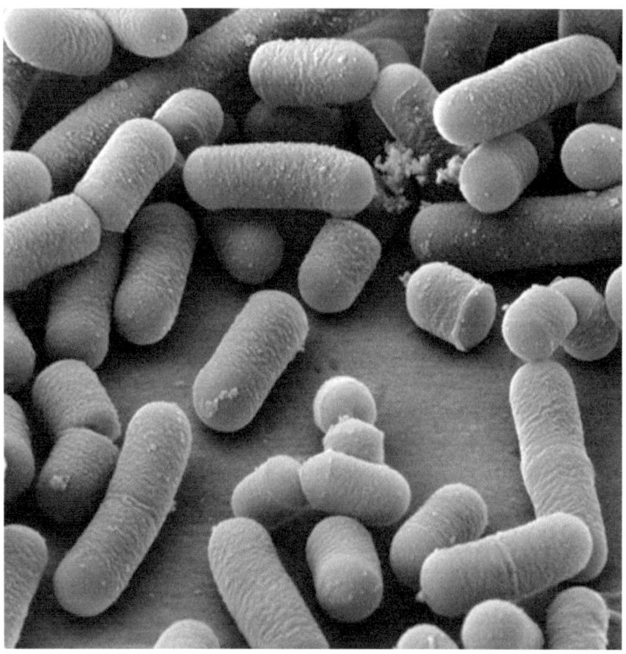

Fig. 9.21 *Lactobacillus plantarum* is a member of the genus *Lactobacillus*, commonly found in many fermented food products as well as anaerobic plant matter. *L. plantarum* can survive in the human gastrointestinal tract, which makes it an ideal delivery vector for vaccine antigens (SEM image kindly provided by G. Wanner, Faculty of Biology, Plant Sciences, LMU Munich, Germany)

Live attenuated pathogenic bacteria, such as derivatives of *Mycobacterium*, *Salmonella*, and *Bordetella* spp., are the most popular live delivery vectors used currently. They are particularly well adapted to interact with mucosal surfaces as they have specialized machinery to initiate the infection process. The major disadvantages of live vaccines include inadequate attenuation and the potential to revert to virulence.

GRAS. Lactic acid bacteria-based vaccines act as live attenuated vaccines but without the safety concern. LAB have a *generally recognized as safe* (GRAS) status and thus are not likely to cause harm.

The production of a desired antigen by LAB can occur in three different cellular locations:

- *Intracellular*, which allows the protein to escape harsh external environmental conditions (such as gastric juices in the stomach) but requires cellular lysis for protein release and delivery
- *Extracellular*, which allows the release of the protein into the external medium, resulting in direct interaction with the environment (food product or the digestive tract)
- *Cell wall anchored*, which combines the advantages of the other two locations (i.e., interaction between the cell wall-anchored protein and the environment, in addition to protection from proteolytic degradation)

In this context, several studies have compared the production of different antigens in LAB, using all three locations, and evaluated the subsequent immunological impact. These studies demonstrated that the highest immune response was obtained with cell wall-anchored antigens exposed on the surface of LAB. Therefore, most of the recent LAB vaccination studies have selected surface exposure of the antigen of interest, rather than intra- or extracellular production [68].

Dendritic cells (DCs) play a central role in bridging the innate immune system with the adaptive immune system. DCs are found throughout the body and are especially common at mucosal surfaces. With only a single layer of epithelial cells separating the external from the internal world amid the constant need for particle exchange, intestinal dendritic cells (DCs) play a key role in maintaining intestinal homeostasis as well as governing protective immune responses against invading pathogens. To avoid activation of self-reactive T cells and to limit unnecessary responses, such as those against commensal flora, DCs can imprint tolerance onto T cells (Fig. 9.22).

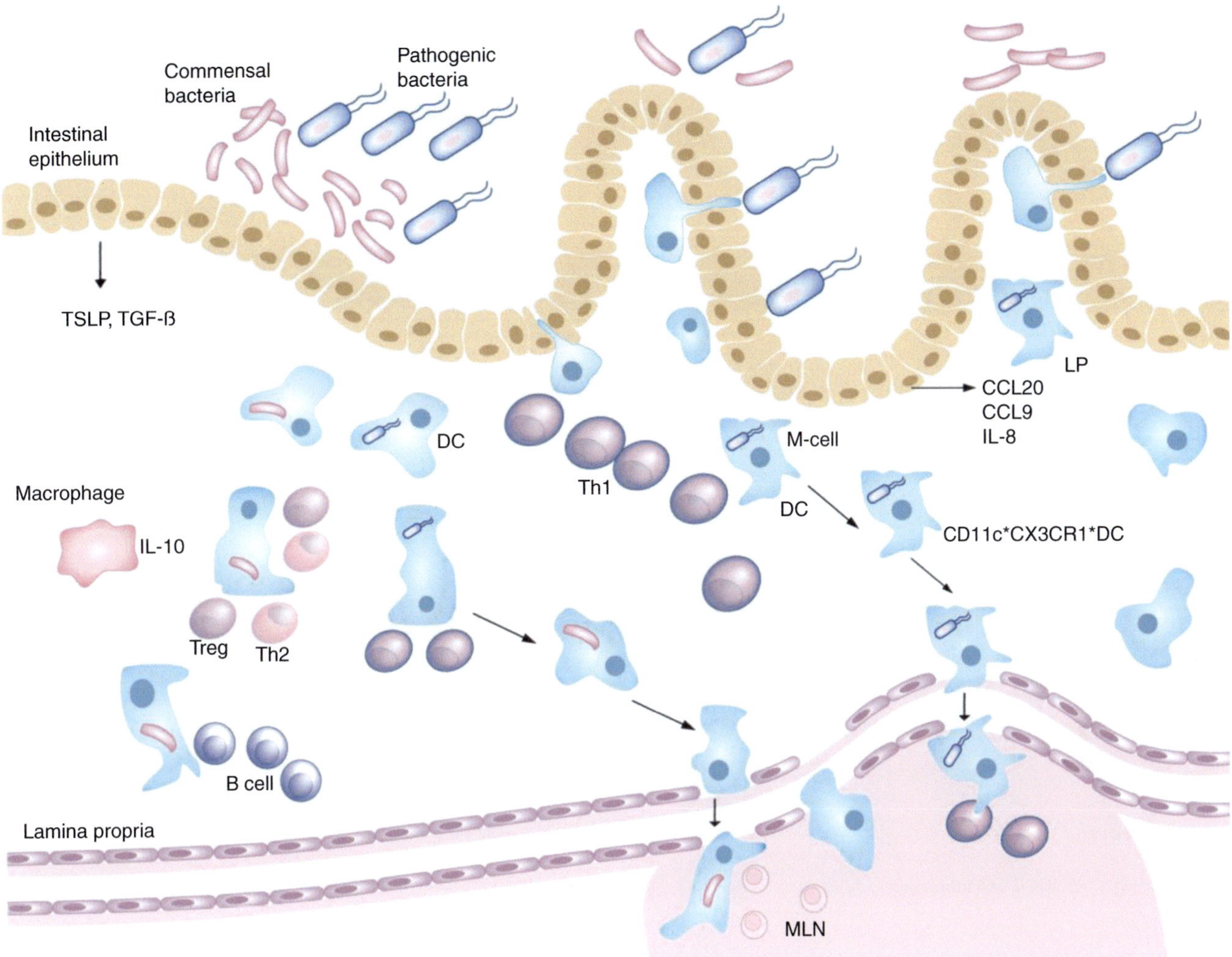

Fig. 9.22 Sampling bacteria and their products by gut DCs

Immature-type DCs are enriched underneath the epithelium of mucosal inductive sites and are poised to capture antigens. They extend protrusions between epithelial cells, enabling direct sampling of luminal antigens [69]. Through upregulation of MHC and co-stimulatory molecules, matured DCs convert into highly efficient antigen-presenting cells. Successful antigen presentation to CD4+ T cells requires recognition of cognate peptide in the context of MHC class II molecules, whereas epitopes presented on MHC class I molecules stimulate Ag-specific CD8+ T cells. When antigen uptake occurs, these DCs change their phenotype by expressing higher levels of co-stimulatory molecules and move to T cell areas of inductive sites for antigen presentation. Thus, DCs and their derived cytokines play key roles in the induction of antigen-specific effector Th cell responses. In this regard, targeting mucosal DCs is an effective strategy to induce mucosal and systemic immune responses.

LAB Persistence. The ability of some LAB to persist in the gastrointestinal tract may be critically important in the effectiveness of LAB-based vaccines. A comparison of a persisting LAB strain, *L. plantarum*, with a nonpersisting LAB strain, *L. lactis*, identified *L. plantarum* to be more effective at eliciting antigen-specific immunity, suggesting that persistence promoted immunogenicity [70]. Furthermore, it has been shown that particular *Lactobacillus* species induced critical inflammatory cytokines and induced activation and maturation of dendritic cells [71]. It has also been shown that immature DCs efficiently capture *Lactobacillus* species, and these bacteria activated human DCs, resulting in the production of pro-inflammatory cytokines like IL-12, increased proliferation of CD4+ and CD8+ cells, and skewed T cell response toward a Th1 pathway believed to be involved in effective clearance of microbial pathogens [72, 73] (Fig. 9.23).

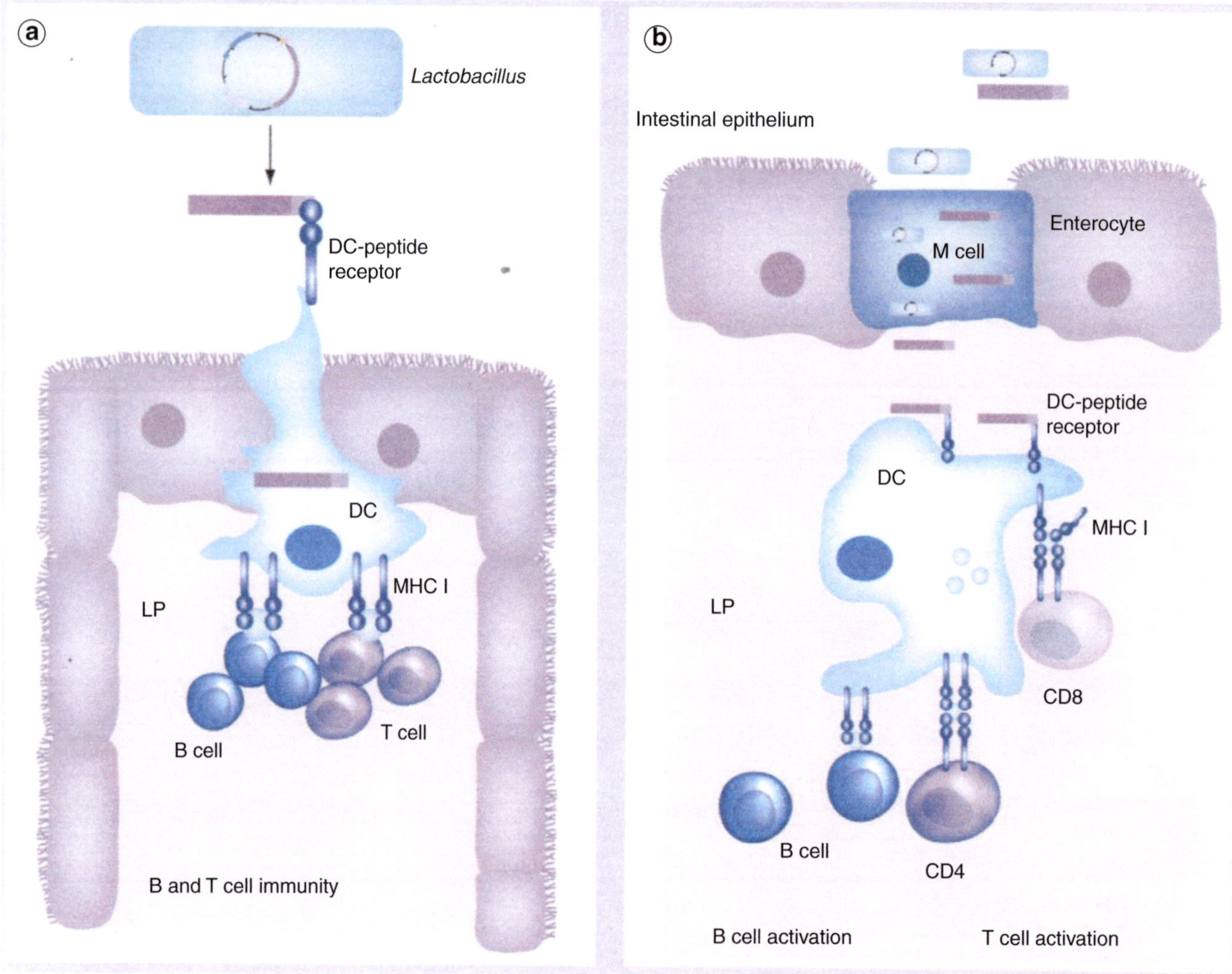

Fig. 9.23 Delivery of immunogenic subunits to gut DCs by probiotic lactobacilli

Evidence suggests that the peptidoglycan layer of some LAB promote natural immuno-adjuvanticity [74], and antigen localization on the cell wall makes it more accessible to the immune system as compared to intracellular or secreted proteins. Leader peptides mark proteins for translocation across the cytoplasmic membrane, and lipid modification is of major importance both for anchoring exported proteins to the membrane and for protein function [75]. It has been shown that lipidation at the first amino acid of the mature *Borrelia burgdorferi* OspA protein is essential to induce an immune response via TLR2 [76]. The leader peptide of OspA targets the protein to the cell envelope of *Lactobacillus* and that the Cys [17] is recognized by the *L. plantarum* cell wall-sorting machinery that lipidates and anchors the protein to the cell envelope. The end result is a delivery system that exerts a potent adjuvant effect [77].

9.6 Virus-like Particles: Norovirus Gastroenteritis[5]

Gastroenteritis (GE) and its associated diarrheal diseases remain as one of the top causes of death in the world. Noroviruses (NoVs) are a group of genetically diverse RNA viruses that cause the great majority of nonbacterial gastroenteritis in humans. However, there is still no vaccine licensed for human use to prevent NoV GE. The lack of a tissue culture system and a small animal model further hinders the development of NoV vaccines.

[5]Virus-like Particle Vaccines for Norovirus Gastroenteritis by *Qiang Chen* in Molecular Vaccines – From Prophylaxis to Therapy, Volume 2, Springer-Verlag Wien, 2013, Ed. Matthias Giese.

Virus-like Particles (VLPs) that mimic the antigenic architecture of authentic virions, however, can be produced in insect, mammalian, and plant cells by the expression of the capsid protein. The particulate nature and high-density presentation of viral structure proteins on their surface render VLPs as a premier vaccine platform with superior safety, immunogenicity, and manufacturability. Therefore, this chapter focuses on the development of effective NoV vaccines based on VLPs of capsid proteins. The expression and structure of NoV VLPs, especially VLPs of Norwalk virus, the prototype NoV, are extensively discussed. The ability of NoV VLPs in stimulating a potent systemic and mucosal anti-NoV immunity through oral and intranasal delivery in mice is presented.

Gastroenteritis (GE) is a worldwide health problem that affects people of all ages. As its name implies, GE is characterized by inflammation of the gastrointestinal tract and often associated with symptoms of diarrhea, nausea, vomiting, and abdominal cramping and pain. GE and its associated diarrheal diseases remain as one of the top causes of death in the world especially in developing countries and in young children with an estimated death toll of four to six million per year [78]. GE can be caused by a variety of pathogens including viruses, bacteria, and parasites and by ingestion of noninfectious toxins or medications, with viruses as the most common offending agents. Norovirus (NoV) and rotavirus are the most common viruses that cause viral GE, while adenovirus, astrovirus, coronavirus, and parechovirus are also known to cause GE in humans.

Noroviruses. NoVs are a group of genetically diverse RNA viruses that belong to the genus of *Norovirus* in the *Caliciviridae* family [79]. They were first discovered and characterized in their prototype virus, the Norwalk virus (NV), in 1972 [80]. Studies of NV revealed that NoVs are non-enveloped viruses with a RNA genome surrounded by a round capsid protein shell approximately 38 nm in diameter.

NoVs are divided into 5 genogroups and 29 clusters with 8 clusters in genogroup I (GI), 17 in GII, 2 in GIII, and 1 each in GIV and GV. Within the five genotypes, GI and GIV strains are found to infect humans exclusively and GII are found in both humans and pigs, while GIII and GV strains are animal viruses that infect cattle and murine species, respectively [81]. Currently, strains in cluster 4 of GII (GII 4) are the most prevalent NoVs in human population [82].

The genome of NoVs, which was first characterized in NV, contains a single-stranded positive-sense RNA of 7.5–7.7 kb with three open reading frames (ORFs) and a poly A tail at its 3′ end [83] (Fig. 9.24). ORF1 encodes a polyprotein that is processed by viral protease 3CLpro into the RNA-dependent RNA polymerase and approximately five other nonstructural proteins including p48, the nucleoside triphosphatase, p22, VPg, and 3CLpro. The two structural proteins, the major (VP1) and minor (VP2) capsid proteins, are encoded by ORF2 and ORF3, respectively [84]. Structural analysis of NoV has revealed that each viral capsid is composed of 90 dimers of VP1 in a $T=3$ icosahedral symmetry. VP1 folds into two domains: a shell (S) domain that is responsible for initiating capsid assembly and icosahedral contacts and a protruding domain (P), containing two subdomains of P1 and P2, that enhance the stability of the capsid by providing intermolecular contacts between VP1 dimers. Studies of NV also indicate that the VP2 protein enhances the expression level of VP1 and stabilizes the VP1 in the viral capsid.

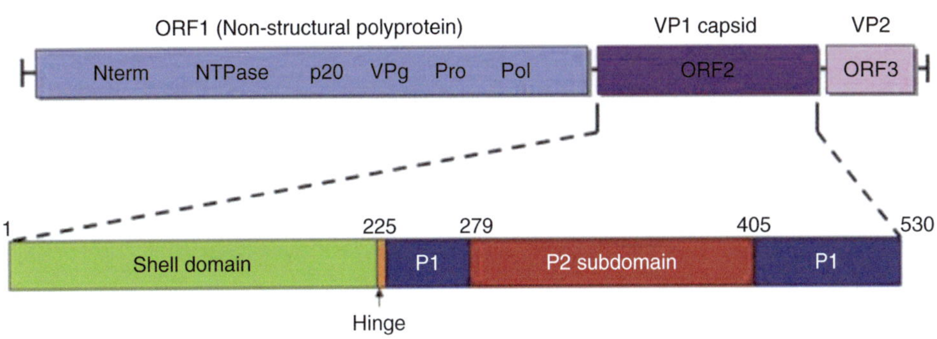

Fig. 9.24 Genome map of norovirus and capsid domains. The NoV genome is composed of 3 open reading frames (ORFs). ORF1 encodes the nonstructural proteins of an NTPase, and RNA-dependent RNA polymerase (Pol). ORF2 encodes the 57 kDa major structural capsid protein of viral protein 1 (VP1). VP1 is divided into the shell domain (S) and the protruding domain (P). The P domain contains two subdomains, known as P1 and P2. ORF3 encodes a minor structural protein VP2 (http://emedicine.medscape.com/article/224225-overview)

Transmission and Infection Cycle of NoVs. NoVs require an extremely low infectious dose, as challenge studies with NV have suggested that the probability of infection with a single virus particle is approximately 50 % among susceptible human populations. They can be transmitted by several routes including fecal-contaminated food or water, direct person to person contact, indirect exposure through droplets, or contaminated objects of infected persons.

NoVs are highly contagious and spread rapidly, and their outbreaks commonly occur in various social places and settings where people share common food and water sources or are in close physical proximity, such as cruise ships, schools, military units, nursing homes, daycare centers, hospitals, restaurants, and catered events .

The life cycle of NoV has not been fully understood due to the lack of an in vitro cell culture system and a small animal model of infection. The failure of NoV replication in mammalian cell cultures is not due to the lack of host factors to support intracellular expression of NoV RNA. Instead, the problem may lie in the steps of viral binding to cellular receptors, virus entry into cells.

Current Diagnostic Methods and Therapeutics for NoV GE. Various diagnostic methods have been developed for NoV [85]. While serum antibodies to NoV can be readily detected, this method has little clinical relevance due to the cross-reactivity of antibodies. Since there is no culture system available for NoV, the detection of virus in stool samples has become the preferred method of diagnosis. Traditionally, NoV infection was diagnosed by detecting the virus by immune transmission electron microscopy (TEM). TEM offers the advantage of direct visualization of any potentially responsible virus particles in stool samples. However, it does have the disadvantage of requiring sophisticated and expensive equipment and highly specialized technicians for its operation.

Several enzyme-linked immunosorbent assays (ELISAs) that detect NoV antigens were later developed for NoV diagnosis. Studies have shown that NoV antigen-detecting ELISAs have high specificity (94–96 %) but poor sensitivity (40–60 %), most likely due to the antigenic diversity of NoV strains [86].

Similar to ELISA-based assays, RT-PCR is rapid and robust, because it can process large numbers of samples simultaneously and results can be obtained within a working day. However, it requires RNA extraction from fecal samples and needs expensive equipment and skilled workers to operate. Therefore, RT-PCR is more labor intensive and less economical than ELISAs.

Overall, TEM, ELISA, and RT-PCR-based methods all have their advantages and challenges. The three methods detect different components of the virus and therefore are complementary to each other.

Immunology of NoV Infection. The immunological knowledge of NoV is mostly obtained from human challenge studies and natural outbreaks due to the lack of small animal models. Observations of repeat infections in adults suggest the scarcity of long-term immunity against these viruses. However, other studies showed that close to 50 % of the genetically susceptible subjects were not infected by NoV challenge, which support the possibility of long-term immunity [87].

Virus-like Particles as an Effective Vaccine Against NoV. The lack of a tissue culture system also impedes the development of vaccines against NoV. Fortunately, the discovery of the spontaneous assembly of expressed VP1 into virus-like particles (VLPs) that are morphologically and antigenically similar to the native viruses has facilitated vaccine development. VLPs combine the best traits of whole-virus and subunit antigens for vaccine development.

VLPs are noninfectious, therefore, safer than inactivated or attenuated virus due to the lack of viral nucleic acid genome. Importantly, VLPs can induce potent cellular and humoral immune responses without adjuvants and are more effective vaccines than other subunit antigens because their architectures mimic infectious viruses. VLPs can be produced by recombinant technology in heterologous expression systems without requiring the ability to support viral replication. This is particularly important for NoV because no such culture system has been developed to support the growth of these viruses.

Studies have demonstrated that viruses and corresponding VLPs have a particle size ideal for DC and macrophage uptake to initiate antigen processing [88]. Thus, the particulate nature of VLPs favors their targeting to relevant APCs for optimal induction of T cell-mediated immune responses.

VLPs can also be presented efficiently to B cells and induce strong antibody responses. Like live viruses, the quasicrystalline surface of VLPs, with its arrays of repetitive epitopes, presents a prime target that vertebrate B cells have evolved to specifically recognize. This recognition triggers the cross-linking of surface membrane-associated immunoglobulins (Ig) on B cells and leads to their proliferation and migration, T helper-cell activation, antibody production and secretion, and the generation of memory B cells. Thus, VLPs can directly activate B cells at much lower concentrations than other subunit antigens and induce high titer and durable B cell responses in the absence of adjuvants.

These inherent advantages of VLPs have made them one of the most successful recombinant vaccine platforms. For example, five VLP-based vaccines for hepatitis B virus

(HBV) and human papillomavirus (HPV) have been commercially licensed, and all have demonstrated excellent safety profiles and long-term protection against infection in humans.

Characterization of NoV VLPs. VLPs of NoVs were first produced in insect cells using baculovirus vectors [89] and then in plants using tobamovirus and geminivirus vectors and in mammalian cells using the Venezuelan equine encephalitis (VEE) replicon system [90]. These studies demonstrated that expression of the major capsid protein VP1 alone can drive the self-assembly of VLPs that morphologically and antigenically resemble native virus particles (Fig. 9.25). VLPs generated by all three expression systems are similar to each other.

The structure of NoV VLPs is exemplified by the VLP of NV capsid protein (NVCP). Studies of insect cell-baculovirus-derived NVCP VLPs by cryo-electron microscopy and X-ray crystallography reveal that the NV capsid is a 38 nm icosahedral arrangement of 180 copies of the 58 kDa capsid protein VP1 organized into 90 dimers in a $T=3$ symmetry. While all dimers are formed from two identical NVCP monomers, two different dimer configurations are required to correctly form the complete assembled capsid [91].

As in native NV particles, the NVCP also folds into two distinctive domains in VLPs, with S domain forming the inner core of the shell and P domain protruding out from the capsid [92]. Similarly, the P2 subdomain is also the most surface-exposed region in NV VLPs and may contain HBGA and neutralizing antibody-binding sites and determinants of strains specificity [93, 94]. The similarity between VLPs of NV and other NoVs including GII.4 viruses has been demonstrated [95].

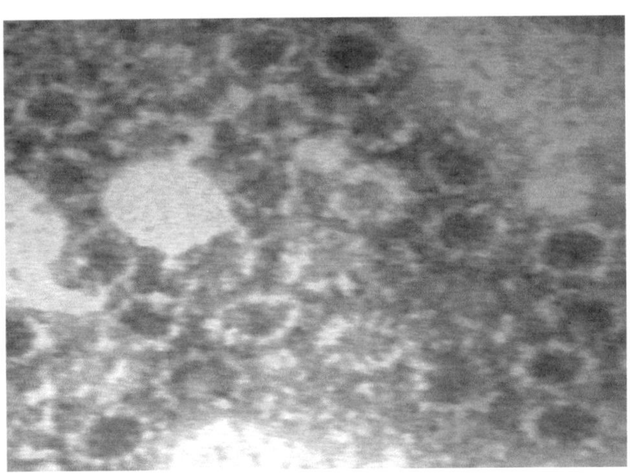

Fig. 9.25 NVCP VLPs produced in plants. NVCP was expressed in lettuce leaves with a geminiviral replicon vector. NVCP VLPs were purified from plants, negatively stained with 0.5 % uranyl acetate, and examined by electron microscopy. Bar = 50 nm. One representative experiment of three is shown

Insect Cell-Baculovirus Vector-Produced NVCP VLPs. It was shown that four oral doses of as little as 5 μg NVCP VLPs without any adjuvant triggered serum NV-specific anti-IgG response in the majority (8/11) of VLP-fed iCD1 outbred mice [90]. Systemic IgG response was observed after two oral dosages and the highest titer was induced by four doses of 200 μg VLPs. Moreover, mice in the 200 μg dosage group developed NV-specific intestinal IgA in a level up to 0.1 % of total IgA. Inclusion of the mucosal adjuvant cholera toxin (CT) did not significantly change the number of positive responders of serum IgG or intestinal IgA but significantly enhanced the amplitude of serum IgG response, especially for higher doses of VLPs. Thus, NVCP VLP is clearly a potent oral immunogen and can induce both systemic and gut mucosal antibody responses.

9.7 Nanovaccines: GAS Infections[6]

Group A streptococcus (*Streptococcus pyogenes*) (GAS) is an important human mucosal pathogen that is responsible for a wide spectrum of diseases with varying clinical manifestations and severity [96, 97]: Pharyngitis (strep throat) is a common minor complication of GAS infection but when left untreated can lead to life-threatening diseases including the autoimmune sequelae rheumatic fever (RF) and rheumatic heart disease (RHD). RHD results in permanent damage to the heart tissues and valves.

GAS infections cause >500,000 deaths each year mostly in developing countries and indigenous populations within developed nations where poor socioeconomic conditions and overcrowding contribute to the high rates of GAS diseases. In developing countries, RF is the leading cause of heart disease among children [6]. There is currently no available vaccine to prevent infection with GAS and consequently prevent GAS diseases.

A successful mucosal GAS vaccine would need to stimulate the appropriate humoral and cellular immunity for protection against GAS infection (Fig. 9.26). This is especially difficult due to a lack of human-compatible mucosal vaccine adjuvants that are essential to boost immune responses. Researchers have therefore focused mainly on parenteral GAS vaccine delivery approaches, for which suitable adjuvants are available, designed to provide protection against systemic infection via the induction of opsonic IgG antibodies.

GAS M Antigen. An effective GAS vaccine needs to have broad antigenic reach because of the many different GAS strains (>150 different M types) circulating in a population

[6]Development of subunit vaccines for group A streptococcus by Colleen Olive in Molecular Vaccines – From Prophylaxis to Therapy, Volume 2, Springer-Verlag Wien, 2013, Ed. Matthias Giese.

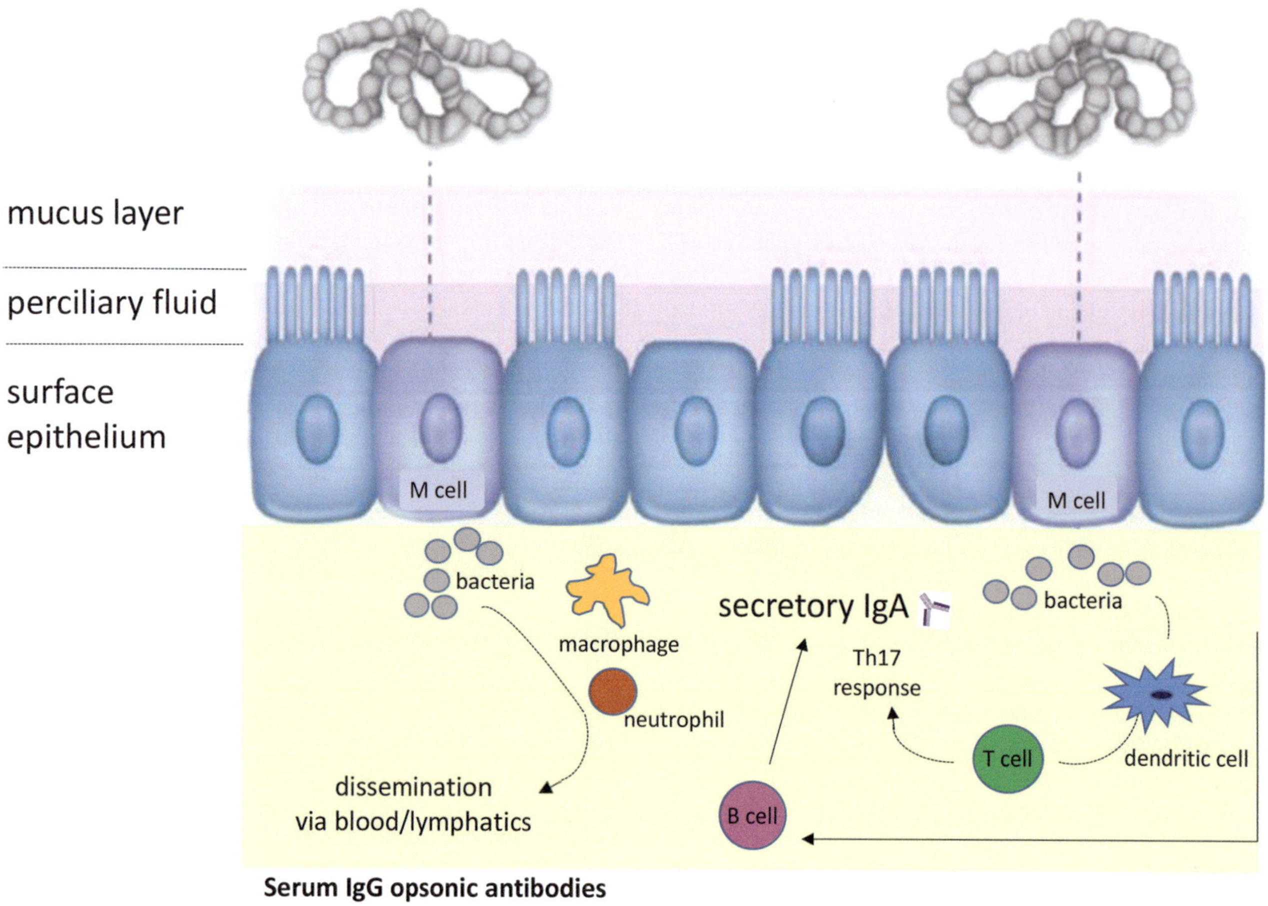

Fig. 9.26 GAS vaccination approaches. GAS that breaches the physical barrier of the mucosal epithelium of the nasal-associated lymphoid tissue, functionally analogous to human tonsils, is purported to be transported to the underlying lymphoid tissue via association with membranous (M) cells. Cells of the innate immune system sense GAS and produce cytokines and chemokines to contain the infection to the mucosa. GAS antigens are delivered to antigen-presenting cells such as DCs and B cells. IgA-committed B cells are activated and initiate antigen-specific IgA responses. DCs play a fundamental role in the development of immunity to GAS and present antigen to T cells to induce a Th17 response that is integral along with IgA for mucosal defense against pharyngeal GAS colonization. Mucosal vaccination is designed to mimic these responses and effectively clear GAS from the mucosal surface upon infection to prevent GAS colonization and carriage. GAS that escapes the host's defense mechanisms can disseminate into the lymphatics and blood, leading to systemic infection. Mucosal vaccination is also able to induce a systemic immune response characterized by the induction of opsonic IgG antibodies, which destroy the pathogen by opsonophagocytosis. Parenteral GAS vaccination induces serum IgG but is not able to induce mucosal immunity

and should not induce immune responses that are potentially cross-reactive with self tissue proteins. The GAS M protein is the major protective antigen and an ideal target for vaccine development; however it contains heart tissue cross-reactive epitopes particularly in the conserved region [98]. Evidence suggests that cross-reactive T cells especially play a pivotal role in the pathogenesis of RHD.

The M protein is an α-helical coiled-coil surface protein consisting of a hypervariable amino-terminal region and a highly conserved (>98 % sequence identity) carboxy-terminal C-repeat region [99] (Fig. 9.27). Functionally, the M protein is important in preventing bacterial clearance by complement-mediated phagocytosis, which limits host defense mechanisms. Previous studies indicate that protective immunity to GAS can be evoked by opsonic antibodies to serotypic epitopes at the amino-terminal region that are M-type specific [100].

Nanovaccine. Combined vaccine/adjuvant delivery systems offer the potential of mucosal vaccine delivery. For example, the lipid-core-peptide (LCP) system is a novel, synthetic, self-adjuvanted vaccine delivery system that incorporates

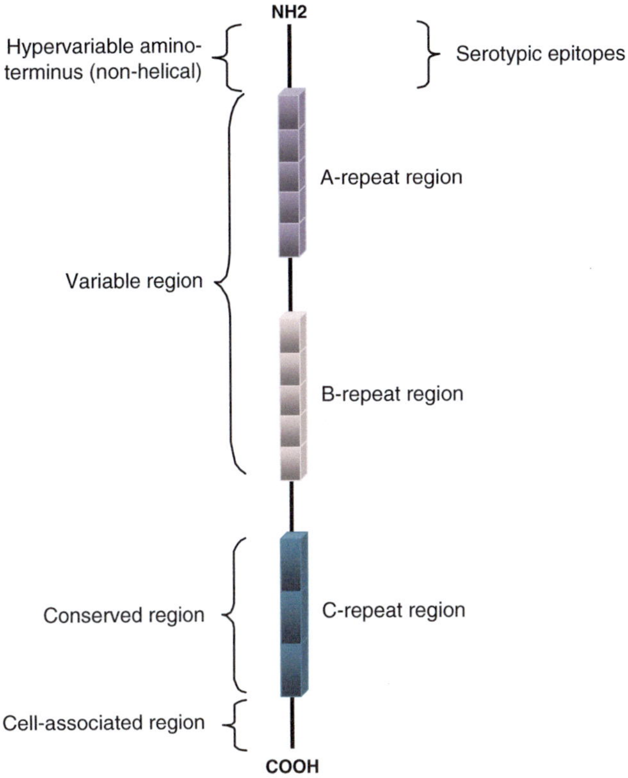

Fig. 9.27 Diagrammatic representation of the GAS M protein illustrating the different repeat regions (*A*, *B*, and *C*), location of serotypic epitopes, and increasing conservation from the amino-terminal to the carboxy-terminal region

the adjuvant (PRR agonist), carrier, and antigenic peptides of a vaccine into a single molecular entity (Fig. 9.28). This system has been previously shown to efficiently deliver GAS vaccines and induce immunity [101]. Evidence suggests the adjuvant activity of LCP involves the induction of DC activation.

Preclinical Developments. Three approaches are currently being investigated in the development of a subunit GAS vaccine based on the M protein:

1. *Multivalent GAS vaccine.* A multivalent approach employs a combination of amino-terminal protein fragments representing different M types and is designed to target prevalent GAS strains in a population. Using this approach, a recombinant multivalent GAS vaccine containing M protein peptides from 26 different GAS serotypes prevalent in North America was demonstrated to evoke opsonic antibodies in animals [102]. From epidemiological data, the 26-valent vaccine would cover the majority of pharyngitis and invasive GAS diseases, including RF, invasive fasciitis, and toxic shock syndrome. Recently, a new 30-valent GAS vaccine was shown to be immunogenic in rabbits and evoked opsonic antibodies against "non-vaccine" serotypes [103] potentially creating a vaccine with much broader coverage. This type of vaccine is population specific and therefore may not be effective universally. It may also need to be re-designed periodically to reflect changes in the epidemiology of GAS infections.

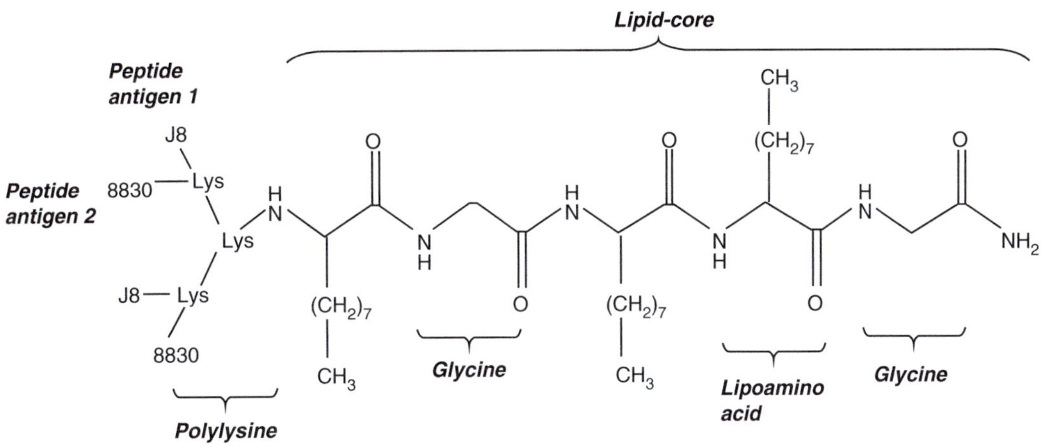

Fig. 9.28 The lipid-core-peptide (LCP) system. The LCP system contains an adjuvant component (lipid-core made of lipoamino acids) and a polylysine carrier onto which peptide epitopes are attached. The example shows a GAS vaccine candidate containing J8 and an amino-terminal serotypic epitope called 8830. The adjuvant has three 2-amino-dodecanoic ($n=9$) lipoamino acids separated by glycine amino acid spacers

2. *J8 vaccine*. A GAS vaccine that employs peptide epitopes from the conserved C-repeat region of the M protein is the second approach and has the potential in theory for greater coverage of M types. Immunization of mice with a C-region peptide GAS vaccine candidate called J8 conjugated to the carrier protein diphtheria toxoid (dT) and co-delivery with an appropriate adjuvant led to protection against systemic and mucosal GAS infection [104] (Fig. 9.29).

   J8 also elicited protective immunity against GAS when linked to lipopeptides [105, 106]. Other studies have shown that intranasal immunization of mice with C-region peptides conjugated to the experimental mucosal adjuvant cholera toxin B subunit (CTB) evoked protective immunity against GAS at the mucosal level [107]. CTB could possibly enter olfactory regions of the central nervous system and cause neuronal damage following intranasal delivery [108] and therefore is not suitable for human use. Vector delivery approaches have included expressing the C-repeat region on vaccinia virus [109], the commensal bacterium *Lactococcus lactis* [110], or *Streptococcus gordonii* [111].
3. *J14*. The third combination vaccine approach uses both serotypic and conserved M protein peptide epitopes. Initially, a heteropolymer GAS vaccine construct was synthesized by free radical-induced polymerization of acryloyl peptides to combine seven serotypic epitopes and a highly conserved C-region peptide epitope called J14 [112]. The M types that were targeted in the heteropolymer represented GAS infections prevalent in the Northern Territory of Australia – a region highly endemic for GAS. Immunization of mice with the heteropolymer demonstrated excellent immunogenicity and protection

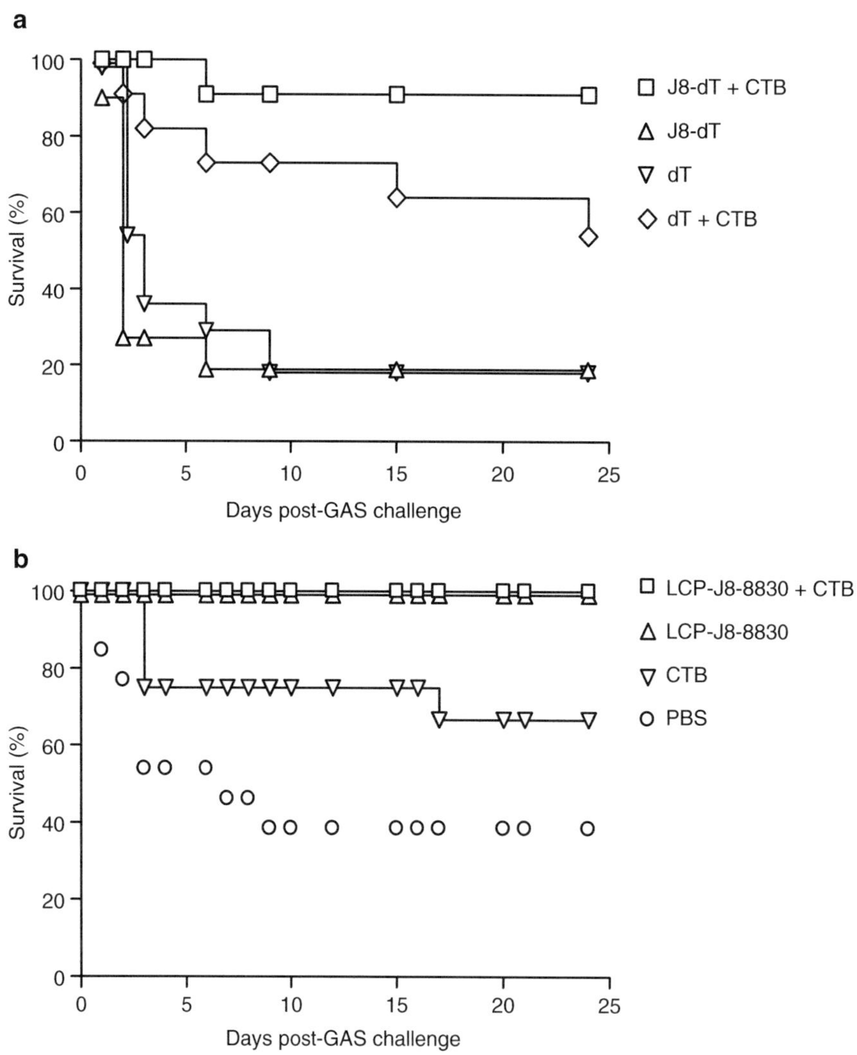

Fig. 9.29 Preclinical evaluation of GAS vaccine candidates. Intranasal immunization of mice with the J8-dT vaccine candidate led to significantly greater survival after intranasal challenge with GAS versus control groups but the mucosal adjuvant CTB was essential for protection (**a**). A multiepitope LCP-based GAS vaccine candidate elicited protective immunity against mucosal GAS infection even in the absence of CTB (**b**)

against homologous and heterologous GAS strains, indicating its potential to provide broad coverage.

However, batch-to-batch variation led to altered immune responses, which limited its applicability for human use. The vaccine also required the addition of an adjuvant to be effective, further limiting its use as a mucosal vaccine due to a lack of safe and effective mucosal adjuvants. Later, multiepitope GAS vaccine candidates were synthesized based on the LCP system that induced highly opsonic antibodies following parenteral delivery to mice [113], as well as protection against mucosal GAS infection following intranasal immunization [114] (Fig. 9.29).

Safety and Efficacy. The main concern when using large regions of the M protein in a GAS vaccine is the potential for inducing an autoimmune response due to immunological cross-reactivity with host proteins. It is therefore important to identify protective antigenic determinants and to separate the biological relevant epitopes from those that are host tissue cross-reactive and potentially harmful. Epitope mapping studies were used to identify the conserved GAS vaccine candidate J8, which contains a conformational protective B cell epitope and was designed to lack a human heart cross-reactive T cell epitope [115, 116].

References

1. Rodrigo Ferracine, R., Rogério Silva, R., Fabiani Gai, F., Frederico Gonzalez Colombo, A., Gaziola de la Torre, L., Celio Lopes, S.: TB vaccines – state of the art and progresses. In: Matthias, G. (ed.) Molecular Vaccines – From Prophylaxis to Therapy, vol. 2. Springer, Wien (2013)
2. Giese, M.: DNA-antiviral vaccines: new developments and approaches – a review. Virus Genes **17**, 219–232 (1998)
3. Davis, B.S., et al.: West Nile virus recombinant DNA vaccine protects mouse and horse from virus challenge and expresses in vitro a noninfectious recombinant antigen that can be used in enzyme-linked immunosorbent assays. J. Virol. **75**, 4040–4047 (2001). doi:10.1128/JVI.75.9.4040-4047.2001
4. Giese, M., et al.: Stable and long-lasting immune response in horses after DNA vaccination against equine arteritis virus. Virus Genes **25**, 159–167 (2002)
5. Liao, J.C., et al.: Vaccination with human tyrosinase DNA induces antibody responses in dogs with advanced melanoma. Cancer Immun. **6**, 8 (2006)
6. Saksida, S.M.: Infectious haematopoietic necrosis epidemic (2001 to 2003) in farmed Atlantic salmon Salmo salar in British Columbia. Dis. Aquat. Organ. **72**, 213–223 (2006). doi:10.3354/dao072213
7. Traxler, G.S., et al.: Naked DNA vaccination of Atlantic salmon Salmo salar against IHNV. Dis. Aquat. Organ. **38**, 183–190 (1999). doi:10.3354/dao038183
8. Garver, K.A., LaPatra, S.E., Kurath, G.: Efficacy of an infectious hematopoietic necrosis (IHN) virus DNA vaccine in Chinook Oncorhynchus tshawytscha and sockeye O. nerka salmon. Dis. Aquat. Organ. **64**, 13–22 (2005). doi:10.3354/dao064013
9. Garibaldi, L.A., et al.: Wild pollinators enhance fruit set of crops regardless of honey bee abundance. Science (2013). doi:10.1126/science.1230200
10. Cox-Foster, D.L., et al.: A metagenomic survey of microbes in honey bee colony collapse disorder. Science **318**, 283–287 (2007). doi:10.1126/science.1146498
11. Vanengelsdorp, D., et al.: Colony collapse disorder: a descriptive study. PLoS One **4**, e6481 (2009). doi:10.1371/journal.pone.0006481
12. Garrido, C., Rosenkranz, P.: The reproductive program of female Varroa destructor mites is triggered by its host, Apis mellifera. Exp. Appl. Acarol. **31**, 269–273 (2003)
13. Maggi, M., et al.: Brood cell size of Apis mellifera modifies the reproductive behavior of Varroa destructor. Exp. Appl. Acarol. **50**, 269–279 (2010). doi:10.1007/s10493-009-9314-7
14. Bowen-Walker, P.L., Martin, S.J., Gunn, A.: The transmission of deformed wing virus between honeybees (Apis mellifera L.) by the ectoparasitic mite varroa jacobsoni Oud. J. Invertebr. Pathol. **73**, 101–106 (1999). doi:10.1006/jipa.1998.4807
15. Benjeddou, M., Leat, N., Allsopp, M., Davison, S.: Detection of acute bee paralysis virus and black queen cell virus from honeybees by reverse transcriptase pcr. Appl. Environ. Microbiol. **67**, 2384–2387 (2001). doi:10.1128/AEM.67.5.2384-2387.2001
16. Di Prisco, G., et al.: Varroa destructor is an effective vector of Israeli acute paralysis virus in the honeybee, Apis mellifera. J. Gen. Virol. **92**, 151–155 (2011). doi:10.1099/vir.0.023853-0
17. Chen, Y.P., Pettis, J.S., Collins, A., Feldlaufer, M.F.: Prevalence and transmission of honeybee viruses. Appl. Environ. Microbiol. **72**, 606–611 (2006). doi:10.1128/AEM.72.1.606-611.2006
18. Mondet, F., Goodwin, M., Mercer, A.: Age-related changes in the behavioural response of honeybees to Apiguard(R), a thymol-based treatment used to control the mite Varroa destructor. J. Comp. Physiol. A Neuroethol. Sens. Neural Behav. Physiol. **197**, 1055–1062 (2011). doi:10.1007/s00359-011-0666-1
19. Hoffmann, J.A.: The immune response of Drosophila. Nature **426**, 33–38 (2003). doi:10.1038/nature02021
20. Williams, M.J.: Drosophila hemopoiesis and cellular immunity. J. Immunol. **178**, 4711–4716 (2007)
21. Honeybee Genome Sequencing, C: Insights into social insects from the genome of the honeybee Apis mellifera. Nature **443**, 931–949 (2006)
22. Liu, B., et al.: Structure and genetics of Shigella O antigens. FEMS Microbiol. Rev. **32**, 627–653 (2008). doi:10.1111/j.1574-6976.2008.00114.x
23. West, N.P., et al.: Optimization of virulence functions through glucosylation of Shigella LPS. Science **307**, 1313–1317 (2005). doi:10.1126/science.1108472
24. Ashkenazi, S., Levy, I., Kazaronovski, V., Samra, Z.: Growing antimicrobial resistance of Shigella isolates. J. Antimicrob. Chemother. **51**, 427–429 (2003)
25. Niyogi, S.K.: Shigellosis. J. Microbiol. **43**, 133–143 (2005)
26. Wassef, J.S., Keren, D.F., Mailloux, J.L.: Role of M cells in initial antigen uptake and in ulcer formation in the rabbit intestinal loop model of shigellosis. Infect. Immun. **57**, 858–863 (1989)
27. Zychlinsky, A., et al.: IpaB mediates macrophage apoptosis induced by Shigella flexneri. Mol. Microbiol. **11**, 619–627 (1994)
28. Schroeder, G.N., Hilbi, H.: Molecular pathogenesis of Shigella spp.: controlling host cell signaling, invasion, and death by type III secretion. Clin. Microbiol. Rev. **21**, 134–156 (2008). doi:10.1128/CMR.00032-07
29. Martino, M.C., et al.: Mucosal lymphoid infiltrate dominates colonic pathological changes in murine experimental shigellosis. J. Infect. Dis. **192**, 136–148 (2005). doi:10.1086/430740
30. Sereny, B.: Not available. Acta Microbiol. Acad. Sci. Hung. **4**, 367–376 (1957)
31. Rabbani, G.H., et al.: Development of an improved animal model of shigellosis in the adult rabbit by colonic infection with Shigella flexneri 2a. Infect. Immun. **63**, 4350–4357 (1995)

32. Shipley, S.T., et al.: A challenge model for Shigella dysenteriae 1 in cynomolgus monkeys (Macaca fascicularis). Comp. Med. **60**, 54–61 (2010)
33. Orr, N., Robin, G., Cohen, D., Arnon, R., Lowell, G.H.: Immunogenicity and efficacy of oral or intranasal Shigella flexneri 2a and Shigella sonnei proteosome-lipopolysaccharide vaccines in animal models. Infect. Immun. **61**, 2390–2395 (1993)
34. Orr, N., et al.: Enhancement of anti-Shigella lipopolysaccharide (LPS) response by addition of the cholera toxin B subunit to oral and intranasal proteosome-Shigella flexneri 2a LPS vaccines. Infect. Immun. **62**, 5198–5200 (1994)
35. Turbyfill, K.R., Hartman, A.B., Oaks, E.V.: Isolation and characterization of a Shigella flexneri invasin complex subunit vaccine. Infect. Immun. **68**, 6624–6632 (2000)
36. Turbyfill, K.R., Kaminski, R.W., Oaks, E.V.: Immunogenicity and efficacy of highly purified invasin complex vaccine from Shigella flexneri 2a. Vaccine **26**, 1353–1364 (2008). doi:10.1016/j.vaccine.2007.12.040
37. Oaks, E.: V. & Turbyfill, K. R. Development and evaluation of a Shigella flexneri 2a and S. sonnei bivalent invasin complex (Invaplex) vaccine. Vaccine **24**, 2290–2301 (2006). doi:10.1016/j.vaccine.2005.11.040
38. Riddle, M.S., et al.: Safety and immunogenicity of an intranasal Shigella flexneri 2a Invaplex 50 vaccine. Vaccine **29**, 7009–7019 (2011). doi:10.1016/j.vaccine.2011.07.033
39. Norton, E.B., Lawson, L.B., Freytag, L.C., Clements, J.D.: Characterization of a mutant Escherichia coli heat-labile toxin, LT(R192G/L211A), as a safe and effective oral adjuvant. Clin. Vaccine Immunol. **18**, 546–551 (2011). doi:10.1128/CVI.00538-10
40. Martinez-Becerra, F.J., et al.: Broadly protective Shigella vaccine based on type III secretion apparatus proteins. Infect. Immun. **80**, 1222–1231 (2012). doi:10.1128/IAI.06174-11
41. Pore, D., et al.: Purification and characterization of an immunogenic outer membrane protein of Shigella flexneri 2a. Vaccine **27**, 5855–5864 (2009). doi:10.1016/j.vaccine.2009.07.054
42. Pore, D., Mahata, N., Pal, A., Chakrabarti, M.K.: Outer membrane protein A (OmpA) of Shigella flexneri 2a, induces protective immune response in a mouse model. PLoS One **6**, e22663 (2011). doi:10.1371/journal.pone.0022663
43. McCosker, P.J.: Global aspects of the management and control of ticks of veterinary importance. In: Rodriguez, J. (ed.) Recent Advances in Acarology. Academic, New York (1979)
44. Jongejan, F., Uilenberg, G.: The global importance of ticks. Parasitology **129**(Suppl), S3–S14 (2004)
45. George, J.E., Pound, J.M., Davey, R.B.: Chemical control of ticks on cattle and the resistance of these parasites to acaricides. Parasitology **129**, S353–S366 (2004)
46. Foil, L.D., Coleman, P., Eisler, M., Fragoso-Sanchez, H., Garcia-Vazquez, Z., Guerrero, F.D., Jonsson, N.N., Langstaff, I.G., Li, A.Y., et al.: Factors that influence the prevalence of acaricide resistance and tick-borne diseases. Vet. Parasitol. **125**, 163–181 (2004)
47. Willadsen, P.: The molecular revolution in the development of vaccines against ectoparasites. Vet. Parasitol. **101**, 353–368 (2001)
48. de la Fuente, J., Kocan, K.M., Almazán, C., Blouin, E.F.: RNA interference for the study and genetic manipulation of ticks. Trends Parasitol. **23**, 427–433 (2007)
49. Steen, N.A., Barker, S.C., Alewood, P.F.: Proteins in the saliva of the Ixodida (ticks): pharmacological features and biological significance. Toxicon **47**, 1–20 (2006)
50. Wang, H., Nuttall, P.A.: Comparison of the proteins in salivary glands, saliva and haemolymph of *Rhipicephalus appendiculatus* female ticks during feeding. Parasitology **109**(Pt 4), 517–523 (1994)
51. Wang, H., Nuttall, P.A.: Immunoglobulin-binding proteins in ticks: new target for vaccine development against a blood-feeding parasite. Cell. Mol. Life Sci. **56**, 286–295 (1999)
52. Jasinskas, A., Jaworski, D.C., Barbour, A.G.: *Amblyomma americanum*: specific uptake of immunoglobulins into tick hemolymph during feeding. Exp. Parasitol. **96**, 213–221 (2000)
53. Peconick, A.P., Sossai, S., Girão, F.A., Rodrigues, M.Q., Souza, E.S., Guzman, Q.F., Patarroyo, V.A.M., Vargas, M.I., Patarroyo, J.H.: Synthetic vaccine (SBm7462) against the cattle tick *Rhipicephalus (Boophilus) microplus*: preservation of immunogenic determinants in different strains from South America. Exp. Parasitol. **119**, 37–43 (2008)
54. Azhahianambi, P., De La Fuente, J., Suryanarayana, V.V., Ghosh, S.: Cloning, expression and immunoprotective efficacy of rHaa86, the homologue of the Bm86 tick vaccine antigen, from *Hyalomma anatolicum anatolicum*. Parasite Immunol. **31**, 111–122 (2009)
55. Kamau, L., Skilton, R.A., Odongo, D.O., Mwaura, S., Githaka, N., Kanduma, E., Obura, M., Kabiru, E., Orago, A., et al.: Differential transcription of two highly divergent gut-expressed Bm86 antigen gene homologues in the tick *Rhipicephalus appendiculatus* (Acari: Ixodida). Insect Mol. Biol. **20**, 105–114 (2011)
56. Rand, K.N., Moore, T., Sriskantha, A., Spring, K., Tellam, R., Willadsen, P., Cobon, G.S.: Cloning and expression of a protective antigen from the cattle tick *Boophilus microplus*. Proc. Natl. Acad. Sci. U. S. A. **86**, 9657–9661 (1989)
57. Cunha, R.C., et al.: Bovine immunoprotection against Rhipicephalus (Boophilus) microplus with recombinant Bm86-Campo Grande antigen. Rev. Bras. Parasitol. Vet. **21**, 254–262 (2012)
58. de la Fuente, J., Kocan, K.M., Blouin, E.F.: Tick vaccines and the transmission of tick-borne pathogens. Vet. Res. Commun. **31**(Suppl 1), 85–90 (2007)
59. de la Fuente, J., Rodríguez, M., Montero, C., Redondo, M., García-García, J.C., Méndez, L., Serrano, E., Valdés, M., Enríquez, A., et al.: Vaccination against ticks (Boophilus spp.): the experience with the Bm86-based vaccine Gavac. Genet. Anal. **15**, 143–148 (1999)
60. Pipano, E., Alekceev, E., Galker, F., Fish, L., Samish, M., Shkap, V.: Immunity against *Boophilus annulatus* induced by the Bm86 (Tick-GARD) vaccine. Exp. Appl. Acarol. **29**, 141–149 (2003)
61. Sun, W., Roland, K.L., Curtiss 3rd, R.: Developing live vaccines against plague. J. Infect. Dev. Ctries. **5**, 614–627 (2011)
62. Perry, R.D., Fetherston, J.D.: Yersinia pestis--etiologic agent of plague. Clin. Microbiol. Rev. **10**, 35–66 (1997)
63. Straley, S.C., Starnbach, M.N.: Yersinia: Strategies That Thwart Immune Defenses, pp. 71–92. Lippincott Williams & Wilkins, Philadelphia (2000)
64. Poland, J. D. a. A. M. B.: Plague. In: CRC Handbook Series in Zoonoses. Section A. Bacterial, Rickettsial, Chlamydial and Mycotic Diseases, vol. I, pp. 515–559. CRC Press, Boca Raton, Florida, USA (1979)
65. Wells, J.M., Mercenier, A.: Mucosal delivery of therapeutic and prophylactic molecules using lactic acid bacteria. Nat. Rev. Microbiol. **6**, 349–362 (2008). doi:10.1038/nrmicro1840
66. Peters, C., Peng, X., Douven, D., Pan, Z.K., Paterson, Y.: The induction of HIV Gag-specific CD8+ T cells in the spleen and gut-associated lymphoid tissue by parenteral or mucosal immunization with recombinant Listeria monocytogenes HIV Gag. J. Immunol. **170**, 5176–5187 (2003)
67. Lee, J.S., et al.: Mucosal immunization with surface-displayed severe acute respiratory syndrome coronavirus spike protein on Lactobacillus casei induces neutralizing antibodies in mice. J. Virol. **80**, 4079–4087 (2006). doi:10.1128/JVI.80.8.4079-4087.2006
68. Bermudez-Humaran, L.G., Kharrat, P., Chatel, J.M., Langella, P.: Lactococci and lactobacilli as mucosal delivery vectors for therapeutic proteins and DNA vaccines. Microb. Cell Fact. **10**(Suppl 1), S4 (2011). doi:10.1186/1475-2859-10-S1-S4
69. Rescigno, M., et al.: Dendritic cells express tight junction proteins and penetrate gut epithelial monolayers to sample bacteria. Nat. Immunol. **2**, 361–367 (2001). doi:10.1038/86373

70. Grangette, C., et al.: Protection against tetanus toxin after intragastric administration of two recombinant lactic acid bacteria: impact of strain viability and in vivo persistence. Vaccine **20**, 3304–3309 (2002)
71. Christensen, H.R., Frokiaer, H., Pestka, J.J.: Lactobacilli differentially modulate expression of cytokines and maturation surface markers in murine dendritic cells. J. Immunol. **168**, 171–178 (2002)
72. Kalina, W.V., Mohamadzadeh, M.: Lactobacilli as natural enhancer of cellular immune response. Discov. Med. **5**, 199–203 (2005)
73. Mohamadzadeh, M., et al.: Lactobacilli activate human dendritic cells that skew T cells toward T helper 1 polarization. Proc. Natl. Acad. Sci. U. S. A. **102**, 2880–2885 (2005). doi:10.1073/pnas.0500098102
74. Maassen, C.B., et al.: Instruments for oral disease-intervention strategies: recombinant Lactobacillus casei expressing tetanus toxin fragment C for vaccination or myelin proteins for oral tolerance induction in multiple sclerosis. Vaccine **17**, 2117–2128 (1999)
75. Navarre, W.W., Schneewind, O.: Surface proteins of gram-positive bacteria and mechanisms of their targeting to the cell wall envelope. Microbiol. Mol. Biol. Rev.: MMBR **63**, 174–229 (1999)
76. Sellati, T.J., et al.: Treponema pallidum and Borrelia burgdorferi lipoproteins and synthetic lipopeptides activate monocytic cells via a CD14-dependent pathway distinct from that used by lipopolysaccharide. J. Immunol. **160**, 5455–5464 (1998)
77. del Rio, B., Seegers, J.F., Gomes-Solecki, M.: Immune response to Lactobacillus plantarum expressing Borrelia burgdorferi OspA is modulated by the lipid modification of the antigen. PLoS One **5**, e11199 (2010). doi:10.1371/journal.pone.0011199
78. Clark, B., McKendrick, M.: A review of viral gastroenteritis. Curr. Opin. Infect. Dis. **17**, 461–469 (2004)
79. Patel, M.M., Hall, A.J., Vinje, J., Parashar, U.D.: Noroviruses: a comprehensive review. J. Clin. Virol. **44**, 1–8 (2009)
80. Dolin, R., et al.: Biological properties of Norwalk agent of acute infectious nonbacterial gastroenteritis. Proc. Soc. Exp. Biol. Med. **140**, 578–583 (1972)
81. Zheng, D.P., et al.: Norovirus classification and proposed strain nomenclature. Virology **346**, 312–323 (2006)
82. Lindesmith, L.C., et al.: Mechanisms of GII.4 norovirus persistence in human populations. PLoS Med. **5**, e31 (2008)
83. Jiang, X., Wang, M., Wang, K., Estes, M.K.: Sequence and genomic organization of Norwalk virus. Virology **195**, 51–61 (1993)
84. Jiang, X., Graham, D.Y., Wang, K.N., Estes, M.K.: Norwalk virus genome cloning and characterization. Science **250**, 1580–1583 (1990)
85. Gallimore, C.I., et al.: Methods for the detection and characterisation of noroviruses associated with outbreaks of gastroenteritis: outbreaks occurring in the north-west of England during two norovirus seasons. J. Med. Virol. **73**, 280–288 (2004)
86. Gray, J.J., et al.: European multicenter evaluation of commercial enzyme immunoassays. Clin. Vaccine Immunol. **14**(10), 1349–55 (2007)
87. Lindesmith, L., et al.: Human susceptibility and resistance to Norwalk virus infection. Nat. Med. **9**, 548–553 (2003)
88. Fehr, T., Skrastina, D., Pumpens, P., Zinkernagel, R.M.: T cell-independent type I antibody response against B cell epitopes expressed repetitively on recombinant virus particles. Proc. Natl. Acad. Sci. U. S. A. **95**, 9477–9481 (1998)
89. Prasad, B.V., Rothnagel, R., Jiang, X., Estes, M.K.: Three-dimensional structure of baculovirus-expressed Norwalk virus capsids. J. Virol. **68**, 5117–5125 (1994)
90. Baric, R.S., et al.: Expression and self-assembly of norwalk virus capsid protein from venezuelan equine encephalitis virus replicons. J. Virol. **76**, 3023–3030 (2002)
91. Ausar, S.F., Foubert, T.R., Hudson, M.H., Vedvick, T.S., Middaugh, C.R.: Conformational stability and disassembly of norwalk virus like particles: Effect of pH and temperature. J. Biol. Chem. **281**, 19478–19488 (2006). doi:10.1074/jbc.M603313200
92. Prasad, B.V.V., Hardy, D., Estes, M.: Structural studies of recombinant Norwalk capsids. J. Infect. Dis. **181**, S317–S321 (2000). doi:10.1086/315576
93. Tan, M., Zhong, W., Song, D., Thornton, S., Jiang, X.: E. coli-expressed recombinant norovirus capsid proteins maintain authentic antigenicity and receptor binding capability. J. Med. Virol. **74**, 641–649 (2004)
94. Tan, M., Meller, J., Jiang, X.: C-terminal arginine cluster is essential for receptor binding of norovirus capsid protein. J. Virol. **80**, 7322–7331 (2006)
95. Cao, S., et al.: Structural basis for the recognition of blood group trisaccharides by norovirus. J. Virol. **81**, 5949–5957 (2007)
96. Cunningham, M.W.: Pathogenesis of group A streptococcal infections. Clin. Microbiol. Rev. **13**, 470–511 (2000)
97. Bisno A. L.Group: A streptococcal infections and acute rheumatic fever. N. Engl. J. Med. **325**, 783–793 (1994)
98. Dale, J.B., Beachey, E.H.: Multiple cross reactive epitopes of streptococcal M proteins. J. Exp. Med. **161**, 113–122 (1985)
99. Fischetti, V.A.: Streptococcal M protein: Molecular design and biological behavior. Clin. Microbiol. Rev. **2**, 285–314 (1989)
100. Dale, J.B., Beachey, E.H.: Localization of protective epitopes of the amino terminus of type 5 streptococcal M protein. J. Exp. Med. **163**, 1191–1202 (1986)
101. Olive, C., Moyle, P.M., Toth, I.: Towards the development of a broadly protective group a streptococcal vaccine based on the Lipid-Core Peptide system. Curr. Med. Chem. **14**, 2976–2988 (2007)
102. Hu, M.C., Walls, M.A., Stroop, S.D., Reddish, M.A., Beaull, B., Dale, J.B.: Immunogenicity of a 26-valent group A streptococcal vaccine. Infect. Immun. **70**, 2171–2177 (2002)
103. Dale, J.B., Penfound, T.A., Chiang, E.Y., Walton, W.J.: New 30-valent M protein-based vaccine evokes cross-opsonic antibodies against non-vaccine serotypes of group A streptococci. Vaccine **29**, 8175–8178 (2011)
104. Batzloff, M.R., Hayman, W.A., Davies, M.R., Zeng, M., Pruksakorn, S., Brandt, E.R., Good, M.F.: Protection against group A streptococcus by immunization with J8-diptheria toxoid: Contribution of J8- and diphtheria toxoid-specific antibodies to protection. J. Infect. Dis. **187**, 1598–1608 (2003)
105. Batzloff, M.R., Hartas, J., Zeng, W., Jackson, D.C., Good, M.F.: Intranasal vaccination with a lipopeptide containing a minimal, conformationally constrained conserved peptide, a universal T-cell epitope and a self-adjuvanting lipid protects mice from *Streptococcus pyogenes* and reduces throat carriage. J. Infect. Dis. **194**, 325–330 (2006)
106. Olive, C., et al.: Immunisation of mice with a lipid core peptide construct containing a conserved region determinant of group A streptococcal M protein elicits heterologous opsonic antibodies in the absence of adjuvant. Infect. Immun. **70**, 2734–2738 (2002)
107. Bronze, M.S., Courtney, H.S., Dale, J.B.: Epitopes of group A streptococcal M protein that evoke cross-protective local immune responses. J. Immunol. **148**, 888–893 (1992)
108. van Ginkel, F.W., Jackson, R.J., Yuki, Y., McGhee, J.R.: Cutting edge: the mucosal adjuvant cholera toxin redirects vaccine proteins into olfactory tissues. J. Immunol. **165**, 4778–4782 (2000)
109. Fischetti, V.A., Hodges, W.M., Hruby, D.E.: Protection against streptococcal pharyngeal colonization with a vaccinia: M protein recombinant. Science **244**, 1487–1490 (1989)
110. Mannam, P., Jones, K.F., Geller, B.L.: Mucosal vaccine made from live, recombinant *Lactococcus lactis* protects mice against pharyngeal infection with *Streptococcus pyogenes*. Infect. Immun. **72**, 3444–3450 (2004)

111. Kotloff, K.L., Wasserman, S.S., Jones, K.F., Livio, S., Hruby, D.E., Franke, C.A., Fischetti, V.A.: Clinical and microbiological responses of volunteers to combined intranasal and oral inoculation with a *Streptococcus gordonii* carrier strain intended for future use as a group A streptococcus vaccine. Infect. Immun. **73**, 2360–2366 (2005)
112. Brandt, E.R., et al.: New multi-determinant strategy for a group A streptococcal vaccine designed for the Australian Aboriginal population. Nat. Med. **6**, 455–459 (2000)
113. Olive, C., Ho, M.-F., Dyer, J., Lincoln, D., Barozzi, N., Toth, I., Good, M.F.: Immunization with a tetraepitopic lipid core peptide vaccine construct induces broadly protective immune responses against group A streptococcus. J. Infect. Dis. **193**, 1666–1676 (2006)
114. Olive, C., Kuo Sun, H., Ho, M.-F., Dyer, J., Horvath, A., Toth, I., Good, M.F.: Intranasal administration is an effective mucosal vaccine delivery route for self-adjuvanting lipid core peptides targeting the group A streptococcal M protein. J. Infect. Dis. **194**, 316–324 (2006)
115. Relf, W.A., et al.: Mapping a conserved conformational epitope from the M protein of group A streptococci. Pept. Res. **9**, 12–20 (1996)
116. Hayman, W.A., Brandt, E.R., Relf, W.A., Cooper, J., Saul, A., Good, M.F.: Mapping the minimal murine T cell and B cell epitopes within a peptide vaccine candidate from the conserved region of the M protein of group A streptococcus. Int. Immunol. **9**, 1723–1733 (1997)

Delivery Technologies 10

Contents

10.1 Invasive and Non-invasive Vaccine Delivery

Most vaccines are administered parenterally via the intradermal, subcutaneous, or intramuscular route, the choice largely dependent on whether the antigen is in the adsorbed or non-adsorbed state.

The major drawbacks of these classical invasive routes include pain associated with the use of syringes, the possibility for needle contamination, and the need for trained medical personnel. There is now a particular focus on the development of mucosal vaccines, designed for direct application to mucosal surfaces such as those present in the mouth and nose.

Modern delivery strategies include microspheres, liposomes, nanoparticles, and virus-like particles and are being actively investigated. The vagina and rectum are also possible sites for mucosal vaccination, but due to cultural, ethical, or religious reason, these are not accepted everywhere.

The incorporation of DNA/RNA antigens or protein and carbohydrate subunits into viral or bacterial vectors, liposomes, and virus-like particles as delivery systems offers a kind of protection for these biological sensitive products against physicochemical and enzymatic degradation resulting in vaccine inefficacy. In addition, modern delivery technologies result in an improved efficacy by immune system modulation, e.g., through sustained release and controlled longer antigen presentation.

Together with noninvasive delivery methods, vaccination practice would become safer, more acceptable, and more suitable for mass immunization. Spray-dried/freeze-dried vaccines would also avoid the need for cold chain.

Another innovative focus is the development of vaccine patches: microneedles penetrate through the stratum corneum and targets Langerhans cells (LCs), skin's dendritic cells.

10.2 Mucosal Delivery: Nasal Powder

As discussed in Chap. 3, the mucosal NALT system is an ideal target for the noninvasive delivery of vaccines.

M. Giese, *Introduction to Molecular Vaccinology*, DOI 10.1007/978-3-319-25832-4_10

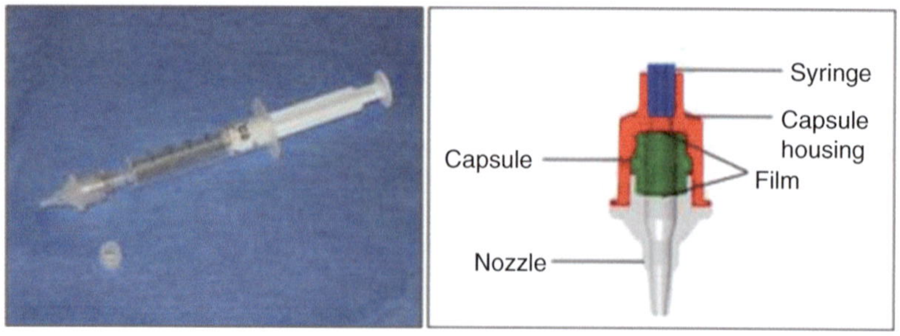

Fig. 10.1 The BD Solovent® device for nasal vaccine administration. This device depends on "burstable membranes" that rupture under syringe air pressure during use. This results in a gentle pop and the expulsion of the dose

The ciliated surfaces of the nasal turbinates deliver mucus to the floor of the nasal cavity and from there to the throat, site of the Waldeyer's ring, consisting notably of adenoids and tonsils. Mucociliary clearance disposes of ambient particulates that deposit on the nasal epithelium. Normal mucociliary clearance rates are approximately 45–90 min from the proximal to distal points in the nasopharynx. The intent of any nasal vaccine delivery system is to achieve a residence time at the nasal mucosa sufficient to elicit the desired immunological and hopefully protective response.

Nasal vaccine delivery proposes to target the nasal associated lymphoid tissue (NALT). The principle on which this approach depends is to present the selected antigen to the NALT and Waldeyer's ring and ultimately to the immunologically important M cells and dendritic cells. These cells are responsible for producing an immune response through antigen presentation to circulating lymphocytes. The Waldeyer's ring is de facto no ring but an aggregation of lymphoid tissues located at the openings of the respiratory and digestive tract.

The two most common (and effective) nasal delivery devices are either multiple- or single-dose pumps, examples of which deliver calcitonin, to treat osteoporosis, and corticosteroids, to treat allergic rhinitis, respectively. However, these FDA-approved products require solution or suspension formulations which are not the most desirable preparations for vaccines.

Dry powders produced by spray freeze drying (SFD) liquid vaccine formulations also provide a vaccine adjuvant strategy to enhance the immunogenicity of nasally delivered vaccines when compared to nasal immunization with liquid vaccine formulations. Since other studies have demonstrated that increased nasal retention of vaccine formulations correlates with increased immunogenicity of the vaccine, it is possible that dry powder vaccine formulations augment the immunogenicity of nasally delivered vaccines by increasing antigen retention in the nasal cavity to ultimately improve antigen delivery to the nasal dendritic cells for better induction of antigen-specific adaptive immunity (Fig. 10.1).

10.3 Mechanisms of Intramuscular Immunization[1]

10.3.1 The Skeletal Muscle

Skeletal muscle is the most abundant tissue of the human body. It consists of myofibers, a class of large syncytial multinuclear cells, which are terminally differentiated permanent cells. Several kinds of resident macrophages are also present within muscle tissue, and recently also monocyte-derived and conventional DCs residing in skeletal muscle before and after intramuscular (i.m.) immunization have been well characterized in mice [1].

TLRs in Muscle Tissue. Microbial proteins, lipids, carbohydrates, and nucleic acids contain common structural patterns collectively called PAMPs (pathogen-associated molecular patterns), that bind to innate immune receptors (Toll-like receptor (TLR)) present on cell surface or endosomal membrane of responding cells. The TLR family includes ten members, with different ligand specificities and differential expression among cell types.

In the last few years, evidence has been accumulating that muscle cells can respond to several kinds of such molecules and actively participate to several steps of the innate and adaptive immune responses, by expressing membrane molecules and cytokines. Stimulation of TLR2 and TLR4, in particular, induces the mRNA of the CCL2 and CXCL1 chemokines in C2C12 mouse myoblasts [2]. Similarly, the stimulation of TLR3 in cultured human myoblasts activates the transcription factor NF-κB and elicits IL-8 secretion, while the binding of unmethylated CpG dinucleotides to TLR9 triggers the release of IL-12, TNF-α, and IFN-α, critical step in cellular immune response. Characteristics of the main TLRs and their expression in muscle are summarized in Table 10.1.

[1] Why does an i.m. immunization work? by *Emanuela Bartoccioni* in Molecular Vaccines - From Prophylaxis to Therapy, Volume 2, Springer-Verlag Wien, 2013, Ed. Matthias Giese.

Table 10.1 The subcellular localization of several Toll-like receptors (TLR), their natural ligands, their synthetic agonist, and the presence in muscle are shown

	Subcellular localization	Natural ligand(s)	Synthetic agonist(s)	Expression in muscle cells	Ref.
TLR2	Plasma membrane	Lipoproteins/lipopeptides/peptidoglycan	BPPcysMPEG Pam3CSK4	Yes (not in myoblasts)	[3, 4, 8]
TLR3	Endosomes	dsRNA	Poly-IC, PolyICLC, Poly-IC_{12}-U	Yes	[7]
TLR4	Plasma membrane	LPS	MPL	Yes	[5, 8]
TLR5	Plasma membrane	Flagellin	Flagellin-antigen fusion proteins	Yes (not in myoblasts)	[8]
TLR 7/8	Endosomes	ssRNA	Imiquimod, resiquimod	?	[6]
TLR9	Endosomes	Bacterial/viral DNA	CpG oligodeoxynucleotides	Yes	[8]

10.3.2 First Trigger for Inflammation

Thus, in the context of i.m. immunization, the injury caused by the needle is by itself the first trigger for inflammation, but it is only in the presence of foreign biological molecules able to bind to TLRs that the adaptive response may begin. When DNA vaccination is used, bacterial DNA from the plasmid backbone, which includes sequence motifs like the CpG dinucleotide, may directly activate bystander cells through TLR9.

Immune Response. Vaccination with protein antigens mostly induces humoral response. Instead, DNA vaccination is able to stimulate both kinds of response because injected plasmid DNA may induce both extracellular and/or intracellular antigen expression (Figs. 10.2 and 10.3). Injected plasmid DNA may enter muscle cells as well as resident professional antigen-presenting cells (APCs), like macrophages and DC. Whichever the producing cells, the protein antigen, if secreted, may induce the normal humoral response (like an extracellular microbe).

In particular, transfected APC may present the antigen to CTL through two distinct routes: either directly, through MHC class I molecules as any other endogenous protein, or

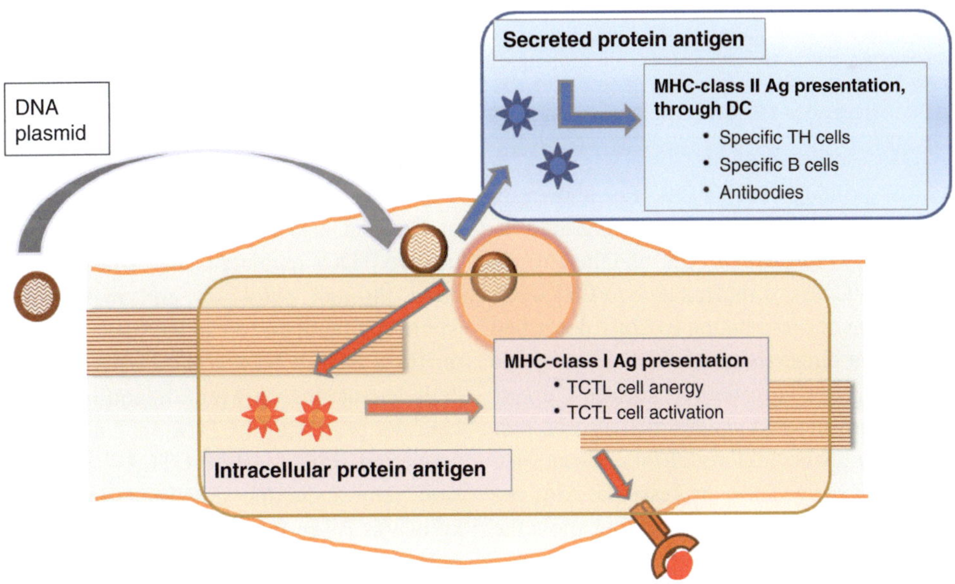

Fig. 10.2 Expression of plasmid DNA-encoded antigens in muscle fibers. Different potential outcomes for DNA-driven antigen expression in muscle cells are depicted. Secretory proteins (i.e., proteins harboring a signal peptide) are released in the extracellular space, where they behave as soluble antigens; thus, they can be taken up by DC and presented through the MHC II route, leading to CD4+ T cell activation and antibody production by B cells. Not secreted proteins (*red pathway*) enter the MHC I route, and their surface exposure can elicit either CD8+ T cell anergy or activation, based on the concurrent expression of co-stimulatory molecules as induced by an inflammatory microenvironment. Note that presentation of secretory proteins through the MHC I route can also occur (not shown)

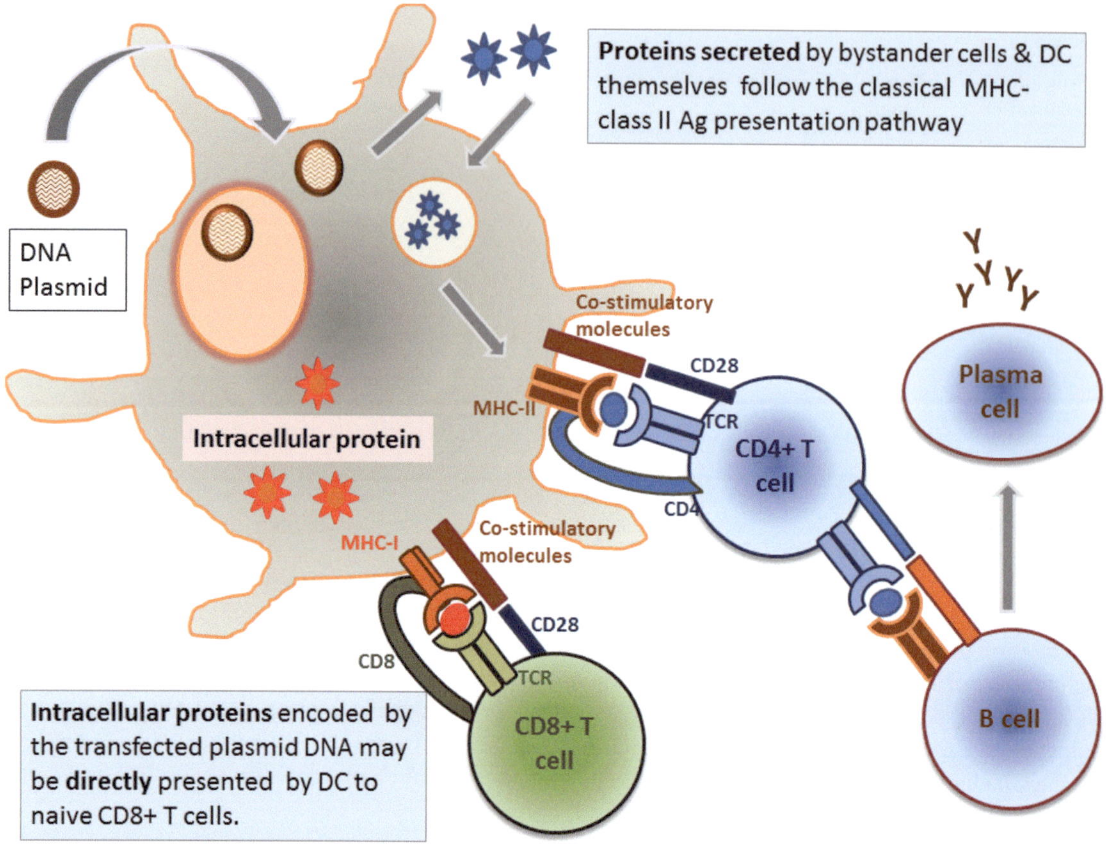

Fig. 10.3 Central role of professional APCs in DNA vaccination. APC (dendritic cells) are also targeted by injected DNA and express DNA-encoded antigens. Proteins secreted by DC and by surrounding cells (muscle fibers, stromal cells) are taken up and exposed for presentation to CD4+ T cells through the MHC II route. Intracellular protein antigens ("pseudoinfection") are presented through the MHC I route to naive CD8+ T lymphocytes. Successful antigen-specific priming of both CD4+ and CD8+ T cells requires the presence of co-stimulatory molecules (B7-1, B7-2) expressed at the surface of professional APC and co-engaged with MHC molecules by T cell receptors co-receptors (TCR and CD28, respectively). This complex and highly specialized multimolecular contact between APC and T lymphocytes has been named, by analogy with connections between neuronal cells, "immunological synapse." The interaction between B and T cells is also depicted. B cells express MCH II and co-stimulatory molecules and can present secreted antigens (once recognized and captured through the BCR) to T cells. Contact with T helper lymphocytes fully primes B cells for antibody production (T cell-dependent response)

by a so-called cross-priming mechanism, (as shown in Fig. 2.7) whereby muscle cell fragments containing the protein would be taken up by professional APC and the antigen presented – through MHC class I molecules – to CTL cells (Fig. 10.4). Another form of presentation recently described may be mediated by the direct transfer of MCH I-peptide complexes from bystander cells to the DC surface ("cross-dressing") [9]. Moreover, captured antigen will also be presented to T helper (Th) lymphocytes through the conventional MCH-class II-dependent route. These professional APC are DCs that migrate to draining lymph nodes, to bring about the adaptive immune process.

10.3.3 Dendritic Cells as Professional APC

Dendritic cells, when activated by foreign antigens via the TLR, start an adaptive immune response to these antigens. The kind of immune response initiated depends on the type of DC and also on the particular innate immune signals received. DCs regulate CD4+ T-helper (Th)-cell differentiation through cytokines and membrane B7 molecules. There is a family of these molecules, with different characteristics. Both B7-1 and B7-2 activate or suppress CD4+ T cells, depending on which ligand is expressed on CD4+ T cell: the presence of CD28 on T cells is able to transduce activating signals, while CTLA-4 induces T cell suppression. The inducible co-stimulator ligand (ICOSL, also known as B7-h, B7-H2) stimulates not only the effector or memory T cell responses but also the generation of regulatory T (Treg) cells.

It is well established that in response to intracellular microbes, Th cells may differentiate into Th1 cells, required for the generation of memory CD8+ T cells, or into Th2 cells in response to extracellular microbes. This different polarization is function of the different set of cytokines produced

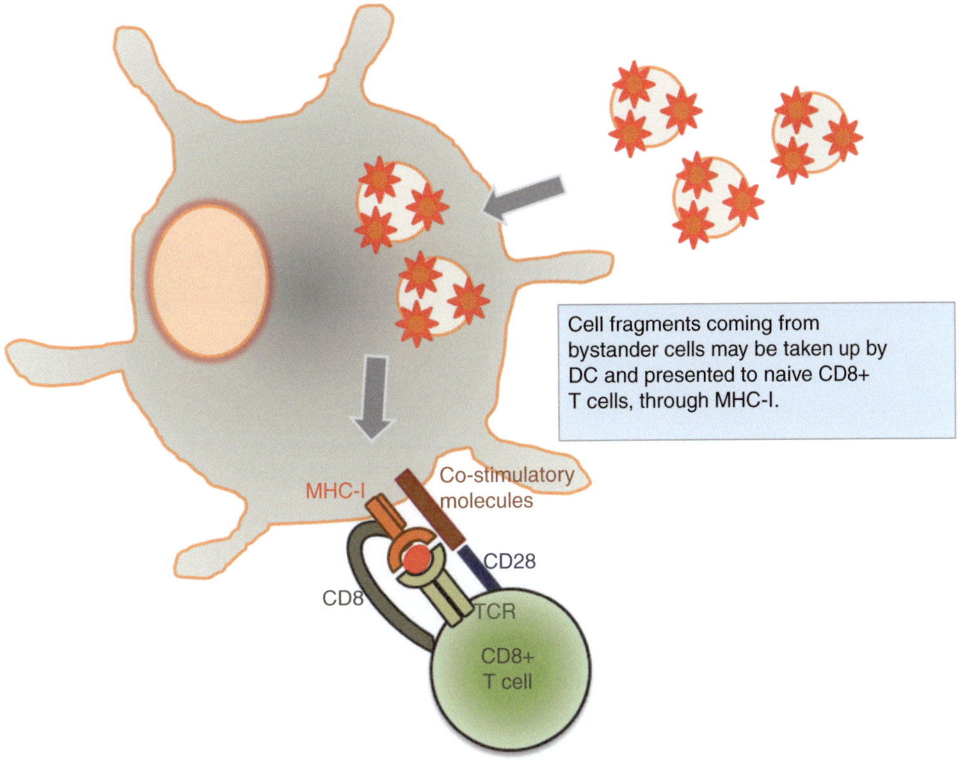

Fig. 10.4 Cross-presentation by dendritic cells. DCs can prime CD8+ cells, other than with endogenous antigens (including those encoded by transfected DNA), also with exogenous antigens taken up as part of cell fragments or microvesicles or from surrounding cells. This modality of antigen presentation, called "cross-presentation," involves the intracellular processing of the antigen. Cross-priming describes the stimulation of naive cytotoxic CD8$^+$ T cells by this process

by DC that in turn reflect the different TLR-mediated innate signal received from the pathogen.

Immature DCs are present into the tissues under steady-state conditions, while TLR agonists stimulate their maturation and promote their migration to draining lymph nodes.

Immature and mature DCs are characterized by different sets of membrane molecules, like MHC class II and B7 family molecules and chemokine receptors. There are two major DC subsets: myeloid (or conventional or classical) DC and plasmacytoid DC, which are not completely overlapping in mouse and man. Recently, human CD141+ DCs have been identified as the human counterpart of mouse CD8+ DCs; they are particularly interesting as being able to capture exogenous antigens and present them through MHC class I molecules (cross-presentation) to CD8+ CTL cells.

A recent interesting study on the characterization of dendritic cells present within the mouse muscle during i.m. immunization has shown that large numbers of resident interstitial DC were able to capture Ag in the muscle, migrate to draining LN, and efficiently activate naive T cells (Fig. 10.5), while DC arising from blood monocytes achieved these abilities largely only after the addition of LPS to sterile alum-adjuvanted antigen.

10.3.4 Muscle Cells as Non-professional APC

Even if transfected DCs play a dominant role in DNA vaccine-mediated immunity, they account for only a part of the total induced response, with local nonprofessional APC having a significant role in adaptive immune response.

Muscle cells are able to actively participate in the induction of immunity and to behave as non-professional APC. Muscle cells express receptors for cytokines and PAMPs that enable them to respond to an inflammatory *milieu*, by secreting cytokines and chemokines and expressing adhesion molecules [10]. In particular, some membrane protein necessary to the APC function, like class I and class II MHC molecules and co-stimulatory molecules, have been observed in several experimental systems [11, 12]. Importantly, following plasmid transfection, muscle cells express several molecules necessary to antigen presentation such as MHC class I and co-stimulatory molecules like BB-1

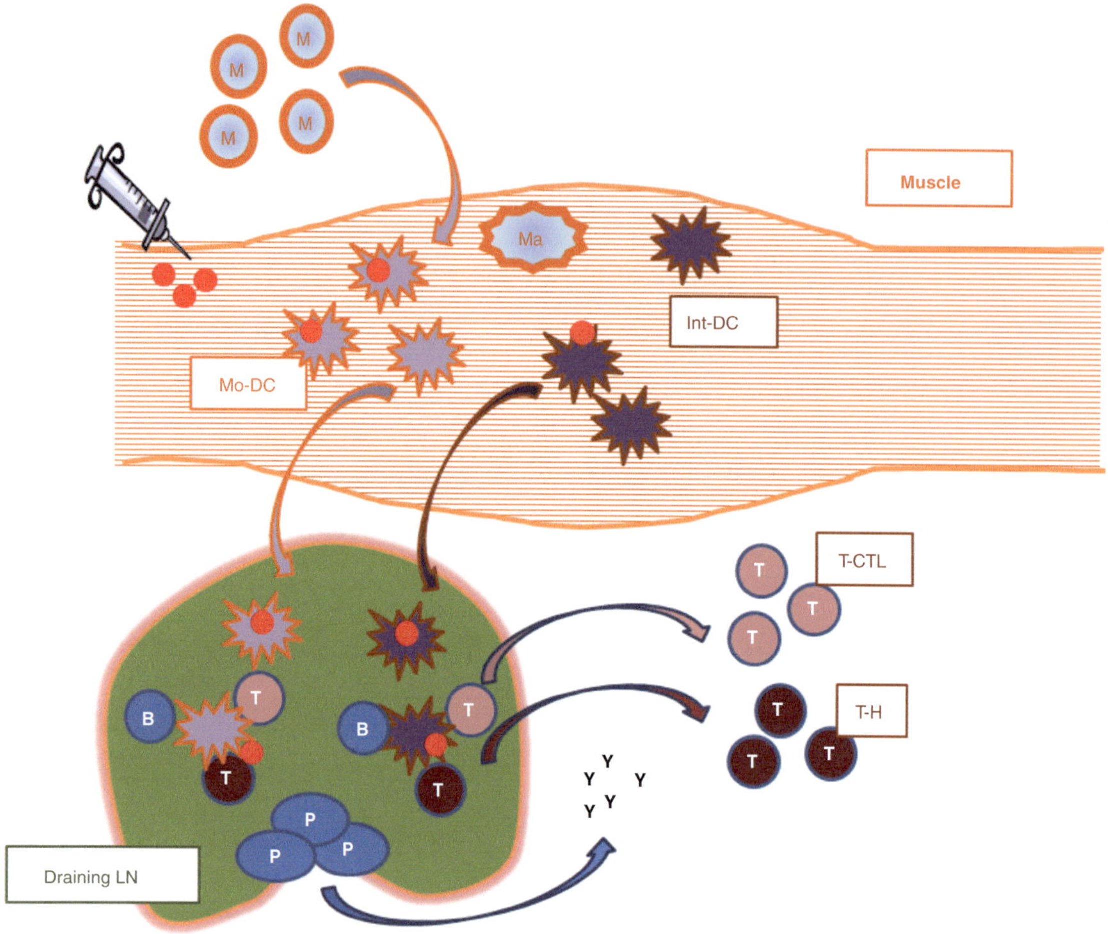

Fig. 10.5 Different classes of DCs involved in muscle response to injected antigens. Muscle contains interstitial/resident dendritic cells (*Int-DC*) that monitor the immunological status of the tissue and transport injected antigens to lymph nodes (*draining LN*) in order to activate specific B- and T cell response. Of note, mobilization of resident DC requires also the presence of inflammatory stimuli (LPS, adjuvants?); another class of DCs differentiates from monocytes (*M*) that migrate to muscle in the context of inflammatory response (*Mo-DC*), capture the antigen, and transport it to LN to fulfill APC duties. These different classes of muscle DC have just begun to be molecularly characterized. B cell-derived plasma cell (*P*) secreting antibodies (*Y*) are depicted. Macrophages (*Ma*) may derive from monocytes or be resident

and B7-1, gaining the ability to present immunogenic DNA-encoded antigens to CTL cells [13].

The idea that muscle fibers act as APC faces a number of important problems:

- First, muscle cells expressing new antigen proteins should appear to the immune system like infected "different" cells and be destroyed by the same cytotoxic specific T cells they induce: however, muscle fibers are large syncytial post-mitotic cells that are unlikely to undergo immune killing by lymphocytes, as it is also suggested by evidence that antigens transfected by DNA electrotransfer extensively diffuse in muscle tissue and are still expressed after 9 months, thus confirming long-term survival of producing cells.
- Second, although antigen production by muscle cells seems to be durable, the APC function conferred by DNA transfection is expected to be transient in nature, due to the extinction of the inflammatory activity that accompanies DNA transfer (see above). Nevertheless, a variety of model systems has shown that both memory T and B cells can persist in the absence of the antigen, ensuring the effectiveness of vaccination even in the absence of active antigen presentation.
- Third, antigen-presenting muscle cells may induce tolerance instead of immunity.

Tolerance. Thus appears that the skeletal muscle may be easily manipulated to express many immunologically relevant molecules, and this makes it a promising target for DNA vaccination. However, the immune system is able to induce tolerance at the level of this tissue, as appears from the rarity of autoimmune diseases directed against the muscle. Understanding the mechanisms involved in the induction and maintenance of immune tolerance, as well as anergy (a state of unresponsiveness to antigen), is essential to efficiently address i.m. vaccination.

In general, in non-inflammatory conditions, the expression of neoantigens could induce tolerance instead of immunity. This may be the case in which the antigen is expressed in transgenic animals.

Very recently, it has been shown that immunological tolerance to muscle autoantigens involves peripheral deletion of autoreactive CD8+ CTL cells [14].

In this model, transgenic mice expressed a membrane-bound form of ovalbumin (OVA) neoantigen specifically in skeletal muscle (SM-OVA). In these animals, there were no signs of autoimmunity, but the immunization with OVA protein induced CD4+-dependent response and anti-OVA IgG antibody production, indicating that OVA-specific CD4+ cells where present in OVA mice and where not intrinsically tolerant to OVA, but simply ignored the antigen unless presented in the appropriate inflammatory context. Conversely, when immunization with vesicular stomatitis virus encoding OVA (VSV-OVA) was used to elicit an OVA-specific CTL response, no cytotoxic activity was observed; moreover, adoptively transferred OVA-specific CD8+ CTL cells were selectively deleted from the periphery of SM-OVA mice. This process, that is not related to regulatory T cells, probably involves both the partial T cell activation in absence of co-stimulatory molecules at the surface of APC and the inadequacy of cytokine presence in noninflammatory conditions. Interestingly, it appears that, when the antigen is permanently expressed by the myofibers, the peripheral tolerance is stronger than immune response.

10.4 Microneedle Patches[2]

Breaching the skin's *stratum corneum* barrier raises the possibility of administration of vaccines, gene vectors, antibodies, photosensitizers, and even nanoparticles, all of which have at least their initial effect on populations of skin cells. Intradermal vaccine delivery, in particular, holds enormous potential for improved therapeutic outcomes for patients, particularly those in the developing world.

The majority of vaccines are delivered either into subcutaneous fat or muscle. Delivery vaccines into the dermis are rare [15], and even topical or transcutaneous applications to the surface of the skin [16, 17], also termed *epicutaneous application* [17], are rarer still. The above routes of application are each effective only because of the ability of dendritic cells (DCs) to uptake, process, and present the antigen to T lymphocytes in the draining lymphoid organs.

[2]Vaccine delivery using microneedles by *Ryan F. Donnelly, Sharifa Al-Zahrani, Marija Zaric, Cian M. McCrudden, Cristopher J. Scott, and Adrien Kissenpfenning* in Molecular Vaccines - From Prophylaxis to Therapy, Volume 2, Springer-Verlag Wien, 2013, Ed. Matthias Giese.

Whereas subcutaneous fat and muscle tissue contain relatively few DCs, the dermis and the epidermis are densely populated by different subsets of DCs. Consequently, antigen delivery by hypodermic injection will bypass the skin's immune cells leading to less efficient vaccination. For this reason, the skin represents an ideal site for vaccine delivery, as vaccination at this site will evoke strong immune responses at much lower doses of antigen than intramuscular vaccines [18].

The potential of skin immunization was observed in a clinical trial where epidermal influenza vaccination induced influenza-specific CD8 T cell response, while classical intramuscular route did not [19]. Dose-sparing approaches are critical to ensuring a sufficient supply of certain vaccines, especially in pandemic diseases [20].

10.4.1 Skin Structure and Function

As the largest and one of the most complex organs in the human body, the skin (Fig. 10.6) is responsible for a varied range of functions. The barrier properties of the skin afford protection against physical, microbial, or chemical invasions. The skin is made up of three layers: the epidermis, dermis, and subcutaneous tissue. The epidermis consists of the viable epidermis and the *stratum corneum*. The viable epidermis consists of four histologically distinct layers: the *stratum germinativum, stratum spinosum, stratum granulosum,* and *stratum lucidum*. The epidermis is not of uniform thickness, varying from 60 μm on the eyelids to 800 μm on the palms. The layers of the epidermis are avascular and receive nutrients by diffusion of substances from the underlying dermal capillaries.

The dermis (or corium) resides atop the subcutaneous fat layer and is approximately 2–4 mm thick and consists of a mucopolysaccharide matrix within which exists a network of elastin and collagen fibers, providing both elasticity and structure to the skin. The dermis is maintained physiologically by a network of nerve endings, lymphatics, and blood vessels. The cutaneous blood supply delivers nutrients and oxygen to the skin and allows waste products to be removed. Beneath the dermis lies the subcutaneous fat layer, subcutis, subdermis, or hypodermis. The hypodermis, consisting mainly of adipose tissue, acts as an insulator (due to the high content of adipose tissue), as well as supporting the dermis and epidermis physically and nutritionally. The hypodermis also carries the main blood vessels and nerves to the skin and may contain sensory organs. Resting beneath the vascular dermis, the role of the hypodermis in drug delivery is not considered to be major [21].

The *stratum corneum*, or horny layer, is the outermost layer of the epidermis, and thus the skin. It has now well accepted that this layer constitutes the principal barrier for penetration of most drugs. The horny layer represents the final stage of epidermal cell differentiation. The thickness of this layer is typically 10 μm, but a number of factors, including the degree of hydration and

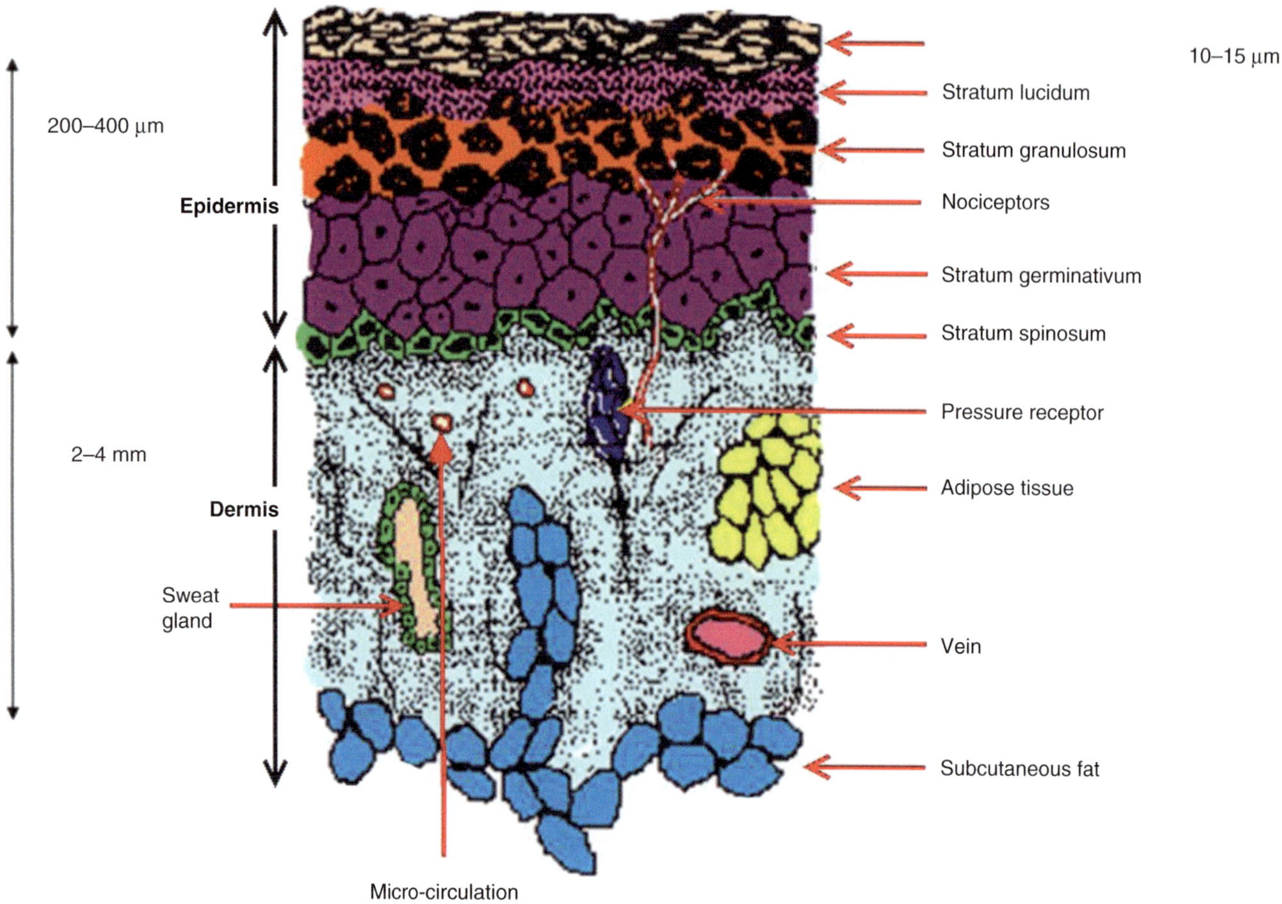

Fig. 10.6 Diagrammatic representation of the major features of skin anatomy

skin location, influence this. For example, the stratum corneum on the palms and soles can be, on average, 400–600 μm thick while hydration can result in a fourfold increase in thickness.

The stratum corneum consists of 10–25 rows of dead keratinocytes, now called corneocytes, embedded in the secreted lipids from lamellar bodies. The corneocytes are flattened, elongated, dead cells, lacking nuclei and other organelles. The cells are joined together by desmosomes, maintaining the cohesiveness of this layer. The heterogeneous structure of the *stratum corneum* is composed of approximately 75–80 % protein, 5–15 % lipid, and 5–10 % other substances on a dry weight basis.

The majority of protein present in the stratum corneum is keratin and is located within the corneocytes. The keratins are a family of α-helical polypeptides. Individual molecules aggregate to form filaments (7–10 nm diameter and many microns in length) that are stabilized by insoluble disulfide bridges. These filaments are thought to be responsible for the hexagonal shape of the corneocyte and provide mechanical strength for the stratum corneum. Corneocytes possess a protein-rich envelope around the periphery of the cell, formed from precursors, such as involucrin, loricrin, and cornifin. Transglutaminases catalyze the formation of γ-glutamyl cross-links between the envelope proteins that render the envelope resistant and highly insoluble. The protein envelope links the corneocyte to the surrounding lipid-enriched matrix.

The main lipids located in the *stratum corneum* are ceramides, fatty acids, cholesterol, cholesterol sulfate, and sterol/wax esters. These lipids are arranged in multiple bilayers called lamellae (Fig. 10.7). Phospholipids are largely absent, a unique feature for a mammalian membrane. The ceramides are the largest group of lipids in the stratum corneum, accounting for approximately half of the total lipid mass, and are crucial to the lipid organization of the *stratum corneum.*

The bricks and mortar model of the *stratum corneum* are a common representation of this layer. The bricks correspond to parallel plates of dead keratinized corneocytes, and the mortar represents the continuous interstitial lipid matrix. It is important to note that the corneocytes are not actually brick shaped, but rather are polygonal, elongated, and flat (0.2–1.5 μm thick and 34.0–46.0 μm in diameter). The "mortar" is not a homogenous matrix. Rather, lipids are arranged in the lamellar phase (alternating layers of water and lipid bilayers), with some of the lipid bilayers in the gel or crystalline state. The extracellular matrix is further complicated by the

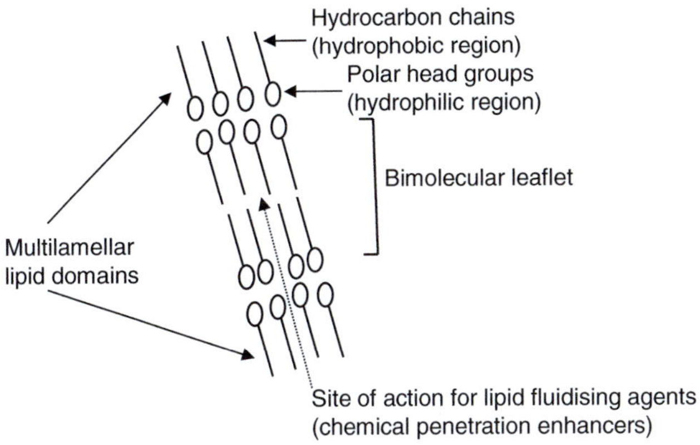

Fig. 10.7 Arrangement of lipids in the *stratum corneum*

presence of intrinsic and extrinsic proteins, such as enzymes. The barrier properties of the stratum corneum have been assigned to the multiple lipid bilayers residing in the intercellular space. These bilayers prevent desiccation of the underlying tissues by inhibiting water loss and limit the penetration of substances from the external environment.

10.4.2 Immune Function of Skin

The concept of delivery of vaccines through or into the skin has been gathering momentum in the past decade, largely due to the increasing recognition that a tight semi-contiguous network of immunoregulatory cells that reside in the different skin layers is an ideal target for vaccine administration. Dendritic cells (DCs), macrophages, and neutrophilic granulocytes are the principal phagocytes in the skin (Fig. 10.8) while numerous cells of the adaptive immune system, such are CD8+ T cells and the full spectrum of CD4+ T cells can be found in normal skin [15, 17, 22]. A detailed description of dendritic cells is provided in Chap. 2 of this book.

10.4.3 Vaccination via the Skin Using Microneedles

Intradermal (ID) vaccination using microneedles (MNs) is one of the most attractive approaches for delivering an antigen to the dermal layer of the skin without using hypodermic injections, which are associated with transmission of infec-

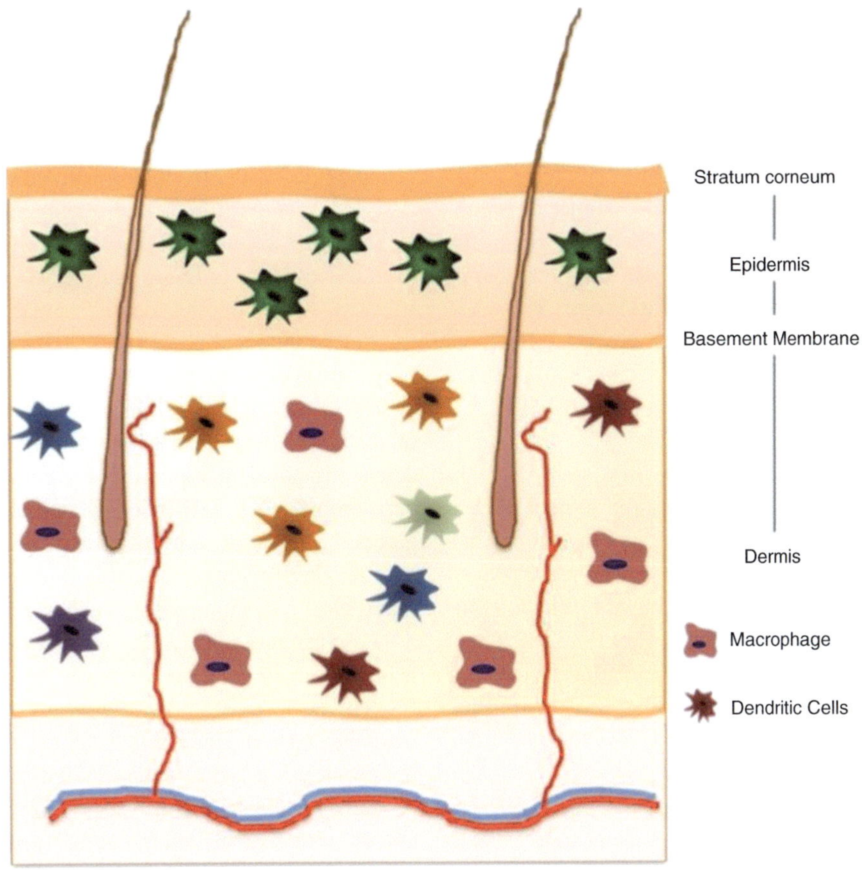

Fig. 10.8 Immune structure of skin

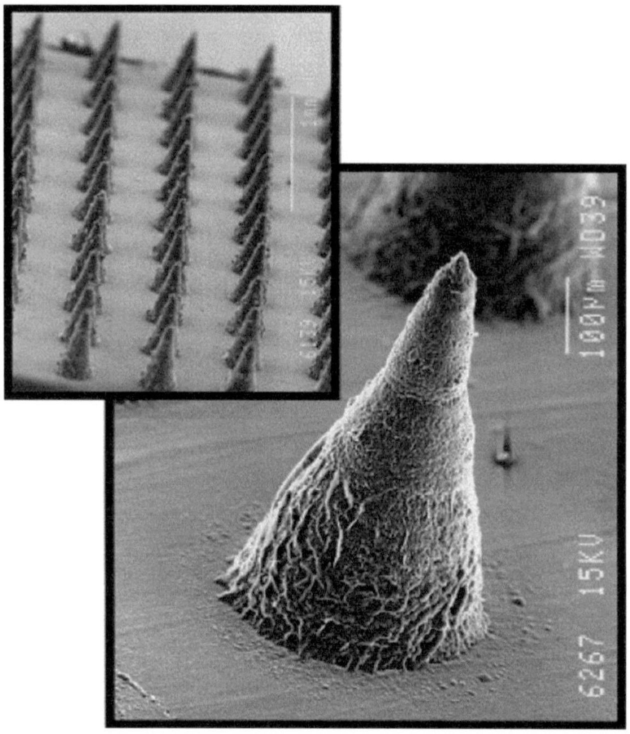

Fig. 10.9 Laser engineered, micromolded, microneedle array prepared from aqueous blends of the structure-forming copolymer poly(methylvinylether-co-maleic acid)

tion and inappropriate disposal in the developing world. MN arrays (Fig. 10.9) consist of a multiplicity of microprojections ranging from 25 to 2000 μm in height, attached to a base support [23]. These microprojections can create aqueous transport pathways at the micron scale, painlessly breaking through the *stratum corneum* barrier when the microneedles are applied to the skin surface [24]. The micropores created by MNs readily permit transport of a wide range of micromolecules and macromolecules, such as immunotherapeutic agents, including vaccines and proteins [25]. Importantly, MN insertion does not cause bleeding.

1998 and Microneedles. MNs were first described by Henry et al. in 1998 and have since been the subject of continuous research [26]. MNs are fabricated from various materials such as metals, glass, silicon, and FDA-approved polymers [27]. Donnelly et al. detail a range of methods for the development and fabrication of various MNs [28]. There are four main modes of action of MNs, which are poke and patch, coat and poke, poke and release, and poke and flow [29] (Fig. 10.10).

10.4.3.1 Poke and Patch

The poke and patch approach is based on using solid MNs to puncture the skin followed by applying antigen to the treated area in order to diffuse antigen into the skin. Substantial work using this approach has been carried out by the Bouwstra Group, where microneedles are inserted into the skin in order to increase its permeability, after which the vaccine is applied.

The Bouwstra Group, in one report, studied mouse immune responses after transcutaneous immunization (TCI) using two model antigens: diphtheria toxoid (DT) and influenza subunit vaccine [30]. Stainless steel MN arrays (16 × 300 μm MNs) were used to perforate the mouse skin followed by application of a DT formulation with or without cholera toxin (CT). The application of DT to MN-treated skin resulted in significantly higher serum IgG and toxin-neutralizing antibody titers than in unperforated skin. The presence of CT increased the immune response to similar levels as observed after subcutaneous injection of AlPO4-adsorbed DT (DT-alum). Unlike in the DT case, MN array pretreatment showed no effect on the immune response to the influenza vaccine alone. The addition of CT strongly improved the immune response, independent of MN treatment. The conclusion drawn by the authors of the study was that that TCI of DT in the presence of CT after MN treatment results in similar protection to injection of DT-alum.

A study investigated the effect of coadministration of various adjuvants with DT in the modulation of the immune response in TCI mice after the application of MN arrays [31]. Mice were treated with DT coadministered with lipopolysaccharide (LPS), Quil-A, CpG oligodeoxynucleotide (CpG), or CT as adjuvants. The MN array pretreatment group displayed high serum IgG levels, and these were remarkably improved by coadministration of adjuvants. The group treated with DT coadministered with CT showed similar IgG levels to those treated subcutaneously with DT-alum. N-Trimethyl chitosan also proved beneficial in boosting the immune response to DT following MN pretreatment when in solution with the antigen, although no improvement in immune response was seen from DT-loaded nanoparticles of N-trimethyl chitosan [32].

The impact of transdermal vaccination on the development of melanoma was reported by Bhowmik et al. (2011), who delivered a novel microparticulate vaccine to the skin following puncture using of MN-based Dermaroller® [33]. Mice were grouped into four groups: group one was treated using Dermaroller® microneedles, followed by application of microparticles containing encapsulated antigen obtained from S-91 melanoma cancer cells. Group two was injected subcutaneously with the same dose of microparticles containing encapsulated vaccine. Group three was given blank microparticles administered in the same way as for the transdermal group. The last group was injected with saline subcutaneously.

Eight weeks following vaccination, the mice were challenged with live melanoma cells. In the group which was treated using Dermaroller® MNs and SC injection of vaccine, there was no measurable tumor growth 35 days after

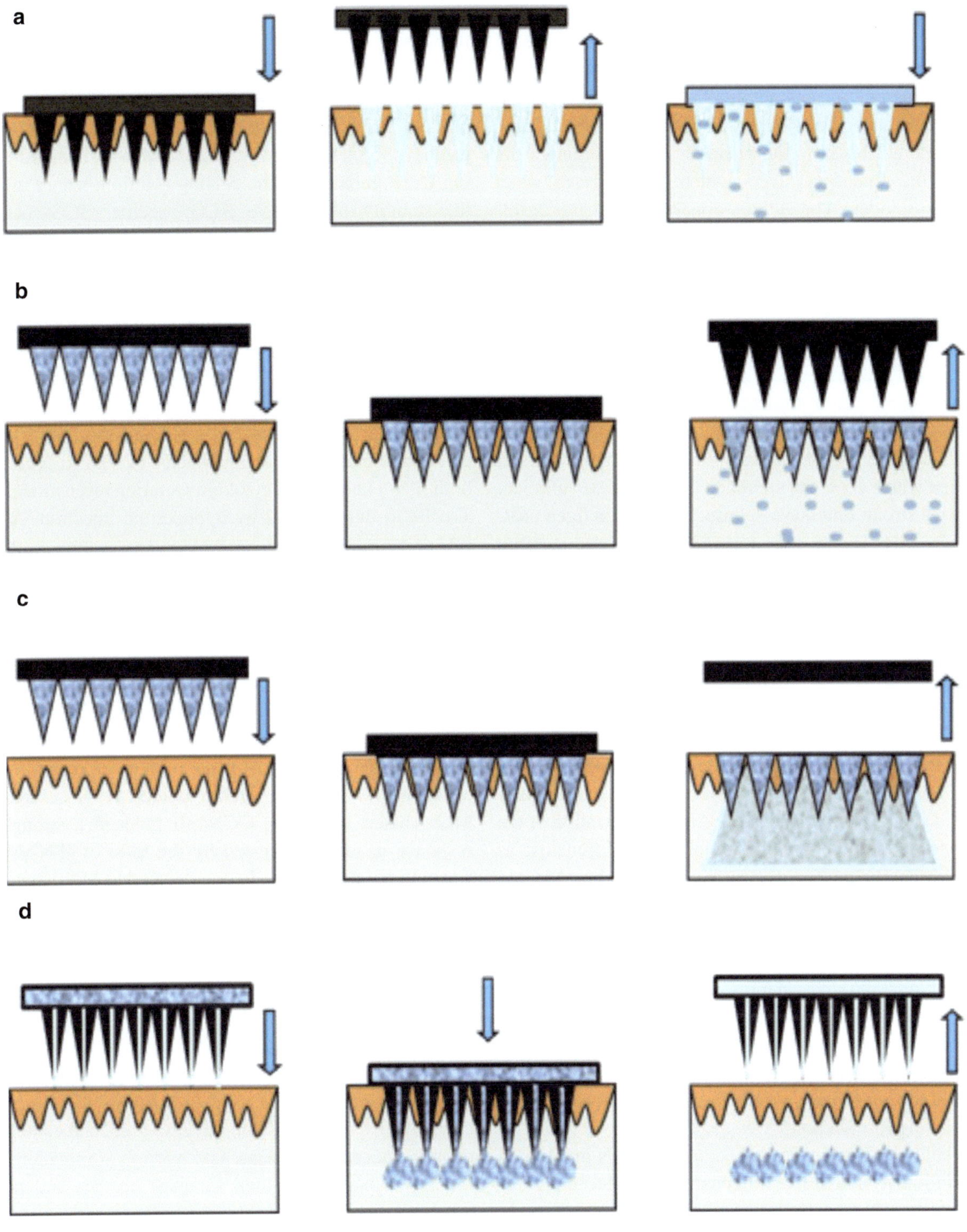

Fig. 10.10 Schematic representation of methods of MN application to the skin to achieve enhanced transdermal drug delivery. (**a**) (Poke and patch) shows solid MNs that are applied and removed to create transient micropores, followed by application of a traditional transdermal patch. (**b**) (Coat and poke) shows solid MN coated with drug for instant delivery. MNs are removed after the coating material dissolves. (**c**) (Dissolving microneedles) show soluble polymeric/carbohydrate MN containing drugs that dissolve in skin interstitial fluid over time, thereby delivering the drug. (**d**) (Poke and flow) shows hollow MN for delivery of fluids containing drug

tumor injection. A significant increase in IgG antibody levels was seen for both transdermal and subcutaneous vaccinated groups when compared with control groups. However, slightly increased IgG antibody levels were seen in the transdermally vaccinated group when compared to the SC group. This can be attributed to the presence of Langerhans cells (LCs) in the epidermis layers which are activated when exposed to antigen. The authors concluded that the developed formulation for melanoma cancer which can be administered using MNs technology gives rise to new approaches to the prevention of melanoma cancer.

10.4.3.2 Coat and Poke

The coat and poke approach involves the coating of solid MNs with an antigen of choice, which can be delivered in a one-step process. This could be a very attractive approach for mediating ID vaccine delivery since the smaller amount of antigen which coats the microneedles should be sufficient to induce a strong immune response. Since the antigen coating on the MNs is in a solid form [34], long-term stability should be improved, ensuring optimal shelf life [35].

The Prausnitz group at the Georgia Institute of Technology has carried out immunization studies using stainless steel monument-shaped arrays of 5 MNs dip coated in vaccine. The MNs used were approximately 700 μm in length, and their manufacture was achieved by laser-cutting stainless steel sheets. Plasmid-encoding hepatitis C virus, seasonal influenza: H1N1, H3N2, inactivated virus, influenza virus-like particles, and recently BCG were engaged successfully in MN-mediated ID immunization. After optimization of the coating formulation that led to the inclusion of trehalose as an antigen stabilizer [36], MNs were coated and inserted into the skin of mice. The results showed that the coated MNs stimulated a robust immune response, providing complete protection against the lethal influenza virus challenge similar to conventional intramuscular injection.

The study concluded that effective vaccination was achieved due to the inclusion of the stabilizing agent in the coating formulation, as this acted to protect antigen activity. In light of this, in subsequent studies, trehalose was included in the coating formulation.

In a study by Koutsonanos et al., a single MN immunization with inactivated H3N2 influenza virus induced significantly higher hemagglutination inhibition (HI) titers in comparison with that observed by i.m. injection. Solid metal MNs coated with inactivated influenza virus were found to be at least as effective as the conventional IM route in inducing similar levels of functional antibodies at low or high antigen concentrations, in clearing the virus from the lungs of infected mice, in conferring protection, and in inducing short-lived as well as memory B immune responses. While serum IgG responses in i.m. injection were seen to be dependent upon dose, this was not the case with MN delivery, which produced similar responses at low or high antigen loadings.

This finding suggests that the skin has a higher capacity to produce an immunologic response. The same system was used to evaluate the potential of BCG-coated MN vaccine patches [37]. The viability of BCG was maintained by adding 15 % trehalose to the coating solution, which improved the stability of the live BCG vaccine. BCG-coated ten microneedle patches (5×10^4 CFUs of BCG) were applied to the skin of guinea pigs. Another group of guinea pigs were injected intradermally with BCG (5×10^4 CFUs) using a 26 gauge needle and 1 ml tuberculin syringe. The results of this study indicated that BCG vaccine-coated MNs can induce a strong antigen-specific cellular immune response in both the lung and spleen of guinea pigs, comparable to that induced by using a 26 gauge needle. It was found that MN BCG vaccination elicited similar frequencies of TNF-α secreting or both IFN-γ and TNF-α cytokine secreting bifunctional CD4+ T cells to that induced by hypodermic injection. A strong IgG response was produced by both vaccination methods.

The capacity to produce a protective immune response of modified recombinant trimeric soluble influenza virus hemagglutinin (sHA GCN4pII)-coated MNs was assessed by the group [38]. Comparison was made between results from the modified and unmodified protein (sHA). Mice vaccinated with MN-coated sHA trimeric induced fully protective immune response against influenza virus challenge. Both sHA and sHA GCN4pII-coated MNs induced improved clearance of replicating virus compared to the s.c. route. The MNs coated with sHA GCN4pII induced a stronger Th1 response in mice suggested by the ratio of IFN-γ+CD4+ T cell to IL- 4+. The study concluded that MNs coated with stabilized sHA trimers were as effective in inducing a protective immune response and afforded equal level of protection as conventional subcutaneous administration.

Nanopatch™. Mark Kendall's research has pioneered the development of Nanopatch™ technology. Nanopatch™ devices are fabricated from silicon using a process of deep reactive ion etching. The projections are solid silicon, sputter coated with a thin (~100 nm) layer of gold, and contain 3364 densely packed projections. These arrays are smaller, by two orders of magnitude, than standard needles and are also much smaller than typical microneedle arrays.

The Nanopatches™ have been used to target ID vaccination against West Nile virus and chikungunya virus in mice. The efficiency of Nanopatch™ immunization was demonstrated using an inactivated whole chikungunya virus vaccine and a DNA-delivered attenuated West Nile virus vaccine [39]. Nanopatch™ technology was also used as an alternative delivery system to the i.m. prophylactic vaccine against cervical cancer Gardasil® and succeeded in delivering up to 300 ng of vaccine to the ears of mice. Moreover, in terms of virus-neutralizing response, results were found equal to those of a control group of i.m. vaccinated mice in mouse serum samples from mice vaccinated using Nanopatch™ technology [40]. Similarly impressive results have also been reported when Nanopatch™ coating was used with the influenza vaccine, Fluvax® [41].

Macroflux®. Research at Zosano Pharma (formerly ALZA Corporation) assessed the performance of the Macroflux®, another device containing an array of microprojections, for intracutaneous delivery of a model antigen, ovalbumin. The findings revealed that at all antigen doses, administration of OVA-coated Macroflux® resulted in immune response comparable to that observed after intradermal administration of the same doses of antigen. In addition, it was observed that application of 1 μg and 5 μg of antigen via Macroflux® resulted in 10- and 50-fold increases in anti-ovalbumin levels in comparison to delivery of equivalent doses via intramuscular or subcutaneous routes [42]. Follow-up mechanistic studies revealed that the immunologic response was unaffected by MN height (225–600 μm) and density (140 and 657/cm^2), but was dependent on the dose of antigen delivered [43].

10.4.3.3 Poke and Flow

The poke and flow approach is based on diffusion of vaccine through conduits of solid MNs. The antigen can be delivered either by passive diffusion, pressure, or electrical driven flow. However, this approach is vulnerable to some of the same problems as conventional vaccination techniques including the requirement of a cold chain and possible need for trained personnel. The narrow bore of MNs and the dense elastic nature of the skin may also limit fluid flow. Partial retraction of the MN array before the introduction of fluid was found by Wang et al. to partially compensate for this limitation however [44]. Frost suggested that the coadministration of the enzyme hyaluronidase, which degrades hyaluronic acid in the extracellular matrix of the skin, might reduce skin resistance [45]. Martanto et al. provided many explanations of the factors affecting the flow rate through hollow MNs. Hollow MNs are the subject of increasing interest because of their potential for use for TCI or ID vaccination [46].

MicronJet®. MicronJet® is a novel device developed by NanoPass specifically for intradermal delivery, consisting of an array of four MNs, each 450 μm in length. The needles are of silicon crystal bonded to a plastic adapter which can be mounted on any standard syringe. Van Damme et al. investigated the safety and efficacy of this device for dose-sparing intradermal influenza vaccination in healthy adults [47]. α-RIX® (GSK Biologicals) influenza vaccines were delivered using a hollow MN device (MicronJet®), and their safety and immunogenicity assessed. In the trial, which was carried out with a group of 180 healthy adult subjects, low-dose influenza vaccines delivered by MicronJet® elicited immune responses similar to those elicited by 15 μg HA per strain injected i.m. in human volunteers.

The prevalence of local reaction presented a limitation, however, although such reactions were transient in nature. Similar developments have been made at BD Technologies. A 34 gauge stainless steel MN with an inner diameter of 76 μm, an outer diameter of 178 μm, and an exposed length of 1 mm was used to deliver three distinct influenza vaccines. Results suggested that this mode of delivery was capable of producing the full immunological response at a dose at least tenfold lower than with i.m. administration and up to 100-fold more potent, depending on the nature of the antigen. The same researchers went on to uncover dose-sparing benefits of MN-delivered anthrax vaccinations over intramuscular administration in a subsequent study [48].

10.4.3.4 Dissolving/Soluble Microneedles

Dissolving MNs may present an innovative approach for vaccine delivery. Such MNs are based upon water-soluble polymers or carbohydrate material which encapsulates the drug within the needle matrix. On piercing the skin, the MNs dissolve completely to deliver their contents. Dissolvable MNs show promise in vaccine delivery breakthrough for many reasons. Since the MNs will dissolve after insertion into the patient's skin, the possibility of cross infection is eliminated. Also, the approach eliminates the necessity of any special disposal mechanism, as no sharp biohazardous waste is produced.

The solid-state nature of the contained/encapsulated vaccine should also reduce the need for cold chain storage and transport. In addition, MN patches offer the possibility of self-administration of vaccine during pandemics as well as rendering mass immunization programs in developing countries. As these self-disabling MNs lack many of the disadvantages of conventional vaccination techniques, and also some of those associated with the MN strategies mentioned to this point, poke and patch MNs are receiving increasing attention for their value in vaccination applications.

Dissolvable MN patches were first taken up for the administration of vaccines by the Prausnitz group. Sullivan et al. manufactured MN patches and investigated possibilities for influenza vaccination using a simple patch-based system. Patches based on 650 μm poly(vinylpyrrolidone) MNs containing 3 μg lyophilized inactivated influenza virus vaccine generated robust antibody and cellular immune responses which gave complete protection against lethal influenza challenge. In fact, in comparison with IM vaccination, MN delivery displayed better results following vaccination in terms of lung virus clearance and cellular recall responses.

The Kendall group described the micromolding of dissolving MN arrays from master templates of one of their Nanopatch™ designs [49]. Replica MNs were formed from carboxymethylcellulose by means of multiple castings into poly(dimethylsiloxane) molds. Dual-layer MNs containing both the model antigen ovalbumin and the adjuvant Quil-A elicited postimmunization schedule antibody levels in mice which were similar to an IM ovalbumin/Quil-A immunization group at day 28 and superior to the IM group at day 102, despite using a lower antigen dose in the MNs. Research using an influenza vaccine gave similar findings.

10.4.4 Intradermal Gene Delivery

Gene therapy may be defined as the insertion, alteration, or removal of genes from an individual's cells and biological tissues to treat disease. Replacement of a mutated gene via the insertion of functional genes into an unspecified genomic location is the most frequently used gene therapy. Other approaches exist however which may involve either directly correcting the mutation or modifying normal genes. While the technology has yet to be developed to its full potential, it has been used with some success.

The most common form of genetic engineering involves insertion of a functional gene into host cells. This is accomplished by isolating and copying the gene of interest, generating a construct containing all the genetic elements for correct expression, and then inserting this construct into the host organism.

Localized delivery and expression of gene therapeutics within the skin may provide novel treatment options for a number of pathological conditions, including skin disorders of genetic origin, as well as nonsurgical management of malignancy. If genetic manipulation could be used to influence epidermal cells to produce and secrete antigenic molecules, then the potent immunostimulatory properties of the skin could be harnessed to provide efficient protection from the disease concerned.

The Birchall Group at Cardiff University in Wales has pioneered epidermal gene delivery using various microneedle arrays to penetrate the stratum corneum, which would form a barrier to intradermal delivery of genetic constructs. The group initially set out to establish whether silicon-based microneedles (150 μm in height, base width 45–50 μm), microfabricated via an isotropic etching/BOSCH reaction process, were capable of creating microchannels in the skin large enough to permit the passage of lipid-polycation-plasmid DNA (LPD) nonviral gene therapy vectors [50]. Scanning electron microscopy was used to visualize the microconduits created in heat-separated human epidermal sheets after application of the microneedles.

Following confirmation of particle size and particle surface charge by photon correlation spectroscopy and microelectrophoresis, respectively, the diffusion of fluorescent polystyrene nanospheres and LPD complexes through heat-separated human epidermal sheets was established in vitro using a Franz-type diffusion cell. In vitro cell culture with quantification by flow cytometry was used to determine gene expression in human keratinocytes (HaCaT cells). Membrane treatment with microneedles was found to notably enhance the diffusion through epidermal sheets of 100 nm diameter fluorescent polystyrene nanospheres, used as a readily quantifiable predictive model for LPD complexes. The delivery of LPD complexes either into or through the membrane microchannels was also demonstrated. In both cases, considerable interaction between the particles and the epidermal sheet was observed. LPD complexes were shown through in vitro cell culture to mediate efficient reporter gene expression in human keratinocytes in culture when formulated at the appropriate surface charge.

The group's next study made use of platinum-coated silicon microneedles. These were used to produce microconduits, approximately 50 μm in diameter and extending through the stratum corneum and viable epidermis. Following optimization of skin explant-culturing techniques and confirmation of tissue viability, it was demonstrated that gene expression could be mediated through use of the microneedles to transmit the beta-galactosidase reporter gene. Preliminary studies confirmed localized delivery, cellular internalization, and subsequent gene expression of pDNA following microneedle disruption of skin.

Following this result, it was decided to establish whether microfabricated silicon microneedle arrays could effectively achieve localized delivery of charged macromolecules and plasmid DNA (pDNA) [51]. Microconduits of 10–20 μm in diameter were found in human epidermal membrane following treatment with the microneedles. The delivery of the marker biomolecule beta-galactosidase, and of a "nonviral gene vector mimicking" charged fluorescent nanoparticle to the viable epidermis of microneedle-treated tissue, was demonstrated using light and fluorescent microscopy.

Track-etched permeation profiles, generated using "Franz-type" diffusion cell methodology and a model synthetic membrane showed that >50 % of a colloidal particle suspension permeated through membrane pores in approximately 2 h. These findings were taken by the group to indicate cutaneous delivery of lipid-polycation-pDNA (LPD) gene vectors, and other related vectors, to the viable epidermis, could be achieved via microneedle treatment. Preliminary gene expression studies confirmed that naked pDNA can be expressed in excised human skin following microneedle disruption of the SC barrier. The presence of a limited number of microchannels, positive for gene expression, points to the value of further investigation aimed at optimization of the morphology of the microneedle device, its method of application, and the pDNA formulation.

Aqueous solutions loaded with gene delivery vehicles would not remain in situ on the surface of the skin and therefore would be of limited use in clinical practice. For this reason, the group then examined the possibility of using sustained-release pDNA hydrogel formulations with their microneedle delivery system to improve delivery of plasmid DNA (pDNA) in skin [52]. Microneedles were again fabricated by wet etching silicon in potassium hydroxide. Hydrogels based on Carbopol® polymers and thermosensitive PLGA-PEG-PLGA triblock copolymers were prepared. Freshly excised human skin was used to characterize microneedle penetration (microscopy and skin water loss), gel residence in microchannels, pDNA diffusion, and reporter gene (beta-galactosidase) expression. Upon application of the microneedles, channels of approximately 150–200 μm depth increased transepidermal water loss in skin. pDNA hydrogels were shown to harbor and gradually release pDNA. Following microneedle-assisted delivery of pDNA hydrogels to human skin, expression of the pCMV beta reporter gene was displayed in the viable epidermis proximal to the microchannels. It was concluded that targeted pDNA hydrogels can potentially provide sustained gene expression in the viable epidermis.

Microneedle-mediated intradermal gene delivery has also been recently explored by The Prausnitz Group [53]. In this study, specific cytotoxic T lymphocytes (CTLs) were effectively primed through vaccination with a plasmid-encoding hepatitis C virus nonstructural 3/4A protein using coated microneedles. Importantly, the minimally invasive microneedles were as efficient in priming CTLs as more complicated or invasive delivery techniques, such as gene guns and hypodermic needles. The Kendall Group has also investigated gene delivery using coated Nanopatches™, as described above.

Microneedles and Electroporation. Although Prausnitz had proposed the use of microneedles in combination with electroporation in 2005, it was in 2007 that this was first achieved, when it was reported by Hooper et al. the efficient delivery of an experimental smallpox DNA vaccine consisting of four vaccinia virus genes (4pox) by means of a novel method involving skin electroporation using plasmid DNA-coated microneedle arrays [54]. Electroporation is a process where cells are transiently permeabilized using high-intensity electric field pulses (see next chapter). The EasyVax® delivery system employed consisted of 80 electrically conducting microneedles each around 1 mm in height coated with dried vaccine DNA.

The pulse protocol consisted of six pulses of 100 V, 100 mS pulse duration, and 125 mS pulse interval. Four arrays, each coated with 30 μg of a separate plasmid, were used to deliver the 4pox DNA vaccine to mice. A separate site used for each array was administered to a separate site (inner and outer right and left thigh). Mice vaccinated with the negative control plasmids were administered using one array to an inner thigh. The smallpox DNA vaccine stimulated robust antibody responses against the four immunogens of interest, including neutralizing antibody titers which were greater than were produced by the conventional live virus vaccine administered by scarification. Furthermore, complete protection was found in the vaccinated mice against a lethal intranasal challenge with vaccinia virus strain IHD-J.

This study represented the first demonstration of a protective immune response being elicited by microneedle-mediated skin electroporation and suggests that there is scope for further exploration of this area. Indeed, Daugimont et al. [55] followed up on this by investigating the potential of hollow conductive microneedles for needle-free intradermal injection and electric pulse application in order to generate an electric field in the superficial layers of the skin sufficient for electroporation.

Microneedle arrays along with a vibratory inserter were employed to disrupt the stratum corneum, thus piercing the skin. Effective injection of proteins into the skin was achieved, resulting in an immune response directed to the model antigen ovalbumin. However, the dual function of microneedle electrode seemed to pose certain drawbacks for DNA electrotransfer. This could be due to the distribution of the electric field in the skin as shown by numerical calculations and/or the low dose of DNA injected.

10.4.5 Microneedle-Mediated Delivery of Antigen Nanoparticles

In the past few years, particle-based vaccines have been proposed for successful immunization. They have been used to protect antigen stability in vivo and to deliver it in a controlled and sustained manner to the site of action.

Drug-loaded nanoparticles (NPs) are colloidal systems, typically 10–1000 nm in diameter, with a therapeutic payload entrapped, adsorbed, or chemically coupled to an orbicular matrix. Nanoparticles are widely used for controlled delivery of small molecule drugs, oligonucleotides, and protein antigens to a variety cell types, including dendritic cells. Among the different parameters that need to be considered in design of particle-based vaccines, the particle size and their physicochemical properties are particularly important for skin vaccination. It has been demonstrated that polymeric nanoparticles <500 nm in diameter have high rate of intracellular uptake by variety of APC [56].

Nanoparticles have been extensively studied for oral and parenteral administration owing to their sustained drug release. This property of nanoparticles could also be utilized for topical antigen administration to target skin DCs with antigen over a prolonged period. Researchers had attempted to use nanoparticles for topical drug delivery, and they found that the drug permeation was enhanced by gradual drug release from the nanoparticles on the skin surface, but did not optimize way to deliver nanoparticles inside the skin [57–59]. This suggested that as a drug delivery vehicle, the nanoparticle could sustain drug release, but if it was applied as a drug reservoir to treat the skin disease, it must be delivered into the skin layers instead of remaining on the skin surface.

Some other researchers tried to verify the penetration of nanoparticles across the skin, but found that only small numbers of NPs were able to permeate into the skin passively through the hair follicles, while most NPs were restricted by stratum corneum and unable to penetrate the skin [60, 61]. In the penetration experiments in vitro using the full-thickness skin, it was found that NPs could diffuse into the dermis as well as into the epidermis [62]. To investigate if the micro-conduits on the epidermis produced by microneedles could be the channels for NPs to penetrate the skin, the researches in vitro have been designed and proved that nanoparticles could pass through the human epidermal membrane and get into skin layers [63, 64]. Moreover, Bal and colleagues showed that in intradermal antigen delivery in vivo to skin pretreated by metal MNs antigen was more efficiently taken up by skin DCs when it was encapsulated into polymeric NPs, comparing when delivered in a soluble form [65]. All of the studies above indicated that microneedles may be an effective vehicle for the intradermal delivery of antigen-encapsulated nanoparticles in vivo.

10.4.6 Needles and Safety

From a regulatory point of view, currently little is known about the safety aspects that would be involved with long-term usage of microneedle devices. In particular, studies will need to be conducted to assess the effect that repeated microporation has upon recovery of skin barrier function. However, given the minimally invasive nature of the micropores created within the skin following microneedle application, especially in comparison to the use of a hypodermic needle, and the fact that statistically it is highly unlikely that microneedles would be inserted at exactly the same sites more than once in a patient's lifetime, it is envisaged that microneedle technology will be shown to have a favorable safety profile.

Infection is an issue that has long been discussed in relation to use of microneedle-based systems, since they, by necessity, puncture the skin's protective *stratum corneum* barrier. However, microbial penetration through microneedle-induced holes is minimal. Indeed, there have never been any reports of microneedles causing skin or systemic infections.

10.5 Electroporation[3]

10.5.1 Cell Membrane Electroporation

Application of an external electric field to a single cell, cell suspensions, or biological tissue generates a change in the cell transmembrane potential. At the cell membrane level, applying electric fields above the threshold value of the transmembrane potential (~1.5 V) [66] results in changes to the membrane structure that renders the membrane permeable to otherwise non-permeant molecules [67], a phenomenon termed electroporation or electropermeabilization resulting in temporary appearance of aqueous pores within the cell membrane (Fig. 10.11).

By modulating applied electric field parameters within a definite window, it is possible to temporarily permeabilize the membrane, allowing the cell to return to its natural state and thus preserving its viability: this process has been historically named reversible electroporation [68] and has been used in combination with chemotherapeutic agents, a procedure termed electrochemotherapy, or as a delivery method for nucleic acids, gene electrotransfer [69].

The application of electric fields of higher intensity and/or for longer times can cause a permanent disruption of cell membrane permeability, leading to cell death. This process is commonly referred to as irreversible electroporation and represents a novel soft tissue ablation modality currently under clinical investigation.

10.5.2 Electrochemotherapy

Electrochemotherapy is the local potentiation, by means of local reversible electroporation of tumor tissues, of the antitumor activity of non permeant (i.e., bleomycin), or poorly permeant (i.e., cisplatin) drugs already possessing intrinsic cytotoxic activity [70]. The first clinical studies on electrochemotherapy date to the early 1990s [71] and reported effectiveness in local disease control on head and neck squamous cell carcinoma nodules. Following the first heterogeneous clinical trials, reviewed elsewhere by Sersa [72] up to 2006, a prospective, multicenter, international clinical trial, the ESOPE (European Standard Operating Procedures of Electrochemotherapy) study, was conducted to evaluate the efficacy and safety of electrochemotherapy on cutaneous and subcutaneous tumor nodules showing an objective response rate of 85 % (73.7 % complete response rate) on treated tumor nodules [73]. Within the study, treatment protocol was

[3]Electroporation-based gene transfer by *Mattia Ronchetti, Michela Battista, Claudio Bertacchini, and Ruggero Cadossi* in Molecular Vaccines - From Prophylaxis to Therapy, Volume 2, Springer-Verlag Wien, 2013, Ed. Matthias Giese.

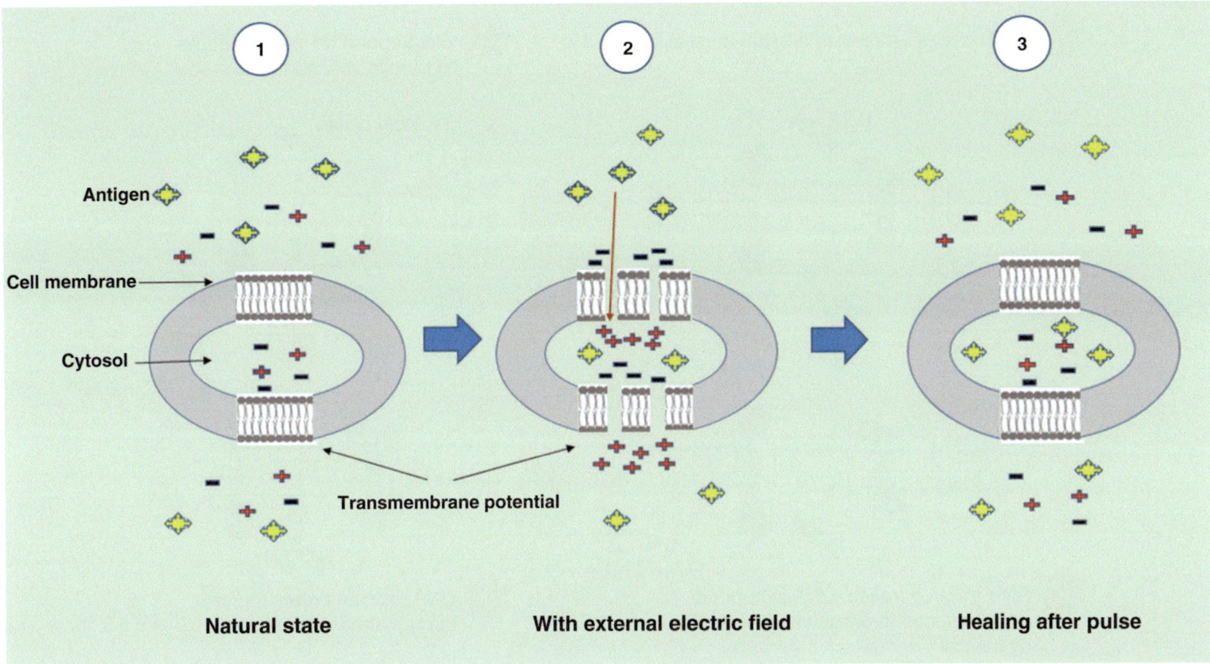

Fig. 10.11 (**1**) Under natural conditions, large molecules and charged ions cannot simply cross the cell membrane. (**2**) Application of an external electric field to a single cell generates a change in the cell transmembrane potential resulting in changes to the membrane structure that render the membrane permeable to otherwise non-permeant molecules. (**3**) When the electric field is deactivated, all pores are closed, and the cell membrane is healed (Figure by M. Giese, Heidelberg/Germany)

unified through the definition of electrochemotherapy standard operating procedures [74]. Recently, a systematic review and formal meta-analysis of all relevant published literature further confirmed the effectiveness of electrochemotherapy along with potential predictors of tumor response to electrochemotherapy with respect to various treatment conditions [75].

10.5.3 Gene Electrotransfer

Gene therapy is a promising field of medicine in which genes are introduced into the body to treat diseases especially those caused by genetic anomalies or deficiencies. The main obstacle for gene therapy has been the safe, effective, and reliable delivery of genes to target tissue. Nevertheless, DNA electrotransfer has proved to be an efficient and safe method for delivery of naked DNA in nonviral gene therapy approaches. Following the pioneering in vitro studies in 1982 that demonstrated that DNA could be introduced into living cells by means of electric pulses, several studies on the use of electroporation for delivery of molecules to eukaryotic cells and in various tissues have been reported. Over the years, the electroporation devices have been developed and electric pulse generators and applicators have been created to deliver nucleic acids under different condition and in different tissues. Modern generators allow controlling amplitude, pulse length, and number, while investigating the effect of the various electric parameters on transfection and expression levels as well as optimization of gene electrotransfer protocols.

The employment of naked DNA eliminates the limitations and the concerns linked to the use of viruses like coding sequence length in the case of the adenovirus and formation of insertional mutations during their integration into the host genome in the case of the Retrovirus or *Lentivirus*. In addition, naked DNA is safe, is simple to manipulate and generate, and is entirely constituted by double-stranded DNA with no associated proteins, whereas Adenovirus viral proteins can induce immunological responses and prevent the possibility to readminister the viral vectors naked. DNA delivered via gene electrotransfer offers the possibility of multiple administrations.

10.5.3.1 Nonviral Gene Therapy

Other physical approaches for nonviral gene therapy include direct injection; plasmid liposome complexes, still one of the most common techniques for gene delivery in to cells; and the biolistic approach for DNA transfer to superficial tissues, like the skin, which employs a device called gene gun that propels plasmid-coated gold microparticles through the cell membrane into the cytoplasm and the nucleus, bypassing the endosomal compartment where DNA can be damaged.

Limitations of this method include the low efficiency of the metal particles in reaching the entire tissue due to the low penetration of the particles, the deposition of metal particles into

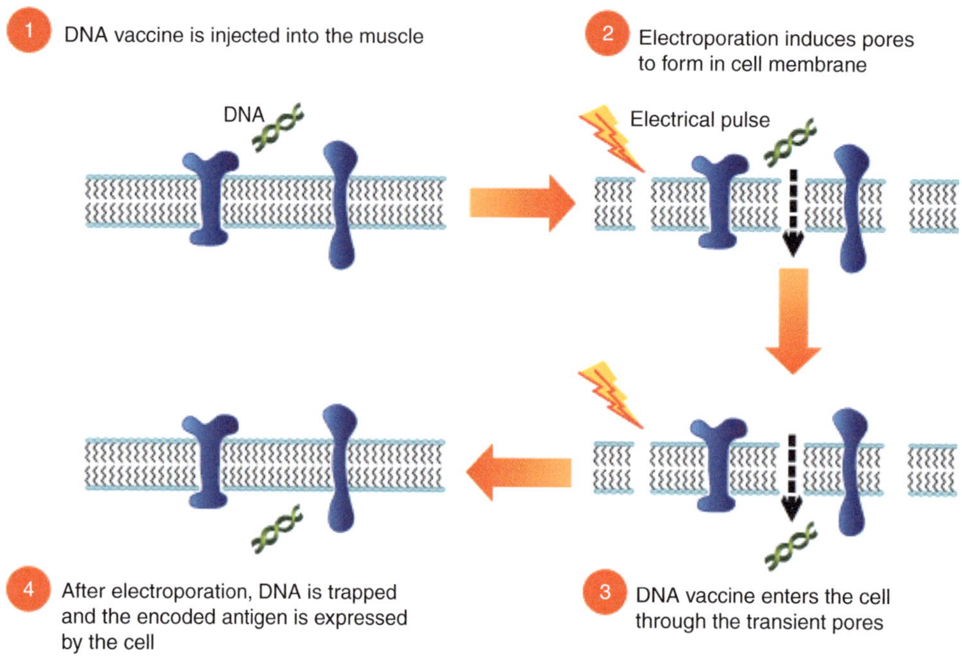

Fig. 10.12 Schematic overview of the effect of electroporation at the cell membrane due to DNA vaccination (Reprinted by permission from Macmillan Publishers Ltd: Molecular Therapy, 17, "Tolerability of Two Sequential Electroporation Treatments Using MedPulser DNA Delivery System (DDS) in Healthy Adults" by Mark Wallace et al. copyright (2015))

the body with the potential for long-term consequences, and sonoporation that applies ultrasound to increase the permeability of cell membrane to macromolecules including plasmid DNA. Indeed, enhancement of gene expression was observed by irradiating ultrasonic wave to the tissue after injection of DNA. In mice, hydrodynamic injection gene transfer is a technique achieved by means of the rapid intravenous injection of a high volume of solution in just a few seconds. Because of the high volume injected, the liquid accumulates in the inferior vena cava and the injected DNA is captured by the internal organs that are perfused by it, mainly the liver. However, because of the very large amount of liquid injected, this approach seems to have limited clinical translation potential.

10.5.3.2 DNA Electrotransfer Principles

Because of its ease of application, safety, and efficiency, DNA electrotransfer has rapidly expanded and advanced to an efficient methodology for nonviral gene delivery. Several experiments showed that in DNA electrotransfer, intake of exogenous DNA by the cell is controlled by different factors. The major role of high voltage, short duration electric pulses is membrane permeabilization. Subsequently, the DNA is moved by electrophoretic forces toward, as well as across, the permeabilized cell membrane by lower voltage and longer duration pulses and enters the cell cytosol [76, 77].

Moreover, it has been shown that when applying the electric field, the presence of DNA facilitates pore formation through direct interaction with the membrane; therefore, DNA must be injected before the electric pulse delivery (Fig. 10.12).

The role of electric pulses in DNA electrotransfer has been studied using combination of pulses, and three ways to deliver pulses for DNA transfer have been identified:

- Delivery of solely short, high-amplitude pulses (e.g., six pulses, 100 μs and 1.4 kV cm^{1}) [78], resulting in a reasonable efficacy and a low mortality.
- Long, low-amplitude pulses delivery (e.g., eight pulses, 20 ms, 200 kV cm^{-1}) [79]. The longer pulses have a better electrophoretic effect and therefore transfection rates can be increased.
- Short, high-amplitude pulse followed by long, low-amplitude pulses [80]. This pulse combination is based on the concept that the high-amplitude pulse induces permeabilization while the following long duration low-voltage pulses can drive the DNA across the destabilized membrane.

Finally, further experiments demonstrated the importance of the lag between high-voltage and low-voltage pulses: the shorter the lag between HV e LV, the higher the transfection efficiency obtained.

10.5.3.3 Gene Electrotransfer to Target Tissues

Gene transfer into muscle has been studied extensively since the observation of Wolff et al. [81] showed that plasmid DNA can be taken up and expressed in mouse skeletal muscle cells. Skeletal muscles are an attractive target for gene transfer due to abundant presence, easy accessibility, high vascularization, and prolonged preservation and expression of introduced

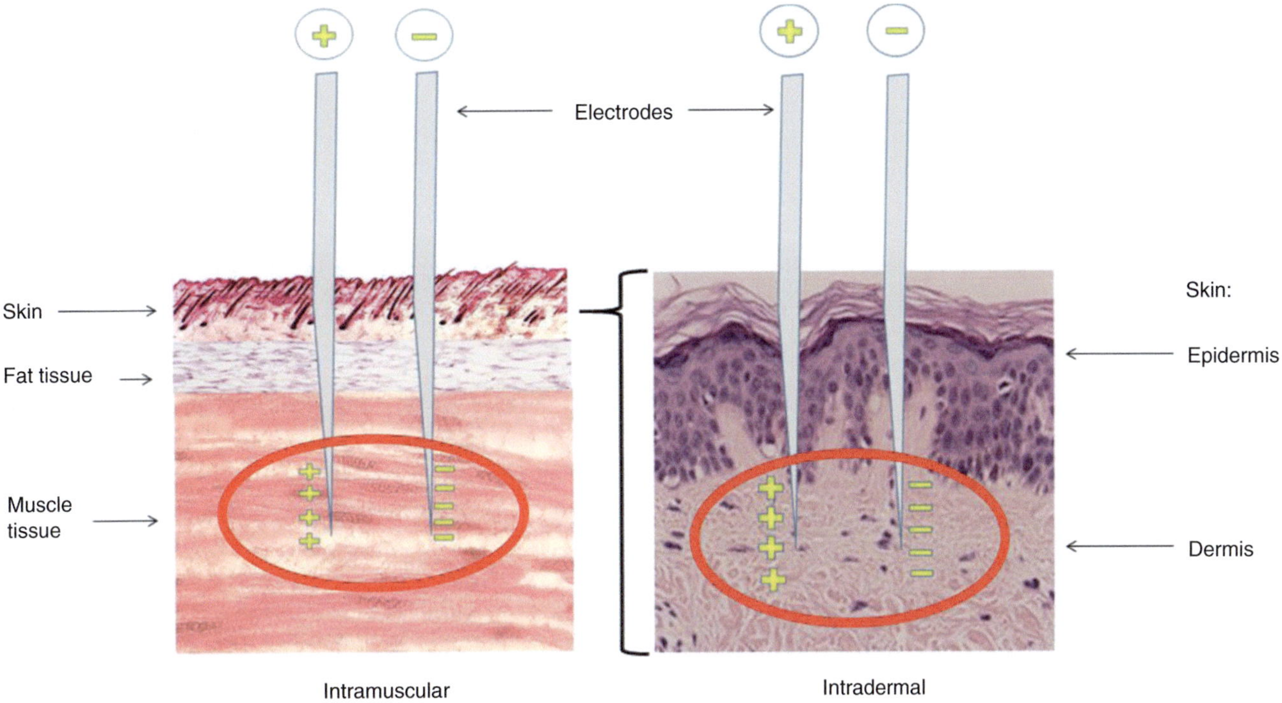

Fig. 10.13 Pair-wise formation needle electrodes are used for intramuscular or intradermal electroporation. Gene transfection to muscle can give long-term expression lasting up to or beyond 1 year, whereas the duration of expression in the skin is approximately 3–4 weeks. Several pulse combinations have been tested; the optimal pulse conditions depend on the type of skin transfected: size, thickness, and age of the skin must be taken into consideration (Figure by M. Giese, Heidelberg/Germany)

genes following mitosis. Nevertheless, the highly variable efficiency of transfection and the unpredictability of the resulting protein synthesis pose important drawbacks of this method. To overcome these limits, several in vivo studies have been focused on the use of electroporation for gene transfer into skeletal muscle. DNA is injected intramuscularly in relative high volumes of an isotonic plasmid solution followed by the application of electrical pulses by means of electrodes that are placed around the injection site. Noninvasive, plate electrodes are used for superficial muscles, while invasive needle electrodes are employed to treat deeper tissues. Figure 10.13 compares the intramuscular with intradermal electroporation.

To ensure a homogenous electric field distribution and a uniform transfection between the electrodes, thus facilitating expression of the plasmid vector, the positioning of the electrodes must be parallel to the muscle fibers. Other factors that are critical for gene expression efficiency include the amount of the injected plasmid, the promoter system, and area of transfection. DNA electrotransfer to muscle tissue has been proven to be highly efficient, and steady gene expression with transgene production has been detected for more than a year overcoming high variability in the level of protein expression.

Following muscle, gene electrotransfer has been successfully applied to several other tissues such as the cornea, testis, lung, liver, kidney, bladder, tumor, and skin. Above all, skin retains several important features that make it an attractive target tissue for gene therapy: it is easy to assess for treatment and for histological and clinical result evaluation, and it contains antigen-presenting cells (Langerhans cells, dendritic cells), which are part of the immune system and make the skin a proper target for DNA vaccination studies.

In order to electroporate the skin, electric pulses must be delivered using appropriate electrodes (noninvasive plate and patch electrodes or invasive array, circular or pair-wise formation needle electrodes). Several pulse combinations have been tested; the optimal pulse conditions depend on the type of skin transfected: size, thickness, and age of the skin must be taken into consideration [82] and also type of electrode and type of DNA [83]. A very extensive number of electrical protocols have been evaluated resolving that the most efficient protocols for gene transfer are combination of high-voltage (HV) and low-voltage (LV) pulses (1HV 1000 V/cm, 100 μs + 1 LV 100 V/cm, 400 ms), several short HV pulses (6 HV 1750 V/CM, 100 μs), and several long LV pulses (8 LV 100 V/cm, 150 ms).

Gene electrotransfer to skin has been employed to achieve the expression of several clinically relevant plasmids. They include local growth factors such as vascular endothelial growth factor (VEGF), keratinocyte growth factor (KGF), and viral targets for the vaccination toward infection diseases as HIV, hepatitis B, smallpox, and malaria. Moreover, the expression of IL-12, for the treatment of melanoma, has been also investigated following delivery in conjunction with electroporation. Preclinical studies employing gene electrotransfer to muscle and to skin have been summarized in Table 10.2.

Table 10.2 Summary of preclinical studies describing in vivo gene electrotransfer to muscle and skin tissues

Electrode type		Animal models	DNA plasmid	Voltage range V/cm	Duration range	Pulse number range	Ref.
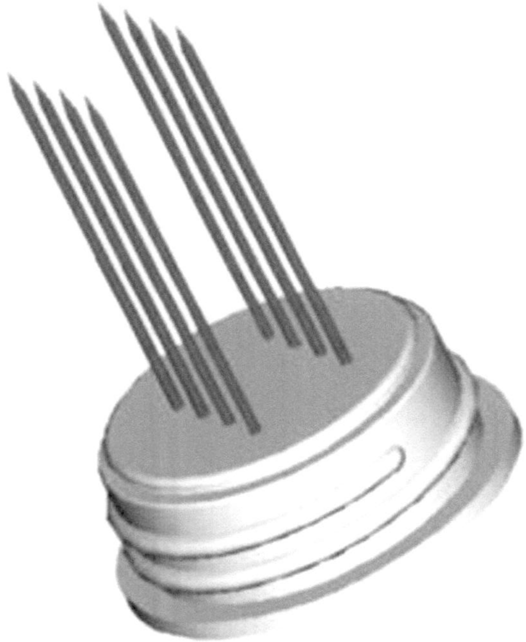 Invasive	Skin	Pig, mouse, rat,	GFP, Luc, hepatitis B, Hif-1α, KGF, VEGF, PSA, CEA, survivin	1125–1800 HV	50–100 μs	2–18	[85–89]
				50–400 LV	10–100 ms	6–10	[90–92]
				1000–10,125 + 80–275 HV + LV	50–100 μs + 275–400 ms	1–2 + 1–8	[89, 93–95]
	Muscle	Mouse, sheep, rat, dog	IL-5, GFP, EPO, GHRH, JEV	100–250	50 ms	5–8	[115–119]

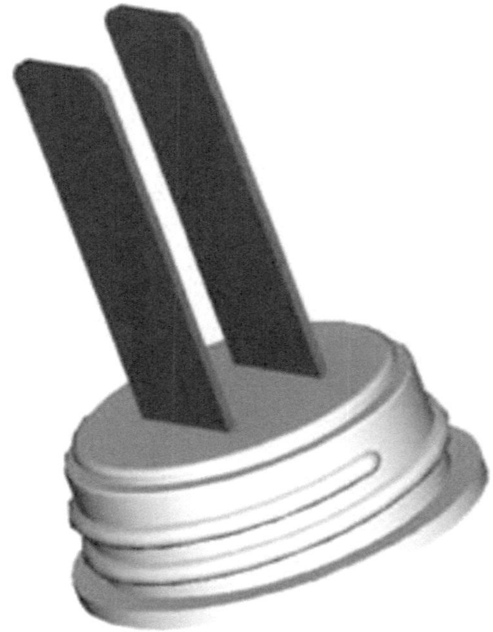 Non-invasive	Skin	Pig, mouse, rat, rabbit	NeoR, LacZ, GFP, OVA, Hepatitis B, IL-12, EPO	400–1750 (HV)	100–300 μs	1–8	[96–98]
				12–800 (LV)	2–400 ms	1–12	[97–103]
				700–1000 + 80–200 (HV + LV)	700–1000 μs + 80–200 ms	1 + 1	[98, 104–107]
	Muscle	Mouse, rabbit, rat	GFP, Luc, IL-4, IL-1Ra, VEGF, EPO	1000 HV	100 μs	8	[110, 111, 114]
				50–600 LV	100 μs – 20- ms	2–8	[108, 109, 112, 113]
				100–2000 + 80 V/cm HV + LV	100 μs + 400 ms	1 + 1	[108, 110]

Invasive needle electrodes and noninvasive plate electrodes have been employed. Needle electrodes have been used to target skin and deeper-lying tissues such as muscles in larger animals, while plate electrodes have been used to treat superficial tissues and rodent muscles. For simplicity, electrical protocols applied are reported as overall ranges

Abbreviations: *V/cm* volt per cm, *HV* high voltage, *LV* low voltage

Gene transfection to muscle can give long-term expression lasting up to or beyond 1 year, whereas the duration of expression in the skin is approximately 3–4 weeks [84]. However, in cases where there is no need for long-term expression of transfected plasmid and continuous production of proteins or antigens is not necessary, or desired, the skin represents an ideal target organ for gene electrotransfer.

10.5.4 Electroporation Devices

Electroporation technology is based on pulse generators that use different applicator electrodes, e.g., matrix of needles or plates to deliver suitable electric pulses to the target tissues. The complete system, pulse generators and applicators, is classified as a medical device. Different systems can have different approaches to the pulse generation. When this technology is developed for use in humans, either for small molecule delivery or gene transfection, specific requirements in terms of safety, reliability, and efficacy must be met. Currently, there are several electroporators available on the market for preclinical and lab testing; however, only few models are certified [120] and bear a CE mark for human clinical use in the European Union. One such example is the Cliniporator™ developed and marketed by IGEA S.p.A., Italy (Fig. 10.14).

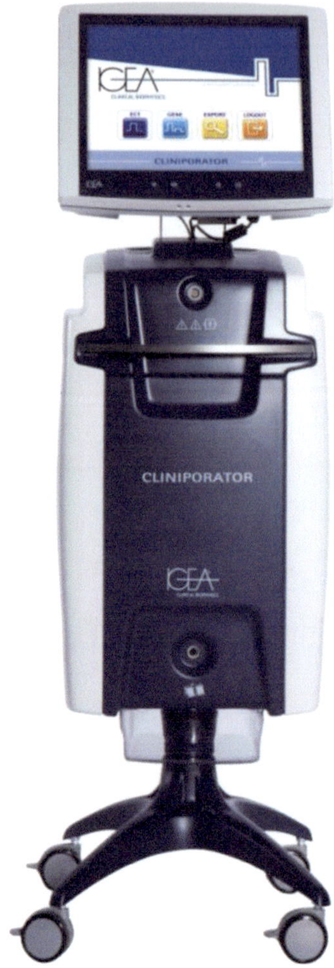

Fig. 10.14 Cliniporator™ for electroporation

Electroporator. It is possible to divide the electroporators considering the characteristics of the pulse and the technology used to generate it. There are several techniques to generate the pulse, all of them having usually a square or an exponential shape. Very short pulses having a length shorter than 1 μs require specific circuits and up to now are used for electroporation research only. Short pulses, having a length between 1 μs up to one thousand μs, and longer pulses, having a length of several milliseconds, are usually generated with different methods: by a direct capacitor discharge, by the pulse transformer, by high-voltage analog generator, or by high-voltage square wave generation [121, 122]. Basic characteristic of an electroporator to be used for gene electrotransfer is to deliver combinations of high-voltage (HV) pulses and low-voltage pulses (LV). This usually requires two different circuitries to ensure an appropriate precision and good control of the pulse shape.

Additionally, sophisticated devices, such as the Cliniporator, can measure in real time voltage and current on the load, providing the user with immediate feedback of the treatment being performed. Real-time measurement of applied pulses is also an ideal way to monitor performances of the device, detecting malfunctions early. Since the high-voltage pulse amplitude has a range between one hundred volts and few thousand volts [123], regulations and safety standards require a very good isolation of the high-voltage circuit to ensure the safety of the patients, of the operator, and of the device. Another very important safety issue is determined by the variability of working environment conditions (e.g., operating theater or clinician office) generally unknown beforehand. Energy delivered is influenced by tissue or cell impedance and can vary from point to point and from tissue to tissue. Thus, since high currents can damage cells, tissues, and even the device itself, the current is the critical parameter to be controlled.

Finally, considering the structure of the device, we see that in some cases the user interface controls directly the power part, but in other cases the power part is controlled by an independent electronic circuit and the user interface simply sends the treatment parameters to the power part. This different approach could have an impact about the reliability and the safety in case of failure of the device. Consequently, the design of a device for electroporation has to keep under close control energy delivered to the patient. Design and implementation should focus on a sturdy and fast pulse generator with a high reactivity in case of failures, using redundancies to improve its safety and providing a very user-friendly interface to minimize the risk of user error.

References

1. Langlet, C., Tamoutounour, S., Henri, S., Luche, H., Ardouin, L., Grégoire, C., Malissen, B., Guilliams, M.: CD64 expression distinguishes monocyte-derived and conventional dendritic cells and reveals their distinct role during intramuscular immunization. J. Immunol. **188**, 1751–1760 (2012)
2. Gurunathan, S., Wu, C.Y., Freidag, B.L., Seder, R.A.: DNA vaccines: a key for inducing long term cellular immunity. Curr. Opin. Immunol. **12**, 442–447 (2000)
3. Lombardi, V., Van Overtvelt, L., Horiot, S., Moussu, H., Chabre, H., Louise, A., Balazuc, A.M., Mascarell, L., Moingeon, P.: Toll-like receptor 2 agonist Pam3CSK4 enhances the induction of antigen-specific tolerance via the sublingual route. Clin. Exp. Allergy **38**, 1819–1829 (2008)
4. Prajeeth, C.K., Jirmo, A.C., Krishnaswamy, J.K., Ebensen, T., Guzman, C.A., Weiss, S., Constabel, H., Schmidt, R.E., Behrens, G.M.: The synthetic TLR2 agonist BPPcysMPEG leads to efficient cross-priming against co-administered and linked antigens. Eur. J. Immunol. **40**, 1272–1283 (2010)
5. Casella, C.R., Mitchell, T.C.: Putting endotoxin to work for us: monophosphoryl lipid a as a safe and effective vaccine adjuvant. Cell. Mol. Life Sci. **65**, 3231–3240 (2008)
6. Gorden, K.B., Gorski, K.S., Gibson, S.J., Kedl, R.M., Kieper, W.C., Qiu, X., Tomai, M.A., Alkan, S.S., Vasilakos, J.P.: Synthetic TLR agonists reveal functional differences between human TLR7 and TLR8. J. Immunol. **174**, 1259–1268 (2005)
7. Schreiner, B., Voss, J., Wischhusen, J., Dombrowski, Y., Steinle, A., Lochmuller, H., Dalakas, M., Melms, A., Wiendl, H.: Expression of toll-like receptors by human muscle cells in vitro and in vivo: TLR3 is highly expressed in inflammatory and HIV myopathies, mediates IL-8 release and up-regulation of NKG2D-ligands. FASEB J. **20**, 118–120 (2006)
8. Boyd, J.H., Divangahi, M., Yahiaoui, L., Gvozdic, D., Qureshi, S., Petrof, B.J.: Toll-like receptors differentially regulate CC and CXC chemokines in skeletal muscle via NF-kappaB and calcineurin. Infect. Immun. **74**, 6829–6838 (2006)
9. Wakim, L.M., Bevan, M.J.: Nature **471**, 629–632 (2011)
10. Marino, M., Scuderi, F., Provenzano, C., Bartoccioni, E.: Skeletal muscle cells: from local inflammatory response to active immunity. Gene Ther. **18**, 109–116 (2010)
11. Goebels, N., Michaelis, D., Wekerle, H., Hohlfeld, R.: Human myoblasts as antigen presenting cells. J. Immunol. **149**, 661–667 (1992)
12. Curnow, J., Corlett, L., Willcox, N., Vincent, A.: Presentation by myoblasts of an epitope from endogenous acetylcholine receptor indicates a potential role in the spreading of the immune response. J. Neuroimmunol. **115**, 127–134 (2001)
13. Shirota, H., Petrenko, L., Hong, C., Klinman, D.M.: Potential of transfected muscle cells to contribute to DNA vaccine immunogenicity. J. Immunol. **179**, 329–336 (2007)
14. Franck, E., Bonneau, C., Jean, L., Henry, J.P., Lacoume, Y., Salvetti, A., Boyer, O., Adriouch, S.: Immunological tolerance to muscle autoantigens involves peripheral deletion of autoreactive CD8+ T cells. PLoS One **7**, e36444 (2012)
15. Nicolas, J., Guy, B.: Intradermal, epidermal and transcutaneous vaccination: from immunology to clinical practice. Expert Rev. Vaccines **7**, 1201–1214 (2008)
16. Warger, T., Schild, H., Rechtsteiner, G.: Initiation of adaptive immune responses by transcutaneous immunization. Immunol. Lett. **109**, 13–20 (2007)
17. Stoitzner, P., Sparber, F., Tripp, C.H.: Langerhans cells as targets for immunotherapy against skin cancer. Immunol. Cell Biol. **88**, 431–437 (2010)
18. Kenney, R.T., Yu, J., Guebre-Xabier, M., Frech, S.A., Lambert, A., Heller, B.A., et al.: Induction of protective immunity against lethal anthrax challenge with a patch. J. Infect. Dis. **190**, 774–782 (2004)
19. Combadiere, B., Vogt, A., Mahe, B., Costagliola, D., Hadam, S.: Preferential amplification of CD8 effector-T cells after transcutaneous application of an inactivated influenza vaccine: a randomized phase I trial. PLoS One **5**, e10818 (2010)
20. Lambert, P.H., Laurent, P.E.: Intradermal vaccine delivery: Will new delivery systems transform vaccine administration? Vaccine **26**, 3197–3208 (2008)
21. Scheuplein, R.J.: Permeability of the skin: a review of major concepts. Curr. Probl. Dermatol. **7**, 172–186 (1978)
22. Teunissen, M.B., Haniffa, M., Collin, M.P.: Insight into the immunobiology of human skin and functional specialization of skin dendritic cell subsets to innovate intradermal vaccination design. Curr. Top. Microbiol. Immunol. **351**, 25–76 (2012)
23. Donnelly, R., Majithiya, R., Singh, T., Morrow, D., Garland, M., Demir, Y.: Design, optimization and characterisation of polymeric microneedle arrays prepared by a novel laser-based micromoulding technique. Pharm. Res. **28**, 41–57 (2011)
24. Chen, X., Fernando, G.J.P., Crichton, M., Flaim, C., Yukiko, S., Corbett, H.J., et al.: Improving the reach of vaccines to low-resource regions, with a needle-free vaccine delivery device and long-term thermostabilization. J. Control. Release **152**, 349–355 (2011)
25. Henry, S., McAllister, D.V., Allen, M.G., Prausnitz, M.R.: Microfabricated microneedles: a novel approach to Transdermal drug delivery. J. Pharm. Sci. **87**, 922–925 (1998)
26. Prausnitz, M., Mikszta, J., Cormier, M., Andrianov, A.: Microneedle-based vaccines. Curr. Top. Microbiol. Immunol. **333**, 369–393 (2009)
27. Donnelly, R., Raj Singh, T.R., Woolfson, A.D.: Microneedle-based drug delivery systems: microfabrication, drug delivery, and safety. Drug Deliv. **17**, 187–207 (2010)
28. Zhou, C., Liu, Y., Wang, H., Zhang, P., Zhang, J.: Transdermal delivery of insulin using microneedle rollers in vivo. Int. J. Pharm. **392**, 127–133 (2010)
29. Ding, Z., Verbaan, F.J., Bivas-Benita, M., Bungener, L., Huckriede, A., Kersten, G., et al.: Microneedle arrays for the transcutaneous immunization of diphtheria and influenza in BALB/c mice. J. Control. Release **136**, 71–78 (2009)
30. Ding, Z., Van Riet, E., Romeijn, S., Kersten, G.F.A., Jiskoot, W., Bouwstra, J.A.: Immune modulation by adjuvants combined with diphtheria toxoid administered topically in BALB/c mice after microneedle array pretreatment. Pharm. Res. **26**, 1635–1643 (2009)
31. Bal, S.M., Slütter, B., van Riet, E., Kruithof, A.C., Ding, Z., Kersten, G.F.A., et al.: Efficient induction of immune responses through intradermal vaccination with N-trimethyl chitosan containing antigen formulations. J. Control. Release **142**, 374–383 (2010)
32. Bhowmik, T., D'Souza, B., Shashidharamurthy, R., Oettinger, C., Selvaraj, P., D'Souza, M.: A novel microparticulate vaccine for melanoma cancer using transdermal delivery. J. Microencapsul. **28**, 294–300 (2011)
33. Cleary, G.: Microneedles for drug delivery. Pharm. Res. **28**, 1–6 (2011)
34. Shah, U.U., Roberts, M., Orlu Gul, M., Tuleu, C., Beresford, M.W.: Needle-free and microneedle drug delivery in children: a case for disease-modifying antirheumatic drugs (DMARDs). Int. J. Pharm. **416**, 1–11 (2011)
35. Kim, Y., Quan, F., Compans, R.W., Kang, S., Prausnitz, M.R.: Formulation and coating of microneedles with inactivated influenza virus to improve vaccine stability and immunogenicity. J. Control. Release **142**, 187–195 (2010)
36. Hiraishi, Y., Nandakumar, S., Choi, S., Lee, J., Kim, Y., Prausnitz, M.R., et al.: Bacillus Calmette-Guérin vaccination using a microneedle patch. Vaccine **29**, 2626–2636 (2011)

37. Weldon, W., Martin, M., Zarnitsyn, V., Wang, B., Koutsonanos, D., Skountzou, I.: Microneedle vaccination with stabilized recombinant influenza virus hemagglutinin induces improved protective immunity. Clin. Vaccine Immunol. **18**, 647–654 (2011)
38. Prow, T.: Nanopatch-targeted skin vaccination against West Nile Virus and Chikungunya virus in mice. Small **6**, 1776–1784 (2010)
39. Corbett, H., Chen, X., Frazer, I.: Skin vaccination against cervical cancer associated human papillomavirus with a novel microprojection array in a mouse model. PLoS One **5**, e13460 (2010)
40. Fernando, G.J.P., Chen, X., Prow, T., Crichton, M., Fairmaid, E.: Potent immunity to low doses of influenza vaccine by probabilistic guided micro-targeted skin delivery in a mouse model. PLoS One **5**, e10266 (2010)
41. Matriano, J., Cormier, M., Johnson, J., Young, W., Buttery, M., Cormier, M., et al.: Macroflux microprojection array patch technology: a new and efficient approach for intracutaneous immunization. Pharm. Res. **19**, 63–70 (2002)
42. Widera, G., Johnson, J., Kim, L., Libiran, L., Nyam, K., Daddona, P.E., et al.: Effect of delivery parameters on immunization to ovalbumin following intracutaneous administration by a coated microneedle array patch system. Vaccine **24**, 1653–1664 (2006)
43. Escobar-Chvez, J., Bonilla- Martinez, D., Villegas-González, M.A., Molina Trinidad, E., Casas Alancaster, N., et al.: Microneedles: a valuable physical enhancer to increase transdermal drug delivery. J. Clin. Pharmacol. **51**, 964–977 (2011)
44. Wang, P., Cornwell, M., Hill, J., Prausnitz, M.: Precise microinjection into skin using hollow microneedles. J. Invest. Dermatol. **126**, 1080–1087 (2006)
45. Frost, G.I.: Recombinant human hyaluronidase (rHuPH20): an enabling platform for subcutaneous drug and fluid administration. Expert Opin. Drug Deliv. **4**, 427–440 (2007)
46. Bal, S., Ding, Z., van Riet, E., Jiskoot, W., Bouwstra, J.: Advances in transcutaneous vaccine delivery: do all ways lead to Rome? J. Control. Release **148**, 266–282 (2010)
47. Van Damme, P., Oosterhuis-Kafeja, F., Van der Wielen, M., Almagor, Y., Sharon, O., Levin, Y.: Safety and efficacy of a novel microneedle device for dose sparing intradermal influenza vaccination in healthy adults. Vaccine **27**, 454–459 (2009)
48. Mikszta, J., Dekker, J., Harvey, N., Dean, C., Brittingham, J., Huang, J., et al.: Microneedle-based intradermal delivery of the anthrax recombinant protective antigen vaccine. Infect. Immun. **74**, 6806–6810 (2006)
49. Raphael, A., Prow, T., Crichton, M., Chen, X., Fernando, G.J.P., Prow, T.: Targeted, needle-free vaccinations in skin using multilayered, densely-packed dissolving microprojection arrays. Small **6**, 1785–1793 (2010)
50. Chabri, F., Bouris, K., Jones, T., Barrow, D., Hann, A., Allender, C., et al.: Microfabricated silicon microneedles for nonviral cutaneous gene delivery. Br. J. Dermatol. **150**, 869–877 (2004)
51. Birchall, J., Coulman, S., Pearton, M., Allender, C., Brain, K., Coulman, S., et al.: Cutaneous DNA delivery and gene expression in ex vivo human skin explants via wet-etch micro-fabricated micro-needles. J. Drug Target. **13**, 415–421 (2005)
52. Coulman, S.A., Barrow, D., Anstey, A., Gateley, C., Morrissey, A., Wilke, N., et al.: Minimally invasive cutaneous delivery of macromolecules and plasmid DNA via microneedles. Curr. Drug Deliv. **3**, 65–75 (2006)
53. Pearton, M., Allender, C., Brain, K., Anstey, A., Gateley, C., Wilke, N., et al.: Gene delivery to the epidermal cells of human skin explants using microfabricated microneedles and hydrogel formulations. Pharm. Res. **25**, 407–416 (2008)
54. Hooper, J., Golden, J., Ferro, A., King, A.: Smallpox DNA vaccine delivered by novel skin electroporation device protects mice against intranasal poxvirus challenge. Vaccine **25**, 1814–1823 (2007)
55. Daugimont, L., Baron, N., Vandermeulen, G., Pavselj, N., Miklavcic, D., Jullien, M., et al.: Hollow microneedle arrays for intradermal drug delivery and DNA electroporation. J. Membr. Biol. **236**, 117–125 (2010)
56. Eniola, A.O., Hammer, D.A.: Artificial polymeric cells for targeted drug delivery. J. Control. Release **87**, 15–22 (2003)
57. Alvarez-Roman, R., Naik, A., Kalia, Y.N., Guy, R.H., Fessi, H.: Enhancement of topical delivery from biodegradable nanoparticles. Pharm. Res. **21**, 1818–1825 (2004)
58. Alvarez-Roman, R., Naik, A., Kalia, Y.N., Guy, R.H., Fessi, H.: Skin penetration and distribution of polymeric nanoparticles. J. Control. Release **99**, 53–62 (2004)
59. Luengo, J., Weiss, B., Schneider, M., Ehlers, A., Stracke, F., Konig, K., et al.: Influence of nanoencapsulation on human skin transport of flufenamic acid. Skin Pharmacol. Physiol. **19**, 190–197 (2006)
60. Lademann, J., Richter, H., Teichmann, A., Otberg, N., Blume-Peytavi, U., Luengo, J., et al.: Nanoparticles – an efficient carrier for drug delivery into the hair follicles. Eur. J. Pharm. Biopharm. **66**, 159–164 (2007)
61. Toll, R., Jacobi, U., Richter, H., Lademann, J., Schaefer, H., Blume-Peytavi, U.: Penetration profile of microspheres in follicular targeting of terminal hair follicles. J. Invest. Dermatol. **123**, 168–176 (2004)
62. Coulman, S.A., Anstey, A., Gateley, C., Morrissey, A., McLoughlin, P., Allender, C., et al.: Microneedle mediated delivery of nanoparticles into human skin. Int. J. Pharm. **366**, 190–200 (2009)
63. McAllister, D.V., Wang, P.M., Davis, S.P., Park, J.H., Canatella, P.J., Allen, M.G., et al.: Microfabricated needles for transdermal delivery of macromolecules and nanoparticles: fabrication methods and transport studies. Proc. Natl. Acad. Sci. U. S. A. **100**, 13755–13760 (2003)
64. Bal, S.M., Slutter, B., Jiskoot, W., Bouwstra, J.A.: Small is beautiful: N-trimethyl chitosan-ovalbumin conjugates for microneedle-based transcutaneous immunisation. Vaccine **29**, 4025–4032 (2011)
65. Ueno, H., Schmitt, N., Klechevsky, E., Pedroza-Gonzalez, A., Matsui, T., Zurawski, G., et al.: Harnessing human dendritic cell subsets for medicine. Immunol. Rev. **234**, 199–212 (2010)
66. Kotnik, T., Bobanovic, F., Miklavcic, D.: Sensitivity of transmembrane voltage induced by applied electric fields – a theoretical analysis. Bioelectrochem. Bioenerg. **43**, 285–291 (1997)
67. Miklavcic, D., Semrov, D., Mekid, H., Mir, L.M.: A validated model of in vivo electric field distribution for electrochemotherapy and for DNA electrotransfer for gene therapy. Biochim. Biophys. Acta **1523**, 73–83 (2000)
68. Rubinsky, B.: Irreversible electroporation in medicine. Technol. Cancer Res. Treat. **6**, 255–260 (2007)
69. Neumann, E., Schaefer-Ridder, M., Wang, Y., Hofschneider, P.H.: Gene transfer into mouse lyoma cells by electroporation in high electric fields. EMBO J. **1**, 841–845 (1982)
70. Silve, A., Mir, L.M.: Cell electropermeabilization and cellular uptake of small molecules: the electrochemotherapy concept. In: Kee, S.T., Gehl, J., Lee, E.W. (eds.) Clinical aspects of electroporation, vol. 1, pp. 69–82. Springer, New York (2011)
71. Mir, L.M., et al.: Electrochemotherapy, a new antitumour treatment: first clinical trial. C. R. Acad. Sci. III **313**, 613–618 (1991)
72. Sersa, G.: The state of the art of electrochemotherapy before ESOPE study. Advantages and clinical use. EJC Suppl. **4**, 52–59 (2006)
73. Marty, M., et al.: Electrochemotherapy – an easy, highly effective and safe treatment of cutaneous and subcutaneous metastases. Results of ESOPE (European Standard Operating Procedures of Electrochemotherapy) study. EJC Suppl **4**, 3–13 (2006)
74. Mir, L.M., et al.: Standard operating procedures of the Electrochemotherapy: instructions for the use of bleomycin or cisplatin administered either systemically or locally and electric

pulses delivered by the Cliniporator by means of invasive or non-invasive electrodes. EJC Suppl. **4**, 14–25 (2006)

75. Mali, B., Jarm, T., Snoj, M., Sersa, G., Miklavcic, D.: Antitumor effectiveness of electrochemotherapy: a systematic review and meta-analysis. Eur. J. Surg. Oncol. **39**(1), 4–16 (2013). http://dx.doi.org/10.1016/j.ejso.2012.08.016
76. Sukharev, S.I., Klenchin, V.A., Serov, S.M., Chernomordik, L.V., Chizmadzhev, Y.A.: Electroporation and electrophoretic DNA transfer into cells. The effect of DNA interaction with electropores. Biophys. J. **63**(5), 1320–1327 (1992)
77. Klenchin, V.A., Sukharev, S.I., Serov, S.M., Chernomordik, L.V., Chizmadzhev, Y.A.: Electrically induced DNA uptake by cells is a fast process involving DNA electrophoresis. Biophys. J. **60**(4), 804–811 (1991)
78. Heller, R., Jaroszeski, M., Atkin, A., et al.: In vivo gene electroinjection and expression in rat liver. FEBS Lett. **389**, 225–228 (1996)
79. Mir, L.M., Bureau, M.F., Gehl, J., et al.: High efficiency gene transfer into skeletal muscle mediated by electric pulses. Proc. Natl. Acad. Sci. U. S. A. **96**, 4262–4267 (1999)
80. Bureau, M.F., Gehl, J., Deleuze, V., Mir, L.M., Scherman, D.: Importance of association between permeabilization and electrophoretic forces for intramuscular DNA electrotransfer. Biochim. Biophys. Acta **1474**, 353–359 (2000)
81. Wolff, J.A., et al.: Direct gene transfer into mouse muscle in vivo. Science **247**, 1465–1468 (1990)
82. Chesnoy, S., Huang, L.: Enhanced cutaneous gene delivery following intradermal injection of naked DNA in a high ionic strength solution. Mol. Ther. **5**(1), 57–62 (2002)
83. Gothelf, A., Mahmood, F., Dagnaes-Hansen, F., Gehl, J.: Efficacy of transgene expression in porcine skin as a function of electrode choice. Bioelechem. **82**(2), 95–102 (2011)
84. Gothelf, A., Eriksen, J., Hojman, P., Gehl, J.: Duration and level of transgene expression after gene electrotransfer to skin in mice. Gene Ther. **17**(7), 839–845 (2010)
85. Glasspool-Malone, J., Somiari, S., Drabick, J.J., Malone, R.W.: Efficient nonviral cutaneous transfection. Mol. Ther. **2**, 140–146 (2000)
86. Byrnes, C.K., et al.: Electroporation enhances transfection efficiency in murine cutaneous wounds. Wound Repair Regen. **12**, 397–403 (2004)
87. Marti, G., et al.: Electroporative transfection with KGF-1 DNA improves wound healing in a diabetic mouse model. Gene Ther. **11**, 1780–1785 (2004)
88. Lin, M.P., et al.: Delivery of plasmid DNA expression vector for keratinocyte growth factor-1 using electroporation to improve cutaneous wound healing in a septic rat model. Wound Repair Regen. **14**, 618–624 (2006)
89. Roos, A.K., et al.: Enhancement of cellular immune response to a prostate cancer DNA vaccine by intradermal electroporation. Mol. Ther. **13**, 320–327 (2006)
90. Kang, J.H., Toita, R., Niidome, T., Katayama, Y.: Effective delivery of DNA into tumor cells and tissues by electroporation of polymer- DNA complex. Cancer Lett. **265**, 281–288 (2008)
91. Liu, L., et al.: Age-dependent impairment of HIF-1alpha expression in diabetic mice: Correction with electroporation-facilitated gene therapy increases wound healing, angiogenesis, and circulating angiogenic cells. J. Cell. Physiol. **217**, 319–327 (2008)
92. Ferraro, B., Cruz, Y.L., Coppola, D., Heller, R.: Intradermal delivery of plasmid VEGF(165) by electroporation promotes wound healing. Mol. Ther. **17**, 651–657 (2009)
93. Brave, A., et al.: Late administration of plasmid DNA by intradermal electroporation efficiently boosts DNA-primed T and B cell responses to carcino embryonic antigen. Vaccine **27**, 3692–3696 (2009)
94. Lladser, A., et al.: Intradermal DNA electroporation induces survivin-specific CTLs, suppresses angiogenesis and confers protection against mouse melanoma. Cancer Immunol. Immunother. **59**, 81–92 (2009)
95. Roos, A.K., Eriksson, F., Walters, D.C., Pisa, P., King, A.D.: Optimization of skin electroporation in mice to increase tolerability of DNA vaccine delivery to patients. Mol. Ther. **17**, 1637–1642 (2009)
96. Titomirov, A.V., Sukharev, S., Kistanova, E.: In vivo electroporation and stable transformation of skin cells of newborn mice by plasmid DNA. Biochim. Biophys. Acta **1088**, 131–134 (1991)
97. Lucas, M.L., Jaroszeski, M.J., Gilbert, R., Heller, R.: In vivo electroporation using an exponentially enhanced pulse: a new waveform. DNA Cell Biol. **20**, 183–188 (2001)
98. Pavselj, N., Preat, V.: DNA electrotransfer into the skin using a combination of one high- and one low-voltage pulse. J. Control. Release **106**, 407–415 (2005)
99. Maruyama, H., et al.: Skin-targeted gene transfer using in vivo electroporation. Gene Ther. **8**, 1808–1812 (2001)
100. Zhang, L., Nolan, E., Kreitschitz, S., Rabussay, D.P.: Enhanced delivery of naked DNA to the skin by non-invasive in vivo electroporation. Biochim. Biophys. Acta **1572**, 1–9 (2002)
101. Lee, P.Y., Chesnoy, S., Huang, L.: Electroporatic delivery of TGFbeta1 gene works synergistically with electric therapy to enhance diabetic wound healing in db/db mice. J. Invest. Dermatol. **123**, 791–798 (2004)
102. Thanaketpaisarn, O., Nishikawa, M., Yamashita, F., Hashida, M.: Tissue- specific characteristics of in vivo electric gene: transfer by tissue and intravenous injection of plasmid DNA. Pharm. Res. **22**, 883–891 (2005)
103. Heller, L.C., et al.: Optimization of cutaneous electrically mediated plasmid DNA delivery using novel electrode. Gene Ther. **14**, 275–280 (2007)
104. Vandermeulen, G., et al.: Optimisation of intradermal DNA electrotransfer for immunisation. J. Control. Release **124**, 81–87 (2007)
105. Vandermeulen, G., et al.: Skin-specific promoters for genetic immunisation by DNA electroporation. Vaccine **27**, 4272–4277 (2009)
106. Vandermeulen, G., et al.: Effect of tape stripping and adjuvants on immune response after intradermal DNA electroporation. Pharm. Res. **26**, 1745–1751 (2009)
107. Gothelf, A., Hojman, P., Gehl, J.: Therapeutic levels of erythropoietin (EPO) achieved after gene electrotransfer to skin in mice. Gene Ther (2010). doi:10.1038/gt.2010.46
108. Ho, S.H., et al.: Protection against collagen-induced arthritis by electrotransfer of an expression plasmid for the interleukin 4. Biochem. Biophys. Res. Commun. **321**, 759–766 (2004)
109. Cukjati, D., Batiuskaite, D., André, F., Miklavcic, D., Mir, L.M.: Real time electroporation control for accurate and safe in vivo non-viral gene therapy. Bioelectrochemistry **70**, 501–507 (2007)
110. Hojman, P., et al.: Physiological effects of high- and low-voltage pulse combinations for gene electrotransfer in muscle. Hum. Gene Ther. **19**, 1249–1260 (2008)
111. Hojman, P., Zibert, J.R., Gissel, H., Eriksen, J., Gehl, J.: Gene expression profiles in skeletal muscle after gene electrotransfer. BMC Mol. Biol. **8**, 56 (2007)
112. Jeong, J.G., et al.: Electrotransfer of human IL-1Ra into skeletal muscles reduces the incidence of murine collagen-induced arthritis. J. Gene Med. **6**, 1125–1133 (2004)
113. Abruzzese, R.V., et al.: Ligand-dependent regulation of vascular endothelial growth factor and erythropoietin expression by a plasmid-based autoinducible Gene-Switch system. Mol. Ther. **2**, 276–287 (2000)
114. Bettan, M., et al.: High level protein secretion into blood circulation after electric pulse mediated gene transfer into skeletal muscle. Mol. Ther. **2**, 204–210 (2000)
115. Aihara, H., Miyazaki, J.: Gene transfer into muscle by electroporation in vivo. Nat. Biotechnol. **16**, 867–870 (1998)

116. Scheerlinck, J.P., et al.: In vivo electroporation improves immune responses to DNA vaccination in sheep. Vaccine **22**, 1820–1825 (2004)
117. Terada, Y., et al.: Efficient and ligand-dependent regulated erythropoietin production by naked dna injection and in vivo electroporation. Am. J. Kidney Dis. **38**, S50–S53 (2001)
118. Tone, C.M., Cardoza, D.M., Carpenter, R.H., Draghia-Akli, R.: Long-term effects of plasmid-mediated growth hormone releasing hormone in dogs. Cancer Gene Ther. **11**, 389–396 (2004)
119. Wu, C.J., Lee, S.C., Huang, H.W., Tao, M.H.: In vivo electroporation of skeletal muscles increases the efficacy of Japanese encephalitis virus DNA vaccine. Vaccine **22**, 1457–1464 (2004)
120. European Standard EN60601-1 Medical electrical equipment – part 1: general requirements for basic safety and essential performance, 3rd edn (2007). The International Electrotechnical Commission, Geneva
121. Bertacchini, C., et al.: Design of an irreversible electroporation system for clinical use. Technol. Cancer Res. Treat. **6**, 313–320 (2007). Num. 1 Adenine Press
122. Rebersek, M., Miklavcic, D.: Advantages and Disadvantages of different concepts of electroporation Pulse generation. ATKAFF **52**, 12–19 (2011)
123. Puc, M., Rebersek, S., Miklavcic, D.: Requirements for a clinical electrochemotherapy device – electroporator. Radiol. Oncol. **31**, 368–373 (1997)

Formulation and Manufacturing 11

Contents

11.1 From Antigen to Active Ingredient

It's a long way for an antigen from the discovery to the final product with application to the patient.

The first step begins with a feasibility study: the experimental evaluation and analysis of the viability of an idea. Questions of biological and technical feasibility are in the focus. Both criteria must be met. It makes no sense to develop a candidate vaccine if there is no safe but also profitable way of production. Not every protein can be expressed in standard industrial systems. Not every virus can be propagated in cell cultures. Also the patent situation has to be respected.

The only mission of a feasibility study is to generate and accumulate information. The conclusions of the feasibility study outline in depth the strengths and the weakness of the vaccine idea. A feasibility study allows the vaccine manufacturer to investigate the possible positive and negative outcomes of project before investing too much time and money. The go/no-go decision is one of the most critical in business development. Make or stop it or buy it.

Active Ingredient. The go decision has made the antigen now an active ingredient (AI), also known as active pharmaceutical ingredient (API). This is the part that challenges the immune system. But an AI is no final vaccine. Lots of various steps and additional compounds are necessary to produce a safe, stable, and biological active vaccine. This process is called formulation and can be only briefly described here for the development of a subunit protein vaccine (Fig. 11.1).

Summary of Product Characteristics (SmPC). This summary is required before marketing authorization of any medicinal product and describes the product both in terms of its physicochemical and/or biological properties, hazardous properties, pharmaceutical form, and the clinical use to which it can put. The patient information leaflet is a patient-friendly condensate of SmPC.

M. Giese, *Introduction to Molecular Vaccinology*, DOI 10.1007/978-3-319-25832-4_11

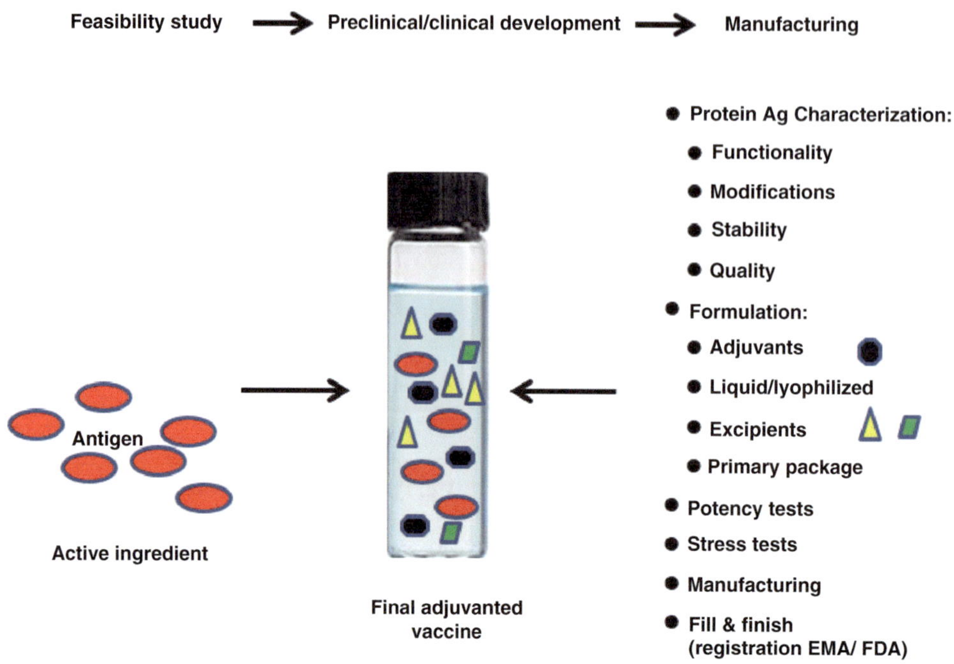

Fig. 11.1 A feasibility study is finished with the presentation of a suitable antigen as active ingredient. But first by a time-consuming formulation process, the antigen is created as a medicine ready for use. Most antigens are sensitive biological entities, and the formulation must ensure that the drug doesn't lose its biological activities. The vaccine must be stable and effective during the complete process of manufacturing, storage, and distribution and be effective in the patient. Stress and potency tests are necessary to investigate the influence of adjuvants and excipients on the stability and effectiveness of the antigen

11.2 Formulation Strategy

The goal of each formulation is to develop pharmaceutical dosage forms. Formulation has to fulfill a complex set of diverse operations that aim to create a biophysical system to facilitate vaccine delivery in such a way that the quality specifications (a list of tests and references to analytical procedures) are met and efficacy, bioavailability, and safety of the AI are ensured. Finally, a large-scale reproducible production of vaccines should be technically feasible. During the complete process of manufacturing, storage, and shipping, the quality of the product must remain unchanged.

A formulation strategy includes a detailed description of the planned dosage form, a preformulation, and a panel of formulation experiments:

1. Target product profile (TPP)
   - Preferred dosage and concentration
   - Preferred primary packaging
   - Route of administration
   - Frequency of administration
2. Preformulation
   - All protein data available
   - Selection of adjuvant
   - Selection of excipients
   - Selection of manufacturing process
3. Evaluating the formulations
   - Degradation pathways
   - Stress and potency tests
   - Stability
   - Primary packaging
   - Sterile filtration and filling

11.2.1 Protein Antigen Characterization

The major hurdles of protein-based vaccines regarding stability and bioavailability are degradation, photooxidation, and aggregation. The package insert must contain a short warning that the vial should be not shaken, must be protected from light, and must be stored at 2–8 °C because of the fragile protein nature. A typical formulation strategy begins with the collection of all protein data as shown in Fig. 11.2.

Only protein antigens can be recognized by T cells and induce T helper cell response. The biological function of a protein antigen depends on its physicochemical properties, such as solubility, hydrophobicity, net surface charge, and molecular weight. Protein antigens are large, macromolecules with more than 10.0 kDa molecular weight. Small molecules (<1000 Da) behave as incomplete antigens and cannot alone induce an antibody response. Proteins are constituted from amino acids (aa), covalently linked together to form the primary structure and subsequently higher structures, secondary, tertiary, and quaternary, which finally determine the biological activities. Proteins range between 50 and 25,000 aa, most proteins are constituted from 200 to 500 aa, and monoclonal antibodies are about 1000–1500 aa.

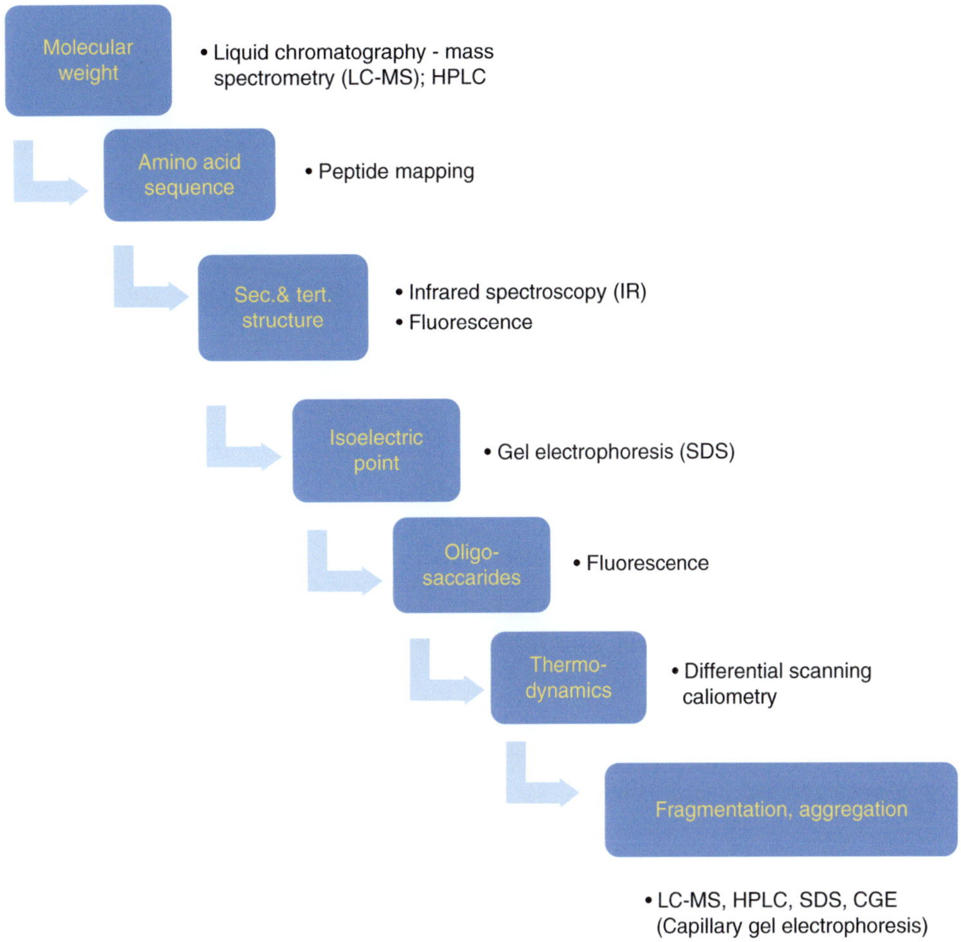

Fig. 11.2 Protein antigen characterization. Proteins are highly sensitive biological entities. For a well-adapted formulation, all protein characteristics, from molecular weight to thermodynamical states, have to be measured. A major challenge is to prevent the denaturation by fragmentation or aggregation

The physicochemical and functional properties are reflected by the basic composition of aa sequence.

11.2.2 Selection of Excipients

The main ingredient in vaccines is water. Injectable vaccines contain 0.5 ml on average. The weight of all ingredients in a vaccine dose together is a few mg.

Beyond the adjuvant (e.g., aluminum gels or salts), protein vaccines contain stabilizer and preservatives. These substances shall prevent the chemical degradation of the protein (by hydrolysis, disulfide reduction, oxidation, deamidation), or the physical degradation (by adsorption, i.e., to the primary package, aggregation, precipitation, heat). Stabilizers help the vaccine remain unchanged when the vaccine is exposed to heat, light, acidity, or humidity.

Depending on the manufacturing process, also traces of the culture medium, or antibiotics (e.g., neomycin, kanamycin, streptomycin, but not penicillin), can be present in the final product. Egg proteins are found in egg-based vaccine production. Traces of formaldehyde, used for inactivation of toxoid vaccines and for killing of viruses, can also contaminate the vaccine. Multidose vials can contain thimerosal, a mercury-containing preservative to prevent contamination and growth of bacteria.

All excipients, which are present in the product, should be listed, even those present in small amounts. Excipients that are of human or animal origin (animal by-products) must include information on country of origin, sources, specifications, and viral safety data.

Table 11.1 gives an overview of a collection of excipients, and Table 11.2 shows examples of licensed vaccine compositions for influenza.

The formulation development is finished with the decision for the dosage form (liquid or lyophilized), the adjusted protein concentration with the correct pH, the selection for the excipients, and the selection for the type and quality of the primary packaging (adsorption!).

11.2.3 Potency and Stress Tests

Has the formulation any influence on the performance of potency and stress tests?

Potential interactions between different components in the vaccine may occur and cause significant problems during product development. But also process failures, improper storage, antigen purity and concentration, etc. influence the potency of the product.

Table 11.1 Overview of standard excipients for parenteral application of protein formulations

Purpose	Examples	Type of excipient
pH maintenance	Citrate, acetate, (potassium-) phosphate Hydrochloric acid	Buffer
Disinfectant and detoxification	β-propiolactone Cetyltrimethylammonium bromide Formaldehyde Phenol Glutaraldehyde	Antimicrobial and detoxifier
Stabilizer, tonicity Cryopreservation	Sucrose, trehalose, lactose	Sugar
Stabilizer, tonicity	Mannitol, sorbitol	Polyalcohol
Stabilizer, tonicity	Chloride Monosodium glutamate	Salt
Stabilizer, tonicity	Glycine, arginine, leucine	Amino acids
Stabilizer	Polysorbate 20 Polysorbate 80 Triton X-100	Surfactant
Preservative	Benzyl alcohol Ethylenediaminetetraacetic acid sodium (EDTA) Monosodium glutamate Thimerosal (mercury)	Preservative
Antioxidant	Methionine Benzyl alcohol	Antioxidant
Stabilizer	Human serum albumin (porcine-) gelatin	Various
Manufacturing residues	Egg proteins Host cell proteins Yeast proteins Cellular DNA Baculovirus Antibiotics Unspecified vitamins	Various

Table 11.2 Examples of final influenza vaccine compositions of USA-licensed flu vaccines and their different production technologies

Vaccine	Manufacturer	Manufacturing process	Excipients	Year
Flucelvax	Novartis Vaccines and Diagnostics, Inc.	Cell-based vaccine: Inactivated	Madin Darby Canine Kidney (MDCK) cell protein, MDCK cell DNA, polysorbate 80, cetyltrimethlyammonium bromide, β-propiolactone, phosphate buffer	2012
Agriflu	Novartis Vaccines and Diagnostics Inc.	Egg-based vaccine: Inactivated	Egg proteins, formaldehyde, polysorbate 80, cetyltrimethylammonium bromide, neomycin sulfate, kanamycin	2012
FluMist	MedImmune	Egg-based vaccine: Live attenuated influenza vaccine (LAIV) as nasal spray	Ethylenediaminetetraacetic acid (EDTA), monosodium glutamate, hydrolyzed porcine gelatin, arginine, sucrose, dibasic potassium phosphate, monobasic potassium phosphate, gentamicin sulfate, egg protein	2013
Flublok	Protein Sciences Corporation	Recombinant vaccine	Monobasic sodium phosphate, dibasic sodium phosphate, polysorbate 20, baculovirus and host cell proteins, baculovirus and cellular DNA, Triton X-100, lipids, vitamins, amino acids, mineral salts	2012

Source: *CDC* Centers for Disease Control and Prevention, Atlanta, USA

Potency tests, operated over the entire life cycle of the product, monitor the biological activities and are a tool to ensure lot-to-lot consistency of commercial vaccines. The mission of potency tests is to predict the true clinical effectiveness of a vaccine.

For example, the single radial immunodiffusion (SRID) assay has been for many years the accepted method to monitor potency (concentration) of trivalent seasonal influenza vaccines for HA antigen (see also in this chapter under 3). Alternative assays to measure the content of HA are now

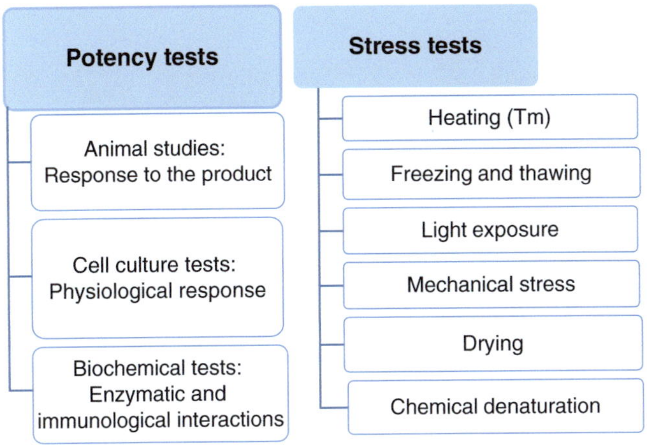

Fig. 11.3 Potency tests are operated over the entire life cycle of the product and monitor the biological activities of the vaccine by a combination of various *in vitro* and *in vivo* tests. Stress tests elucidate the inherent stability characteristics of the final vaccine formulation. Has the formulation influence on the performance of the potency test? (Tm – melting point)

being investigated, and their relative performance is validated against the current SRID. Also tests for the measurement of neuraminidase (NA) content are under consideration.

Stress tests elucidate the inherent stability characteristics of the active ingredient. Stability tests should include all attributes of the final vaccine that influence safety, efficacy, and quality. Potential changes during storage and shipment are also at the focus of stability tests (Fig. 11.3).

11.2.4 Quality by Design

Sterile filtration of the product is the method of choice that follows manufacturing of the formulated vaccines, running over to fill and finish. Other sterilization methods such as heat would ultimately destroy the protein nature. The complete manufacturing process is well controlled when all critical sources of variability are identified and explained, and the variables can be managed by the process. From this follows that the product quality can be accurately and reliably predicted.

The concept behind this manufacturing process is that quality is built into all phases of the product realization. For example, active ingredients, excipients, and primary packing materials should be bought only from approved suppliers. Details of sterilization processes and/or aseptic procedures used must be described. The risks involved in manufacturing the product and how best to mitigate those risks are analyzed. *Critical quality attributes* (CQAs) and *critical process parameters* (CPPs) are to be identified. CQAs are physicochemical and functional attributes that can be measured and continually monitored to ensure final product outputs remain within acceptable quality range. CPPs are key variables affecting the production process such as selection of AI, excipients of other materials, or the definition of the process flow and production parameters.

To summarize this concept, quality starts very early by the accurate design of experiments (planning, conducting, analyzing, and interpreting), the choice of materials and methods, tools for permanent in-process controls, and the awareness of permanent improvement: *the process is the product, what you feed is what you get.*

It's a long, long way for an antigen from the discovery to the final product and application to the patient (Fig. 11.4).

11.2.5 Marketing Authorization

It's a long way for an antigen from the discovery to the final product with application to the patient. This whole process

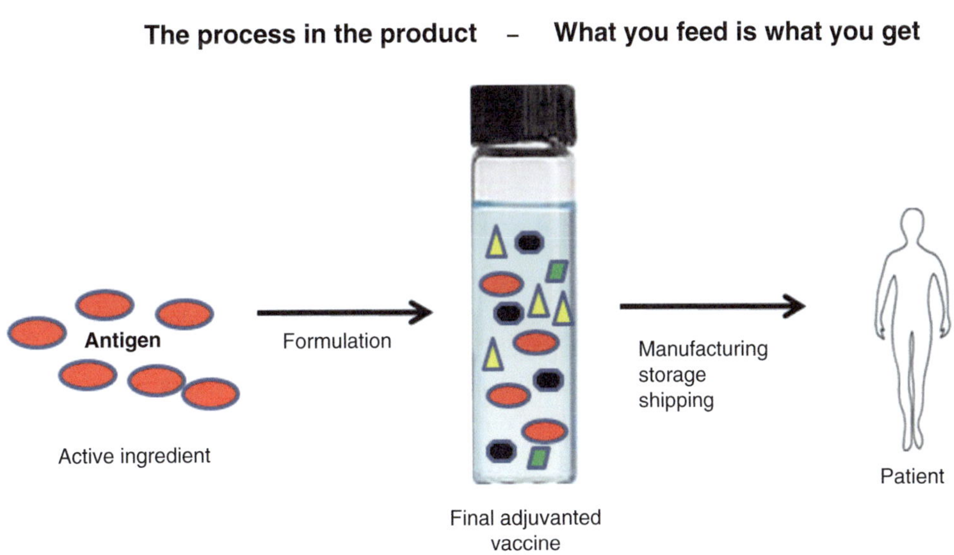

Fig. 11.4 It is the process not just the product that is the yardstick of drug development. To meet this high demand, a change in behavior and understanding is necessary. Quality starts very early by the accurate design of experiments, the choice of materials and methods, tools for permanent in-process controls, and the awareness of permanent improvement…. What you feed is what you get

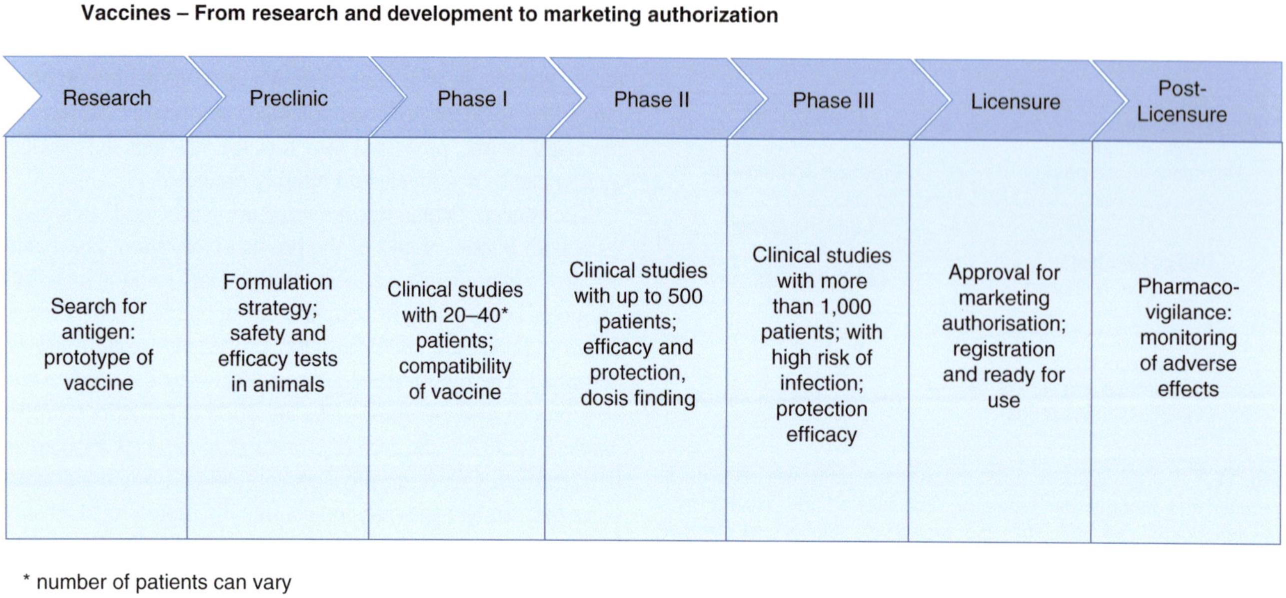

Fig. 11.5 A vaccine development process could take 10 years. Before a new vaccine is approved for release on the market, an evaluation of the risk/benefit ratio of the vaccine is done. Quality, safety, and efficacy of the product are in the focus of evaluation

could take 10 years. Before a new vaccine is approved for release on the market, an evaluation of the risk/benefit ratio of the vaccine is done. Quality, safety, and efficacy of the product are in the focus of evaluation. Compliance with GxP guidelines for laboratory and production and later for clinical testing is also verified by regulatory agencies prior to approval of a marketing authorization. Figure 11.5 summarizes the steps from research to application in the field.

Pharmacovigilance. All vaccines are monitored after release onto the market for adverse events (pharmacovigilance). More than 100 member nations have systems in place for recording and reporting adverse effects of drugs in their patients. These data are collected by the WHO and presented in "International Drug Monitoring Programme."

11.3 Cell Culture Manufacturing: Influenza Vaccine[1]

Influenza vaccination is currently the principal means of reducing or counteracting influenza mortality and morbidity burden in the community. Since the early development of monovalent killed-virus vaccine formulations in the 1940s, different principal strategies were followed by vaccine manufacturers resulting in a variety of influenza vaccines (e.g., inactivated whole virus vaccines, live attenuated vaccines, detergent or solvent "split" vaccines, subunit vaccines, and adjuvanted vaccines).

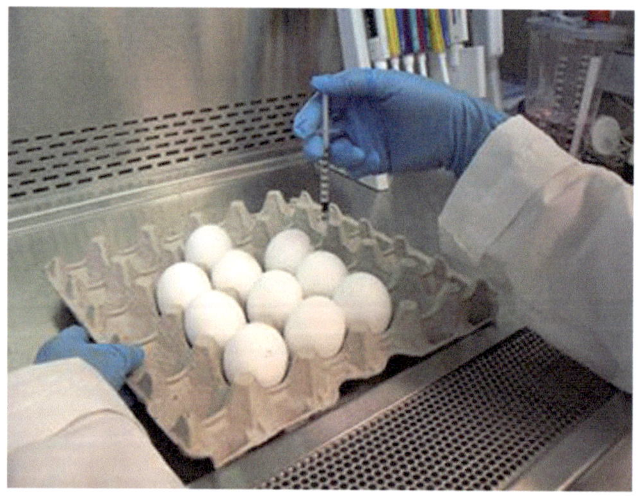

Fig. 11.6 Classical influenza production in eggs. Eggs are injected with virus aliquots, incubated, and harvested. Complex purification steps follow. This production method requires large numbers of specific pathogen-free (SPF) chicken eggs and usually takes a long period of time to produce vaccine (Photo credit: FDA/ USA)

Actually three main production processes, the classical egg-based technology and more recently cell culture based and recombinant manufacturing, can be distinguished. In addition different routes of immunization allow the generation of intramuscular, intradermal, and intranasal influenza vaccines (Fig. 11.6).

The development and the production of influenza vaccines is based on a complex manufacturing process starting

[1] Influenza cell-culture vaccine production by *Markus Hilleringmann*, *Björn Jobst*, and *Barbara C. Baudner* in Molecular Vaccines – From Prophylaxis to Therapy, Volume 2, Springer-Verlag Wien, 2013, Ed. Matthias Giese.

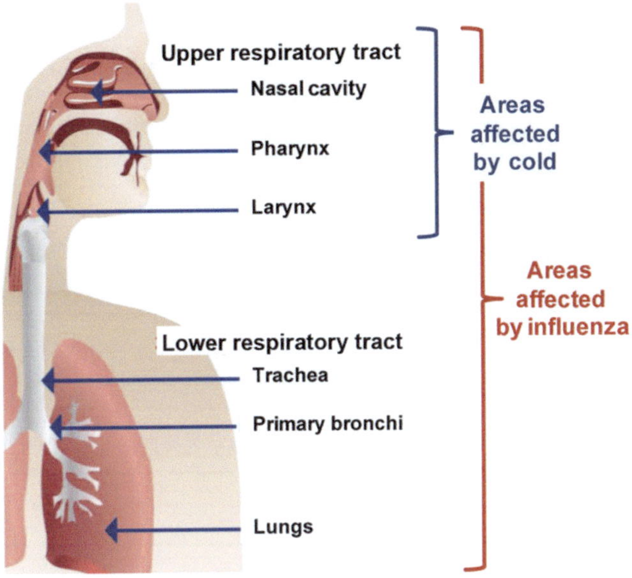

Fig. 11.7 Areas affected by cold and influenza

with the selection and development of optimal candidate vaccine viruses, and it requires various dynamic interactions with regulatory authorities and health-care officials. Planning for vaccine supplies and use and provision of other related health-care resources are essential components of a comprehensive seasonal and pandemic influenza response. Rapid spread of influenza viruses during seasonal epidemics and occasional pandemics tightly frames the whole process if vaccine is to be manufactured and delivered on time. There is a continuous effort to develop new and safe influenza vaccines and improve reagents for strain-specific potency testing to face complex influenza-related challenges better.

11.3.1 Influenza Disease

Influenza has a viral origin and often results in an acute respiratory illness affecting mainly the nose, throat, bronchi, and, occasionally, lungs (Fig. 11.7). The infection is characterized by sudden onset of high fever, aching muscles, headache and severe malaise, nonproductive cough, sore throat, and rhinitis. At the early stage of influenza infection, it might be difficult to distinguish it from the common cold, although influenza could be recognized by a high fever with a sudden onset and extreme fatigue [1].

The virus is transmitted easily from person to person via droplets and small particles produced when infected people cough or sneeze; therefore, influenza tends to spread rapidly in seasonal epidemics occurring yearly during autumn and winter [2].

Most people recover from fever and other symptoms within a week without requiring medical attention. However, mainly among high-risk groups (the very young, elderly, or chronically ill), influenza can result in hospitalizations and deaths. Worldwide, annual epidemics cause about three to five million cases of severe illness and about 250,000–500,000 deaths [3].

11.3.2 Influenza Viruses and Pandemics

There are three types of influenza viruses, A, B (both seasonal), and C. With type A and B, influenza cases occur much more frequently than type C influenza. Type A influenza viruses are further typed into subtypes according to different kinds and combinations of virus surface glycoproteins – hemagglutinin (HA or H, respectively) and neuraminidase (NA or N, respectively) (Fig. 11.8 and Table 11.3) [3, 4].

For example:

- *A/California/7/2004(H3N2)* – for a virus of human origin
- *A/duck/Alberta/35/76 (H1N1)* – for a virus from duck origin

Among many subtypes of influenza A viruses, currently influenza A(H1N1) and A(H3N2) subtypes are circulating among humans. Influenza viruses are well adapted to human populations and have the capacity to evade the immune

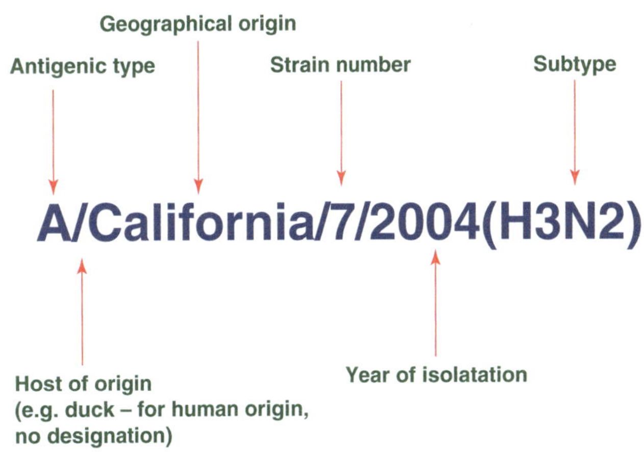

Fig. 11.8 Nomenclature system for influenza viruses (WHO 1980, A revision of the system of nomenclature for influenza viruses: a WHO Memorandum): (1) the antigenic type (e.g., *A*). (2) The host of origin (e.g., swine – for human-origin viruses, no host of origin designation is given). (3) Geographical origin (e.g., *California*). (4) Strain number (e.g., *7*). (5) Year of isolation (e.g., *2004*). (6) For influenza A viruses, the hemagglutinin and neuraminidase antigen description in parentheses (e.g., (*H3N2*)) (Figure by M. Giese Heidelberg/Germany)

Table 11.3 There are 18 known hemagglutinin (HA) subtypes and 11 known neuraminidase (NA) subtypes. Many different combinations of HA and NA proteins are possible. HA-NA combinations in humans are marked by red lines. All subtypes of influenza A virus can infect birds, except subtypes H17N10 and H18N11 which are found only in bats. The natural hosts for all known influenza type A viruses are wild aquatic birds (Table by M. Giese Heidelberg/Germany)

Species	Hemagglutinin	Neuraminidase	Species	Pandemics
man, swine, horse	H1	N1	man, swine	1918 - Spanish Flu: A/H1N1
man	H2	N2	man, swine	
man, horse	H3	N3		1957 - Asian Flu: A/H3N2 1968 - Hong Kong: A/H3N2
seal	H4	N4		
man	H5	N5		
	H6	N6		
man, horse, seal	H7	N7	man, horse, seal	
	H8	N8	horse, dog	
man	H9	N9		
	H10-18	N10-11		

system through mechanisms of mutations (antigenic drift) and swapping of surface protein genes between distantly related virus strains (antigenic shift) [5] (Figs. 11.9, 11.10, and 11.11). When a major change occurs, the risk of a human pandemic arises [6].

Three influenza pandemics occurred during the twentieth century, the most serious being the Spanish influenza. The last pandemic of the past century occurred in 1968, and the responsible virus infected an estimated 1–3 million people throughout the world. The first pandemic of the present century occurred in 2009 and was caused by an H1N1 strain (A/California/07/09).

In 1997, a novel avian influenza virus, H5N1, first infected humans in China. Since its emergence, the H5N1 virus has spread from Asia to Europe and Africa, resulting in the infection of millions of poultry and wild birds. Several hundred human cases and deaths have been reported by the WHO [7].

Genetic Reassortment. Reassortment is the mixing of the genetic material of a species into new combinations. Reassortment is the major basis for genetic shifts and one of the main mechanisms by which pandemic viruses emerge. Coinfection of a single human or animal host by two or more different strains of the influenza virus is the major determinant of reassortment efficiency.

Because pigs can become infected with influenza viruses from a variety of different hosts (birds or humans), they can act as a mixing vessel, facilitating the reassortment of influenza genes. The prerequisite for this mixing is that pigs are animal species with two types of influenza virus receptor, α 2,3 of birds and α 2,6 of swine. But the α 2,6 receptor is also in humans (Fig. 11.11). With that said, it is clear why a bird virus can infect humans. Pigs serve as reservoirs for human flu gene collections. Pigs are not the only animal species with both avian- and human-type receptors.

11.3.3 Influenza Drugs

Antiviral drugs such as adamantanes (amantadine and rimantadine) and the neuraminidase inhibitors zanamivir and oseltamivir (Tamiflu®) [8, 9] have been used to treat influenza; however, some influenza viruses develop resistance to antiviral medicines, limiting the effectiveness of treatment. WHO constantly monitors antiviral susceptibility in the circulating influenza viruses [3].

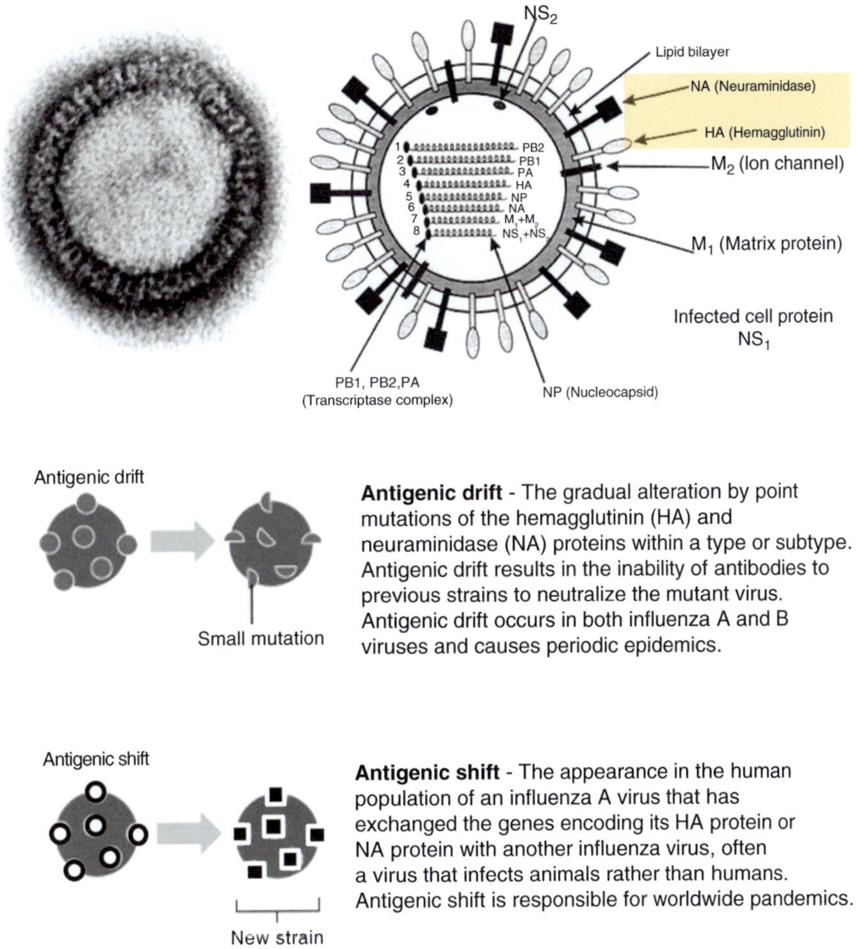

Fig. 11.9 Influenza virus: antigenic drift and shift

11.3.4 Candidate Influenza Vaccine Viruses (CVV)

According to the WHO, vaccination against influenza is the most effective way to prevent infection and severe outcomes caused by influenza viruses. Vaccination is especially important for people at higher risk of serious influenza complications and for people who live with or take care of high-risk individuals.

Various influenza vaccines have been available for many years [10]. Seasonal influenza vaccines are usually trivalent, each dose containing 15 μg of each of two influenza A subtypes (e.g., H1N1 and H3N2) and 15 μg of one influenza B strain. There are currently three predominant types of inactivated influenza vaccine: whole virus, split and subunit vaccines [11, 12] (Fig. 11.12).

The seasonal flu vaccine does not protect against influenza C viruses.

Among healthy adults, influenza vaccine can prevent 70–90 % of influenza-specific illness. Among the elderly, the vaccine reduces severe illnesses and complications by up to 60 % and deaths by 80 % [3].

World Health Organization (WHO) and Influenza Surveillance

Influenza Surveillance

As a result of genetic mutation, influenza viruses evolve frequently, and new strains quickly replace the older ones. Thus, vaccines formulated for 1 year may be ineffective in the following year, and continuous global monitoring and frequent reformulation of influenza vaccines is needed. For this reason, the WHO coordinates an international surveillance system to monitor the epidemiology of influenza viruses [13]. The surveillance system is undertaken year-round, allows for the detailed analysis of circulating influenza viruses isolated from both humans and animals, especially birds (e.g., H5N1) and pigs, and is able to detect newly evolved antigenic variants of the influenza A (H3N2 and H1N1) and B strains to which human populations are likely to be susceptible [14].

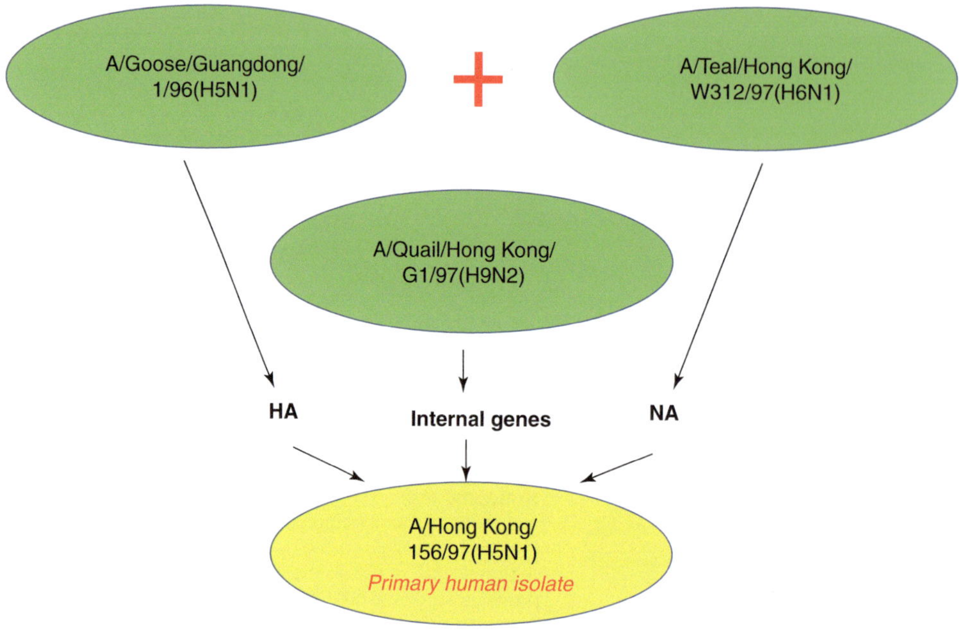

Fig. 11.10 Example of the generation of a new influenza A subtype by antigenic shift. Three different viruses have combined to form a new subtype (*H5N1*) having a mixture of the surface antigens HA and NA of the original strains (Figure by M. Giese Heidelberg/Germany)

The WHO Global Influenza Surveillance and Response System (GISRS)

The GISRS monitors which influenza viruses are circulating in humans around the world throughout the year [13]. GISRS comprises:

- Five WHO Collaborating Centers (Atlanta, Beijing, London, Melbourne, Tokyo)
- 136 National Influenza Centers in 106 countries
- 11 H5 Reference Laboratories
- Four Essential Regulatory Laboratories (ERLs)

The major technical roles of GISRS are to:

- Monitor human influenza disease burden
- Monitor antigenic drift and other changes (such as antiviral drug resistance) in seasonal influenza viruses
- Obtain suitable virus isolates for updating of influenza vaccines
- Detect and obtain isolates of new influenza viruses infecting humans, especially those with pandemic potential

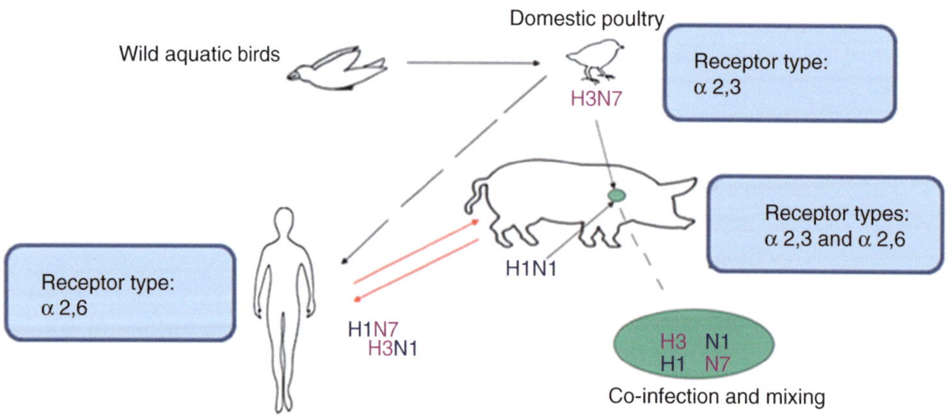

Fig. 11.11 Reassortment of influenza genes in pigs: pigs are susceptible to avian influenza in contrast to humans. By coinfection of respiratory cells in the pig, the influenza viruses undergo adaptation to mammalian hosts (pig as a mixing vessel) and can transmit to humans. Probably humans can also infect pigs. The direct infection of humans by birds is possible and was described in 1997 for A(H5N1) during a poultry outbreak in Hong Kong. It is not known why some avian influenza viruses are better able to cross the species barrier and infect humans than others (Figure by M. Giese Heidelberg/Germany)

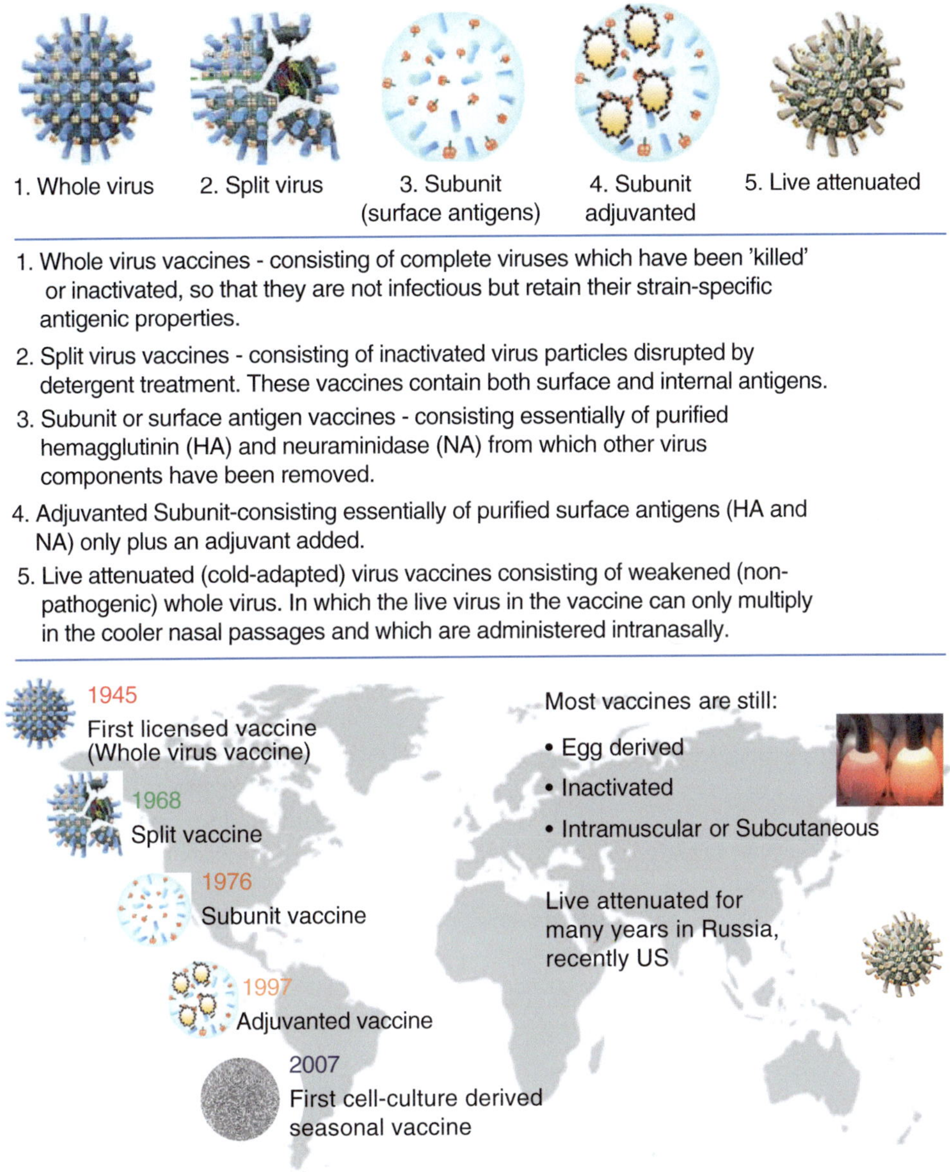

Fig. 11.12 Influenza vaccines

Influenza Vaccine Recommendations

Since 1973, twice a year the WHO convenes technical consultations to recommend which dominant circulating strains should be included in the vaccine – for the northern hemisphere in February and for the southern hemisphere in September. These recommendations are based on information provided by the formerly known WHO Global Influenza Surveillance Network (GISN), now the WHO Global Influenza Surveillance and Response System (GISRS) (Fig. 11.13). Recently, influenza A(H5N1), A(H9N2), and other subtypes of influenza viruses have also been taken into consideration by GISRS for pandemic preparedness purposes [14].

Seed Strains

Once the WHO recommends which dominant circulating strains should be included in the vaccine, WHO Collaborating Centers start to generate and analyze seed strains for vaccine production [14]. Since the 1970s, this has been mainly done by genetic reassortment for influenza A strains. Embryonated eggs are coinfected with the field strain selected for the vaccine and an A/PR8/34 (or similar) donor strain that is known to give good yields on eggs [15]. High-growth progeny virus is analyzed to confirm the presence of surface glycoproteins from the field strain. A second technology is reverse genetics, a patented technology, available to attenuate highly pathogenic viruses and reassort the attenuated HA and NA with backbone virus [16]. Once developed, these candidate reassortants are characterized for their antigenic and genetic properties before being released to interested institutions on request.

Vaccine Potency/Reference Reagents

Antigen standards and sheep antisera are subsequently developed and standardized by Essential Regulatory Laboratories

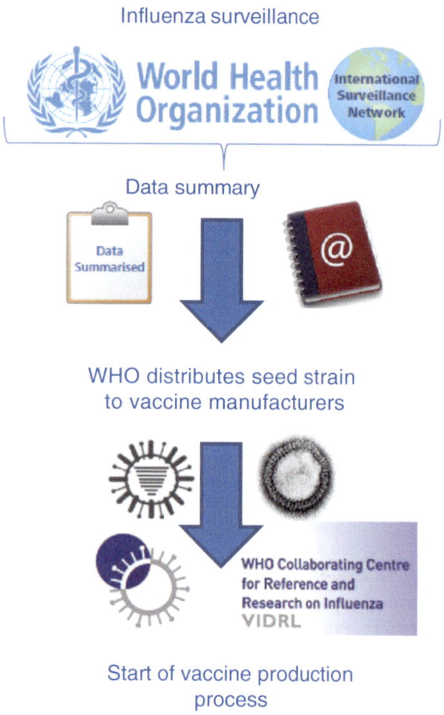

Fig. 11.13 WHO Global Influenza Surveillance and Response System (GISRS)

(ERLs), in collaboration with vaccine manufacturers. Strain-specific reagents are made available to manufacturers worldwide on request. The antigen standard and sheep antisera are needed for single radial immunodiffusion (SRID) testing in order to quantify the produced antigen in the influenza vaccine bulks and release the vaccines [17].

11.3.5 Influenza Vaccine Production

The manufacture of influenza vaccine has several unique aspects that render the production process challenging:

(a) Influenza vaccine composition must match actual global WHO epidemiological surveillance data. Therefore, an updated vaccine formulation is developed each time.
(b) Yearly licensure has to be obtained for every amendment.
(c) There are very tight time slots and short windows of opportunity to adopt processes and respond to changes. The production process is one step of many, involving various institutions.
(d) Seasonal and pandemic influenza vaccines are interrelated with a major impact on production capacities.

Therefore, manufacturers of influenza vaccines are continuously optimizing existing processes and developing new and novel methods of preparing seasonal influenza vaccines, as well as pandemic vaccine candidates. Special efforts are made to increase production capacities and introduce more automated processes, designing more flexible and timesaving manufacturing methods.

11.3.5.1 Egg-Based Production

Most influenza vaccine production is based on classical egg-based technology, a technology that has been used to produce seasonal vaccine for more than 30 years [18, 19].

As of 2011, the production capacity of egg-based technology, according to WHO's Global Action Plan for influenza (GAP), was 1.42 billion doses of trivalent vaccine, with a reported number of actually produced doses of 620 million, thereof 534 million doses for the northern hemisphere. This estimated global annual capacity is based on the information of 28 known vaccine manufacturer. In case of a pandemic, approximately 4260 million doses will be needed to immunize two billion people. This is obviously not possible with the classical egg-based production.

Novel cell-culture technologies can offer various advantages over egg-based manufacturing methods and most likely will supplement the current egg-based technology (Fig. 11.14) [20, 21].

Independent of which production process is used, either egg based or cell-culture based, and the downstream production process could produce a whole virus vaccine, a split vaccine, or a subunit vaccine from the viral harvest. All manufacturing processes must go through extensive testing and validation before licensure, and the production of each batch is tightly controlled. In the current chapter, we will focus on recent cell-culture influenza vaccine production, describing the procedure for a subunit influenza vaccine.

11.3.5.2 Cell-Culture-Based Vaccine Production

Vaccine seed strains are distributed to the vaccine producers by WHO Influenza Reference Centers in order to evaluate their suitability for vaccine production. Factors such as yield when grown in cell culture (or in eggs), antigenic stability, inactivation, and purification process are evaluated. The experiences with the vaccine candidate strains at the manufacturer from all participating companies are considered for the final endorsement of the vaccine strains by the European Medicines Agency (EMA) and the US Food and Drug Administration (FDA). The meetings with the national authorities are typically held 1 month after the initial WHO decision on composition.

Different cell lines can be used to produce the influenza virus such as VERO [22], a kidney cell from the African green monkey and Madin-Darby canine kidney (MDCK) cells [23], which originated in 1958 from the kidney of a healthy dog. Alternative expression systems for recombinant influenza proteins, like insect cells, are under study and evaluation. A MDCK cell line was optimized for the production of influenza vaccine and tested with numerous virus variants. It has proven to be particularly suitable for the production of

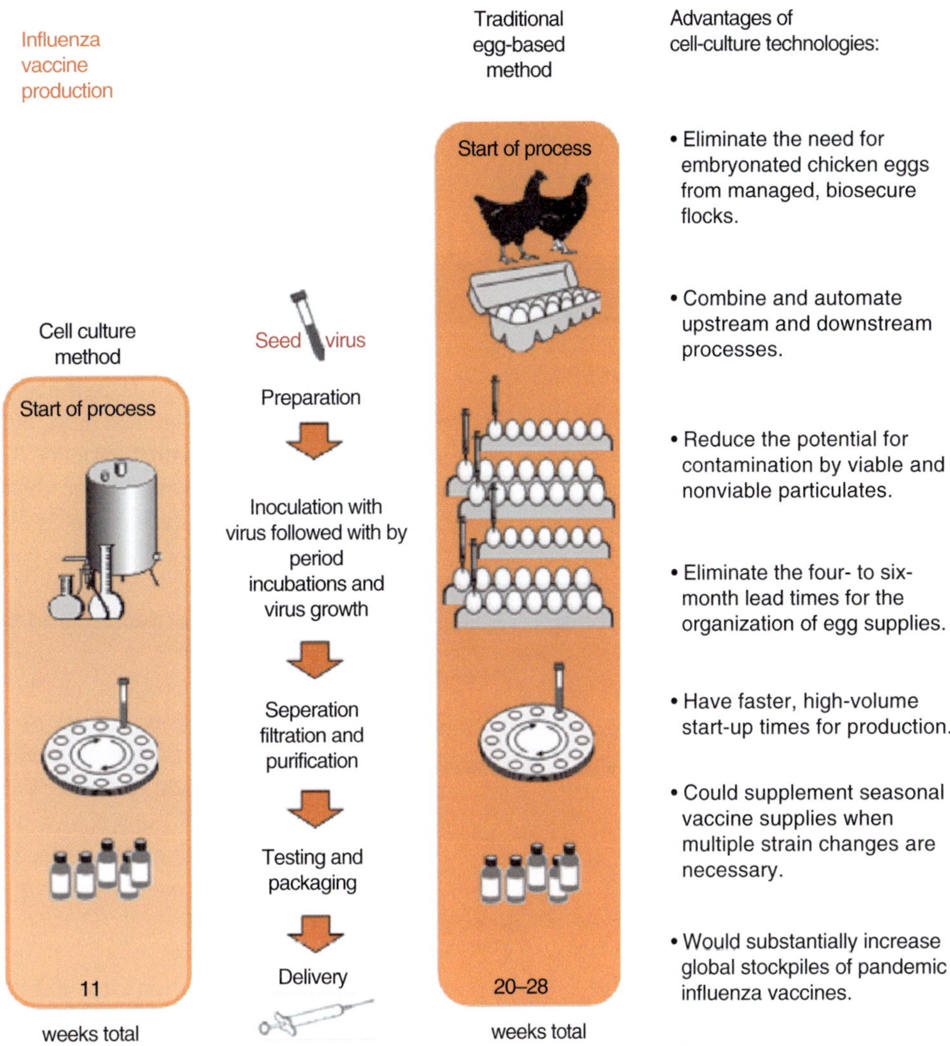

Fig. 11.14 Vaccine production by classical egg-based technology and novel cell culture processes: timeline comparison and advantages of cell-culture-based manufacturing methods

influenza vaccines as it grows in suspension. Thus, it requires no surface to proliferate, simplifying industrial production considerably.

Cell-culture influenza vaccine production resulting in a subunit influenza vaccine can be divided into the following steps (see Figs. 11.15, 11.16, 11.17, 11.18, and 11.19). A summarized scheme is shown in Fig. 11.20.

1. Cell Propagation

Preparation of a cell line for propagation starts with the thawing of the cell line "seed" lot (e.g., MDCK). For a "first-pass" cell line, propagation begins with the small-scale pre-culture propagation of seed cells. The cells are stored in liquid nitrogen at −196 °C. For the production, minimum amounts – a so-called cryo-tube containing 1 ml with approximately 10

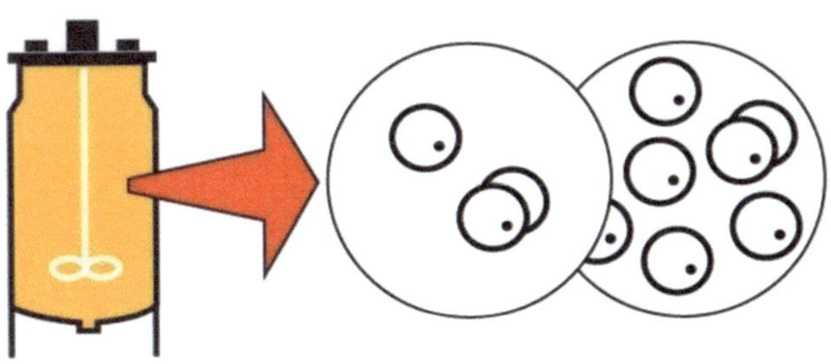

Fig. 11.15 Cell propagation

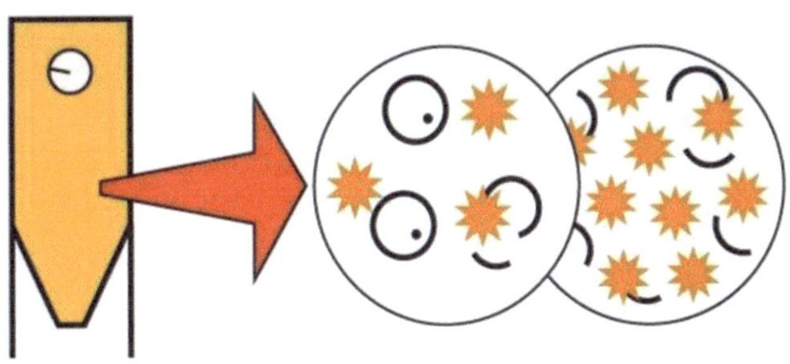

Fig. 11.16 Virus production

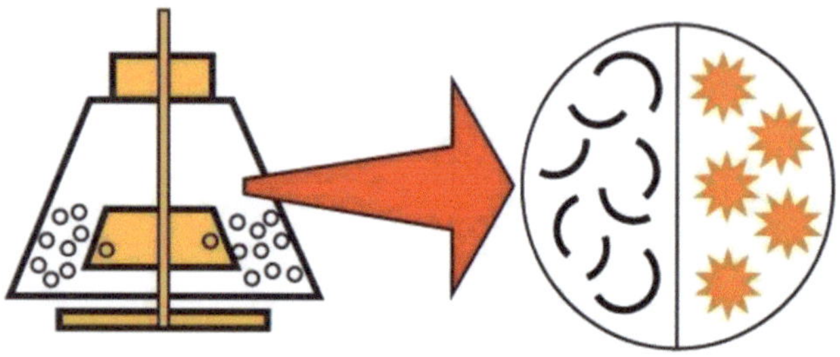

Fig. 11.17 Virus purification

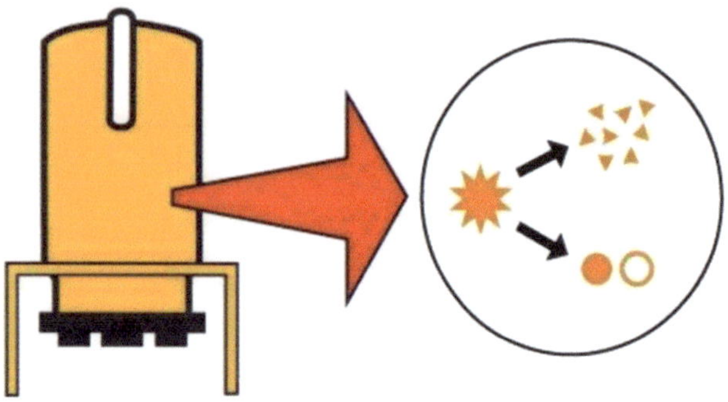

Fig. 11.18 Virus inactivation and splitting and subunit extraction

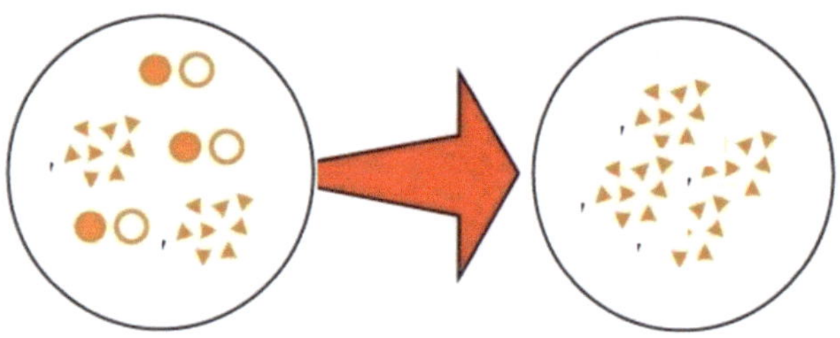

Fig. 11.19 Polishing

million cells – are thawed and proliferated in three steps from a 10 liters volume to 100 liters and then to 1000 liters. At each stage the cells receive the optimum conditions for growth with respect to temperature, oxygen, pH value, and nutrient supplies. The proliferation of the cells in fermenters (stainless steel tanks) is constantly monitored with the aid of a computer system that automatically checks all data and accurately records each step. Cell proliferation takes place in a contained fermenter system in so-called clean rooms, resulting in maximum safety and purity for employees, environment, patient, and product. Approximately 3 weeks after the removal of the cells from the nitrogen refrigeration, sufficient cells have grown in the 1000 liters fermenter. In contrast, it can take up to 6 months to organize the egg supplies, flock setting, etc. for initial inoculation in classical egg-based technology.

2. Virus Production

Upon achieving a certain predetermined density, the cells are transferred to a 2500 liters fermenter via a closed pipe system. The influenza virus is added to the tank to start infecting the mammalian cells. Virus replication in the host cell requires several days (approximately 3 days) until sufficient virus amounts for downstream processing are produced. During the course of this process, the cells die off and viruses are released in the medium/supernatant.

3. Virus Purification

The first step of a long series of purification procedures is so-called separation, by which the virus suspension is separated from the cell residue. In a subsequent chromatography step, the virus is captured and separated from the medium solution. The next step, ultrafiltration, further concentrates the intermediate product. This occurs in an automated and closed system, whereas harvesting of an egg-based virus is largely a manual process that requires extracting infected cells and fluids and then collecting the virus.

4. Virus Inactivation and Splitting and Subunit Extraction

After the purification, the virus is inactivated (rendered unable to cause infection) via a chemical reaction process. Most manufacturers use either beta-propiolactone or formaldehyde for this purpose. Virus splitting/extraction of surface antigens (HA and NA) with detergent follows, because only fractions of specific surface proteins are required for the subsequent subunit influenza vaccine.

5. Polishing

Splitting of the virus is followed by ultracentrifugation for removal of undesired viral core structures that have no role in eliciting neutralizing antibodies. This purification technology is basically similar to the egg-based vaccine process, and the resulting purified subunit vaccine is very similar in composition to egg-based vaccines. After further purification and concentration steps, approximately 10 liters of antigen concentrate of a virus strain is left of the original 2,500 liters coming from infection. Since the seasonal influenza vaccines contain three (or more recently four) viral strains (H1N1, H3N2, and one or two B strains), the production process must be performed three to four times – once for every strain (influenza vaccine monobulk) in order to generate a trivalent or quadrivalent vaccine.

6. Vaccine Characterization and Quality Tests (Bulk Release)

Subsequently the three individual bulks are analyzed for their HA antigen content by a single radial immunodiffusion (SRID) assay (Fig. 11.21) [24, 25]. SRID assay is a technique used in immunology to determine the quantity of an antigen by measuring the diameters of circles of precipitin complexes surrounding samples of the antigen that mark the boundary between the antigen and an antibody suspended in a medium, such as an agar gel. Measurement of

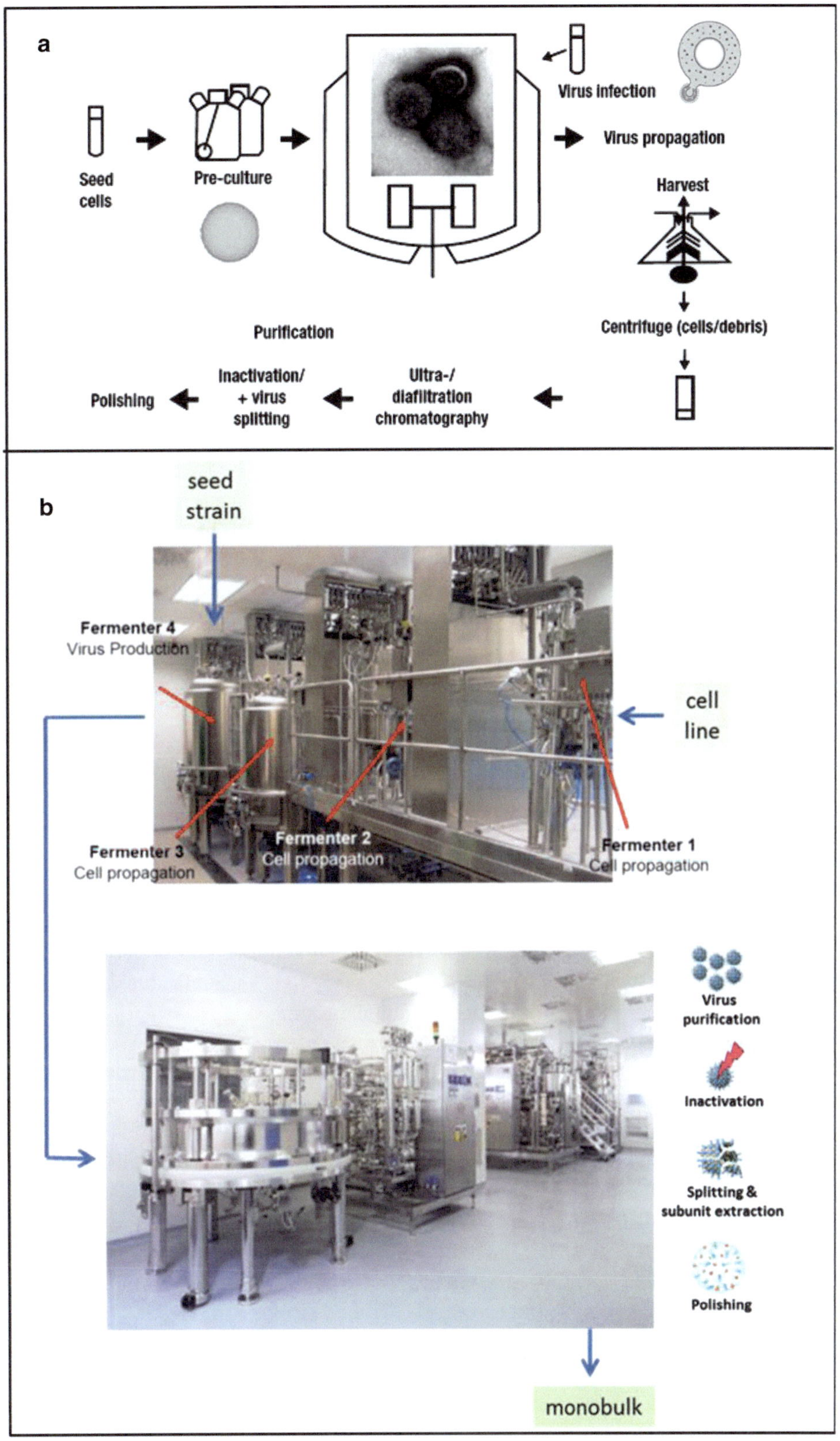

Fig. 11.20 Influenza vaccine monobulk generation. The production of a monovalent bulk containing one virus strain takes approximately 6 weeks from the thawing of the cells to the finished antigen concentrate. For trivalent vaccine, three rounds of monobulk manufacturing are needed. After the monovalent bulks are available, it takes another 10 weeks for mixing, filling, packaging, and regulatory approval before the final vaccine product can be shipped (**a** schematic workflow; **b** process showing examples of manufacturing equipment)

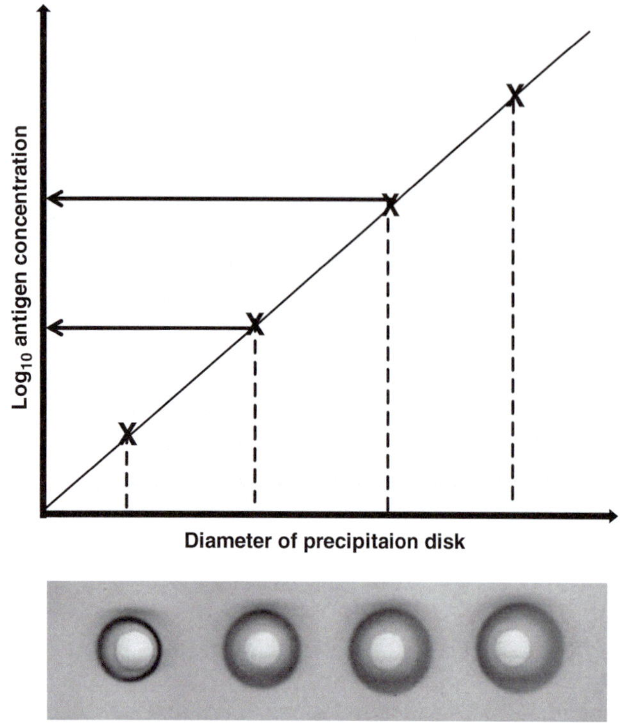

Fig. 11.21 SRID assay

the diameters of the precipitin discs of the unknown solutions allows an estimation of the antigen concentration to be made by simple interpolation to diameters of the precipitin discs of standard antigen solutions with known concentration.

The reagents need to be specific for the strains in the vaccine and take approximately 3 months to be produced and distributed (see above: *Vaccine potency/reference reagents*). This can delay the release of the vaccine. Additional testing for process-related impurities, sterility, and residual infectious virus as well as stability studies is also required for each manufactured bulk and for the release of material [26].

7. Formulation (Mixing and Filling)

The three individual influenza antigen monobulks are subsequently diluted into standard doses using sterile phosphate-buffered salt solutions in a concentration similar to bodily fluids. Final vaccine is then sterile filtered and added to bottles, prefilled syringes, or in nasal spray containers (Fig. 11.22).

8. Final Quality Control and Lot Release

Each trivalent batch or "lot" (like the individual monobulks) undergoes rigorous quality control testing to ensure it meets regulatory agency standards for safety, efficacy, and stability prior to vaccine release [25]. At this point, the development phase of an influenza cell-culture subunit vaccine is complete. All that remains is to complete the licensing process.

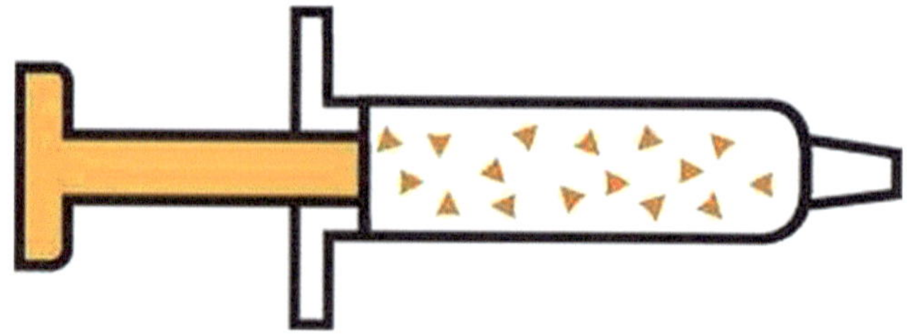

Fig. 11.22 Mixing and filling

11.3.6 Influenza Vaccine Release

Clinical Trials and Regulatory Agency Review

Vaccines are classified as biological products and regulated by both the US Food and Drug Administration (FDA) and the European Medicines Agency (EMA). In Europe clinical trials are requested to demonstrate the safety and immunogenicity of each new influenza vaccine formulation. This is not the case in the United States or the southern hemisphere.

Vaccine lots are also carefully labeled in case problems and are identified after the vaccine has been distributed. Vaccine cannot be delivered until they are formally released by the regulatory agencies [26, 27] (Fig. 11.23).

All in all, it takes about 16 weeks from the extraction of the cells until a finished seasonal influenza vaccine is packaged and ready for delivery. As mentioned above, external factors such as availability of strain-specific reagents can influence the timeline. The complex process of a seasonal influenza vaccine campaign including various dynamic interactions of public health institutions/laboratories and vaccine manufactures is depicted schematically in Fig. 11.24.

11.3.7 Improved Influenza Vaccines

During influenza pandemics, vaccine production faces a race against the time. Although during the 2009 H1N1 influenza pandemic, first vaccines were available approximately 3 months after the declaration of the pandemic, quantities of the vaccine were limited, and only a minority could be vaccinated in time – before the pandemic waves had peaked. More flexible platforms that enable more rapid vaccine production and facilitate regulatory processes are highly desirable, and both manufacturers and governments together with research institutions have encouraged a wave of innovation to develop novel methods in influenza vaccine manufacturing [28], as recently reviewed in detail by Dormitzer et al. [29].

Historically, most efforts have been put on improving already licensed egg-based vaccines and their manufacturing, focusing on increased production capacities and the

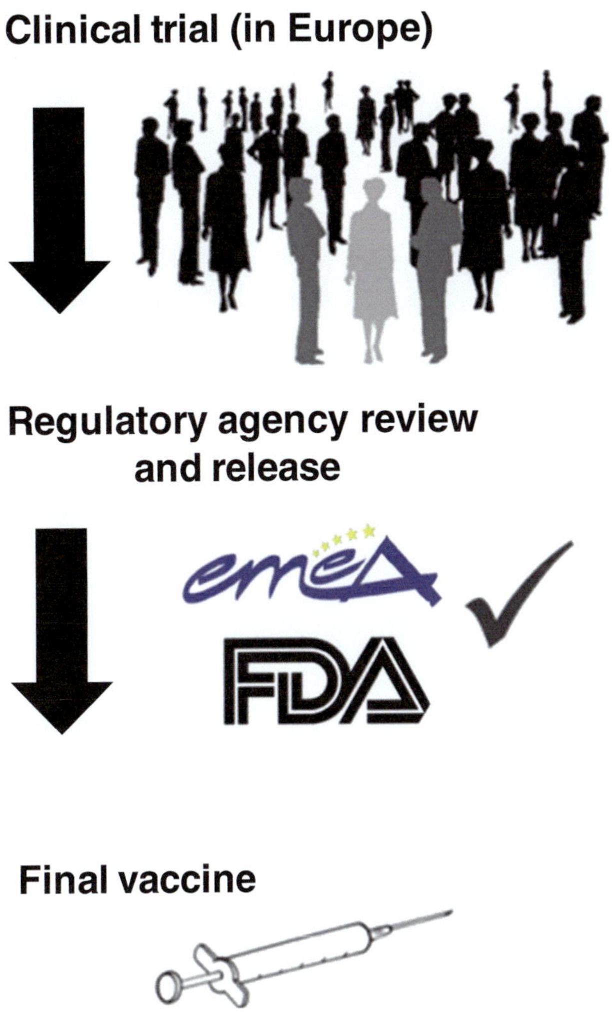

Fig. 11.23 Influenza vaccine release

automation of the production processes [19]. The introduction of cell-culture-based influenza production brings several advantages over egg-based vaccine production, with a high potential to better face future influenza-related challenges [20, 21, 30].

11.4 Making Transgenic Plants

Let food be the medicine and medicine be the food.
– Hippocrates

11.4.1 Basics of Plant Engineering

All organisms, animals, plants, bacteria, viruses, and fungi, have the same 20 different amino acids. Plants are eukaryotic organisms with a complex cell structure and nucleus, in which the genetic material is organized, with a subordinated protein biosynthesis machinery compared to animals:

DNA makes RNA makes protein.

Plant-expressed eukaryotic proteins are properly folded, posttranslational modified, and assembled in a biologically active form. They are naturally free of human or animal microbial toxins and pyrogens and recognized as safe. It is therefore not surprising that genetic engineering very early discovered plants for direct manipulation of genetic material not only for making improvement to plants but for production of recombinant proteins.

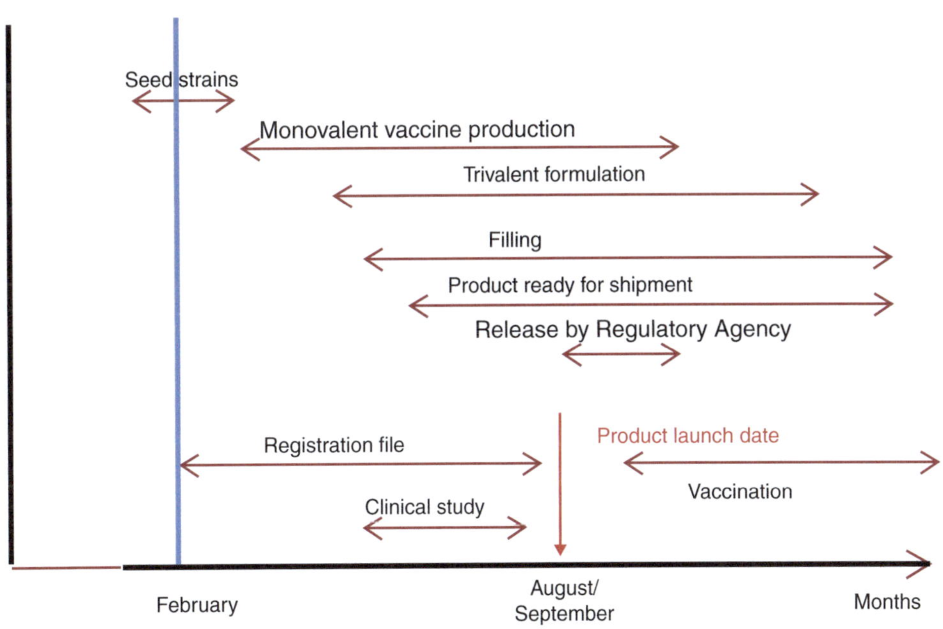

Fig. 11.24 Life cycle of a seasonal vaccination product development for the northern hemisphere starting from influenza vaccine seed strains

Table 11.4 Milestones in transgenic plants for expression of biopharmaceuticals

Year	Recombinant protein	Plant	Ref.
1986	Human growth hormone	Tobacco Sunflower	[31]
1989	Antibodies	Tobacco	[32]
1992	HBsAg (hepatitis)	Tobacco	[33]
1998	E. coli heat-labile enterotoxin (LT-B)	Potato (uncooked as edible vaccine)[a]	[34]
2002	Rabies virus: G-N fusion protein	Tobacco	[35]
2012	VLP *Norovirus*	Tobacco Lettuce	[36]
2012	ZMapp, mAb cocktail	Tobacco	[37]

[a]Edible vaccines are discussed in Chap. 13

11.4.1.1 Host Plants

Transgenic plants are usually divided into food crops and nonfood crops. One of the most used plants is tobacco with a high biomass yield due to its easy and well-established handling of genetic transformation. Transgenic tobacco can be used for the production of antibodies, vaccines, cytokines, etc. (Table 11.4).

11.4.1.2 *Agrobacterium tumefaciens*

To get stable transformation (and expression), a DNA fragment encoding the protein of interest and a selectable marker needs to be inserted into the nuclear or chloroplast genome in cells of leaf explants in culture [38]. The transfer of the heterologous sequence into the nuclear genome is efficiently obtained using the plant pathogen *Agrobacterium tumefaciens* (Fig. 11.25) transformed with binary vectors (i.e., artificial vectors including elements derived from naturally occurring tumor-inducing plasmids originally found in *A. tumefaciens* and required to transfer heterologous DNA into plant cells) [39], while the transfer into the plastid genome needs the use of direct DNA delivery methods, such as particle bombardment or treatment with polyethylene glycol [40].

In both cases, after transformation, the explants are used to regenerate whole plants, relying on the totipotency properties of plant cells, by growth on a selective medium that allows the survival (and plants regeneration) only to cells expressing the selectable marker gene. In order to obtain homozygosity and stable inheritance of the gene, plants transformed into the nuclear genome (and the seeds they produce through self-fertilization) are grown under selective conditions for a couple of generations, while in the case of plastid transformation, the selection process necessary to achieve homoplasmy (the condition in which the transgene is integrated in every plastid genome, i.e., up to 10,000 per leaf cell) takes a longer time [41].

As compared to stable transformation methods, transient transformation is a much more rapid and easy high-throughput procedure to produce large quantities of recombinant proteins in plants, but as suggested by the name, the heterologous sequence is only temporarily expressed and cannot be transmitted to the plant progeny as transformation is performed in vivo on fully developed plants [42].

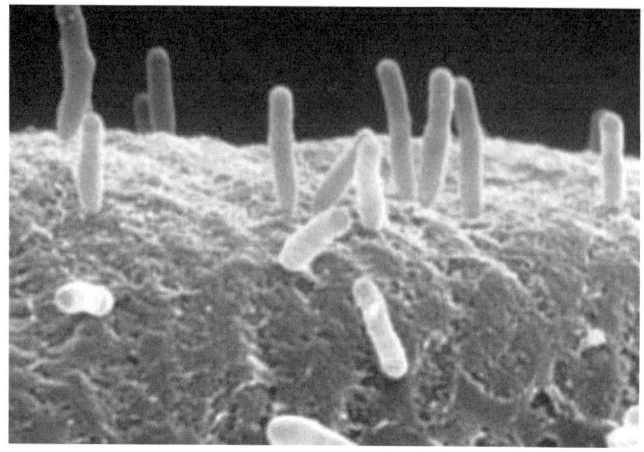

Fig. 11.25 *Agrobacterium tumefaciens* cells attached to a plant cell. It is a rod-shaped, gram-negative soil bacterium. *A. tumefaciens* infects the plant through its Ti plasmid, tumor-inducing plasmid. The modification of this plasmid that has 196 genes is important in the creation of transgenic plants (Photo credit: Martha Hawes, University of Arizona/USA)

Agroinfiltration. One of the methods that can be used to get transient transformation has the same initial step of stable nuclear transformation, i.e., the insertion of the sequence to be expressed into a binary vector that is then used to transform *A. tumefaciens* cells [43] (Fig. 11.26). In transient transformation however, a suspension of the transformed bacteria is then infiltrated onto the abaxial (i.e., underside) surface of leaves attached to the plant using a syringe deprived of needle. This procedure, called agroinfiltration, allows the penetration of the suspension into the leaf air-spaces through stomata or through a tiny incision made on the leaf. Alternatively the whole plant can be submerged upside down into a beaker containing the bacterial suspension and placed in a vacuum chamber.

Instead of agroinfiltration, transient expression can be gained by inserting the heterologous sequence into the genome of a plant virus (or into an expression vector encoding a complete viral genome) and using the genetically modified plant pathogen to infect plants [44]. To this aim, few microliters of a solution containing recombinant

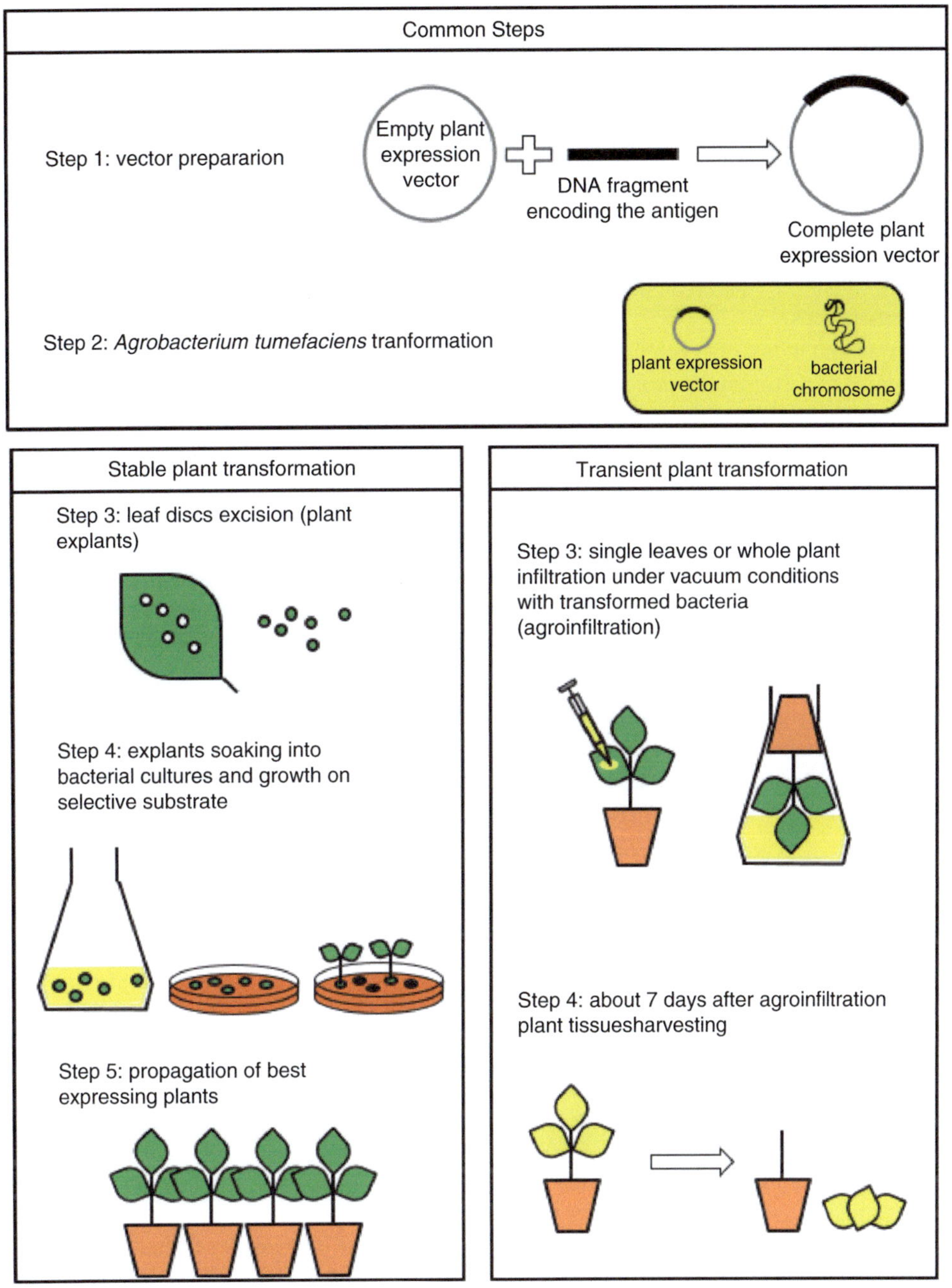

Fig. 11.26 A schematic diagram illustrating the main steps to be followed to stably or transiently transform plants exploiting *Agrobacterium tumefaciens*. In the upper box, initial genetic engineering and bacteria transformation steps common to both transformation procedures (Baschieri [66])

plant virus particles or the expression vector encoding the recombinant viral genome are distributed on the adaxial (i.e., upper) surface of the leaf, and the expression of the heterologous protein proceeds throughout the plant together with viral infection.

Viral Vector Systems. Beside *A. tumefaciens*, which does not infect all plant species, also viral vector systems for transformation are widely used, such as infiltration with the MagnICON system, which is based on a tobacco mosaic virus (TMV) RNA replicon system or a geminiviral DNA replicon system derived from bean yellow dwarf virus (BeYDV), described below in this chapter.

Harvest of Proteins. Harvest dates vary determined by the transformation system used and by the plant species. Generally, if the plant starts turning yellow as a consequence of the bacterial or viral infection, the day for harvest has come. Tubers, grains, leaves, or fruits can be selected for the downstream isolation and purification process.

Advantages and Limitations. Plant expression systems are postulated to be safe, cheap, and simple in the production and logistic sense. Transgenic plants can be produced locally or distributed without a cold chain and can be stored at ambient temperatures, favorable attributes especially for developing countries. Grown in the field, plants require little more than sunlight, water, and basic horticultural input. Their multiplication through inbred seeds is relatively simple and efficient, and they can also be propagated by vegetative means without the use of seeds.

The most important limitations of transgenic plants are their low expression level of recombinant proteins and often a long cultivation time of plants. The low expression levels make it necessary to enlarge the fields for growing.

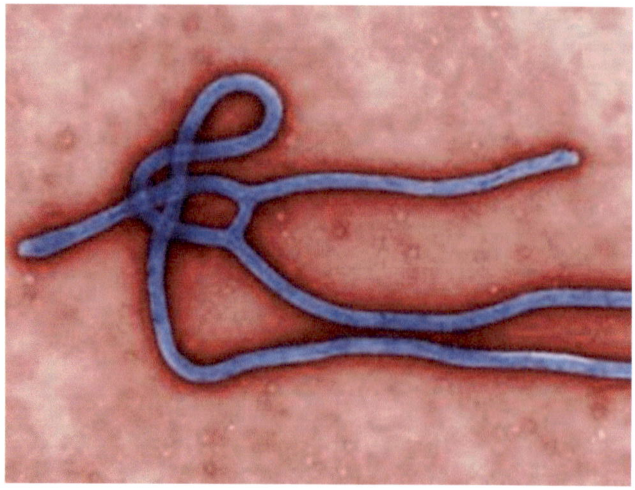

Fig. 11.27 Colorized transmission electron microscopy of Ebola virus. Virion: filamentous, 970 nm long, 80 nm in diameter, and enveloped. It is suggested that the primary natural reservoir of Ebola virus, named after a river in the Democratic Republic of the Congo in Africa, where it was in 1976 first recognized to cause the EV disease, is bats. Ebola can cause disease in humans and nonhuman primates by direct contact (e.g., via blood and other body fluids) (Photo credit: C. Goldsmith, CDC/USA)

11.4.2 Cocktail of Plant-Derived Antibodies against Ebola Virus

11.4.2.1 The Ebola Epidemic

The Ebola Outbreak in 2014 has affected multiple countries in West Africa and was the largest in history. At the beginning of this epidemic, no vaccine was available, but a cocktail of plant-derived antibodies against Ebola virus which was used to cure infected patients. In summer 2015, preliminary results of a phase 3 trial with rVSV-ZEBOV-GP, a vector-based vaccine (vesicular stomatitis virus) in Guinea, indicated that this new vaccine is highly efficacious and safe.

11.4.2.2 The Ebola Virus

The Ebola virus (EV) causes the Ebola virus disease (EVD), formerly known as Ebola hemorrhagic fever, a severe, often fatal illness in humans. EV belongs to the family of *Filoviridae*. Filovirus virions may appear in several shapes. These shapes include long, sometimes branched filaments, or a circle. These filaments may measure up to 14,000 nm in length, have a uniform diameter of 80 nm, and are enveloped in a lipid membrane (Fig. 11.27). The genome has an approximately 19 kb ss(−) RNA, and the proteome is arranged in 7 proteins. The infection is initiated by the attachment of GP glycoprotein to host receptors (Fig. 11.28).

11.4.2.3 The Cocktail Against Ebola

MB-003. Three Ebola virus (EBOV)-specific chimeric (mouse/human) antibodies, c13C6, c13F6, and c6D8, directed against three distinct, nonoverlapping EBOV glycoprotein (GP) epitopes were produced in whole plant (*Nicotiana benthamiana*) cells and in CHO cells [37].

A mixture of these three monoclonal antibodies (mAb), called MB-003, given as a single dose of 16.7 mg/ kg per mAb to macaques, 1 h postinfection (p.i.), followed by the same dose on day 4 and 8, protected 3 of 3 monkeys in a lethal challenge model with 1000 pfu of Ebola virus. Subsequent immunization studies with more animals and MB-003 treatment given 24 h or 48 h p.i. confirmed the protection capacity of these cocktail: four of six animals survived and had little to no viremia and few, if any, clinical symptoms.

ZMAb. This is also mixture of three monoclonal mice/chimeric antibodies, m1H3, m2G4, and m4G7, developed by the National Microbiology Laboratory (Winnipeg, Canada), through the Public Health Agency of Canada (PHAC).

ZMapp. An optimized cocktail comprising of individual monoclonal antibodies selected from the previous antibody cocktails MB-003 and ZMAb, which turned out to be c13C6 from MB-003, and two chimeric mAbs from ZMAb, c2G4 and c4G7.

Results. A remarkable finding was that the tobacco-produced mAbs were three times as potent as the CHO cell-based mAbs.

Production Limits. The calculated ZMapp doses for a human adult of 70 kg are 10.5 g of highly purified monoclonals (three doses × 3.5 g). 1 kg plant biomass results in 100 mg purified mAbs which means the biofarming company has to cultivate 105 kg tobacco plants for only one treatment [45].

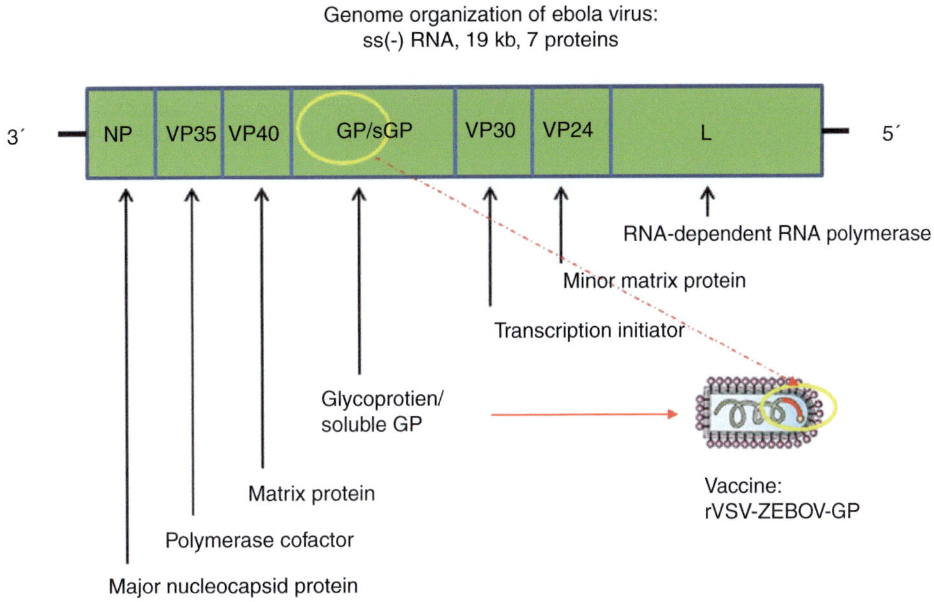

Fig. 11.28 Genome organization of Ebola virus. The genome has an approximately 19 kb ss(−) RNA and is approximately 19,000 nucleotides long. It encodes seven structural proteins: nucleoprotein (*NP*), polymerase cofactor (*VP35*), (*VP40*), GP, transcription activator (*VP30*), VP24, and RNA-dependent RNA polymerase (*L*). The vaccine rVSV-ZEBOV-GP is a live attenuated recombinant vesicular stomatitis virus (*rVSV*) with the glycoprotein (*GP*) antigen from the Zaire Ebola virus (*ZEBOV*). The development for this vaccine begun 10 years ago

11.4.3 *Norovirus* Vaccines from Plants[2]

The development of virus-like particles against *Norovirus* infection is discussed in Chap. 9. The plant-based production is described in detail here:

Noroviruses (NoVs) are a group of genetically diverse RNA viruses that cause the great majority of nonbacterial gastroenteritis in humans. The lack of a tissue culture system and a small animal model further hinders the development of NoV vaccines.

Virus-Like Particles (VLPs). VLPs mimic the antigenic architecture of authentic virions, however, can be produced in insect, mammalian, and plant cells by the expression of the capsid protein. The particulate nature and high-density presentation of viral structure proteins on their surface render VLPs as a premier vaccine platform with superior safety, immunogenicity, and manufacturability.

Plant Production. The advantages of plant expression systems as a novel production platform for VLP-based NoV vaccines are discussed in light of their cost-effectiveness, production speed, and scalability. Recent achievements from the first successful demonstration of NoV VLP production in plant expression system under the current Good Manufacture Practice (cGMP) regulation by the US Food and Drug Administration (FDA) are detailed.

Results of human clinical trials demonstrating the safety and efficacy of insect and plant-derived NoV VLPs are also presented.

Characterization of NoV VLPs. VLPs of NoVs were first produced in insect cells using baculovirus vectors, then in plants using tobamovirus and geminivirus [46] vectors, and in mammalian cells using the Venezuelan equine encephalitis (VEE) replicon system [47]. These studies demonstrated that expression of the major capsid protein VP1 alone can drive the self-assembly of VLPs that morphologically and antigenically resemble native virus particles (Fig. 11.29). VLPs generated by all three expression systems are similar to each other.

The structure of NoV VLPs is exemplified by the VLP of NV capsid protein (NVCP). Studies of insect cell-baculovirus-derived NVCP VLPs by cryo-electron microscopy and X-ray crystallography reveal that the NV capsid is a 38 nm icosahedral arrangement of 180 copies of the 58 kDa capsid protein VP1 organized into 90 dimers in a T=3 symmetry [46]. While all dimers are formed from two identical NVCP monomers, two different dimer configurations are required to correctly form the complete assembled capsid [48].

[2]Virus-like Particle Vaccines for Norovirus Gastroenteritis by *Qiang Chen* in Molecular Vaccines - From Prophylaxis to Therapy, Volume 2, Springer-Verlag Wien, 2013, Ed. Matthias Giese.

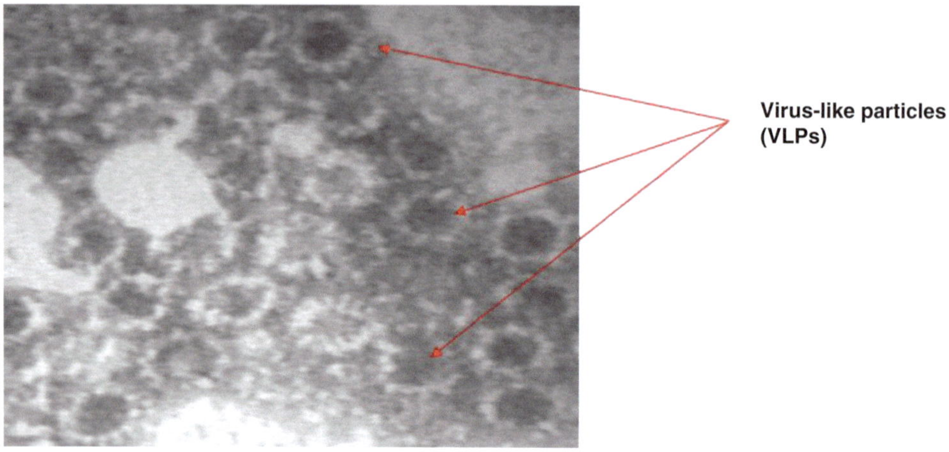

Fig. 11.29 NVCP VLPs produced in plants. NVCP (NV capsid protein) was expressed in lettuce leaves with a geminiviral replicon vector. NVCP VLPs were purified from plants, negatively stained with 0.5 % uranyl acetate, and examined by electron microscopy. Bar = 50 nm. One representative experiment of three is shown

As in native NV particles, the NVCP also folds into two distinctive domains in VLPs, with S domain forming the inner core of the shell and P domain protruding out from the capsid [49]. Similarly, the P2 subdomain is also the most surface-exposed region in NV VLPs and may contain HBGA and neutralizing antibody binding sites and determinants of strains specificity. The similarity between VLPs of NV and other NoVs including GII.4 viruses has been demonstrated [50].

Plants as Production Platform. Plants are considered as an alternative protein vaccine production system because they can produce high levels of vaccine protein at low cost and biomass production does not require expensive investment in cell culture facilities or facility duplication for scale-up production [51]. As a result, the flexibility and capital efficiency for plant biomass generation and scale-up are far more superior to current fermentation-based technologies [52]. In addition, plants possess eukaryotic processing machinery for proper posttranslational modification and assembly of proteins and have low risk of introducing adventitious pathogens to humans. Despite these potential advantages, earlier production of protein vaccines using stable transgenic plants resulted in slow and low levels of target protein accumulation. The long time frame (several months to a year) to generate transgenic plants, the lack of strong promoters, and the position effects from the random insertion of the transgene are responsible for these problems that reduce the cost-saving benefit of plants as a production system.

The challenges of VLP production speed and yield have been overcome by the development of plant virus-based transient plant expression systems [53]. For example, some groups have reported that the cloning and high-level transient expression of plant-derived VLPs can be achieved quickly in 1–2 weeks of vector infiltration with the MagnICON system, which is based on a tobacco mosaic virus (TMV) RNA replicon system or a geminiviral DNA replicon system derived from bean yellow dwarf virus (BeYDV) [54]. These improvements in the speed and yield of VLP expression also provide plant expression systems, an additional advantage in versatility for producing VLP vaccines against NoV and other viruses that have rapid antigenic drift and multiple genogroups and strains with unpredictable epidemics around the world.

11.4.3.1 NoV VLPs Derived from Stable Transgenic Plants

VLP based on NV capsid protein (NVCP) is one of the most investigated VLPs in plants and has been successfully expressed in many plant species including tobacco, potato, *Nicotiana benthamiana*, tomato, and lettuce by our group and collaborators [52].

Tabacco. As for other vaccine proteins, NVCP was first expressed in transgenic tobacco and potato plants [55]. It usually took several months to generate and select transgenic tobacco and potato plants that expressed NVCP. Expression of NVCP in these transgenic plants was approximately 10 μg/g fresh tissue weight, which is rather low compared with the insect or mammalian cell-based expression system. However, assembled virion-sized icosahedral VLPs that resemble insect cell-derived VLPs or native NV particles were observed in transgenic tobacco leaves and in potato tubers. In another experiment, the VP1 gene of NV was codon optimized and expressed in transgenic tomato plants [56]. Comparative studies indicated that VLP yield and assembly varied depending on the codon usage, host plant species, and possibly the target tissue of NVCP accumulation. For instance, NVCP expression level was low, and only 25–50 % of them were assembled into VLP in potato tubers, while at least tenfold higher expression and more efficient VLP assembly were achieved in tomato fruits.

Uncooked Potatoes. To achieve gut mucosal immunity against NV, four doses of 4 g uncooked potato tuber containing 40–80 μg NVCP were fed to mice at days 1, 2, 11, and 28. This immunization regime induced specific serum IgG and intestinal IgA responses in mice. When four doses of 50 μg purified NVCP VLPs were orally delivered to mice in the same immunization regime, serum anti-NV response was fourfold higher than that of mice fed with NVCP expressing. The humoral immune response can be further enhanced to 16-fold higher when adjuvant (CT) was co-delivered. Perhaps the enrichment of assembled VLPs in the purified samples is responsible for the enhancement of humoral immunity because only ~50 % of the NVCP in the potato tubers was assembled into VLPs. It is also possible that NVCP was not efficiently released from the potato tissue to be delivered to GALT for antigen processing and presentation.

Tomatoes Versus Potatoes. Tomato fruits present a more feasible plant material for developing oral NoV vaccines as they are more palatable than raw potato tubers, and their production and processing have been well established by the food industry. Oral delivery of 4 doses of 0.4 g freeze-dried tomatoes (containing 40 μg VLP) stimulated strong serum anti-NVCP IgG and intestinal mucosal IgA responses in more than 80 % of mice [57]. Furthermore, 100 % of mice developed strong systemic and mucosal antibody responses when a higher dosage (0.8 g per dose) of transgenic tomato was used.

Freeze-Drying Versus Air-Drying. The same study also showed that NVCP fed in freeze-dried tomato was more immunogenic than that in freeze-dried potato tubers [56]. The less oxidative environment or the unique tissue structure in tomato fruits may allow better stability or more efficient release of VLPs and, in turn, better immunogenicity. It was also noticed that ingestion of NVCP air-dried tomatoes elicited more potent serum IgG and intestinal IgA responses than that NVCP freeze-dried tomatoes. It is possible that the freeze-drying process altered the assembly status of VLPs in tomato fruits. Alternatively, air-drying may result in better VLP stability by preserving the architecture of VLPs and the tissue structure so that VLPs are better protected from the digestive enzymes in the oral–gastrointestinal tract or more efficiently released from the tissue for uptake by GALT. Overall, these data support the development of oral vaccines for NoV in tomato plants.

Plant Virus-Based Vectors. The major challenges up to this point for NoV VLP production in plants were the slowness of obtaining VLP-expressing plant lines and poor VLP yield. One of the strategies to overcome these challenges was the use of transient expression systems based on vectors developed from plant viruses. In these systems, transgenes are not integrated into one of the plant genomes, but instead they are present in the plant nucleus transiently while being transcribed, and later the transcripts are transported into the cytoplasm, and the transgenic proteins are translated [58].

TMV and Potato Virus. These systems are focused on production speed and yield and gain the flexibility of nuclear gene expression with the speed and expression amplification of viruses. For example, the MagnICON transient expression system based on replication-competent TMV and potato virus X (PVX) allows high levels of recombinant protein production within 7–10 days of vector delivery [59]. Indeed, the results show that the MagnICON system allows to produce fully assembled NVCP VLPs at a level of 0.8 mg/g of fresh leaf weight (FLW) within 12 days of infiltration in *N. benthamiana* plants, at least an 80-fold greater production than in transgenic tobacco and tomato.

Mucosal Delivery. When delivered through the oral route, the partially purified VLPs (100 μg per dose) from transiently expressed plant material provoked potent and balanced systemic IgG1/IgG2a response in the absence of any adjuvant. Significant NVCP-specific vaginal and fecal mucosal IgA responses were also detected in 100 % of immunized mice by the same immunization regime. Moreover, a significant enhancement in NVCP-specific immunity was achieved by the inclusion of adjuvant CT in the oral immunization. Thus, the "destructed" viral–vector-based transient expression system has enabled us to overcome the challenges associated with transgenic plant systems and rendered a robust plant system for NoV production.

Geminiviral BeYDV Replicon. To further optimize the transient expression systems for commercial production of NoV VLP vaccines, another robust expression system based on geminiviral BeYDV DNA replicon vectors and commercially available lettuce was developed [60]. There are two major advantages of this transient expression system: the noncompetitive nature of BeYDV DNA replicon vector and the use of commercially produced lettuce. In contrast to the MagnIcon system, which can produce proteins with maximally two different hetero-subunits, the geminiviral vector allows the production of VLPs with up to at least five hetero-subunits (Fig. 11.30).

Lettuce. Lettuce is cultivated readily and rapidly produced in large quantities in well-established commercial greenhouses. Unlike tobacco and related species of *Nicotiana* such as *N. benthamiana*, lettuce is a palatable plant and can be consumed raw for oral delivery of NoV VLPs. When NVCP was expressed in *N. benthamiana* plants with BeYDV replicon vectors, assembled VLPs were accumulated up to 0.4 mg/g FLW in leaves. This data also indicate that the BeYDV replicon system allows a high level of NVCP VLP expression and assembly in lettuce as those driven by the MagnICON system in *N. benthamiana* [52].

Actually, VLP accumulated to its highest level at day four after vector introduction, indicating that this expression system can produce similar levels of VLPs in lettuce but in a

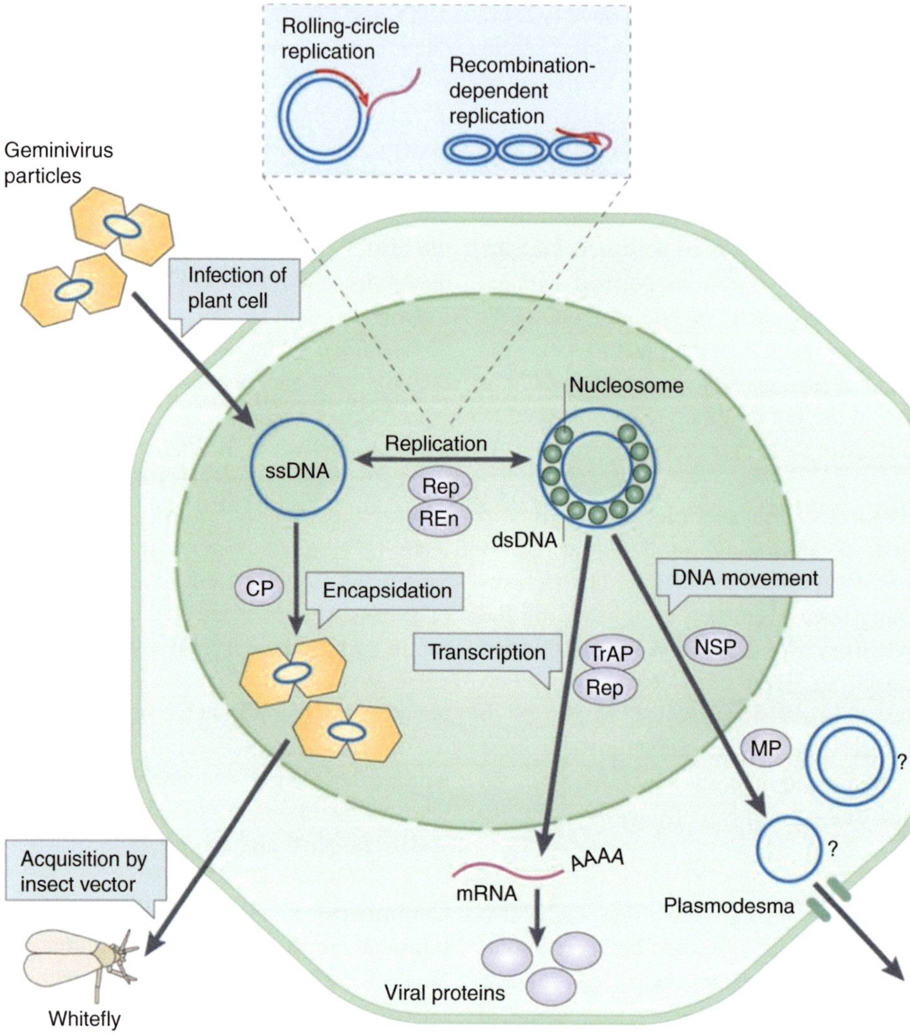

Fig. 11.30 Geminiviral replicon. Infection begins in a plant cell when viral single-stranded DNA (*ssDNA*) is released from virions and copied to generate double-stranded DNA (*dsDNA*). The dsDNA, which assembles with nucleosomes, is transcribed by host RNA polymerase II, allowing production of replication initiator protein (*Rep*). Rep initiates rolling circle replication by introducing a nick into a viral dsDNA molecule to generate a free 3′-hydroxyl end that primes ssDNA synthesis, leading to displacement of the parental strand (inset). The released ssDNA is converted to dsDNA to reenter the replication cycle. Viral replication transitions to recombination-dependent replication, which is initiated by homologous recombination between a partially replicated ssDNA and a closed, circular dsDNA to form a looped molecule that serves as a template for both ssDNA and dsDNA synthesis (inset). Later in infection, Rep represses its own transcription, leading to activation of transcriptional activator protein (*TrAP*) expression, which in turn activates coat protein (*CP*) and nuclear shuttle protein (*NSP*) expression. Circular ssDNA can then be encapsidated by CP into virions, which are available for whitefly acquisition. NSP binds to viral DNA and moves it across the nuclear envelope, where movement protein (*MP*) traffics it across a plasmodesma. It is not known whether viral DNA moves as ssDNA versus dsDNA or as a linear versus a circular molecule (Credit: Hanley-Bowdoin et al. [67], Nature Publishing Group)

much shorter time frame than the MagnICON system in tobacco. Importantly, this study is one of the first demonstrations of using commercially produced lettuce for rapid and high-level production of VLPs [52]. This represents a significant milestone for the eventual commercial production of NoV VLP-based vaccines, as this would allow our production system to have access to unlimited quantities of low-cost material from existing commercial sources. Coupled with the almost unlimited nature of lettuce production, the high efficiency and scalability of our BeYDV replicon vectors provide us a new NoV VLP production platform that is low cost, robust, safe, and amenable to large-scale manufacturing.

11.4.4 Plant Vaccines and Regulatory Conditions

Despite the successes in expressing NVCP VLPs and a variety of other subunit vaccines in plants and the recent improvement of vaccine production levels by transient expression systems, no plant-derived vaccine has been licensed yet for human use. This lack of commercial success lies in several technical and regulatory barriers that remain to be overcome. These challenges include the lack of scalable downstream processing procedures, the uncertainty of regulatory compliance of production processes, and the lack of demonstration to date of plant-derived vaccines that meet the required standards of regulatory agencies in identity, purity, potency, and safety.

While immunization by ingesting plant tissue still presents a viable approach to orally delivering plant-produced VLPs, product regulatory concerns have necessitated the development of downstream processing technologies to produce purified VLP vaccines with a defined unit dosage. Therefore, for the promise of plants as an alternative for vaccine production to become a reality, the technology must be able to produce sufficient quantities of VLPs at a relevant scale and with product qualities that meet all required standards of regulatory agencies such as US Food and Drug Administration (FDA) or the European EMA.

11.4.5 Approved Facilities for Plant Vaccine Production

To overcome these remaining challenges, the regulatory compliance of facilities, materials, and procedures for production of NoV VLPs under current Good Manufacture Practice (cGMP) has to be addressed first. Qiang Chen's group from the Biodesign Institute, Arizona State University, USA, has lead the effort in this area and established the first cGMP-compliant bioprocessing facility in academia for the production of NoV VLPs in plants [61].

As shown in Fig. 11.31, the purposefully built facilities in the Arizona State University permit biomass generation and bioprocessing of plant-derived NoV VLP vaccines under cGMP Quality Management System (QMS). For example,

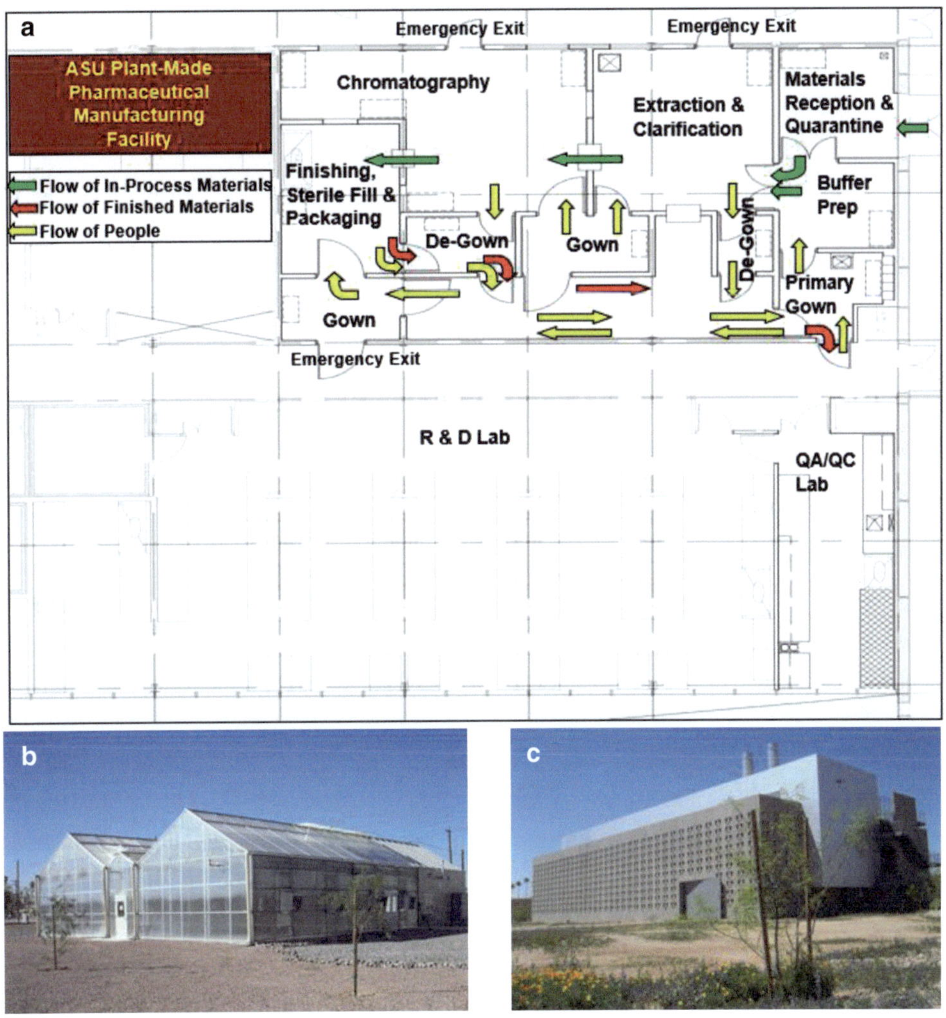

Fig. 11.31 cGMP production facilities for NVCP VLP vaccine. (**a**) The design of the central bioprocessing suite. The arrows indicate the unidirectional flow of in-process materials (*green*), purified final product (*red*), and people (*yellow*). (**b**) The BSL-2 greenhouse facility for plant biomass generation and NVCP expression. (**c**) The Plant Biopharmaceutical Center that houses the central bioprocessing suite, the QA/QC laboratory, and the Process Development Laboratory

separated rooms for buffer preparation, incoming plant samples, chromatography, and sterile fill are purposefully designed in the central bioprocessing suite (Fig. 11.31a).

As indicated by the arrows in the same figure, the suite is operated under differential pressure with the sterile fill room being a class 100 environment and designed to have a separated unidirectional flow of human workers and biological material, so that the products meet the requirements of both US and European Union (EU) regulatory agencies for manufacturing of human pharmaceuticals. As a part of the QMS, the quality control (QC)/Quality Assurance (QA) laboratory is adjacent to the bioprocessing suite for product testing and quality management (Fig. 11.31a). A 3600 ft^2 Biosafety level 2 (BSL-2) greenhouse facility has also been built for plant biomass production under cGMP (Fig. 11.31b).

The BSL-2 greenhouse is equipped with advanced technology for containment of plants or pathogens, which is necessary to maintain the integrity of the plant-derived VLPs and to minimize the risk of accidental genetic contamination of the external environment.

The established bioprocessing facilities and QA/QC laboratories have also been certified for producing human vaccines, which laid a solid foundation for the cGMP compliance of VLP production procedures and the final VLP vaccine product.

11.4.5.1 *A. tumefaciens* and *N. benthamiana* Master and Working Banks

As part of the cGMP compliance of upstream processes, biomaterials including relevant *Agrobacteria* strains and the *N. benthamiana* plant line have to be qualified by the QMS. This process starts with the establishment of master and working banks of *A. tumefaciens* strains that contain the NVCP expression vectors and a seed bank of wild-type *N. benthamiana* for growing biomass for transient expression.

To generate plant material for cGMP-compliant production of NVCP VLPs, three *A. tumefaciens* master banks, each containing the expression cassette for VLP production in TMV 3' module, TMV 5' module, and integrase of the MagnICON system [59], have been established in the bacterial strain of GV3101. The identity of the *A. tumefaciens* host strain and associated functional genes and vectors are fully validated. These banks have been shown to be genetically stable over a 4-year period [31].

A master seed bank for wild-type *N. benthamiana* was also established. Our experiment has shown that this seed bank has a germination rate of 99 % and produced uniform seedlings with typical *N. benthamiana* morphology even after a 4-year storage at 4 ± 2 °C (Fig. 11.32). These results collectively demonstrated that it is feasible to establish master and working banks of *A. tumefaciens* strains and *N.*

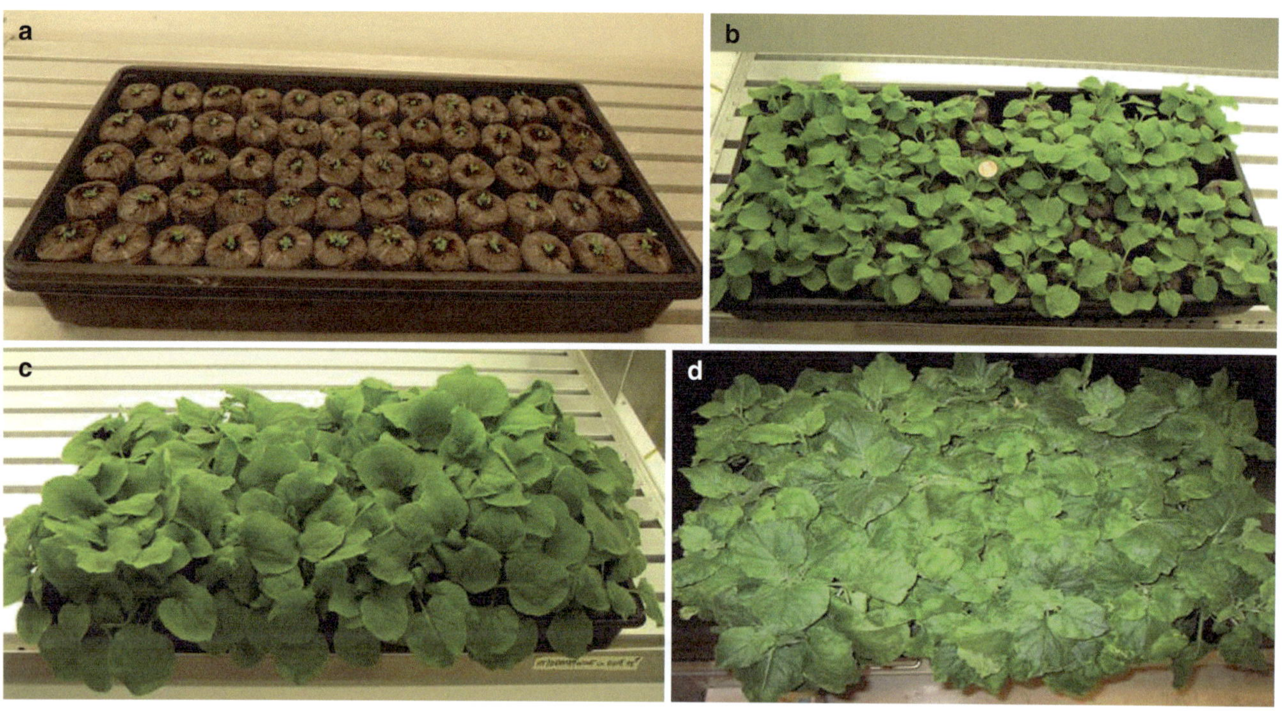

Fig. 11.32 Biomass generation under production conditions. Wild-type *N. benthamiana* plants one (**a**), three (**b**), four (**c**), and five (**d**) weeks after planting

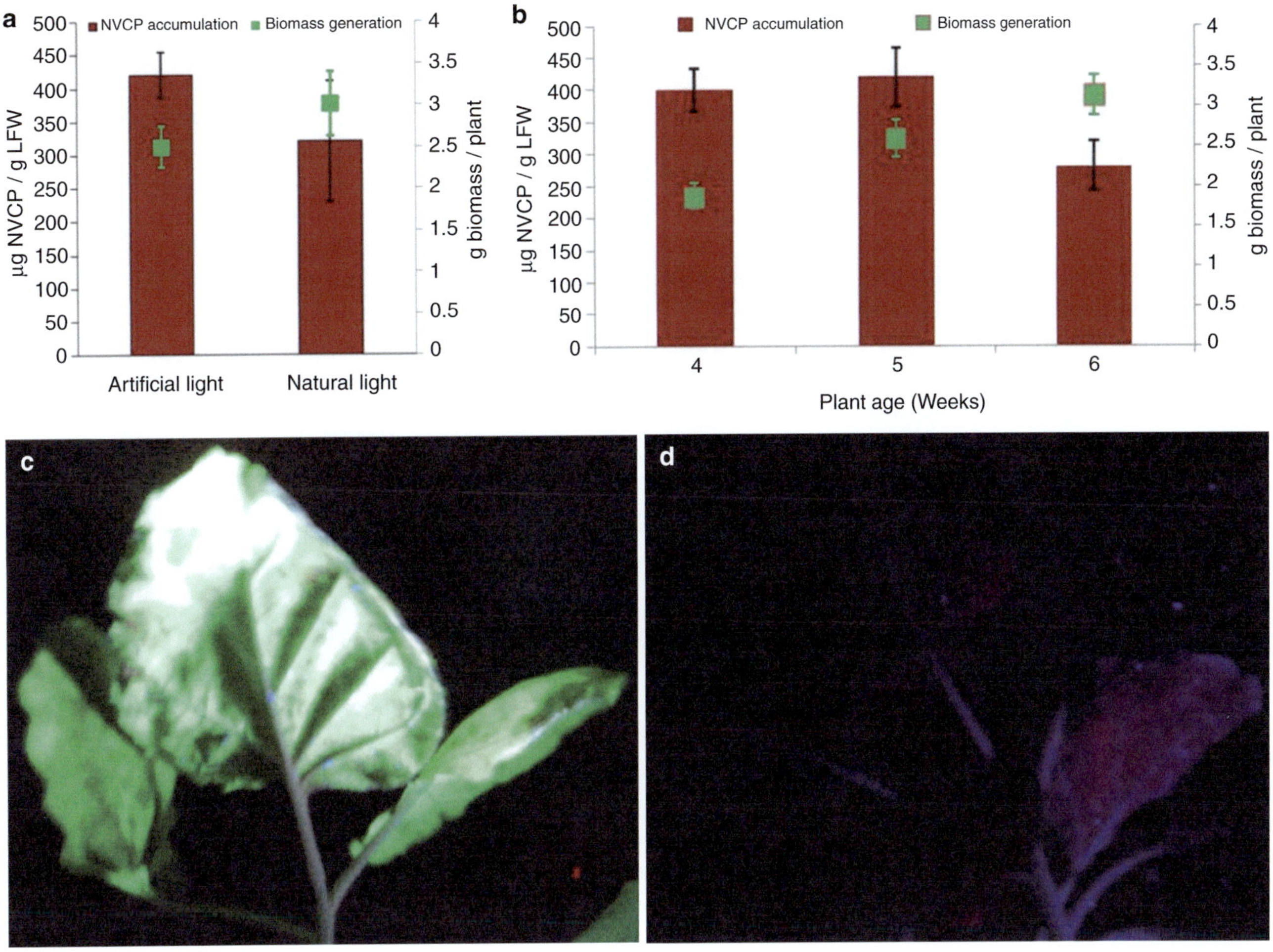

Fig. 11.33 Optimization of biomass and NVCP VLP accumulation. (**a**) Biomass and NVCP yield under natural and artificial light. *N. benthamiana* plants were grown either under natural or artificial light for 5 weeks. Leaf biomass (*green square*) and NVCP expression level (*red column*) were measured by weighing and ELISA, respectively. (**b**) Temporal pattern of biomass yield and NVCP expression. Plants were grown under artificial light for 5 weeks, and biomass production (green square) and NVCP accumulation (*red column*) were examined. For both (**a**) and (**b**), mean ± standard deviation (SD) of samples ($N > 10$) from three independent infiltration experiments (**c**) and (**d**) visualization of GFP expression in agroinfiltrated leaves are presented. *N. benthamiana* plants were infiltrated either with GV3101 cultures that carry the three MagnICON vectors for GFP expression (**c**) or with infiltration buffer as a negative control (**d**). Leaves were examined and photographed 7 dpi under UV light. One representative of at least three independent experiments is shown

benthamiana seeds that meet the qualification standards of identity and stability for cGMP production of NoV VLPs.

11.4.5.2 Biomass Production

In this part of the upstream process, the goal is to optimize conditions that permit the maximal production of leaf biomass and VLPs per square meter of greenhouse space. Studies demonstrated that temperature, light source and intensity, plant age, and incubation time after leaf infiltration all have significant impacts on biomass generation and VLP accumulation. For example, *N. benthamiana* grown under nature light produces more biomass but accumulates much less NVCP VLPs than plants grown under artificial light (Fig. 11.33a). Furthermore, leaves grown under natural light also produce more solid debris during VLP extraction, causing problems for VLP purification. The data also indicate that a 16 h light/8h dark cycle at 25 °C is the optimal condition to generate biomass under such artificial lighting. When *N. benthamiana* plants were grown under these conditions and sampled at various ages for NVCP VLP expression, it was founded that 5-week old plants provided the optimal material for VLP production, because they already accumulated an adequate amount of biomass and produced the highest level of VLPs (Fig. 11.33b). Younger plants produce insufficient biomass, and older plants are too tall for infiltration and start to produce more secondary metabolites that complicate VLP purification. Consequently, 5-week old *N. benthamiana* optimally balance the combined need for biomass generation, filtration operation, and VLP accumulation. The data demonstrated that under these optimized conditions, biomass for producing sufficient amount of purified NVCP VLPs for a phase I clinical trial can be generated in 5.6 square meters of greenhouse space in a 5-week period. The horizontal space requirements for this type of production could be significantly reduced by vertically stacking layers of growth trays vertically.

Methods for efficient introduction of *Agrobacterium* into leaves by vacuum infiltration were also developed [61]. As illustrated by the expression of the GFP and NVCP VLPs, plants infiltrated based on these methods under scale-up conditions allowed efficient infiltration of vector-carrying *Agrobacteria* in the entire leaf area (Fig. 11.33c) and accumulated the highest level of NVCP VLPs in leaves 7 dpi (Fig. 11.33a and b). Moreover, the yield and temporal expression pattern of NVCP VLPs under these scale-up conditions are similar to that of our previous smaller bench-scale experiments. These results clearly indicate that the upstream process for NV VLP production in plants is scalable and can be further scaled up for commercial production.

11.4.5.3 Downstream Processing of NoV VLPs

While eating unprocessed or partially processed NoV VLP-containing plant tissue remains a viable option for vaccine delivery, purified VLPs with a well-defined unit dosage are most likely to be the first generation of successful vaccine candidates for commercialization due to regulatory requirements. Therefore, it is absolutely necessary to have a robust and scalable downstream process that can effectively recover and purify VLPs in place in order for plant-produced NoV VLP vaccines to become commercial reality. An optimized downstream process should be able to preserve the integrity of VLPs and produce highly purified VLPs with a high recovery rate and a minimal number of processing steps.

It should also be scalable, economical, and compliant with the FDA's cGMP regulations. The most common practice for NoV VLP purification is density gradient ultracentrifugation [49]. While these methods are useful for characterizing VLP size and assembly [48], they are not practical for commercial VLP manufacturing as they are difficult to scale up and time-consuming [60]. They may also be problematic for preserving the integrity of VLPs because the hyperosmotic gradient agents and severe centrifugation force can often shear VLPs. To meet the demand for more scalable and robust methods of NoV VLP processing, a new trend has started toward more sophisticated methods like filtration and chromatography. For example, Q. Chen's group has recently developed a robust and scalable downstream processing scheme for recovering NVCP VLPs from plants (Fig. 11.34).

FDA's cGMP Compliance. In this three-step process, plant extracts are processed by low pH precipitation, ultrafiltration, and diafiltration (UF/DF) with tangential flow filtration (TFF) membranes and ion-exchange (IEX) chromatography [61]. Low pH and UF/DF eliminated most plant host proteins and IEX chromatography purified NVCP VLPs to>95 %

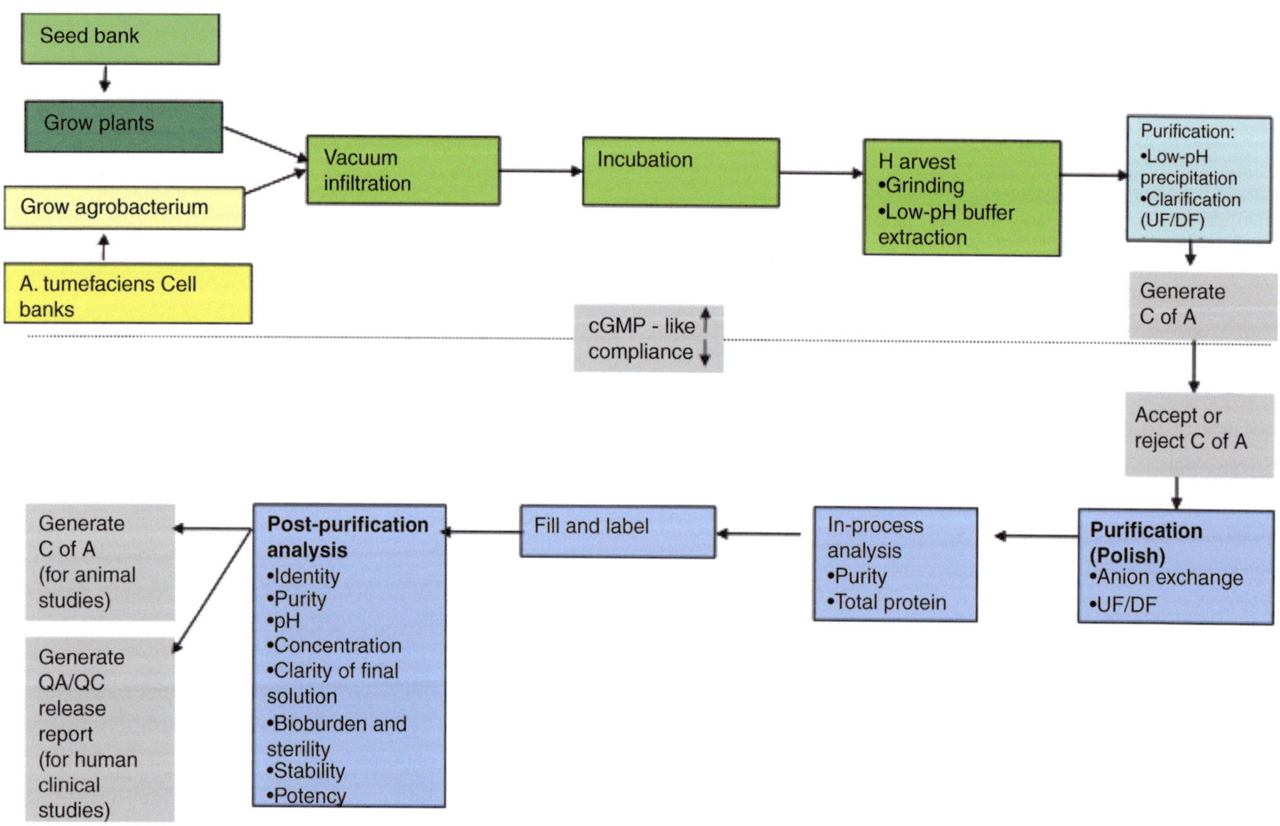

Fig. 11.34 Process flow for the production of NVCP VLP vaccine under cGMP regulations. *C of A* certificate of analysis, *UF/DF* ultrafiltration and diafiltration

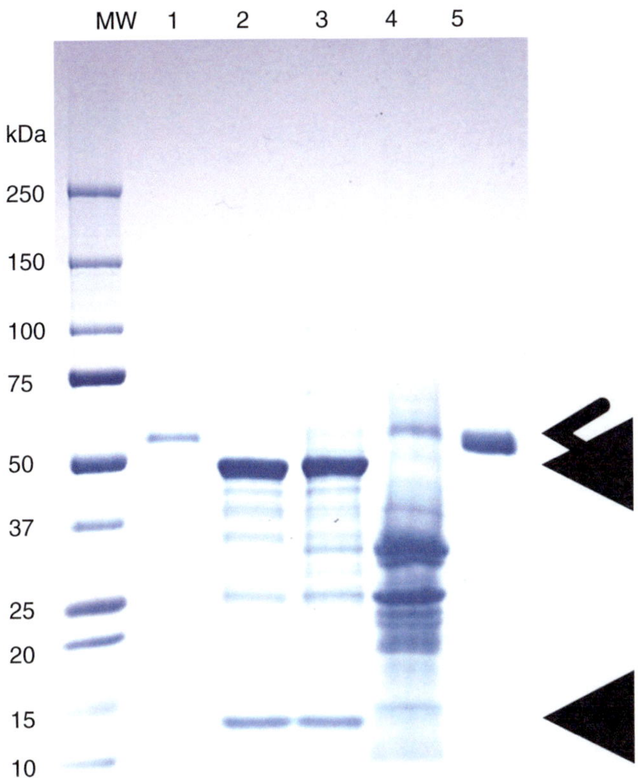

Fig. 11.35 Purification of NVCP from *N. benthamiana* plants. Leaf protein extract was purified and analyzed on a 4–20 % SDS-PAGE gel under reducing condition. *Lane 1* insect cell-produced NVCP as a reference standard, *Lane 2* clarified leaf extract from uninfiltrated plants, *Lane 3* clarified leaf extract from NVCP-producing plants, *Lane 4* supernatant of low-pH precipitation, *Lane 5* purified plant-derived NVCP from DEAE anion-exchange chromatography. ◄: RuBisCo large and small subunits; ←: NVCP

purity (Fig. 11.35, Lane 5). Production runs with various scales of plant biomass demonstrated that this downstream process is highly scalable and can consistently yield highly pure NVCP VLPs with high recovery rates. In contrast to gradient centrifugation that is laborious and time-consuming, the new method is robust, is more scalable, and can be completed within ≤12 h instead of several days [60]. Importantly, this new process is fully cGMP compliant and has produced cGMP grade VLPs for a human clinical trial.

These advantages along with the rapid ligand discovery process and the low cost of peptide production would allow its application to large-scale NoV VLP manufacturing.

11.4.6 Quality Control of Plant-Derived NoV VLPs

One of the remaining challenges for the commercialization of plant-derived vaccines is the lack of examples that meet the required standards of regulatory agencies in identity, purity, potency, and safety. As part of the efforts to overcome this challenge, Chen's laboratory has identified and developed analytical assays to monitor the in-process samples and

Table 11.5 Analytical assays for NVCP VLP in-process samples and the final purified product

Product attribute	Analytical method
Product identity	Western blot
Product identity	N-terminal sequence with automated Edman sequencing
Purity and molecular	SDS-PAGE/profile Coomassie and silver staining
Protein purity and concentration	RP-HPLC
Protein concentration	Absorption at wavelength of 280 nm (A280)
Protein concentration	Amino acid analysis (AAA)
Mass	ESI-TOF mass spectrometry (ESI-TOF MS)
Quaternary structure	SEC HPLC multi-angle laser light scattering (MALLS)
Quaternary structure	Sucrose gradient centrifugation, TEM
Determination of pI	Isoelectric focusing (IEF)-PAGE
Glycan analysis	MALDI-TOF MS
Endotoxin	Limulus amebocyte lysate
Bioburden	Turbidity and colony formation
Residual host DNA	PicoGreen and PCR
Small molecules, Nicotine	LC-MS/MS
Residual host cell protein	Polyclonal Abs to wild-type *N. Benthamiana* plant protein

SDS-PAGE sodium dodecyl sulphate polyacrylamide gel electrophoresis, *RP-HPLC* reverse-phase high-pressure liquid chromatography, *ESI-TOF* electrospray ionization time of flight, *TEM* transmission electron microscopy, *MALDI* matrix-assisted laser desorption–ionization, *PCR* polymerase chain reaction, *LC-MS/MS* liquid chromatography-tandem mass spectrometry

to ensure that the final VLP product meets preset specifications for the release of human pharmaceuticals in identity, purity, concentration, tertiary structure, functionality, and in concentrations of host contaminating molecules essential for the cGMP compliance (Table 11.5). The analyses showed that the identity and assembly of the final VLP product were confirmed, and its purity, concentration, appearance, residual host DNA concentration, and stability all conformed to the insect cell-derived reference standard [61].

The final VLP product elicited strong NVCP-specific systemic, local, and distal mucosal immune responses in mice, demonstrating its potency. These results have provided the first example of plant-derived NoV VLPs from a scale-up process that meets the predetermined release specifications. Preliminary data suggest that mucosal immunization with several adjuvants evoked stronger serum IgG and mucosal IgA responses than with VLP alone.

11.4.7 Human Clinical Trials with NoV VLPs

The successful demonstration of strong systemic and mucosal immunogenicity in preclinical studies has led to several clinical trials to examine the safety and immunogenicity of NoV VLP-based vaccines in humans (Table 11.6).

Table 11.6 Phase I human clinical trials with NVCP VLP-based vaccines

Production system	Number of volunteers	Formulation	Number of doses and dosage range	Delivery route	Immunogenicity
Insect cell /baculovirus	20	Water, no adjuvant	Two doses of 100–250 μg at days 1 and 21	Oral	Serum IgG and IgA responses were dose-dependent and NV-specific tilters increased at least fourfold in 100 % of volunteers in the 250 μg group. Eighty-three percent responded in serum IgG titers after the first VLP dose and showed no increase after the second dose [63]
Insect cell /baculovirus	36	Water, no adjuvant	Two doses of 250, 500, and 2000 μg at days 1 and 21	Oral	Increase of NV-specific IgG titers was detected in 90 % of participants in the 250 μg group. No further increase in the rates of seroconversion or IgG titers for the 500 and 2000 μg groups. Increase of NV-specific IgA ASC numbers in 100 % of vaccinated volunteers was observed, and 30–40 % of volunteers developed salivary, fecal, or genital fluid IgA antibody [62]
Insect cell /baculovirus	28	Dry power with chitosan, MPL as adjuvant	Two doses of 5, 15, and 50 μg at days 0 and 21	IN	Serum IgG and IgA responses were dose dependent with their titers increased to 4.7- and 4.5-folds, respectively, for the 50 μg group. 53 % of subjects developed rises in NV-specific IgA ASCs [64]
Insect cell /baculovirus	61	Dry power with chitosan, MPL as adjuvant	Two doses of 50 and 100 μg at days 0 and 21	IN	63 and 79 % of vaccinated subjects in the 100 μg group increased IgG and IgA titers by 4.8- and 9.1-folds, respectively. The IgG and IgA titers of the 100 μg group are higher than the 50 μg group but not statistically different. All vaccinated individuals in the 50 and 100 μg groups developed IgA ASCs. Homing molecules to mucosal and peripheral lymphoid tissues were detected on these ASCs [64]
Transgenic potato	20	Raw potato tuber[a]	Two or three doses of 215–751 μg in 150 g potato tuber[a] at days 0 and 21 or at days 0, 7, and 21	Oral	20 and 30 % of vaccinated volunteers developed NV-specific serum IgG (12-fold rise) and fecal IgA (17-fold increase), respectively. 95 % of subjects developed NV-IgA ASCs [65]

IN intranasal, *ASCs* antibody-secreting cells

[a]Each 150 g of raw potato tuber contained between 215 and 751 μg variable amounts of NVCP antigen

Insect cell-derived NVCP VLPs were initially tested in two phase I trials [62]. In the first trial, 20 antibody-positive adult volunteers were given two oral doses (days 1 and 21) of 100 or 250 μg of VLPs formulated in water without adjuvant. It was observed that serum IgG responses were dose dependent, and 100 % of vaccinated subjects who received 250 μg of VLPs increased their NV-specific titers at least fourfold. Fifteen out of 18 participants responded in serum IgG titers after the first VLP dose and showed no increase after the second dose. Importantly, no side effects were observed in vaccinated volunteers [63].

In the second trial, the safety and immunogenicity of NVCP VLPs were further tested in 36 adult seropositive healthy individuals between 18 and 40 years of age with two oral doses of increasing amounts (250, 500 and 2000 μg) of antigens without adjuvant using the same immunization regime [62]. Significant increase in the number of NV-specific IgA antibody-secreting cells (ASC) was observed in all vaccinated volunteers, and approximately 30–40 % of volunteers developed salivary, fecal, or genital fluid IgA antibody. An increase of NV-specific IgG titers was also detected in 90 % of participants who received 250 μg of VLPs. However, further increase in VLP doses (500 and 2000 μg) did not increase the rates of seroconversion or IgG titers.

While the results from the first two trials were encouraging, however, the maximal serum IgG titers elicited by oral immunization were lower than those after experimental NV infection. Consequently, two additional phase I studies were conducted to investigate whether the immunogenicity of NVCP VLPs can be further enhanced by using mucosal adjuvants. Insect cell-produced NVCP VLPs were formulated in a dry power containing a TLR4 agonist adjuvant, monophosphoryl lipid A (MPL), and the mucoadherent chitosan and delivered by IN route to healthy subjects [64].

Study 1 was a stepwise dosage escalation trial with 5, 15, and 50 μg of NVCP VLPs. Study 2 was a dose comparison study of the two highest dosages (50 and 100 μg) VLPs. These studies indicate that IN delivery of NVCP VLPs in a dry power formula with MPL and chitosan was well tolerated and no vaccine-related serious adverse events occurred. In study 1, dose-dependent serum IgG and IgA responses were observed with their titers increased 4.7- and 4.5-fold, respectively, for the 50 μg group. In study 2, the 100 μg group developed higher titers of IgG and IgA (4.8- and 9.1-fold increase, respectively) than that of the 50 μg group, but the differences were not significant in statistical terms [64].

All vaccinees in the 50 and 100 μg groups developed IgA ASCs. Furthermore, expression of homing molecules targeting to mucosal and peripheral lymphoid tissues was detected in these ASCs. Compared with the previously described oral nonadjuvanted VLPs, IN delivery of MPL-adjuvanted VLPs induced a higher number of these ASCs. While the correlates of protective immunity against NV disease are still unknown, these mucosally primed ASCs in combination with the serum IgG and IgA antibodies may contribute to protection.

A phase I/II trial has been initiated to assess safety and immunogenicity of NVCP VLPs administered by the IN route, followed by a live virus challenge to determine the effectiveness of this approach in preventing or limiting NV infection in humans.

Safety and Efficacy. To demonstrate the safety and efficacy of plant-derived NoV VLPs, a phase I clinical trial was conducted with potato-produced NVCP VLPs. In this trial, two or three doses of 150 g uncooked NVCP-transgenic potato tubers (215–751 μg VLPs per dose) were orally ingested by 20 human subjects on days 0 and 7, or on days 0, 7, and 21.

All but one of the volunteers responded with a rise in NV-specific IgA ASCs, while the majority responded following the first dose. Four of the volunteers developed NVCP-specific serum IgG, and six developed specific intestinal IgA with a mean titer rise of 12- and 17-fold, respectively. The incidence rates of nausea, vomiting, mild cramps, fever, or diarrhea were similar among volunteers who ate recombinant or control tubers, indicating that the ingestion of VLP-producing potato tubers appeared to be safe [65].

Summary. Together, these results indicate the immunogenicity and safety of using edible VLP-containing plant parts as oral vaccines of NoV in humans. However, the overall antibody response was not as strong as that obtained by orally delivered purified NVCP VLPs (250 μg per dose) produced in insect cells [62]. Perhaps, the variable effective VLP dosage due to inconsistent NVCP content and poor VLP assembly in potato tubers may cause this weak antigenicity. The potency of the plant-derived VLPs may also be further reduced by their poor release from the potato tissue in the gut lumen.

Overall, these clinical studies have demonstrated that NoV VLP-based vaccine candidates produced in insect cells and plants are safe and immunogenic in humans. Since the model of NV infection in human volunteers has been established recently, the efficacy of adjuvanted NVCP VLP vaccines through IN and oral delivery should be further examined in this human challenge model.

References

1. Eccles, R.: Understanding the symptoms of the common cold and influenza. Lancet Infect. Dis. **5**, 718–725 (2005). doi:10.1016/S1473-3099(05)70270-X
2. http://www.who.int/topics/influenza/en/
3. http://www.who.int/mediacentre/factsheets/fs211/en/
4. http://www.cdc.gov/flu/about/viruses/index.htm
5. Webster, R.G., Laver, W.G.: Antigenic variation in influenza virus. Biology and chemistry. Prog. Med. Virol. **13**, 271–338 (1971)

6. Hay, A.J., Gregory, V., Douglas, A.R., Lin, Y.P.: The evolution of human influenza viruses. Philos. Trans. R. Soc. Lond. B Biol. Sci. **356**, 1861–1870 (2001). doi:10.1098/rstb.2001.0999
7. Gasparini, R., Amicizia, D., Lai, P.L., Panatto, D.: Aflunov(®): a prepandemic influenza vaccine. Expert Rev. Vaccines **11**, 145–157 (2012). doi:10.1586/erv.11.170
8. Beigel, J., Bray, M.: Current and future antiviral therapy of severe seasonal and avian influenza. Antiviral Res. **78**, 91–102 (2008). doi:10.1016/j.antiviral.2008.01.003
9. Jefferson, T., et al.: Neuraminidase inhibitors for preventing and treating influenza in healthy adults and children. Cochrane Database Syst. Rev. **18**, 1 (2012). doi:10.1002/14651858.CD008965.pub3
10. Oxford, J., Gilbert, A., Lambkin-Williams, R.: Influenza vaccines have a short but illustrious history of dedicated science enabling the rapid global production of a/swine (H1N1) vaccine in the current pandemic. In: Del Giudice, G., Rappuoli, R. (eds.) Influenza vaccines for the future, pp. 115–147. Birkhauser Inc, Basel (2011)
11. Verma, R., Khanna, P., Chawla, S.: Influenza vaccine: an effective preventive vaccine for developing countries. Hum. Vaccin Immunother **8**, 675–678 (2012). doi:10.4161/hv.19516
12. Ellebedy, A.H., Webby, R.J.: Influenza vaccines. Vaccine **27**(Suppl 4), D65–D68 (2009). doi:10.1016/j.vaccine.2009.08.038
13. http://www.influenzacentre.org/centre_GISRS.htm
14. Gerdil, C.: The annual production cycle for influenza vaccine. Vaccine **21**, 1776–1779 (2003), pii: S0264410X03000719
15. Burnet, F.M.: Growth of influenza virus in the allantoic cavity of the chick embryo. Aust. J. Exp. Biol. Med. Sci. **19**, 291–295 (1941)
16. Hoffmann, E., Neumann, G., Kawaoka, Y., Hobom, G., Webster, R.G.: A DNA transfection system for generation of influenza a virus from eight plasmids. Proc. Natl. Acad. Sci. U. S. A. **97**, 6108–6113 (2000). doi:10.1073/pnas.100133697
17. Expert Committee on Biological Standardization Geneva, 17 to 21 Oct 2011 Proposed Generic Protocol for the Calibration of Seasonal/Pandemic Influenza Antigen Working Reagents by WHO Essential Regulatory Laboratories (WHO/BS/2011.2183). http://www.who.int/biologicals/expert_committee/BS2011.2183_Flu_vax_ERL_calibration_protocol.pdf
18. Hickling, J., D'Hondt, E.: A review of production technologies for influenza virus vaccines, and their suitability for deployment in developing countries for influenza pandemic preparedness – WHO World Health Organization Initiative for Vaccine Research Geneva Switzerland. 20 Dec 2006. www.who.int/entity/vaccine_research/diseases/influenza/Flu_vacc_manuf_tech_report.pdf
19. Matthews, J.T.: Egg-based production of influenza vaccine: 30 years of commercial experience. Bridge **36**, 17–24 (2006)
20. Rappuoli, R.: Cell-culture-based vaccine production: technological options. Bridge **36**, 25–30 (2006)
21. Dormitzer, P.R.: Cell culture-derived influenza vaccines. In: Del Giudice, G., Rappuoli, R. (eds.) Influenza vaccines for the future, pp. 293–312. Birkhauser Inc, Basel (2011)
22. Kistner, O., Barrett, P.N., Mundt, W., Reiter, M., Schober-Bendixen, S., Dorner, F.: Development of a mammalian cell (Vero) derived candidate influenza virus vaccine. Vaccine **16**, 960–968 (1998), pii: S0264-410X(97)00301-0
23. Palache, A.M., Brands, R., van Scharrenburg, G.: Immunogenicity and reactogenicity of influenza subunit vaccines produced in MDCK cells or fertilised chicken eggs. J. Infect. Dis. **176**(Suppl 1), S20–S23 (1997)
24. Schild, G.C., Wood, J.M., Newman, R.W.: A single radial-immunodiffusion technique for the assay of influenza hemagglutinin antigen. Bull. World Health Organ. **52**, 223–231 (1975)
25. Wood, J.M., Schild, G.C., Newman, R.W., Seagroatt, V.: Application of an improved single radial-immunodiffusion technique for the assay of influenza hemagglutinin antigen content of whole virus and subunit vaccines. Dev. Biol. Stand. **39**, 193–200 (1977)
26. Recommendations for the production and control of influenza vaccine (inactivated) © World Health Organization WHO Technical Report Series, No. 927, http://www.who.int/vaccine_research/diseases/influenza/TRS_927_ANNEX_3_Influenza_2005.pdf
27. Wood, J.M., Levandowski, R.A.: The influenza vaccine licensing process. Vaccine **21**, 1786–1788 (2003), pii: S0264410X03000732
28. Sambhara, S., Rappuoli, R.: Improving influenza vaccines. Expert Rev. Vaccines **11**, 871–872 (2012). doi:10.1586/erv.12.79
29. Dormitzer, P.R., Tsai, T.F., Del Giudice, G.: New technologies for influenza vaccines. Hum. Vaccin Immunother **8**, 45–58 (2012). doi:10.4161/hv.8.1.18859
30. Montomoli, E., et al.: Cell culture-derived influenza vaccines from Vero cells: a new horizon for vaccine production. Expert Rev. Vaccines **11**, 587–594 (2012). doi:10.1586/erv.12.24
31. Barta, A., et al.: The expression of a nopaline synthase – human growth hormone chimaeric gene in transformed tobacco and sunflower callus tissue. Plant Mol. Biol. **6**, 347–357 (1986). doi:10.1007/BF00034942
32. Hiatt, A., Cafferkey, R., Bowdish, K.: Production of antibodies in transgenic plants. Nature **342**, 76–78 (1989). doi:10.1038/342076a0
33. Tacket, C.O., et al.: Immunogenicity in humans of a recombinant bacterial antigen delivered in a transgenic potato. Nat. Med. **4**, 607–609 (1998)
34. Mason, H.S., Lam, D.M., Arntzen, C.J.: Expression of hepatitis B surface antigen in transgenic plants. Proc. Natl. Acad. Sci. U. S. A. **89**, 11745–11749 (1992)
35. Yusibov, V., et al.: Expression in plants and immunogenicity of plant virus-based experimental rabies vaccine. Vaccine **20**, 3155–3164 (2002)
36. Lai, H., Chen, Q.: Bioprocessing of plant-derived virus-like particles of Norwalk virus capsid protein under current Good Manufacture Practice regulations. Plant Cell Rep. **31**, 573–584 (2012). doi:10.1007/s00299-011-1196-6
37. Olinger Jr., G.G., et al.: Delayed treatment of Ebola virus infection with plant-derived monoclonal antibodies provides protection in rhesus macaques. Proc. Natl. Acad. Sci. U. S. A. **109**, 18030–18035 (2012). doi:10.1073/pnas.1213709109
38. Newell, C.A.: Plant transformation technology. Mol. Biotechnol. **16**, 53–65 (2000)
39. Lee, L.-Y., Gelvin, S.B.: T-DNA binary vectors and systems. Plant Physiol. **146**, 325–332 (2008)
40. Bock, R., Khan, M.S.: Taming plastids for a green future. Trends Biotechnol. **22**, 311–318 (2004)
41. Meyers, B., et al.: Nuclear and plastid genetic engineering of plants: comparison of opportunities and challenges. Biotechnol. Adv. **28**, 747–756 (2010)
42. Komarova, T.V., et al.: Transient expression systems for plant-derived biopharmaceuticals. Expert Rev. Vaccines **9**, 859–876 (2010)
43. Sheludko, Y.V.: Agrobacterium-mediated transient expression as an approach to production of recombinant proteins in plants. Recent Pat. Biotechnol. **2**, 198–208 (2008)
44. Pogue, G.P., et al.: Making an ally from an enemy: plant virology and the new agriculture. Annu. Rev. Phytopathol. **40**, 45–74 (2002)
45. Rybicki, E.P.: Plant-based vaccines against viruses. Virol. J. **11**, 205 (2014). doi:10.1186/s12985-014-0205-0
46. Prasad, B.V., Rothnagel, R., Jiang, X., Estes, M.K.: Three-dimensional structure of baculovirus-expressed Norwalk virus capsids. J. Virol. **68**, 5117–5125 (1994)
47. Baric, R.S., et al.: Expression and self-assembly of Norwalk virus capsid protein from venezuelan equine encephalitis virus replicons. J. Virol. **76**, 3023–3030 (2002)
48. Ausar, S.F., Foubert, T.R., Hudson, M.H., Vedvick, T.S., Middaugh, C.R.: Conformational stability and disassembly of Norwalk virus like particles: Effect of pH and temperature. J. Biol. Chem. **281**, 19478–19488 (2006). doi:10.1074/jbc.M603313200

49. Prasad, B.V.V., Hardy, D., Estes, M.: Structural studies of recombinant Norwalk capsids. J. Infect. Dis. **181**, S317–S321 (2000). doi:10.1086/315576
50. Cao, S., et al.: Structural basis for the recognition of blood group trisaccharides by norovirus. J. Virol. **81**, 5949–5957 (2007)
51. Faye, L., Gomord, V.: Success stories in molecular farming- a brief overview. Plant Biotechnol. J. **8**, 525–528 (2010)
52. Lai, H., He, J., Engle, M., Diamond, M.S., Chen, Q.: Robust production of virus-like particles and monoclonal antibodies with geminiviral replicon vectors in lettuce. Plant Biotechnol. J. **10**, 95–104 (2012)
53. Komarova, T.V., et al.: Transient expression systems for plant-derived biopharmaceuticals. Expert Rev. Vaccines **9**, 859–876 (2010). doi:10.1586/erv.10.85
54. He, J., Lai, H., Brock, C., Chen, Q.: A novel system for rapid and cost-effective production of detection and diagnostic reagents of west Nile virus in plants. J. Biomed. Biotechnol. **2012**, 1–10 (2012). doi:10.1155/2012/106783
55. Herbst-Kralovetz, M., Mason, H.S., Chen, Q.: Norwalk virus-like particles as vaccines. Expert Rev. Vaccines **9**, 299–307 (2010). doi:10.1586/erv.09.163
56. Zhang, X., Buehner, N.A., Hutson, A.M., Estes, M.K., Mason, H.S.: Tomato is a highly effective vehicle for expression and oral immunization with Norwalk virus capsid protein. Plant Biotechnol. J. **4**, 419–432 (2006)
57. Huang, Z., et al.: Virus-like particle expression and assembly in plants: hepatitis B and Norwalk viruses. Vaccine **23**, 1851–1858 (2005)
58. Huang, Z., et al.: High-level rapid production of full-size monoclonal antibodies in plants by a single-vector DNA replicon system. Biotechnol. Bioeng. **106**, 9–17 (2010)
59. Giritch, A., et al.: Rapid high-yield expression of full-size IgG antibodies in plants coinfected with noncompeting viral vectors. Proc. Natl. Acad. Sci. U. S. A. **103**, 14701–14706 (2006)
60. Chen, Q., He, J., Phoolcharoen, W., Mason, H.S.: Geminiviral vectors based on bean yellow dwarf virus for production of vaccine antigens and monoclonal antibodies in plants. Hum. Vaccin. **7**, 331–338 (2011)
61. Lai, H., Chen, Q.: Bioprocessing of plant-derived virus-like particles of Norwalk virus capsid protein under current Good Manufacture Practice regulations. Plant Cell Rep. **31**, 573–584 (2012)
62. Tacket, C.O., Sztein, M.B., Losonsky, G.A., Wasserman, S.S., Estes, M.K.: Humoral, mucosal, and cellular immune responses to oral Norwalk virus-like particles in volunteers. Clin. Immunol. **108**, 241–247 (2003)
63. Ball, J.M., et al.: Recombinant Norwalk virus-like particles as an oral vaccine. Arch. Virol. Suppl. **12**, 243–249 (1996)
64. El-Kamary, S.S., et al.: Adjuvanted intranasal Norwalk virus-like particle vaccine elicits antibodies and antibody-secreting cells that express homing receptors for mucosal and peripheral lymphoid tissues. J Infect Dis **202**, 1649–1658 (2010). doi:10.1086/657087
65. Tacket, C.O., et al.: Human immune responses to a novel Norwalk virus vaccine delivered in transgenic potatoes. J. Infect. Dis. **182**, 302–305 (2000)
66. Baschieri, S.: Plant heat shock protein-based self-adjuvanted immunogens. In: Giese, M. (ed.) Molecular vaccines – from prophylaxis to therapy, vol. 2. Springer, Wien (2013)
67. Hanley-Bowdoin, L., et al.: From Geminiviruses: masters at redirecting and reprogramming plant processes. Nat. Rev. Microbiol. **11**, 777–788 (2013)

Part III

Therapeutical Vaccines

Cancer Vaccines

12

Contents

12.1 Cancer Immunology

12.1.1 From Immunosurveillance to Editing

The immune system is able to control, at least in part, growth of tumors. In 1863 Rudolf Virchow discovered active leucocytes in tumor tissues. And it was Paul Ehrlich in 1909 who postulated a "body's own protection system" against tumor cells. "The immune surveillance hypothesis" was born and elaborated by Thomas and Burnet in the 1950s and 1960s: T cell-mediated immunity evolved as a specific defense against cancer cells and that T cells constantly patrol the body, searching for abnormal body cells [1]. Until today there are many clinical data demonstrating the correlation between the immune system/surveillance and the development of tumors: spontaneous remission of colon carcinoma, acute myeloid leukemia, or remission of lung and liver metastases of lung cancer (NSCLC). As long as the tumor load is controlled by the immune system and as long as this balance between diseases and innate and acquired immunity works, the life is not threatened. The same is for infectious diseases.

According to the statistics, transplanted and immunosuppressed patients get a three- to eightfold higher risk to develop cancer [2]. The incidence of malignancy in (kidney) cancer patients chronically immunosuppressed over 10 years has been estimated at 20 % [3]. Immunodeficiency in humans is associated with increased cancer risk what is clearly demonstrated in HIV-infected patients. In contrast, melanoma or colorectal patients whose tumors have high levels of tumor-infiltrating lymphocytes have a better prognosis.

Taken together, there are compelling evidences that the immune system is to confer protection not only against foreign pathogens but also against cancer. If this were not so, the body would collapse within a short time. Our live would be a short episode only. Every day abnormal cells are produced somewhere in the body and are recognized by the immune system and eliminated. Whether this elimination is perfect or imperfect is not clear.

M. Giese, *Introduction to Molecular Vaccinology*, DOI 10.1007/978-3-319-25832-4_12

Probably the immune surveillance leads to a balance between normal and abnormal cells. Precancerous cells stimulate an immune response and are destroyed. But if the immune system can't detect every malignant cell and at the same time a suitable tumor microenvironment (TME) is formed by inflammatory processes, a carcinogenesis is not longer to be blocked [1].

The mechanisms leading to immune tolerance against malignant cells are unknown. Precancerous cells are the results of multiple mutations. Lethal mutations induce apoptosis, but other mutated cells might be recognized and destroyed by the immune system, others survive, and their antigenic phenotype is immunologically silent and not recognized as "danger": DAMPs are missing.

DAMPs or Alarmins. Danger signals are defined analogous to PAMPs as endogenous host-encoded proteins that are released after cellular stress, tissue injury, and necrotic cell destruction, in the complete absence of any pathogen. Those molecules are collectively called damage-associated molecular patterns, DAMPs, sometimes also called alarmins. Many DAMPs are nuclear or cytosolic proteins but also extracellular matrix proteins (ECM), which are either upregulated or released following tissue injury. These normally hidden proteins send a signal "danger" resulting in a sterile inflammation. Substances in this process released from damaged cells change now from the intracellular reducing to the extracellular oxidizing milieu, leading to a dramatical change of the extracellular redox milieu (see Chap. 2).

The immune system has successfully edited these cancer cells, and the cancer cells have their "lessons learned" [4]. It is not surprising. The evolutionary mandate of life means to adapt to the environment, to permanently improve the genetic configuration, everything to do for survival only. The MDR (multidrug resistance) pump system in many cancer cells underlines this survival strategy, and immunediting is only another mechanism of the evolutionary survival strategy.

12.1.2 Tumor Microenvironment (TME)

Precancerous cells need a niche in which they can thrive and prosper to cancer cells. This niche is the TME and protects the malignant cells against the immune system. Apart from malignant cells, immune cells, fibroblasts, tube-forming endothelial cells and their surrounding pericytes (for generation of the tumor vasculature and lymphatics), and other cells form the TME. The non-cancerous cell mass can comprise >50 % of the tumor mass (Fig. 12.1).

These non-cancerous cells are suggested to support cancer development and progression. The tumor and its microenvironment are closely related with an intensive intercellular communication. Without the support of normal tissue and stromal cells, cancerous cells would not evolve and would be unable to manifest the disease [5]:

Cancer cells are similar to senescent cells in that they increase expression of microenvironment with pro-survival networks that help them resist apoptosis.

TME Immune Cells. The dual functions of immune cells arise in TME. While outside the TME, T cells, B cells, macrophages, etc. protect the body against invaders, within TME these cells contribute to an immunosuppressive milieu. All solid tumors contain infiltrates of leukocytes. Among these are T cells (Th1, Th2, Th17, Treg, γδ T cells, CTLs) and tumor-associated macrophages (TAMs). Immune cells now stimulate the tumor proliferation and angiogenesis by secretion of mitogenic growth factor such as tumor necrosis factor-α (TNF-α), epidermal growth factor (EGF), transforming growth factor-β (TGF-β), vascular endothelial growth factor (VEGF), chemokines such as CXCL-12, and various cytokines. Tumor cells depend on pro-inflammatory cytokine stimulation. The basis for cytokine production is in the permanent activation of the NF-κB pathway. Permanent activation of the NF-κB pathway of tumor-infiltrating cells represents one mechanism that appears to favor tumor survival.

The NF-κB activation is strongly maintained by the hypoxic environment which favors the influx of cells depending on the glycolytic pathway, macrophages, and granulocytes. These cells also produce many reactive oxygen species (ROS) [6]. The NF-κB pathway is regulated by (mitochondrial) ROS. The sustained NF-κB activation is a direct link between inflammation and cancer.

Dendritic cells found in TME are defective and cannot present (tumor) antigens. Moreover, it seems that many DCs suppress T cell activities.

Antitumor CTL activity is blocked; NK and T cell-mediated killing is blocked – cancer cells can escape – successfully edited by TAMs and others. TAMs are reprogrammed to inhibit lymphocyte functions through release of inhibitory cytokines such as IL-10, prostaglandins, and reactive oxygen. TAMs also recruit Treg cells via the chemokine CCL22, a further contribution to the immune suppressive milieu. In TME, Treg cells expand, downregulate T cell proliferation, and suppress antitumor responses of both $CD4^+$ and $CD8^+$ T cells by production of inhibitory cytokines such as TGF-β, IL-10, and IL-35.

The tumor vascularization is particularly enhanced by TAMs via production of VEGF. The tumor vasculature itself has lost high endothelial venules which support high levels of lymphocyte extravasation. That means that the influx of CTLs, NK cells, T cells, and monocytes from outside the TME into the TME is blocked.

All these support the evolving of neoplastic cells and produce tolerance. The state of TME can be modulated via blockade of immune checkpoints, depletion of immunosuppressive

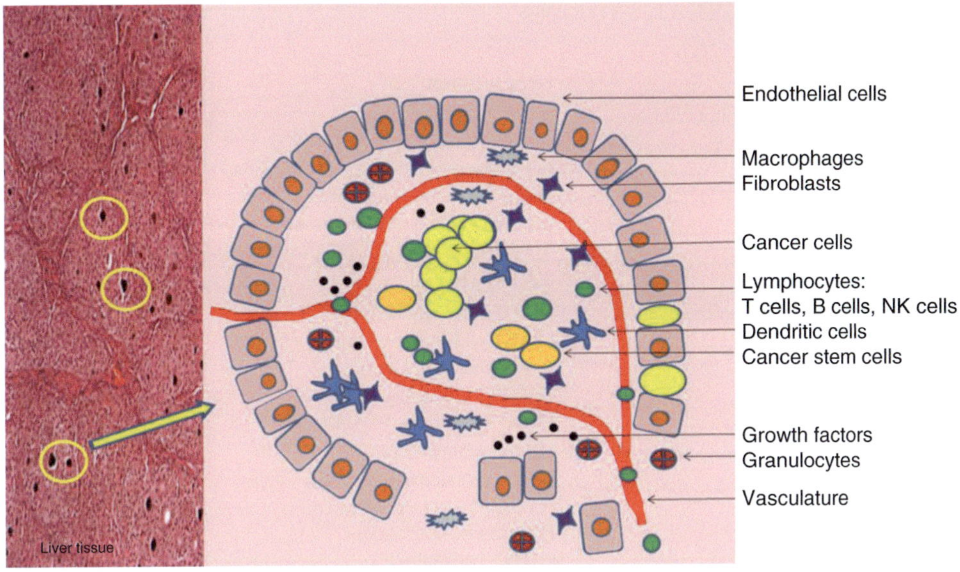

Fig. 12.1 Tumor and its microenvironment are closely related with an intensive intercellular communication. Without the support of normal tissue and stromal cells, cancerous cells would not evolve and would be unable to manifest the disease. Apart from malignant cells, immune cells, fibroblasts, tube-forming endothelial cells and their surrounding pericytes, and other cells form the TME. The noncancerous cell mass can comprise >50 % of the tumor mass. *Yellow circles* on a histological sample of liver tissue on the left side represent tumor cell niches (TME); such a niche is schematically illustrated on the right side of the figure

cells, or neutralization of immunosuppressive cytokines such as TGF-β.

The presence of immune cells within TME is part of the immune surveillance. Why and particularly when these cells are co-opted to promote tumor growth is not understood.

12.1.3 Immunogenicity of Dying Cancer Cells

The programmed cell death (PCD) is a fundamental physiological terminal path for cells of all metazoan mediated by a genetic program (Table 12.1). Unnecessary and obstructive cells during the life cycle of the organism undergo a regulated process of dying. During the normal tissue turnover, necessary to retain the homeostasis, million to billions of cells die per day and will be substituted again. An adult person has about 100 billion cells.

In contrast to PCD, necrosis is an unnatural death of cellular damage.

Apoptosis of rapidly expanding cancer cells is common. But it has long been considered that apoptotic cell death delivers no immunogenic antigens. The positive effect is that this cell death does not cause autoreactivity. On the negative side, an immune response against dying cancer cell is generally missing.

But the simple idea that apoptosis is tolerogenic has been challenged by observations that some types of chemotherapeutic drugs can cause an immunogenic cell death (ICD) of tumor cells (discussed in the next section). Various factors influence the proper outcome of the dying cell such as the nature of the cell death inducer (inclusive oncolytic viruses, described later in this chapter), the availability of immune cells, or the antigenicity. In addition, intracellular stress can be displayed on the cell surface by expression of proteins that are, e.g., ligands for NK cells.

Table 12.1 Different types of programmed cell death (PCD) are described

Type 1: Apoptosis	• programed suicide via caspase actions activated by extrinsic or intrinsic signalling
Type 2: Autophagy	• proteolytic targeted degradation of cytosolic components (autophagosome); activation via intracellular stress signals
Type 3: Necroptosis	• engulfed by macrophages or DCs, in a capase-independent fashion; extrinsic stimulus through TNFα
Type 4: Pyroptosis	• programed form of necrosis, in a caspase-independent fashion; extrinsic stimulus through TNFα

Dying cells are engulfed by macrophages or DCs. The traffic route of activated and primed immune cells probably codetermines the fate of the cancer antigens, tolerogenic or immunogenic. It could be shown that intravenously injected apoptotic cancer cells were engulfed and transported to the spleen leading to a state of immune tolerance [7]. In contrast, subcutaneously injected apoptotic cancer cells are picked up

Table 12.2 Classification of tumor antigens and selected examples

Tumor antigens	Specifications	Gene – tumor	Patients positive for this antigen
1. Unique antigens	1.1 Derived from point mutations	**p53*** – head and neck squamous cell carcinoma	14 %
		bcr-abl – chronic myeloid leukemia	16 %
		K-ras – pancreatic adenocarcinoma	No data available
		hsp70-2 – renal cell carcinoma and bladder	No data available
		ME1 – non-small cell lung carcinoma	No data available
	1.2 Patient specific	**Neoantigens**	No data available
2. Shared antigens	2.1 Tumor-specific antigens	**MAGE-A1** – melanoma	16 %
		MAGE-A3 – melanoma	100 %
		Cyclin-A1 – leukemia	No data available
		BAGE-1 – melanoma	No data available
		HERV-K-MEL – melanoma	100 %
	2.2 Differentiation antigens	**CEA** – gut carcinoma	No data available
		PSA – prostate carcinoma	16 %
		NY-BR-1 – breast cancer	100 %
		tyrosinase – melanoma	100 %
		gp100 – melanoma	100 %
	2.3 Overexpressed antigens	**p53*** – ubiquitous (low level)	100 %
		HER-2/neu – ubiquitous (low level)	11 %
		VEGF – ubiquitous (low level)	No data available
		CD45 – proliferating cells, testis, multiple tissues (low level)	No data available
		MUC1 – glandular epithelia	100 %

p53* can be cancerogenic either by mutations or by overexpression

by Langerhans cells and transported to lymph nodes leading to an immune response. The location of uptake rather the type of DC influences the outcome [8].

Immunogenic apoptosis can be induced, e.g., by anthracylines, oxaliplatin, but also by radiation therapy.

12.1.4 Tumor Antigens and Neoantigens

In principle, every abnormally expressed protein in cancer cells can serve as tumor antigen (TA), based on the recognition by T cells. Since the discovery of the first TA in 1991 [9], MAGE-1 of melanoma cells, a huge plethora of TAs has been described. Today, more than 2000 tumor antigens are identified.

According to Peptide Database/Cancer Immunity (http://cancerimmunity.org/peptide/), four requirements must be fulfilled for TAs:

1. Isolation of stable human T-lymphocyte clones or lines recognizing the peptide
2. Identification of the peptide recognized by the T cells
3. Identification of the HLA/MHC presenting molecule
4. Evidence that the peptide is processed by tumor cells and presented to the specific CTL

Tumor antigens were broadly classified into two categories, unique and shared antigens (Table 12.2).

In 2009 the National Cancer Institute of the United States published a project on prioritization of cancer antigens and defined criteria for the "ideal" cancer antigen [10]. The ranking criteria were based on the likelihood for efficacy in clinical trials and were as follows (Table 12.3):

Seventy-five representative antigens were selected. None of the 75 antigens met all criteria. Forty-six antigens were immunogenic, and only 20 antigens had a therapeutical function and induced immune responses. Therapeutic function was considered the most important criteria.

Cancer Vaccines

Prophylactic cancer vaccines may be an option in case of involvement of viruses such as human papillomavirus (HPV) and cervix carcinoma or other microorganisms. This anti-HPV vaccine is in a classical sense of an antiviral vaccine only and can prevent a chronic inflammation.

Chronic inflammation causes genotoxic stress in form of mutations or genomic instability and is known to enhance angiogenesis and tissue remodeling. Chronic inflammation has a deep impact on tumor initiation. It takes about 20 years from HPV infection to cervical cancer. The typical time course of the infection begins with HPV acquisition in adolescence and early adulthood, around 17–25 of age, and cancer arises around 45–60. During this dark period accompanied with chronic inflammation, innumerable mutations took place finally resulting in cancer. So far, there are no clinical data demonstrating antitumor efficacy of the diverse commercialized anti-HPV vaccines.

Genetic Instability. Prophylactic cancer vaccines may be no option for cancer diseases caused by other agents beside

Table 12.3 Prioritization of ideal cancer antigens

Weighting 100 %	Criteria for ideal cancer antigen	Defined by
32 %	1. Therapeutic function	Clinical trial data showing a vaccine-induced response
17 %	2. Immunogenicity	T cell and/or antibody elicited in clinical trials
15 %	3. Oncogenicity	Associated with oncogenic processes: "self" antigens, viral antigens; tissue differentiation
15 %	4. Specificity	Unique or shared antigens; location of expression
7 %	5. Expression level	Highly expressed to lower level of expression
5 %	6. Stem cell expression	Evidence for expression on putative cancer stem cells
4 %	7. Number of patient with antigen-positive cancer	High to low level expression in *n* patients
4 %	8. Number of antigenic epitopes	Multiple epitopes vs. one/few epitopes
1 %	9. Cellular localization of antigen expression	Cell surface/circulating antigen

microorganisms. The high mutation rate in tumor cells can generate a mutational load of 1–10 mutations per megabase of coding DNA [11]. The prophylactic selection of proper tumor antigens would be a lottery, an endless cycle of trial and error. The genetic instability produces permanent changes of epitopes.

Efficacy. The efficacy of therapeutic cancer vaccines is still disappointing. Since the first scientific report on an experimental autologous (personalized) cancer vaccine (whole tumor homogenate, mixed with Freund's adjuvant and 3× injected intramuscularly in patient) was published in 1964 [12], the clinical efficacy of cancer vaccines was not as expected. Already in the 1890s William B. Coley injected streptococcal organisms in patients with solid tumors ("Coley's toxins") to activate the immune system.

A therapeutical cancer vaccine is confronted with several massive natural barriers:

- The efficacy is limited by the local tolerance of T cells within the immunosuppressive milieu (TME).
- Tumor antigens are often "self" proteins or masked antigens.
- Overall weakness of the immune system (central immunosenescence) due to chronic inflammation accompanying most cancer diseases.
- Also ineffective adjuvants contribute to this failure.

As discussed in Chap. 1, personalized (P-) vaccines – *The 3 B's: Bedside-Bench-Bedside* – use patient's antigens, tissues, or cells which are manipulated ex vivo and re-injected to the same patient as autologous vaccine.

Immunological Profiling. The aim of individual profiling is to understand the patient-specific interplay between disease and immune system and to tailor a vaccine fitting with measured individual biological conditions. The prerequisite for a P-vaccine is the collection of individual data starting with the age, gender, family history, and the analysis of results from (epi-) genomic epidemiology studies to define general genetic variants and combine with the regular monitoring of the physiological state. Because generally the patient come first to the doctor when he/she has fallen ill, the healthy baseline of gene and protein data are missing, and also a longitudinal profile of healthy conditions is not available which limits the use of genomics and proteomics.

Neoantigens. A new class of mutated and patient-specific antigens, present in tumor cells but not in normal cells and with a lack of central tolerance against them

Neoantigens are the result of mutations. So far analyzed neoantigens are missense mutations, a type of nonsynonymous substitution ("missense neoantigens"), in which one DNA nucleotide is switched out with another one in a way that changes the amino acid specified [13]. The so made

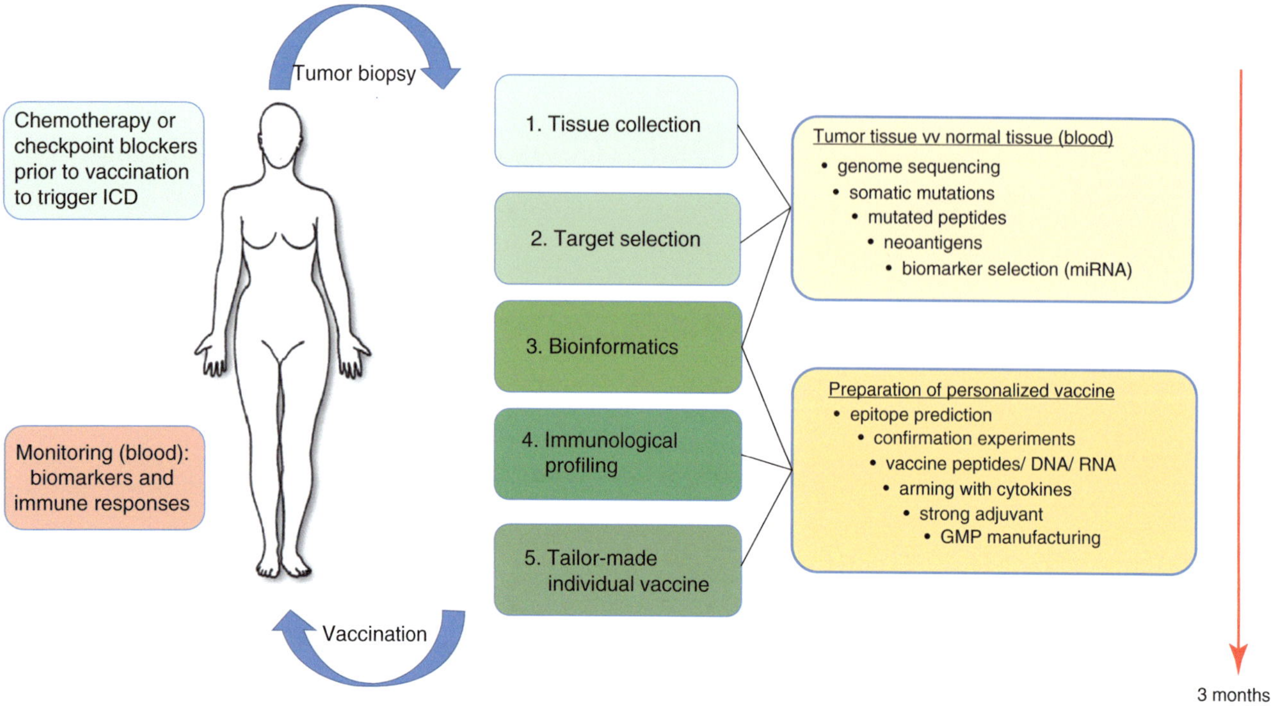

Fig. 12.2 P-vaccine against cancer. The vaccine development begins with an immunological profiling. The aim of individual profiling is to understand the patient-specific interplay between disease and immune system. Tumor tissue is compared to normal tissue, and targets are identified to tailor a vaccine fitting with measured individual biological conditions. A chemotherapy or immunotherapy with antibodies as checkpoint blockers prior to vaccination can trigger the development of immunogenic cell death (ICD) and prime the immune system with released neoantigens, among them should be the vaccine target antigen. Neoantigens additionally stimulate an immune response and thus support checkpoint blockade drugs. The vaccine-induced immune response is monitored by the antibody titer and cytotoxic T cell (CTL) response and specific biomarkers. The whole process of P-vaccine development takes about 3 months

neo-protein looks quite different to the corresponding wild type and may not even be functional but an ideal antigen for a personalized vaccine because it is recognized by the immune system [14]: MHC class I (in humans, HLA class I) molecules bind intracellular antigens and present them to cytotoxic CD8+ T cells, whereas MHC II bind extracellular antigens and present them to CD4+ T helper cells.

A recently published study in melanoma patient with stage III examined the immunogenicity of tumor-derived neoantigens [15]. Surgically excised tumor tissues were investigated for mutations through DNA and RNA sequencing and compared to normal tissues. Tumor-specific mutated *neo*-peptides were in silico translated into predicted proteins and checked for MHC binding. Some immunogenic neoantigens in each patient were identified, synthesized, and finally incorporated into an autologous dendritic cell vaccine. In all patients, a robust neoantigen T cell immunity was detectable.

Of note to comment that in all patients enrolled in this study, pre-existing CTL immunity to the used neoantigens was detectable as confirmed by ex vivo assays. This highlights the relevance of neoantigens for therapeutical vaccination because the immune system is able to find these tumor antigens and to mount a response.

Dominant Neoantigens. But not each neoantigen is a suitable vaccine candidate and able to induce a T cell response. Schumacher et al. [16] used in silico prediction tools to describe 448 neoantigens detected in a patient with melanoma. Only one strong and one weak neoantigen out of 448 were found. Like all other antigens, neoantigens are classified into dominant and subdominant. A third category describes cryptic peptides which have low MHC I affinity. Cryptic peptides are weekly presented at the cell surface and are therefore non-immunogenic. Protein antigens typically contain multiple epitopes capable of binding MHC II molecules, or MHC I, but T cell responses are limited to only a small number of these determinants in each individual. A vaccine that induces responses against subdominant epitopes will be less protective than a vaccine that induces a robust immunodominant response. Immunodominance is evident for both antibody-mediated immunity and cell-mediated immunity (see also Chap. 6).

Figure 12.2 illustrates the development of P-vaccines based on neoantigens.

12.1.5 Immune Checkpoints and Vaccines

The regulation of every immune response is highly balanced by a cascade of stimulatory and inhibitory signals. Any imbalance could lead to uncontrolled infection or autoimmunity. Various checkpoints are widely incorporated into the immune system that are crucial for maintaining self-tolerance

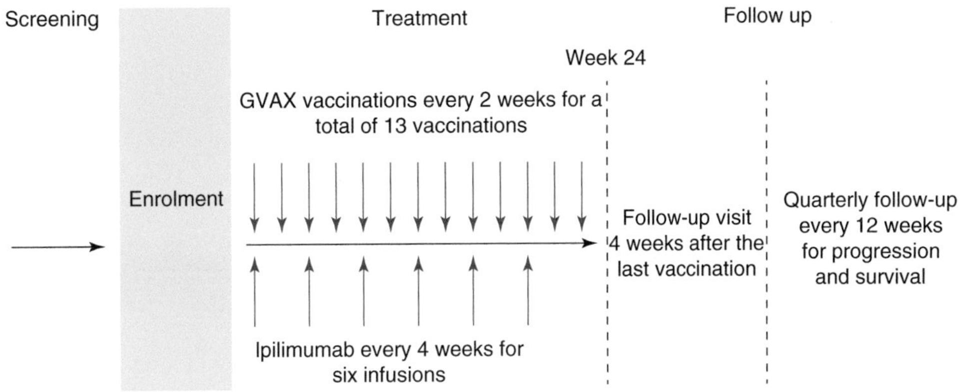

Fig. 12.3 Treatment schedule (Credit: van den Eertwegh et al., VU University Medical Centre Amsterdam/Netherlands, Ref. [18])

and for controlling the duration and amplitude of physiological immune responses. *These checkpoints are generally stop signals for proliferating immune responses and are mainly based on ligand–receptor interactions.*

One major mechanism of immune resistance of many tumors is their hijacking of checkpoints, particularly within regulatory pathways of T cells.

Checkpoint Modifiers. Membrane-bound ligand–receptor interactions can be easily modified by monoclonal antibodies (mAbs), also known as *checkpoint modifiers*. While therapeutical mAbs such as anti-Her2 directly targets epitopes on tumor cells, immune checkpoint mAbs don't target tumor cells but restore the antitumor immune activities of cytotoxic T cells by blocking immune checkpoint molecules on T cells or their ligands on antigen-presenting and tumor cells.

CTLA-4 and Ipilimumab. The first demonstration that the blockade of a T cell-specific receptor, here the cytotoxic T-lymphocyte-associated protein 4 (CTLA-4), can induce a therapeutic antitumor effect was already published in 1996 [17]. CTLA-4 is a receptor exclusively on T cells and highly expressed on Treg cells that downregulate T cell activity and acts as opponent to CD28 that binds to B7.2 and B7.1 molecules. B7.2 (CD86) on APC or cancer cells is the more likely primary ligand for CD28. Once antigen recognition by TCR occurred, CD28 signals amplify T cell activation. The physiological role of CTLA-4 is to control these T cell activities by delivering firstly inhibitory signals and secondly through internal blocking of CD28 by specific ligands. Besides that, CTLA-4 has also a higher affinity for both APC ligands, B7.2 (CD86) and B7.1 (CD80), compared with CD28.

The blockade of CTLA-4 in vivo by mAbs resulted in restoration of T cell activities and finally in an enhancement of immune responses against tumor in a mouse model. In 2011, the US Food and Drug Administration (FDA) approved ipilimumab, an anti-CTLA-4 antibody, for the treatment of metastatic melanoma.

Checkpoint Blockers and Vaccines. The combination of immune checkpoint modifiers with cancer vaccines offers a new strategy to treat cancer diseases. Firstly, checkpoint blockers remove the brakes on T cells that cancer uses to suppress the immune response, and secondly, tumor antigens delivered by the vaccine can meet now revitalized T cells.

In a phase 1b, open-label, randomized study dose-escalation trial, ipilimumab in combination with allogeneic pancreatic tumor cells transfected with a GM-CSF gene (GVAX) was evaluated in patients with a castration-resistant disease, with evidence of PSA (prostate-specific antigen) progression, and radiological evidence of metastatic disease Median Overall Survival (OS) for the all patients was 4.3 months. Median OS was 3.6 months for arm 1 and 5.7 for arm 2. The percent alive after 1 year also favored the combination arm (7 % vs. 27 %) [18].

Composition of the vaccine: GVAX consists of 2 allogeneic pancreatic tumor cell lines, 2.5×10^8 cells each, modified with a plasmid encoding the cDNA for human GM-CSF and subsequently cultured and irradiated and administered into a single vaccine as intradermal injections, 2 each in the right and left thighs and 2 in the nondominant arm. The treatment schedule is shown in Fig. 12.3, and the results are presented in Fig. 12.4.

Results. In this study, the overall survival was improved. The combination of GVAX and ipilimumab was clinically and immunologically active and measurable.

In another large randomized phase III trial, ipilimumab was tested for its efficacy using a 3-arm randomization strategy with ipilimumab alone, together with a gp100 (melanoma antigen) peptide vaccine, or the gp100 vaccine alone [19]. This study showed that ipilimumab alone or in combination with the gp100 vaccine was superior to the gp100 vaccine alone but surprisingly, no benefit was seen from combining ipilimumab with the vaccine. This has also been observed in other studies combining ipilimumab with gp100 vaccination [20].

Programmed Cell Death. PD-1 receptors are other important immune checkpoints on T cells and responsible for immune suppression in peripheral tissues by preventing

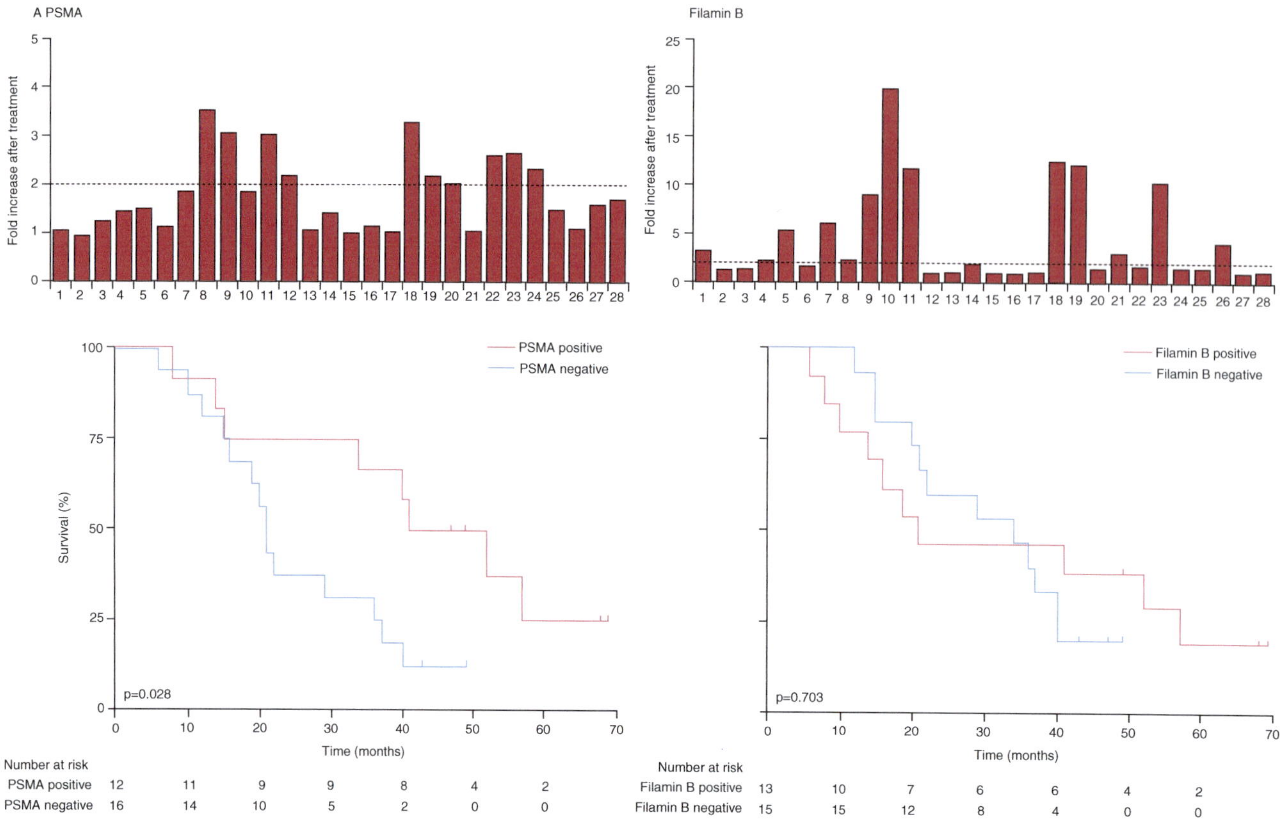

Fig. 12.4 Treatment-induced autoantibodies against PSMA and filamin B. (**a**) Antibody response against PSMA and filamin B measured by ELISA and expressed as fold increase over pretreatment levels. Anti-PSMA and anti-filamin B antibodies were measured before and after treatment (week 24, visit 13 or follow-up). (**b**) Kaplan–Meier curves of overall survival for seroreactivity against PSMA and filamin B after treatment. In this study, the overall survival was improved. The combination of GVAX and ipilimumab was clinically and immunologically active and measurable (Credit: van den Eertwegh et al., VU University Medical Centre Amsterdam/Netherlands, Ref. [18])

T cell activation at the time of an inflammatory response to infection and to limit autoimmunity. PD-1 has dual functions: on the one hand, PD-1 promotes apoptosis (programed cell death) in antigen-specific T cells; otherwise PD-1 reduces apoptosis in Treg cells. Tumor cells express the ligands for PD-1, PD-L1, and PD-L2, both are members of the B7 family. PD-L1 is upregulated in a number of cancers. Anti-PD-1 studies included melanoma, renal cell cancer, non-small cell lung cancer (NSCLC), castration-resistant prostate cancer, and colorectal cancer [21].

Pembrolizumab. In 2014, the US FDA approved pembrolizumab, an anti-PD-1 antibody, for treatment of patients with advanced or unresectable melanoma who are no longer responding to other drugs.

Another strategy is to target the ligand PD-L1. Recently, an interaction between PD-L1 and B7.1 (CD80) was discovered increasing the complexity with blocking antibodies [22]. PD-L1 probably sequesters B7.1 (CD80) but not B7.2 (CD86). Anti-PD-L1 antibodies would block the interaction between PD-L1 and B7.1 as well as between PD-L1 and PD-1 but would not block the interaction between PD-1 and PD-L2. What about the second ligand, PD-L2? Would PD-L2 mediate agonistic signals? Figure 12.5 illustrates the mechanisms of CTLA-4 and PD-1 checkpoint blockers.

12.1.6 Cancer Trial Endpoints and Immunotherapeutics

The cost of cancer treatment is among all other cost for healthcare one of the highest. Some approved drugs in the United States tend to cost around $100,000 for a year's treatment, like Avastin (bevacizumab, colon cancer), $85,000 per year, or Provenge (sipuleucel-T, prostate cancer), $93,000. Studies show these high-price drugs prolong life by only a few months.

RECIST. Before approval each drug must be very carefully evaluated in clinical trials with a large number of patients. In 2000 the European Organization for Research and Treatment of Cancer (EORTC), the National Cancer Institute of the United States, and the National Cancer Institute of Canada defined a set of rules for determination of the effectiveness of new oncology drugs. These rules called Response Evaluation Criteria in Solid Tumors, or RECIST, determine when tumor

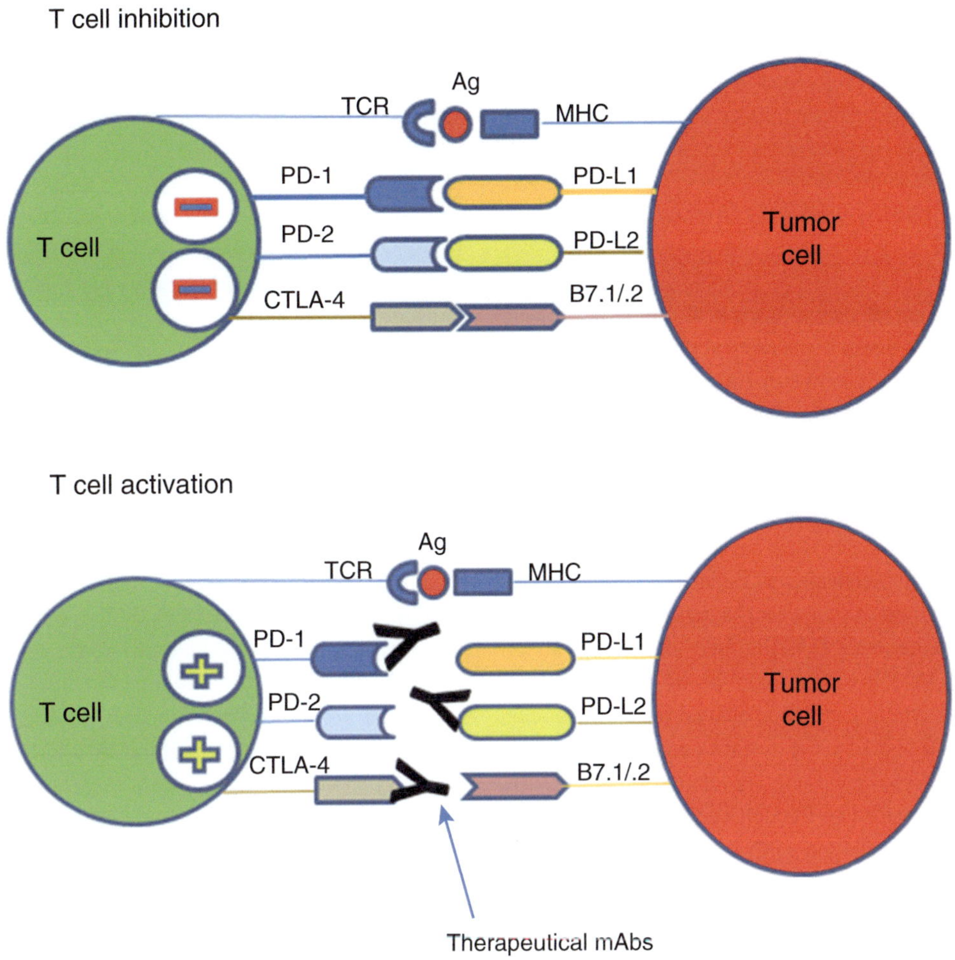

Fig. 12.5 Immune checkpoint interactions between T cell and tumor cell. The T cell activation can start with the presented antigen (TCR-Ag-MHC), combined with co-stimulatory signals (not shown). PD-1 and PD-2 receptors are immune checkpoints on T cells and responsible for immune suppression in peripheral tissues by preventing T cell activation at the time of an inflammatory response to infection and to limit autoimmunity. *T cell inhibition*: tumor cells express the ligands for PD-1, PD-L1, and PD-L2, both are members of the B7 family. Binding of these tumor-derived ligands mediates an inhibitory signal and stops the natural PD-1 and PD-2 action. T cells don't attack tumor cells. Also tumor-derived ligands for the CTLA-4 receptors cause a T cell inactivation. *T cell activation*: immune checkpoint modifiers (therapeutical monoclonal antibodies) against PD-1 or CTLA-4 can prevent the tumor-driven T cell inactivation and restore the natural antitumor response

size in cancer patients changes during treatment: improvement (complete or partial respond, CR or PR), stable disease (SD), or progressive disease (PD). The majority of all clinical trials evaluating cancer drugs use RECIST.

Progressive-Free Survival. The response criteria of RECIST were defined for chemotherapeutic drugs. The clinical response of immunotherapeutic agents, however, is quite different to chemical drugs. The kinetics of antitumor effects is much slower. Whereas a response to a chemical drug commonly occurs within some weeks only after initial administration, the response to an immunological drug can be delayed up to 6 months after initial treatment. In addition, the tumor size can increase, and new lesions (progressive disease) can appear after starting the immunotherapy before a regression begins.

In case of progressive-free survival (PFS) as key endpoint rarely, any immunotherapeutic agent would meet these criteria due to no improvement in PFS.

Overall Survival Time (OS). Novel criteria for evaluation of antitumor responses with immunotherapeutic agents are strongly required focusing on the overall survival time (OS) defined by the date of death from any cause as the most meaningful endpoint.

12.2 Chemo and Radiotherapy Combined with Vaccines[1]

The use of chemotherapy in combination with immunotherapy has been controversial due to the immunosuppressive effects of the chemotherapeutic agents. During the last

[1] Cancer vaccines and the potential benefit of combination with standard cancer therapies *Eva Ellebæk, Mads Hald Andersen and Inge Marie Svane* in Molecular Vaccines – From Prophylaxis to Therapy, Volume 1, Springer-Verlag Wien, 2013, Ed. Matthias Giese.

decade, data have accumulated that point to possible advantages of combining these two treatments. To this end, some chemotherapeutic drugs lead to an immunogenic death of cancer cells and selective depletion of Treg cells.

12.2.1 Chemotherapy and Its Immunological Benefit

Even though the use of chemotherapy in combination with immunotherapy may seem controversial due to the immune-inhibiting potential of chemotherapeutics, evidence arise that this combination may have more beneficial than negative consequences. Several groups have in preclinical models examined the efficacy of different chemotherapeutic agents on the immune cells and the immune defense mechanisms [23–25].

Chemotherapeutics exert their immunomodulating function through multiple mechanisms (Table 12.4). Firstly, when tumor cells undergo apoptosis after the treatment with certain chemotherapeutics, several DAMPs (see also Chap. 2) are released. These DAMPs can be taken up by APC, presented for T cells, and an immune reaction against other cancer cells expressing these antigens on the surface can be initiated.

This immunogenic apoptosis is characterized by the expression of calreticulin on the cell surface and the release of several intracellular factors to the outside of cell such as adenosine triphosphate [26].

Secondly, tumor cells can be more sensitive to T cell-mediated lysis after treatment with certain chemotherapeutics due to a cell membrane more permeable for granzyme B [27]. This can result in increased tumor cell killing.

Thirdly, it has been observed that chemotherapy-induced lymphopenia is often followed by a secretion of cytokines, i.e., IL-7, IL-15, and IL-21. This can lead to a period of T cell proliferation where new antigens are presented to the proliferating T cell clones, and this reaction can be exploited to redirect immunity against a tumor-hostile reaction. Finally, as mentioned above Treg cells play an important role in the regulation of immune reactions induced naturally as well as with immunotherapeutics. It has been shown that chemotherapeutic agents target Treg cells by direct killing and also by reducing the inhibitory function of these cells [28, 29].

Figure 12.6 illustrates the release of DAMPs and traffic to the cell surface or release into the extracellular space after treatment with some anticancer therapeutics. Table 12.5 classifies the nature of these inducers of the immunogenic cell death (ICD). Most of these agents target the endoplasmic reticulum (ER), site of protein synthesis, folding, and transport to the Golgi apparatus, leading to stress and the production of reactive oxygen species (ROS). ROS is one of the key molecules of intracellular pathways that govern ICD. One consequence of the disordered redox milieu is a chronic inflammation. Examples of such substances are different so-called leaderless secretory proteins (LSPs), like high mobility group B 1 molecule, HMGB 1, or IL-18.

12.2.1.1 Combinatorial Chemo-immunotherapy with Low-Dose Immunomodulator Chemotherapy

Cyclophosphamide is one of the chemotherapeutics most investigated for its potential immunomodulatory effects [24]. It has been shown that low/metronomic doses of cyclophosphamide might be able to reduce the number of regulatory T cells and influence the function of dendritic cells with increased expression of maturation markers and enhanced antigen presentation.

In a pilot study, a metronomic dose of cyclophosphamide, 50 mg p.o. daily for 3 months, was tested in 12 metastatic breast cancer patients [30]. The level of Treg was transiently reduced but recovered completely during treatment. The antitumor T cell response on the contrary was increased along with the reduction in Treg and maintained at high levels throughout the treatment. This was found to be due to a reduced suppression of pre-existing tumor-specific T cells as well as to a de novo generation of tumor-specific cells. Furthermore, the number of tumor-reactive T cells correlated with clinical benefit. Thus, even though this dose of cyclophosphamide was not able to constitutively reduce the level and function of Treg, it still had an impact on the antitumor response.

A phase I study of Emens et al. [31] tested the most optimal doses of cyclophosphamide and doxorubicin when combined with a HER2-positive allogeneic GM-CSF-secreting tumor vaccine. Different doses of each drug were tested to determine the chemotherapy doses most optimal for induction

Table 12.4 The immunomodulating functions of chemotherapeutics

Immunogenic apoptosis – the release of tumor-associated antigens after tumor cell apoptosis induced by chemotherapy, characterized by: Expression of calreticulin on the surface of cancer cells Release of adenosine triphosphate Release of high mobility group B 1 molecule (HMGB1) Release of heat shock proteins (HSPs)
Fragile tumor cells – chemotherapy can induce cell membranes permeable for granzyme B → increased sensitization of T cell-mediated killing
Increased T cell proliferation after lymphodepletion → de novo presentation of antigens to the proliferating T cell clones → increased T cell reactivity toward tumor cells
Reduced number and function of regulatory T cells

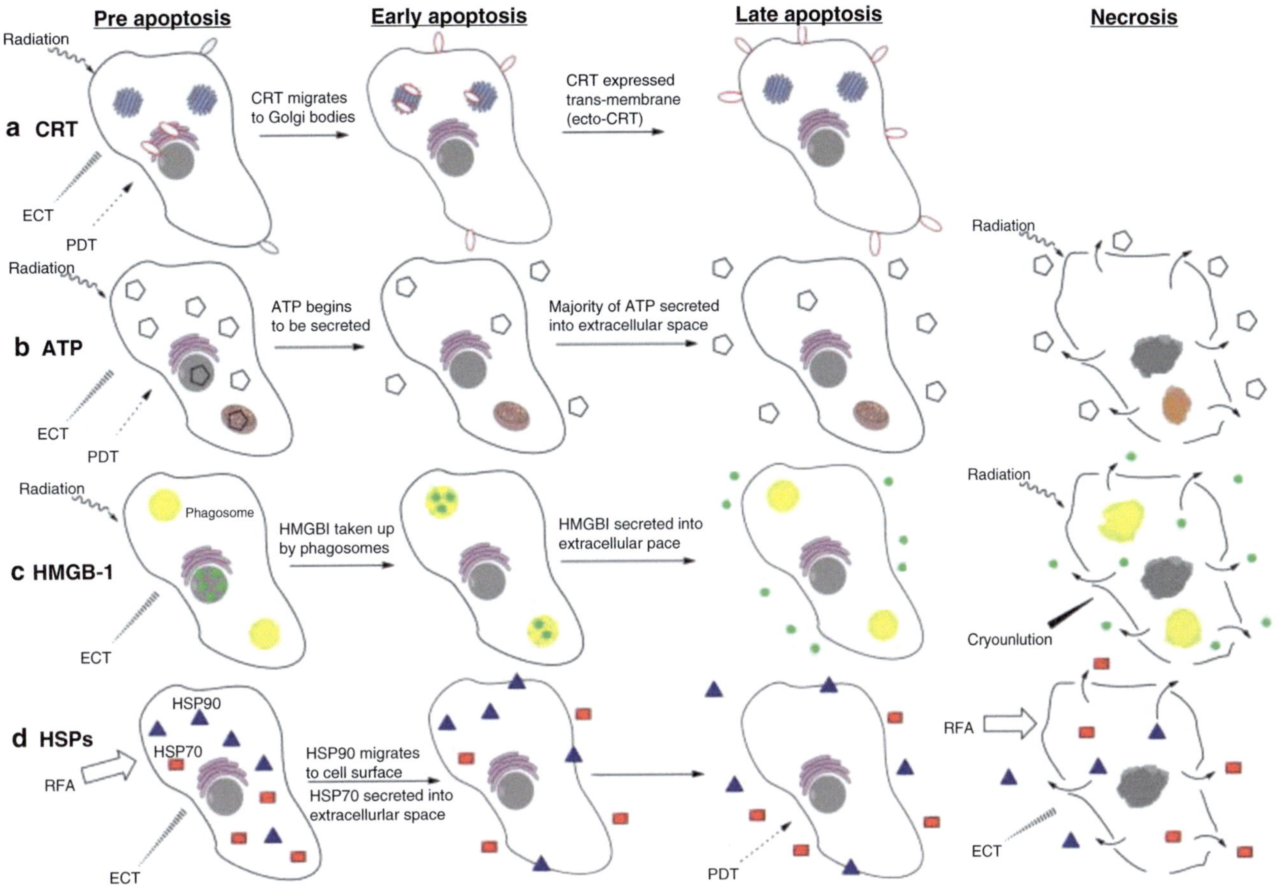

Fig. 12.6 Immunogenic cell death (ICD) caused by ablative modalities and subsequent DAMP release. (**a**) Cellular stress causes CRT (calreticulin) to migrate from ER to Golgi bodies and as apoptosis progresses; CRT is expressed on the plasma membrane (ecto-CRT). This can be induced by radiation and ECT (electroconvulsive therapy). (**b**) During cellular apoptosis, ATP (adenosine triphosphate) is actively secreted from dying cells. The loss of membrane integrity during necrosis allows leakage of ATP into the extracellular space. Radiation and ECT have been proven to cause this ATP release. (**c**) HMGB-1 (high mobility group B 1 molecule) is typically located within the nucleus, but during apoptosis it relocates to phagosomes in the cytoplasm, late stages of apoptosis, and necrosis sees it is expelled in the extracellular space. Ablative techniques that cause this include cryoablation, radiation, and ECT. (**d**) Heat shock proteins move from intracellular compartments to the extracellular space and form complexes on the plasma membrane as the stages of apoptosis advance. Cellular necrosis, as caused by RFA and in some cases ECT, leads to passive diffusion of HSPs into the extracellular space (Credit under CC BY: O'Brien et al. [135])

Table 12.5 Nature of inducers of the immunogenic cell death (ICD)

ICD inducer	Target for ICD	Released DAMP	Induced immunity
Anthracyclines: Doxorubicin, epirubicin, idarubicin	Nucleus DNA or proteins for mitosis	CRT HMGB1 ATP	CD4^{+} and CD8^{+} T cell activation; interferon-γ production
Mitoxantrone	Nucleus DNA or proteins for mitosis	CRT HMGB1 ATP	Suppressed proliferation of tumor cells; NK cell activation
Platinum derivative: Oxaliplatin	Nucleus DNA or proteins for mitosis	CRT HMGB1 ATP	Activation of DCs via TLR4
Cyclophosphamide	Nucleus DNA	CRT HMGB1	Suppression of Treg cells and lymphocytes infiltration in tumor tissue
Bortezomib	Proteasome Inhibitor	HSP90	Activation of DCs and tumor-specific cytotoxic T cells
Specific irradiation	Nucleus DNA	CRT HMGB1 ATP	NK cells attack on irradiated tumor cells
Photodynamic therapy	Nucleus DNA	CRT	Tumor-specific cytotoxic T cells

of HER2-specific immunity. Results showed that 200 mg/m² of cyclophosphamide and 35 mg/m² of doxorubicin could improve the magnitude of HER2-specific humeral immunity and preserve DTH development. It also showed that this was a narrow therapeutic window since larger doses of cyclophosphamide would interfere with immunity and DTH development emphasizing that dosing of chemotherapy is important when immunomodulating effects want to be preserved.

In another study, metastatic renal cell carcinoma patients were treated with an allogeneic dendritic cell vaccination with (10 patients) or without (12 patients) cyclophosphamide in a phase I/II trial [32]. Out of 22 patients treated, two had a mixed response, and one patient had stable disease – all of whom were treated with cyclophosphamide. Very weak or absent immune responses were found, but the two patients with mixed response had the strongest KLH-specific and antigen-independent proliferative response observed which might indicate that cyclophosphamide was able to augment immune and clinical responses.

Finally, Ghiringhelli et al. [33] treated 28 patients with late stage cancer with metronomic doses of cyclophosphamide, 50 mg twice a day in 1 week altering with 1 week off treatment. This regimen resulted in a selective reduction of Treg cells. However, in a clinical trial [34], this cyclophosphamide regimen was used in combination with a dendritic cell vaccine and IL-2, but in this trial the number of Treg cells was not reduced. Whether this was due to the co-treatment with IL-2 will be assessed in a new trial with metronomic doses of cyclophosphamide in combination with DC vaccination but without IL-2 (clinicaltrial.gov Identifier NCT00978913) (Table 12.6).

Table 12.6 Examples of combinatorial chemo-immunotherapy

	Trial examples	Drug/dose	Vaccine	Cancer	No. of patients	Response/efficacy
Low-dose chemotherapy, cyclophosphamide (Cy)	Ge et al. [30]	Cy 50 mg/day	None	Breast cancer	12	Transient reduction in Treg, increased antitumor T cell response
	Emens et al. [31]	Cy 200 mg/m² + doxorubicin 35 mg/m²	HER2⁺ allogeneic GM-CSF-secreting vaccine	Breast cancer	28	Increased HER2-specific humeral immunity
	Holtl et al. [32]	Cy 300 mg/m² day 3–4 prior to vaccination vs. no Cy	Allogeneic DC vaccine	Renal cell carcinoma	10 (+Cy) vs. 12 (−Cy)	2 patients with mixed response – also the ones with highest immune response; both received Cy
	Ghiringhelli et al. [33]	Cy 50 mg × 2/day every 2nd week	None	Late stage cancer	28	Selective reduction in Treg
	Ellebaek et al. [34]	Cy 50 mg × 2/day every 2nd week	Autologous DC vaccine + IL-2	Metastatic melanoma	28	No reduction in Treg – disease stabilization in 58 % of patients
Standard dose chemotherapy	Kyte et al. [35]	Temozolomide	Telomerase peptide vaccine	Metastatic melanoma	25	Increased number of immune responders and long-lasting clinical responses
	Harrop et al. [36]	5-FU, leucovorin, irinotecan	TroVax (5 T4 encoding virus vaccine)	Metastatic colorectal cancer	12	Increased immune responses and the correlation of clinical activity and immune reactivity
	Nistico, et al. [37]	Dacarbazine +/–	Melan-A/MART-1 peptide vaccine	Stage II–IV disease-free melanoma	5 (+ dacarbazine), 5 (– dacarbazine)	Increased number of antitumor T cells in 3 patients treated with the combination who stayed disease-free
	Quoix et al. [38]	Cisplatin and gemcitabine	+/– TG4010 (MUC-1 and IL-2 encoding poxvirus)	Non-small cell lung cancer	74 patients in each group (+/– vaccine)	Improved ORR and prolonged survival among patients treated with the combination

12.2.1.2 Combinatorial Chemo-immunotherapy with Standard Dose Chemotherapy

Several clinical studies have focused on the feasibility of adding cancer vaccination strategies to standard chemotherapy. In a Norwegian study from 2011 [35], Kyte et al. treated 25 metastatic melanoma patients with standard chemotherapy, temozolomide, in combination with a 16-amino acid-long telomerase peptide vaccine. Temozolomide was given in a dose of 200 mg/m^2 for 5 consecutive days every 4 weeks, and vaccine injections were given with increasing intervals with the first 5 injections given during week 2 and 3 after chemotherapy was initiated. Clinical results revealed that five patients obtained a partial response and a further six patients had stable disease. All five clinical responders developed vaccine-specific T cell responses during vaccination, and this lasted throughout the period of tumor regressions. Survival analyses showed that OS was extended compared to matched controls and responders who survived up to more than 5 years.

Two interesting observations were done: Firstly, this group has previously published results from a clinical trial treating melanoma patients with vaccine only, but in the trial combining the vaccine with chemotherapy, an increased number of patients with an immune response toward the vaccine was observed. Secondly, the clinical responses observed were long-lasting (up to 5 years) and developed gradually (up to almost a year) and not shortly after treatment induction as would have been expected with chemotherapy.

These facts indicate that the combination of standard doses of temozolomide and vaccination can have a positive influence on the induction of immune responses as well as the durability of clinical responses. To this end, in three consecutive studies [36], Harrop et al. have treated metastatic colorectal cancer patients with the vaccine TroVax; a tumor-associated antigen 5 T4 engineered into the virus vector modified vaccinia Ankara. As in the above described study, immune responses induced during the vaccination course were of greater magnitude and longevity when administered in combination with standard chemotherapy (5-fluorouracil, leucovorin, and irinotecan) [36] than when given as monotherapy. Also, signs of clinical activity with stable CEA levels after completion of chemotherapy seemed to correlate with the induction of 5 T4-specific immune responses.

Ten patients with disease-free malignant melanoma stage II–IV were randomized to receive dacarbazine plus a Melan-A/MART-1 peptide vaccine or the vaccine alone in a phase I/II pilot study [37]. Immunological analyses revealed that an expansion of peptide-specific effector memory CD8$^+$ T cells capable of killing Melan-A$^+$ tumor cell lines was observed among patients treated with dacarbazine and vaccination but not in the vaccine-only group. Also, an upregulation of immunoregulatory factors in the gene expression profile was seen the day after administration of chemotherapy which could potentially enhance immune responses induced by vaccination. Only one patient with stage II disease in the vaccine alone group remained disease-free after a follow-up of 29 months where as in the combination arm, three patients with stage III/IV disease were without evidence of disease. Interestingly, those three patients showed an impressive expansion of CD8$^+$ antitumor T cells with an effector memory phenotype. Still, conclusions cannot be drawn from this study including only five patients in each arm.

In another phase IIB trial [38], patients with non-small cell lung cancer (NSCLC) who were to receive first-line chemotherapy were randomized to receive either chemotherapy alone or chemotherapy in combination with TG4010, a poxvirus coding for MUC-1 tumor-associated antigen and IL-2. The primary endpoint of this study was 6-month PFS of 40 % or more in the combination arm, which was reached. Clinically, they found that the objective response rate was better in the combination arm and that objective responses were associated with a prolonged overall survival in this group. In addition, analyses of immunophenotypes showed that patients with an increased number of NK cells (CD16$^+$CD56$^+$CD69$^+$) had a worse clinical outcome indicating that response to treatment was conditioned by the patients' immune status.

In conclusion, these studies show that chemotherapy possesses the ability to modulate the immune system and improve the circumstances under which vaccines are given in order to exert their immune-stimulating potential (Fig. 12.7). Still, it is also clear that the optimal dosing and scheduling of chemotherapy and the best chemotherapeutic drug remain unknown and research in this area is therefore highly warranted.

12.2.2 Cancer Vaccines in Combination with Other Cancer Therapies

12.2.2.1 Radiotherapy

Not only chemotherapy can induce changes in the immune system that might be beneficial for combination with cancer vaccines. Radiotherapy (RT) can induce some of the same modulations as do chemotherapy, including the induction of immunogenic apoptosis resulting in increased antigenic presentation by DCs [39]. In addition, if cell death is not induced by irradiation, it can lead to increased expression of MHC I complexes and adhesion molecules by the surviving cancer cells which can increase T cell recognition and killing [40]. This might again result in an increased number of circulating tumor-specific T cells with the potential to mediate tumor regression in other parts of the body than on the irradiated sites.

Abscopal Effect. Tumor regression at sites distant from the locally irradiated site is called an abscopal effect, a phenomenon described only in few cases [41].

Patients with NSCLC in stable disease or response after chemotherapy or chemoradiation were included in a phase IIB study [42] and randomized to vaccination with BLP25

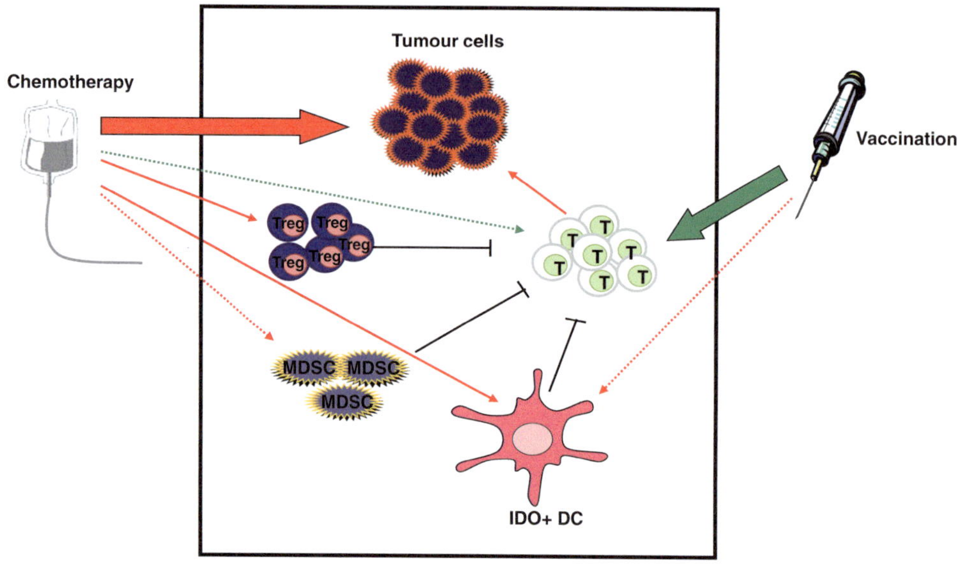

Fig. 12.7 The interaction between tumor cells, effector T cells, and immunoregulatory cell subsets. The effector T cells (*T*) have little cytolytic activity toward the tumor cells in the immunosuppressive tumor milieu. There function is inhibited by regulatory T cells (Treg), myeloid-derived suppressor cells (*MDSC*), and IDO+ dendritic cells (*DC*) as well as the tumor cells' ability to escape from T cell recognition by, e.g., downregulation of MHC molecules. Chemotherapy and cancer vaccinations can work in synergy: the vaccines giving rise to a number of tumor-specific T cells and the chemotherapy killing tumor cells directly and priming the tumor for T cell killing, decreasing the number and functionality of regulatory cell subsets, and inducing cytokine release leading to T cell proliferation. In addition, selective inhibition of, e.g., IDO+ DC by specific immunization against the IDO peptide can further improve T cell activity. Inhibitory activity by chemotherapy/vaccination is indicated by *red arrows* where increasing activity is indicated by *green arrows*

liposome vaccine plus best supportive care (BSC) or BSC alone. A remarkable prolonged survival time for patients in the vaccination arm was shown, most pronounced in the subgroup of patients with stage IIIB locoregional disease (30.6 vs. 13.3 months). It was hypothesized that besides the fact that patients with less immunosuppression and less aggressive disease have more time for development of an immune response, these patients were more often pretreated with RT maybe contributing to the effects of immunotherapy. A new trial has been initiated including only patients with stage IIIB disease pretreated with radiochemotherapy.

Only few clinical studies have been conducted examining the efficacy of RT in combination with cancer vaccines. Gulley and colleagues [43] conducted a clinical phase II trial with prostate cancer patients undergoing local RT and randomized patients to RT alone or RT in combination with a recombinant vaccine encoding PSA. They found a threefold increase in PSA-specific T cells in the combination arm, whereas no increase was observed in the RT alone arm.

Thus, RT seems to have the immunomodulating potential for being combined with immunotherapy, and future clinical trials are being conducted or are in the process of being planned, among these two studies combining RT with ipilimumab (ClinicalTrials.gov identifier: NCT00861614 and NCT01557114) (Table 12.7).

12.2.2.2 Targeted Therapies

Another well-established antineoplastic treatment modality is the targeted therapies of which more and more are being approved for treatment. Targeted therapies have been approved in first-line treatment for chemotherapy-resistant cancers such as renal cell carcinoma [44] and in some cases for melanoma patients [45]. These therapies might very well also have a positive impact on the immune system by the induction of immunogenic cell death and the release of tumor antigens. Furthermore, the fast and impressive but often short-lasting objective responses observed with some of these therapies might benefit from being combined with the slower but more sustained responses seen with immunotherapy.

A prolonged time to disease progression effectuated by the targeted therapies might also expand the time from where a clinically significant immune response can be induced by, e.g., cancer vaccinations [46]. Recent research have found that BRAF gene inhibitors do not negatively influence the function of cytotoxic T cells [47] and that these agents might increase antigen expression on the surface of melanoma cells making them more prone to T cell killing [48]. This suggests that a combination of BRAF inhibitors and immunotherapy could be possible, and discussions on the combination of BRAF inhibitors and anti-CTLA-4 or MEK-inhibitors are ongoing.

Recently, we have shown that blockade with the BRAF inhibitor, vemurafenib, could increase the antitumor reactivity of tumor-infiltrating lymphocytes when cocultured with $BRAF^{V600}$ mutant autologous melanoma cell lines pretreated with vemurafenib. Improved tumor recognition was associated with upregulation of MHC I molecules and heat shock protein on the tumor cells. These data suggest that a combination of

Table 12.7 Examples of cancer vaccines in combination with other cancer therapies

	Trial examples	Drug	Vaccine	Cancer	No. of patients	Response/efficacy
Radiotherapy (RT)	Butts et al. [42]	Chemotherapy/ chemoradiotherapy	+/– Stimuvax (BLP25 liposome vaccine)	Non-small cell lung cancer	88 (+ vaccine) and 83 (–vaccine)	Prolonged survival for patients treated in the vaccination arm – especially those pretreated with chemoradiotherapy
	Gulley et al. [43]	Local RT	+/– PSA encoding vaccine	Prostate cancer	19 (+vaccine) vs. 11 (–vaccine)	Threefold increase in PSA-specific T cells in the combination arm
Targeted therapy	Comin-Anduix et al. [47]	BRAF inhibitor (PLX4032)	None	Malignant melanoma cells BRAF V600E+ (in vitro study)		No negative effects on cytotoxicity of T cells
	Boni et al. [48]	BRAF inhibitor	None	Malignant melanoma cells BRAF V600E+ (in vitro study)		Increased antigen expression
Immunotherapy	Schwartzentruber et al. [49]	High-dose IL-2	+/– gp100 peptide vaccine	Metastatic melanoma patients	94 (IL-2 alone) vs. 91 (IL-2 + vaccine)	Improved clinical response and progression-free survival in the combination arm
	Hodi et al. [51]	+/– ipilimumab (Ipi)	+/– gp100 peptide vaccine	Metastatic melanoma patients	403 (Ipi + vaccine), 137 (Ipi alone), 136 (vaccine alone)	No clinical benefit was seen in the combination arm

vemurafenib and adoptive cell transfer could be beneficial for patients with $BRAF^{V600}$ mutant malignant melanoma, but increased tumor recognition by tumor-specific T cells could also be exploited in a cancer vaccination setup.

12.2.2.3 Other Immunotherapies

In a study from 2011 [49], Swartzentruber and colleagues reported of the findings from a phase III trial randomizing 185 metastatic melanoma patients between treatment with high-dose IL-2 alone and in combination with a gp100 peptide vaccine. Results showed a significant improvement in clinical response with an objective response rate of 16 % in the combination group compared to 6 % in the IL-2 alone group. In addition, progression-free survival was significantly improved, and overall survival was in favor of the combination (17.8 months vs. 11.1 months, $p=0.06$). Only 7 out of 37 immune evaluable patients from the combination arm developed measurable peptide-specific T cells, and immune analyses did not show any correlation between the antitumor response and clinical response. Still, results from this randomized study underline the possible advantages of combining cytokine therapy with cancer vaccination.

The impact on the immune system of the CTLA-4 antibody ipilimumab (Yervoy, BMS) has been investigated by Weber et al. [50] who found that the percentage of activated $CD4^+$ and $CD8^+$ T cells and the percentage of effector memory T cells were increased during treatment. Concomitant with this a decrease in the level of naive T cells was seen. These data suggest that ipilimumab increases T cell activity making it an obvious agent for combination with cancer vaccines. In a large randomized phase III trial [51], ipilimumab was tested for its efficacy using a 3-arm randomization strategy with ipilimumab alone, together with a gp100 peptide vaccine, or the gp100 vaccine alone. This study showed that ipilimumab alone or in combination with the gp100 vaccine was superior to the gp100 vaccine alone, but surprisingly, no benefit was seen from combining ipilimumab with the vaccine. This has also been observed in other studies combining ipilimumab with gp100 vaccination [52].

12.2.3 Perspectives

Drug resistance is the major problem that limits the effectiveness of chemotherapies used in the treatment of cancer. A frustrating property of such acquired resistance is that the tumor not only become resistant to the specific drug in use but may also acquire cross-resistance to other drugs with different mechanisms of action. Cancer-associated defects in apoptosis play a vital role in resistance to chemotherapy and radiotherapy. An important reason for this impaired apoptosis is an overexpression of the antiapoptotic regulators of apoptosis proteins, e.g., the tumor antigen surviving.

Additionally, drug inactivation by the tumor antigen CYP1B1 may represent a mechanism of resistance, influencing the clinical outcome of chemotherapy. Consequently, immunotherapy targeting these antigens in combination with conventional chemotherapy appears to be particularly appealing. In such a setting, conventional therapy would kill the majority of the cancer cells, leaving only cells that express high levels of antigens, which would be particularly vulnerable to killing by vaccination-induced T cells. The synergy of these measures could potentially give a more effective treatment than the added effect of either regime alone, thereby strengthening the already described synergistic effect of anticancer vaccines and chemotherapy. Thus, the synergistic effects of conventional and immunological therapies necessitate re-thinking of the clinical strategies not only with respect to the chosen chemotherapeutics but also considering design of the selected immunotherapy.

Undoubtedly, the combination of cancer vaccines with other antineoplastic treatments has high potential, and the possibilities are numerous. However, interactions between the individual therapies are in general very difficult to predict, and thorough clinical testing is therefore essential. The diversity from immunogenic cell death induced by some chemotherapeutics and radiotherapy regimens to the synergistic effects of cytokines and vaccines points toward number of potential new clinical trials that should be based on reasonable scientific arguments and solid preclinical work.

12.3 Oncolytic Virus as Vaccine: Parvovirus[2]

12.3.1 Cancer Virotherapy

Over the last 20 years, the oncolytic activity of a dozen viruses has been characterized, and several have entered clinical trials. Most of them derive from modified human pathogenic viruses such as herpes simplex and adeno- and poxviruses and possess large cloning capacities. This opens up the possibility of designing multifunctional virus-based products (therapeutic and imaging molecules) to be selectively expressed at high concentrations within human tumors.

The initial idea of an oncolytic virus (OV) infecting the tumor and causing its eradication through successive rounds of infection–replication–oncolysis and reinfection has turned to be rather idealistic due to limitations on the efficiency of intratumoral virus replication and spreading in humans and the presence of a large percentage of normal stromal cells within most tumors. These limitations are however not necessarily

[2]Parvoviruses – the friendly anticancer immunomodulator by *Zahari Raykov, Svitlana P.Grekova, Assia L.Angelova and Jean Rommelaere* in Molecular Vaccines – From Prophylaxis to Therapy, Volume 1, Springer-Verlag Wien, 2013, Ed. Matthias Giese.

Table 12.8 Examples of oncolytic viruses used in clinical trials

Virus	Origin	Cancer	Application	Combination with
HSV-1 + GM-CSF (T-VEC™)	Human	Melanoma	Intratumoral	
Adenovirus 5 + p53[a] (Advexin™)	Human	Head and neck cancer	Intratumoral	
PVS-RIPO[b] (poliovirus modified by rhinovirus 2)	Human	Glioma	Intratumoral	
Coxsackievirus A21 (Cavatak™)	Human	Melanoma, breast, head and neck cancer	Intratumoral	Cisplatin, radiation
Measles virus (MV-NIS)[c]	Human	Multiple myeloma	Intravenous	Cyclophosphamide
Reovirus 3 (Reolysin™)	Human	Pancreatic cancer	Intravenous	Gemcitabine
Newcastle disease virus (strain PV701)	Avian	Breast, ovarian, sarcoma	Intravenous	
Myxoma[d]	Rabbit	Melanoma	Intratumoral or intravenous	
Parvovirus	Rodent	Glioma	Intratumoral/intracerebral[e] or intravenous/intracerebral	

[a]p53 is a tumor suppressor gene found in most cells; in many cancers, and the p53 gene is mutated and cannot stop the growth of the cancer cells. Adenovirus 5 engineered with a "new" p53 reactivate the normal actions of the p53 genes in patients with cancer
[b]PVS-RIPO recognizes Necl-5, an oncofetal cell adhesion molecule and tumor antigen
[c]Measles virus encoding the human thyroidal sodium iodide symporter (iodine-123)
[d]Still in preclinical studies
[e]Intratumoral (via catheter), intracerebral (direct injection at multiple locations of resection wall), intravenous infusion
Table by M. Giese Heidelberg/Germany

reflected in a poor oncosuppressive effect of oncolytic viruses. Engineered viruses, armed with cytokines or not armed, used in oncolytic immunotherapy are listed in Table 12.8.

Indeed, apart from their direct lytic activity, these viruses have the capacity to trigger both the cellular and humoral arm of the immune system within the tumor, representing in this way the perfect vaccine adjuvant (Fig. 12.8). Oncolytic viruses would also support the release of neoantigens out of the tumor. These neoantigens additionally stimulate an immune response and thus support checkpoint blockade drugs. Checkpoints are generally stop signals for proliferating immune responses and are mainly based on ligand–receptor interactions. One major mechanism of immune resistance of many tumors is their hijacking of checkpoints. Therefore, oncolytic viruses combined with checkpoint blockade drugs could be a powerful therapy.

Dual Role of Immune System. The immune system plays a dual role in relation to cancer virotherapy. On one hand, it contributes to defend the organism against infection, thereby antagonizing OV activity. Most OVs trigger a cellular defense mechanism that involves the induction of type I

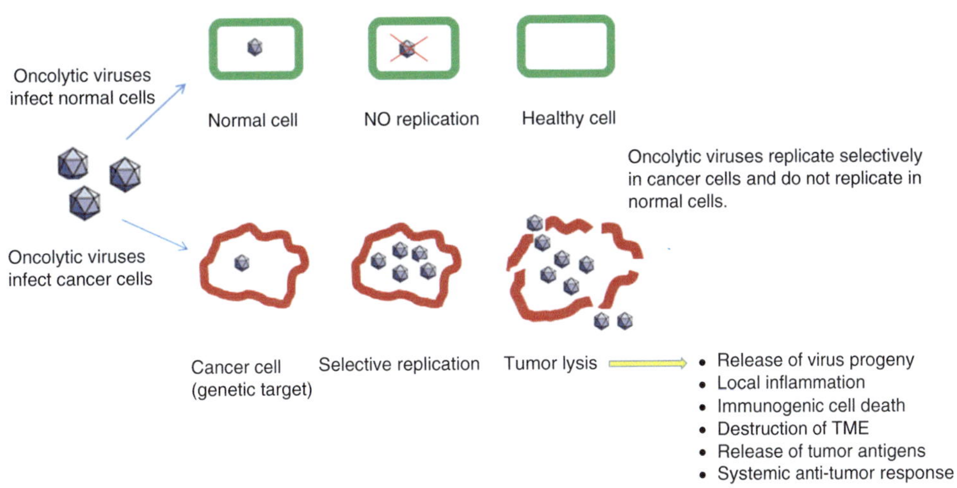

Fig. 12.8 The process of lytic and non-lytic action of oncoviruses in tumor and normal cells (Figure by M. Giese Heidelberg/Germany)

interferons and limits virus replication and propagation. This may not necessarily handicap OVs since IFN signaling is often impaired in tumor cells. The impairment is actually used to design OVs that are unable to block the interferon pathway and as a consequence replicate preferentially in tumors.

Furthermore, the early innate immune responses mediated by NK cells, monocytes, macrophages, and neutrophils provide the initial line of defense of the host to limit OV infection, replication, and spread, while facilitating the maturation of viral antigen-presenting cells and setting the stage for the subsequent adaptive immune response [53]. In particular, the recruitment of NK cells to infected tumors correlates with the production of IFN-γ that plays an essential role in the activation of macrophages that contribute to both OV clearance and later induction of T and B cell-mediated adaptive responses.

On the other hand, this pro-immune microenvironment arising from tumor infection with OVs is also favorable to the activation of anticancer innate response, cross-presentation of tumor-associated antigens, and induction of tumor-specific adaptive immunity [54]. In this regard, oncolytic viruses may act as in situ personalized vaccine adjuvants by revealing the patient own tumor antigens to the immune system. This immune component of OV activity is especially important since it should contribute to the destruction of noninfected tumor cells which may represent the majority of malignant cells in an OV-treated tumor. It should also be stated that the immunostimulating activity of OVs can be enhanced by arming them with appropriate regulating motifs or transgenes. This can be exemplified by the herpes- and vaccinia-based OncoVEX and JX594 vectors supplemented with a GM-CSF-encoding transgene, which can be assumed to play a role in the recently reported ability of these OVs to affect metastatic cancers after i.v. inoculation [55].

12.3.2 Parvoviruses

Parvoviridae are small (25 nm) icosahedral particles containing a single-stranded DNA genome of about 5 kb. Members of rodent origin belonging to the genus *Parvovirus* (PV) are of special interest due to their oncolytic properties. Among oncolytic viruses, rodent PVs fall in the category of the non-engineered (naturally oncolytic) animal viruses, together with *Newcastle disease virus* (NDV) (bird), myxoma (rabbit) *Semliki Forest virus*, and others [56–58]. These viruses can cause diseases in their natural hosts but are not pathogenic to humans. Furthermore, they show oncotropic and oncolytic features [59] in both animal and human cancer cells. The natural oncoselectivity of PVs appears to result, at least in part, from the dependence of viral DNA replication gene expression and nonstructural protein cytotoxic activity on the proliferation and transformation of host cells. In particular, it has been shown that the rat parvovirus H-1PV selectively kills a panel of human tumor-derived cell lines [60]. Moreover, H-1PV systemic or intratumoral injection leads to the suppression of various human carcinomas, lymphomas, and nervous system tumors in animal models [61]. Importantly, H-1PV is infectious but devoid of significant pathogenicity for humans [62].

H-1PV. Studies of PV infection through different routes in animal models show that the viremia is transient and followed by a wave of virus-specific antibody production within 7–10 days p.i. A similar sequence of events was observed in humans experimentally infected with H-1PV. Anti-PV antibodies are, at least in part, neutralizing and can thereby be expected to impede viral oncosuppression. Indeed, the ability of H-1PV to suppress hepatoma metastases in adult ACI rats upon virus administration shortly after tumor cell injection was impaired when animals were pre-infected with H-1PV several weeks prior to treatment [63]. However, no or little pre-existing natural immunity against PVs was found in the human population and even in laboratory personnel working routinely with these agents, unpublished observations. Table 12.9 gives an overview on current clinical trials on parvovirotherapy.

12.3.2.1 Activation of the Immune System by PVs

The possibility of PVs triggering anticancer vaccination was raised by the pioneering studies of Mc Kisic et al. with the mouse parvovirus MPV-1. These authors showed that animals cured of a tumor upon virus infection are protected against subsequent challenges with the same tumor cells. This virus was shown to persistently infect mouse lymphoid tissues and to accelerate rejection of sarcoma allografts without directly infecting tumor cells.

Another hint as to the involvement of the immune system in PV oncosuppression was given by the comparison of mice differing in their immune status for their responsiveness to parvovirus MVMp-induced suppression of transplanted syngeneic gliomas. Immunocompetent mice were fully protected from tumoral outgrowth of GL261 glioma cells infected *ex vivo* with MVMp. In contrast, immunodeficient ($RAG2^{-/-}$) animals were less competent for MVMp-dependent tumor inhibition, with only 20 % of the recipients being protected, arguing for an additional adaptive immune component to allow full tumor suppression [64].

In a syngeneic immunocompetent rat model of pancreatic ductal adenocarcinomas (PDAC), parvovirus H-1PV could achieve striking tumor suppression under conditions where only a relatively minor fraction of the tumor cells underwent direct virus-induced lysis. In this system, the virus appears to act mainly as trigger of an anticancer immune response. Indeed, adoptive transfer of splenocytes from H-1PV-treated tumor-bearing

Table 12.9 Current clinical trials on parvovirotherapy

Model	Description and effects
Glioma	Single intranasal instillation of H-1PV was sufficient to reach the brain and induce efficient regression of rat glioma. In rats with xenografts of human glioma, oncolytic activity of H-1PV was less pronounced, however, leading to significant prolongation of survival
Pancreas carcinoma (PDAC)	H-1PV monotherapy had strong anticancer effect both in vitro (human PDAC cells) and in vivo in rats and SCID mice (human xenotransplants) with reduction of tumor growth, prolonged survival of the animals, and absence of metastases on CT scans. H-1PV + Gemzar combination had synergistic effect
Burkitt lymphoma	H-1PV productively infected and efficiently killed through necrosis, cell cultures originating from Burkitt lymphoma (BL) including resistant to apoptosis induction by rituximab cells. Parvovirus-based monotherapy efficiently suppressed established human BL at an advanced stage in a severe combined immunodeficient (SCID) mouse model of the disease
Cervical carcinoma	H-1PV caused a dose-dependent regression of subcutaneous tumors from human cervical carcinoma (HeLa) cells into immunodeficient rats and SCID mice
Breast carcinoma	Injection of parvovirus H-1PV at the site of human tumor cells' implantation in adult nude mice drastically inhibited tumor growth (greater than 80 %). When injected i.v. in animals bearing preformed tumors, H-1 virus was able to slow down and even in some cases to revert neoplastic growth
Metastatic cancer (lung, peritoneum)	Lung metastases from rat hepatoma were successfully treated with subcutaneous injection of a virus-infected (wild-type H-1PV or CpG-enriched) autologous vaccine Concomitant i.p. treatment of H-1PV with recIFN-γ immunotherapy resulted in improved therapeutic effect on peritoneal carcinosis from rat pancreatic cancer
Phase I Clinical trial Glioma (GBM) (ongoing)	ParvOryx01 is an open, noncontrolled, two-group, intragroup dose escalation, single-center, phase I/IIa trial. 18 patients with recurrent GBM will be treated in 2 groups of 9 patients each. Treatment group 1 will first receive H-1PV by intratumoral injection and second by administration into the walls of the tumor cavity during tumor resection. In group 2 the virus will initially be injected intravenously and afterward, identical to group 1, into the surrounding brain tissue during tumor removal. The primary objective of the trial is local and systemic safety and tolerability and to determine the maximum tolerated dose (MTD). Secondary objectives are proof of concept (PoC) and progression-free survival (PFS) up to 6 months

donors resulted in tumor regression in naive recipients bearing preestablished orthotopic pancreatic cancers. In another setup, H-1PV-induced oncolysis of an infected pancreatic tumor was found to lead to the regression of a noninfected distant tumor in the same animal. In both types of experiments, the regression of the recipient or distant tumor, respectively, occurred in the absence of virus transfer, presumably via a virus-triggered antitumor immune response. Another line of evidence for the role of the immune system in PV oncosuppression comes from immunodepletion experiments showing that the selective removal of CD8+ cells from immunocompetent rats correlates with reduced effectiveness of H-1PV to eradicate transplanted gliomas and hepatoma metastases [63].

12.3.2.2 Indirect Activation of the Immune System by PVs through Killing of Tumor Cells

A number of experimental observations support the notion that PV-mediated oncosuppression is immunogenic (see Fig. 12.9, upper left panel). As mentioned above, the oncotropism of PVs is not due to a better virus uptake by transformed cells but rather to the dependence of intracellular steps of the viral life cycle on the presence, absence, or activation of factors that are regulated as function of cell cycling and oncogenic transformation. Due to small size and limited coding capacity of their genome, PVs exploit their nonstructural proteins to perform multiple functions. In particular, the activities of the major nonstructural protein NS1 are timely regulated through posttranslational modification and/or subcellular distribution. Phosphorylation of distinct NS1 domains controls both enzymatic (ATPase, helicase) and nonenzymatic (DNA and protein binding) functions of the viral product and varies during infection. Cell death and eventual lysis are the final outcome of the infection of permissive malignant cells with PVs. Depending on the cell type and metabolic status, PV-infected cells can die through different mechanisms, namely, apoptosis, necrosis, or cathepsin spillage from lysosomes.

Several studies show evidence of an enhanced capacity of PV-infected versus noninfected tumor cells for activating APCs in human and rodent in vitro systems. This effect does not merely result from the PV-induced killing of tumor cells. Indeed, in vitro matured dendritic cells (DCs) were found to be more efficiently activated by H-1PV-infected human melanoma cells than by melanoma cell lysates obtained by freezing/thawing. When DCs were cocultured with PV-infected SK-29MEL cells, phagocytosis and cross-presentation of tumor-associated antigens by the DCs led to effective activation of melanoma-specific CTLs [65]. Mouse glioma cells (GL261) infected with the parvovirus MVMp (minute virus of mice) were also tested for their ability to activate dendritic cells (DCs) and microglia (MG), two distinct cell types that can act as APCs. Microglia and discrete DC subsets were

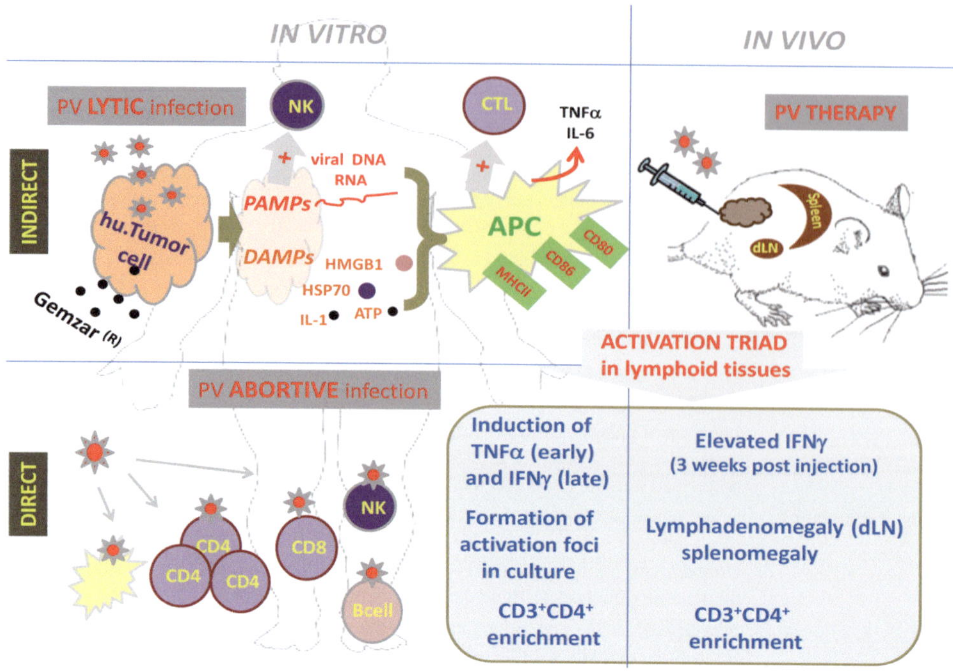

Fig. 12.9 Immunomodulation by PVs. *Upper panel* – indirect in vitro (*left*) immunomodulation by PVs in combination with standard pancreatic carcinoma chemotherapeutic. Tumor cells undergo immunogenic cell death (ICD), and the contribution of H-1PV-derived PAMPs (*DNA*, *RNA*) and H-1PV–Gemzar-induced DAMPs (*HMGB1*, *HSP70*, *ATP*, *IL-1*) to activate antigen-presenting cells (*APC*) is indicated. Immunomodulation in vivo in PDAC model (*right*); tumor-draining lymph node (*dLN*). *Lower panel* direct in vitro (human PBMCs) immunomodulation. The PV activation triad is observed in both systems; *CD4* T helper, *CD8* cytotoxic T cells, *NK* natural killers

activated after coculture with MVMp-infected glioma GL261 cells, as evidenced by the upregulation of specific activation markers (CD80, CD86) and the release of pro-inflammatory cytokines (tumor necrosis factor-α and interleukin-6).

Immunogenic Cell Death (ICD). Apoptosis and necrosis as anti- and pro-inflammatory dying modalities, respectively, has been amended to relate immunogenicity of cell death to the induction of the above three key ICD determinants. Display of calreticulin (CRT) and release of HMGB1 and ATP appear sufficient to enable paracrine maturation and activation of dendritic cells and consequent CTL priming – the cornerstone event of an adaptive immune response. Surface exposure of CRT mediates the uptake of dying tumor cells by dendritic cells, while the releases of HMGB1 and ATP are, respectively, involved in the activation of TLR2/TLR4/RAGE-mediated signaling and in the initiation of P2X7/inflammasome-mediated activation of caspase 1 (CASP1) leading to processing and secretion of matured interleukin-1 (IL-1).

H-1PV is a potent inducer of HMGB1 release from pancreatic carcinoma cells. In some of these cells, the combination of H-1PV with the standard PDAC chemotherapeutic gemcitabine can stimulate the full panel of ICD determinants including even IL-1. In an earlier study, H1-induced apoptotic killing was reported to correlate with strong release of the immunogenic signal heat shock protein (HSP72) of SK29-Mel-1 melanoma cells [66]. In this system also, the combination of H-1PV infection and treatment with cytotoxic agents or sunitinib resulted in enhanced immunogenicity of melanoma cells, as revealed by their higher ability to induce the maturation of cocultured DCs compared to singly treated tumor cells [67].

In addition to the cell-derived danger signals, viral elements such as double-stranded RNA or unmethylated CpG-containing DNA have been shown to serve as pathogen-associated molecular patterns (PAMPs) and trigger immune activation through pathogen recognition receptors (PRRs) (PKR, TLR 3, TLR 9). In the case of autonomous PVs, this issue is still under investigation, considering also the peculiar single-stranded nature of the viral genome, which offers unique opportunities to increase the genuine adjuvant effect of these viruses (see below).

Beside DCs, important effectors of innate immunity, namely, NK cells, also appear to "sense" PV-mediated killing of PDAC cells, resulting in IFN-γ, TNF-α, and MIP-1α/β production. This activation was recently observed in cell cultures and may play an important role especially at the early stages of the immune response. NK cell-dependent killing of infected tumor cells in vitro could be traced back to the upregulation of the DNAM-1 ligand, CD155, and to the downregulation of MHC class I expression [68].

12.3.3 Direct Effects of PVs on the Immune System

There is evidence that PVs may also have a direct impact on the immune system, as demonstrated in vitro in human

PBMCs (see Fig. 12.9, lower left panel). Early work has shown that long-term cultured lymphocytes, monocytes, and immature and mature dendritic cells were not susceptible to the cytotoxic effect of H-1PV. Furthermore, direct inoculation of H-1PV to human PBMC cultures caused only abortive infection [69]. The virus could enter into the cells and achieve different levels of replication according to the nature and activation status of the cells, but no virus production could be detected. Upon mitogenic activation, the infection pattern (predilection of the virus to particular cell types) shifted from monocytes and B and NK cells toward T cells and especially CD4+ lymphocytes.

However, CD4 T cells were quite stable, showing no impairment of proliferation and viability upon infection, in agreement with their low capacity for expressing the cytotoxic PV protein NS1. The fraction of CD4 T cells was even increased in infected nonstimulated PBMCs correlating with the formation of activation foci in the cultures. These changes were accompanied by early TNF-α (24 h) and late IFN-γ (72 h) production upon PBMC infection. Monocytes were identified as the source of TNF-α, as established through isolation and separate infection of the adherent fraction of the cultures. CD4+ T cells also got activated in infected PBMC cultures, as revealed by activation marker expression and Th1 and Th2 cytokine secretion. In addition, the immunosuppressive properties of Treg cells were reduced as a result of H-1PV infection, while the virus did not affect the viability of these cells.

Besides these in vitro data, some observations indicate that PVs can also interact in a direct way with immune cells under in vivo conditions. Significant MVMp gene expression was detected in lymphoid tissues from infected mice, whether or not with tumors (melanoma, lymphoma, hemangiosarcoma) [70]. This expression was especially obvious in lymph nodes draining virus-injected tumors (dLNs). In the hemangiosarcoma model, tumor cells could be easily identified using the transforming polyoma middle T oncogene (PymT) as specific tumor marker. The tumors of hemangiosarcoma-bearing mice showed strong accumulation of PymT, whereas this marker was barely detectable in spleens and not detectable in dLN. Therefore, MVMp expression in lymph nodes is unlikely to be due to their invasion with infected metastasizing tumor cells and can be assigned to the infection of lymphoid cells instead. Indeed, myeloid DCs and B-1 lymphocytes were found to be the major source of viral mRNA expression in dLN, providing evidence for direct interaction of the parvovirus with immune cells.

Analysis of H-1PV-treated pancreatic carcinoma in a rat model (see above) confirmed that within the first days following intratumoral inoculation, PV expression is predominant in the tumor but can also be detected in lymphatic tissues and most abundantly in tumor-draining lymph nodes. In both glioma and pancreas cancer models, immunocompetent animals treated with PVs showed spleno- and lymphadenomegaly, accompanied by an increase in the T cell compartment with elevated CD4/CD8 ratios and induction of IFN-γ in dLNs and splenocytes. The fact that this same triad of changes was also observed upon direct infection of PBMC cultures suggests that in whole organisms, PV infection of immune cells takes place and results in a Th1 bias.

12.3.4 PVs as Part of Novel Immunotherapeutic Combinations

The fact that intratumoral injection of an oncolytic virus generates an autologous in situ vaccine with the virus acting as an adjuvant may provide a basis for designing a more effective virus. The silent immunomodulating features of H-1PV call for a certain increase in its immunogenicity, in order to create a more "dangerous" virus that can more potently revert the tolerogenic conditions prevailing in tumors.

12.3.4.1 Arming Propagation-Deficient Parvoviral Vectors with Immunostimulating Transgenes

Historically, the first attempts to increase the adjuvant properties of PVs were made by generating capsid replacement vectors from parvoviruses MVMp, H-1PV, and LuIII. These vectors were supplemented with transgenes encoding for toxic (Apoptin) or immunostimulatory (cytokines/chemokines) products [71–73]. Using an appropriate helper system, recombinant viruses transducing these heterologous genes were produced. Pilot animal experiments showed that recombinant PVs carrying the interleukin-2 (IL-2) cytokine gene have a reinforced anticancer capacity, in comparison with empty vectors [74]. Strong anticancer effects of recombinant parvoviruses expressing interferon-gamma-inducible protein 10 (IP-10) and monocyte chemotactic protein 3 (MCP-3) were also observed against established hemangiosarcomas and melanomas in immunocompetent mice, respectively. Interestingly, MVMp vectors transducing TNF-α and IP-10 were found to act synergistically in the suppression of mouse glioma [75].

12.3.4.2 Use of Replication-Competent Parvoviral Vectors as Vaccine Adjuvants

Knowing that CpG motifs are underrepresented in the genomes of virtually all small eukaryotic viruses, including PVs, we assumed that enriching the genome of H-1PV with immunostimulatory CpG patterns would improve its immunomodulating properties. The oncospecific replication of H-1PV should result in the selective amplification of these motifs within tumor cells, followed by their oncolytic release in the context of tumor antigens. This is expected to lead to a higher level of dendritic cell activation through the TLR9 receptor, with cross-presentation of viral and tumor antigens to prime CTLs for killing both infected and noninfected tumor cells.

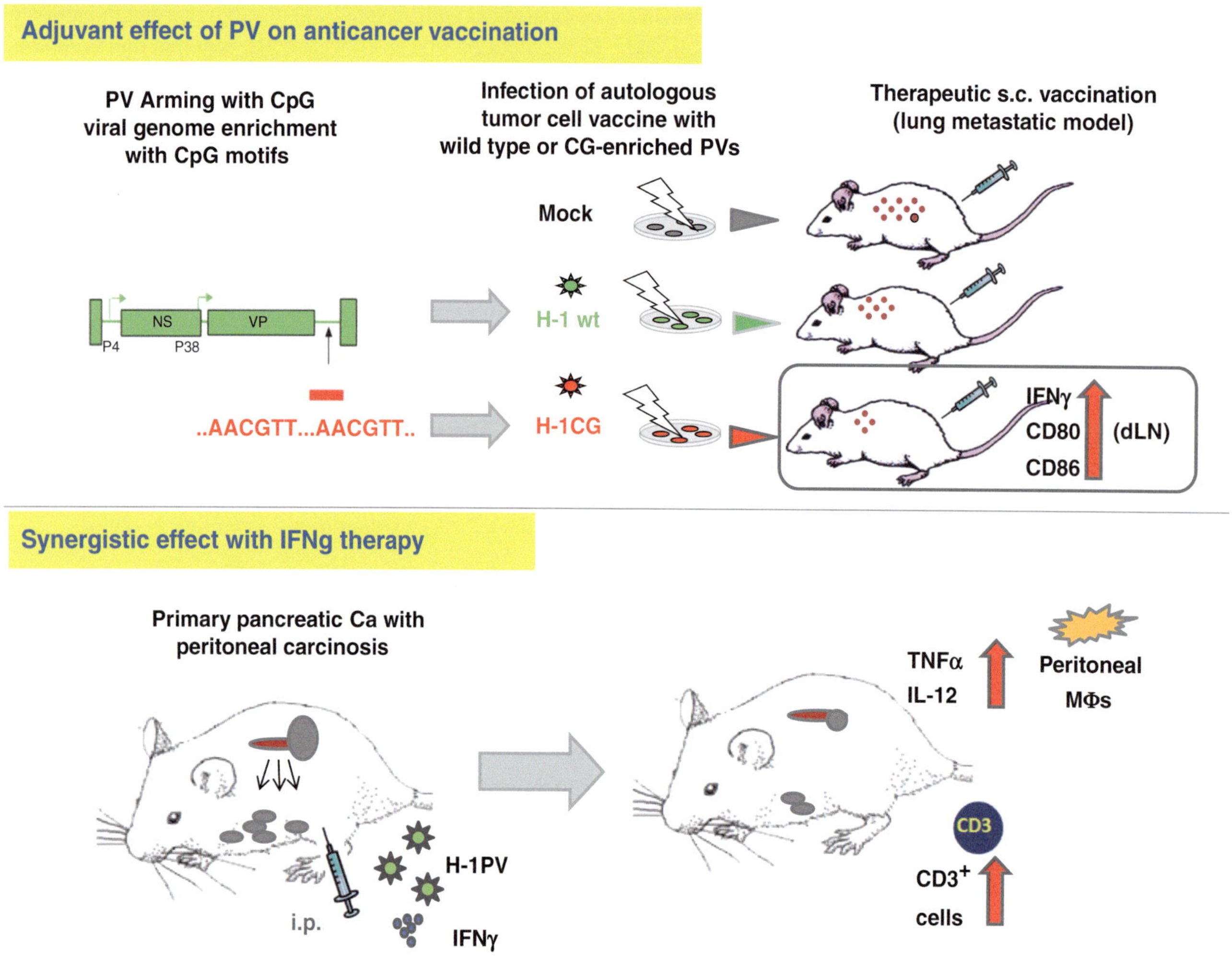

Fig. 12.10 Immunotherapy using PVs. *Upper panel* – improved vaccination approach with TLR9 engagement. Treatment of established hepatoma lung metastasis using subcutaneous application of an autologous PV-infected vaccine. Infecting the vaccine with an engineered H-1PV virus genomically enriched with immunostimulatory CpG sequences improves the vaccination effect by reducing metastasis. IFN-γ, CD80, and CD86 expression in mediastinal lymph nodes is boosted when the H-1PVCpG-inoculated vaccine is applied. *Lower panel* – combined immunotherapy (H-1PV with IFN-γ). Orthotopic pancreatic tumors complicated with peritoneal metastasis were treated by intraperitoneal injection of H-1PV + IFN-γ. IFN-γ enhanced peritoneal macrophage activation and CD3+ lymphocyte proliferation in spleens leading to retardation of primary tumor growth and carcinosis and prolonged survival

Fully infectious CpG-armed H-1PV vectors were produced and tested for their adjuvant capacity in a typical therapeutic vaccination protocol (see Fig. 12.10, upper panel). Rat hepatoma cells with a known predisposition to metastatically settle in the lungs were intravenously injected in syngeneic immunocompetent ACI rats. The established lung metastases were treated by subcutaneous injection of irradiated autologous tumor cells infected with wild-type or modified H-1PVs. Under these conditions, the viruses did not reach the target metastases to exert direct oncolytic effects but replicated in and served as adjuvant to the autologous vaccine.

In keeping with the above evidence of parvoviral immunomodulation, infection with wild-type H-1PV (or GpC-supplemented control vector) improved the efficacy of the cell vaccine. This viral adjuvant effect was significantly enhanced by the H-1PV armed with CpG motifs, resulting in suppression of most metastases by the H-1PV-CG-infected autologous vaccine. This therapeutic vaccination effect was accompanied by strong induction of markers of cell-mediated immune response (IFN-γ) and particularly of DC activation (CD80 and CD86) in the mediastinal lymph nodes draining metastases-harboring lungs. This is an exciting result, showing for the first time that non-defective parvoviral vectors can be engineered and used to generate oncolysates enriched in immunostimulatory CpG motifs and to boost vaccination against distant metastases even in the absence of virus spread [76]. The same strategy (CpG genomic integration) was recently followed to modify oncolytic adenoviruses, improving significantly therapeutic effects.

12.3.4.3 Combining PVs with Interferon-Gamma

Our abovementioned studies of PDAC suppression by H-1PV strongly suggested that the immune system plays a major role in the therapeutic effect of the parvovirus in this system. Most PDAC patients have already distant (liver, peritoneum) metastasis at the time of diagnosis and are in need of aggressive chemotherapy at this stage. We assumed that a local application of PVs into the peritoneal cavity can be effective under these conditions. The production of IFN-γ in tumor-dLNs was found to systemically accompany the therapeutic effect of PVs, implying the importance of this potent cytokine in mediating PV immunomodulation. Intraperitoneal application of IFN-γ has been shown to achieve surgically documented responses as both first- and second-line therapy in randomized phase III clinical trials for ovarian cancer (Fig. 12.10, lower panel).

Altogether these data led to reason that the therapeutic properties of H-1PV may be boosted with IFN-γ for the treatment of late incurable stages of PDAC such as peritoneal carcinomatosis. Rats bearing established orthotopic pancreatic carcinomas with peritoneal metastases were treated through a single or intraperitoneal (i.p.) injection of H-1PV with or without concomitant IFN-γ application (see Fig. 12.10, lower panel). This co-treatment with H-1PV and recIFN-γ resulted in an improved therapeutic effect (prolonged animal survival), compared with i.p. injection of H-1PV alone. Interestingly, the co-treated group could also be distinguished by its immunological parameters, namely, (i) the proneness of isolated peritoneal macrophages to TNF-α production, (ii) the enhanced proliferation of spleen T cells in presence of tumor cells under ex vivo conditions, and (iii) a significant reduction in the titers of H-1PV-neutralizing antibodies in ascitic fluid.

12.4 Lung Cancer Immunotherapy[3]

Lung cancer is the most common cancer worldwide and accounts for 1.3 million deaths annually, which is more than the next three most common cancers combined (colon, breast, and prostate). The insidious nature of lung cancer renders the vast majority of cases to advanced stage at the time of diagnosis. Since stage is most strongly associated with prognosis, late diagnosis is primarily responsible for the 15 % 5-year survival [77, 78].

Nearly half of the patients that can undergo potentially curative surgical resection ultimately succumb to their disease. The rate of second primary lung cancer following first cancer diagnosis is 1–2 % per year. Early detection and prevention initiatives may help reduce overall disease mortality, but the burden of improving outcomes following diagnosis falls more squarely on treatment.

12.4.1 Conventional Therapies

Lung cancer is divided into two main histologic subtypes, non-small cell (NSCLC) and small cell (SCLC), which describes distinct somatic origin, behavior, phenotype, and prognosis. Relative frequency of NSCLC: SCLC is 4:1 (80 % vs. 20 %). Conventional therapies are tailored to both stage and histologic cell type (NSCLC vs. SCLC); more recently, molecular phenotyping has been used to direct therapy toward the most effective regimen.

SCLC. For practical purposes, all cases of this aggressive tumor type are assumed metastatic at the time of diagnosis. Chemotherapy is the mainstay of therapy and surgery does not offer any therapeutic advantage. Radiation is added for local control in limited thoracic disease. SCLC mortality is roughly 95 %.

NSCLC. Surgery is the primary treatment modality for early stage cancer and chemotherapy and radiation for more advanced disease. Combinations of surgical and nonsurgical therapies have incrementally increased survival rates over the past decade.

Early Stage Disease. Surgical resection continues to offer the best chance of cure for the minority of patients diagnosed with early stage NSCLC. Cure rates approach 80 % for small cancers and steadily decrease commensurate with tumor burden. Adjuvant chemotherapy is now conventionally offered to individuals with >35 % chance of recurrence following potentially curative resection [stage II and III disease] providing a 4–15 % survival advantage at 5 years. Other than pathological stage, there are no clinically validated predictive measures of recurrence to aid in the selection of appropriate candidates for adjuvant chemotherapy.

Advanced-Stage Disease. 80 % of patients with non-small cell lung cancer (NSCLC) present with locally advanced or metastatic disease, and an additional 10 % develop mortal recurrence following potentially curative surgical resection. Median survival with treatment ranges from 7 to 12 months. Only 60 % of patients with advanced NSCLC will have clinical response to first-line chemotherapy, typically lasting 3–6 months; newer agents have reduced toxicities but have done little to produce durable responses. Maintenance chemotherapy is conceptually appealing, but only pemetrexed has yet

[3] Lung Cancer Immunotherapy: Programmatic Development, Progress and Perspectives by *Edward A. Hirschowitz, Terry H. Foody and John R. Yannelli* in Molecular Vaccines – From Prophylaxis to Therapy, Volume 1, Springer-Verlag Wien, 2013, Ed. Matthias Giese.

proven effective in delaying time to progression in patients with adenocarcinoma. Upon progression second-line chemotherapies offer 8-month increase in median survival over best supportive care.

12.4.2 Cancer Immunotherapy

Disease characteristics have certainly influenced developmental strategies for lung cancer. Antigenic heterogeneity, which is somewhat dependent on tumor histology, is a defining characteristic and significant challenge for antigen-specific therapies. Other considerations include the notable disparity in stage distribution, spectrums of conventional therapy, and poor prognosis. Targeting microscopic residual disease that leads to recurrence in nearly half the patients with surgically resected non-small cell lung cancer (NSCLC) is a logical application.

The risk to benefit ratio is especially relevant for these patients since recurrence cannot yet be predicted beyond statistical probability. Conversely, efficacy trials are encumbered by variable rates of recurrence and protracted clinical endpoints. Patients with advanced-stage disease have not been widely viewed as likely to benefit from immunotherapy, although slowing disease progression with minimal added risk is a meritorious objective.

The terminal prognosis of advanced-stage NSCLC and the ability to accurately define tumor progression and survival make this population a logical choice for clinical trials. With the majority of those cases being diagnosed by scant cytological sampling, limited access to intrathoracic sites of disease presents secondary hurdles. Apart from being an obvious barrier to in situ approaches, availability of lung tumor tissue is an impediment to autologous vaccine production, antigen characterization, and immune monitoring; the risks of repeated sampling by invasive procedures can rarely be justified.

Immunotherapy for small-cell lung cancer (SCLC) has not been as widely investigated. The disease tends to be very aggressive, and immunotherapy has not been regarded as having significant potential to affect outcomes. The lack of pathologic specimens has also slowed preclinical investigation (in the same way readily available NSCLC specimens have facilitated study) because SCLC is not available for in vitro study or xenogeneic tumor modeling, and there is no appropriate SCLC animal model. Regardless, the poor prognosis associated with SCLC makes it a rational choice for further investigation.

12.4.2.1 Choosing an Immune Adjuvant

A multitude of agents, ranging from nonspecific to highly selective, effectively promote antigen uptake, presentation, and/or recognition through a variety of intersecting mechanisms [79]. The innate capacity of dendritic cells (DCs) to fully orchestrate an adaptive response has led to their characterization as "nature's adjuvant" [80]. At the time, techniques for generating large numbers of dendritic cells (DCs) from peripheral blood had been established, and the ability to generate potent vaccines by loading cultured DC ex vivo with antigen was just being translated from laboratory to the clinics. Promising preclinical data and apparent reliability of immune induction in a few early human studies suggested this approach was an emerging standard for cancer vaccines. With collective experience in NSCLC limited to a handful of patients bearing antigens common to other cancers, the open niche of DC vaccines for NSCLC seemed a logical entry to clinical investigations [81].

12.4.2.2 Antigen

Beyond constraints of antigenic relevance, there is no ideal source of antigen. Distinctions between autologous versus allogeneic, monovalent versus multivalent, and whole cell versus recombinant preparations are part theoretical and part pragmatic. Autologous tumor antigen would offer the advantage of a patient-specific vaccine that circumvents the need to know the antigens patient's cancer expresses, but the volume of tumor tissue generally required to produce autologous tumor vaccines restricts that approach to individuals with a surgically resectable tumor.

Monovalent approaches utilizing allogeneic recombinant protein (including gene therapy derived) or synthetic peptides would restrict usage to a subset of individuals bearing relevant antigens and introduce a secondary hurdle for antigen characterization, with or without HLA restrictions. Allogeneic whole-cell preparations offer an array of well-described antigens, as well as a complement of minor determinants and mismatch antigens to enhance cross-priming [82]. Cell lines are a renewable source of tumor protein that provide a standardized, multivalent antigen preparation. Recipient APCs process and present the most relevant epitopes via class I and class II pathways, thus generating the potential for both immune effector and immune memory responses.

12.4.2.3 Immune Monitoring

Immunological assays are measures of vaccine potency and immune competence. IFN-gamma ELISPOT is a mainstay of immune monitoring. This highly sensitive and reliable assay quantifies the number of CD4+ and CD8+ T cells, in mixed lymphocyte or fractionated populations, which recognize specific antigens. Cytotoxic T-lymphocyte (CTL) assays by contrast are highly specific functional measures of adaptive immunity but have only moderate sensitivity and require cell numbers greater than that recovered from routine clinical blood draws. Tetramer assays that quantify HLA-matched T cells bearing selected antigen receptors are most widely

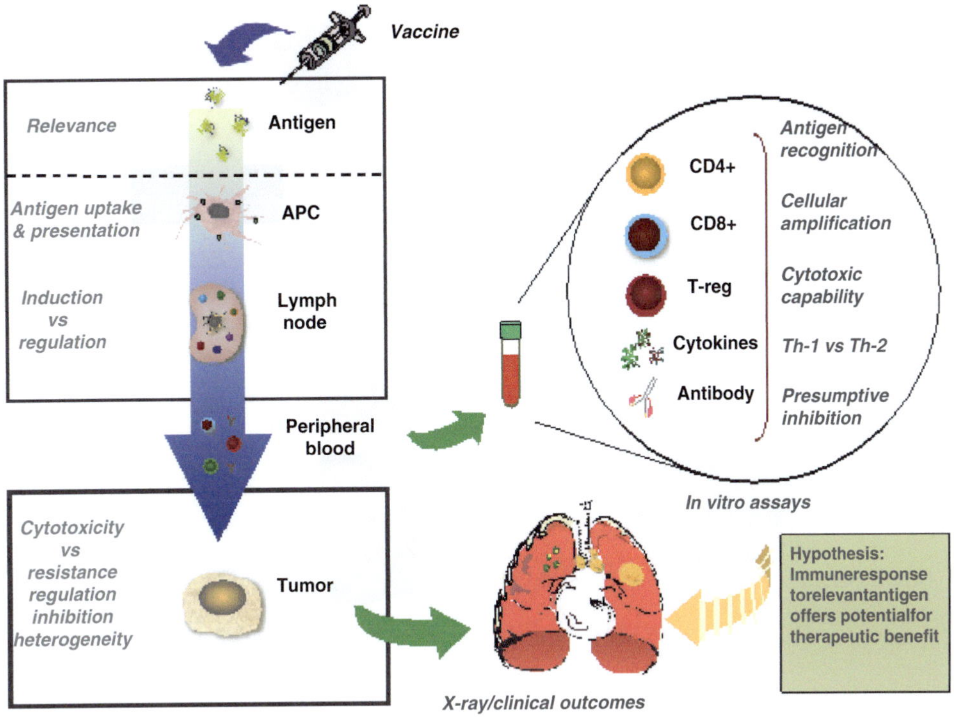

Fig. 12.11 Immune monitoring. The accompanying schematic characterizes the myriad of known, measurable, and unknown elements of immune monitoring, including the somewhat speculative link between measurable immunological criteria and clinical outcomes. Putative mechanisms of adaptive immunity are depicted on the *left of the diagram*: sequential sites of antitumor immune induction and actions of competing pathways are shown in black boxes. Vaccines, produced either with assumed or known antigenic relevance, are delivered into a biological crucible. Windows to the biologic and therapeutic effects of vaccine delivery are shown *on the right*: immunologic and clinical endpoints offer quantifiable metrics. Immune status is extrapolated from batteries of in vitro assays that characterize the constituents of peripheral blood. Serial changes in measures are the fundamental basis of immune "response." Radiographic changes and clinical outcomes reflect the sum of cytotoxicity, inhibition, and resistance in the tumor microenvironment. The relationship of immune monitoring assays and therapeutic efficacy are recapitulated in the hypothesis that *immunological response to relevant antigens offers potential for therapeutic benefit*

used for monitoring HLA-restricted peptide vaccines. Delayed-type hypersensitivity (DTH) responses to intradermal antigen are commonly used to monitor allogeneic approaches, where antigens characteristically vary between individual vaccines [83].

It is generally accepted that a statistical increase in measureable reactivity following immunization reflects the mobilization of T cells to one or more antigens delivered by the vaccine. The clinical relevance of "immunological response" continues to be speculative [84, 85]. Problematically, assays are multiple, varied, and not standardized across laboratories. Further, in the notable absence of viable tumor from individual patients for assay production, most immune monitoring extrapolates antigenic relevance and specificity from allogeneic surrogates.

Notwithstanding antigenic relevance to an individual's tumor, there are multiple downstream elements that can modulate effector function following induction. Nonetheless, at the current level of maturity in the field, immunological assays are the only practical measures of comparative potency and metrics of success during developmental phases of vaccines. Although it must be emphasized that immunological responses do not directly translate into therapeutic efficacy, multiple immunotherapy studies have observed an association of clinical response and induced immunity. The ability of most vaccines to induce measurable immunological responses suggests that many vaccines could have similar efficacy. Once efficacy is defined in NSCLC and the relevance of monitoring assays to outcomes better defined, standardized monitoring could facilitate development, provide comparative analysis, promote optimal study design, and support strategies that enhance response rates (Fig. 12.11).

12.4.3 Autologous DC Vaccines

Rationale and Trial Design. A clinical trial with DC vaccines was initiated to determine feasibility, to gain information with which to build future studies, and to work toward optimizing vaccines in NSCLC [86]. Vaccine production and mechanisms of action are reasonably well understood

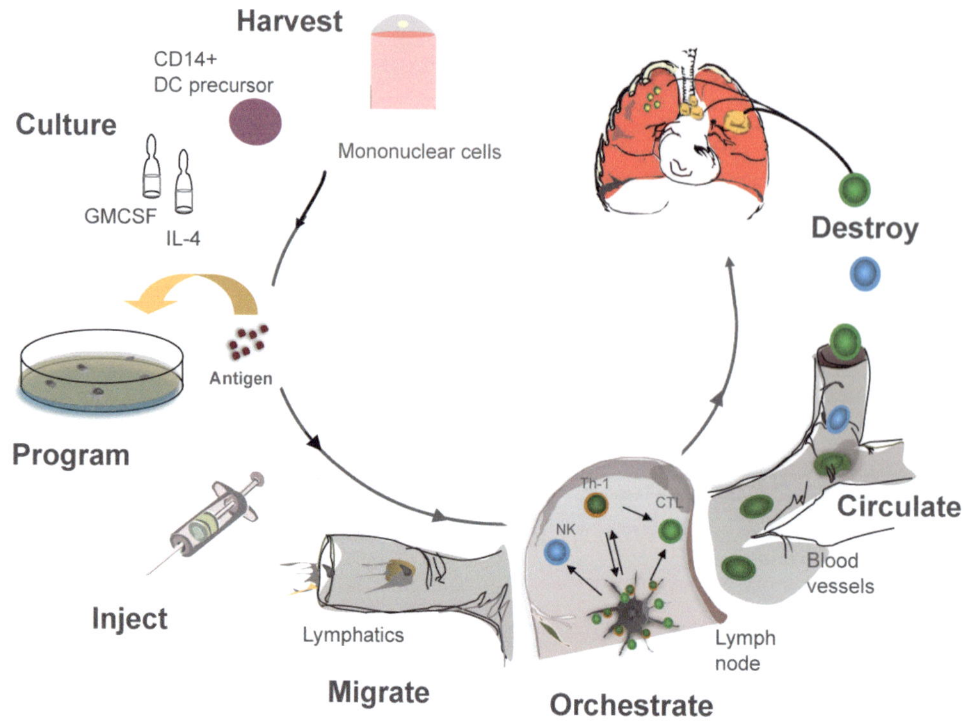

Fig. 12.12 Dendritic cell (*DC*) vaccines. Peripheral blood mononuclear cells from a patient are cultured in GM-CSF and IL-4 to drive differentiation of CD14+ DC precursors to immature myeloid DCs. Immature DCs are phagocytic and readily take up particulate antigen in culture. DCs process antigen into smaller peptides that are presented on the cell surface in context of MHC class I or class II molecules. Full antigen-presenting capacity is achieved when DCs are driven to maturity by addition of bioactive molecules in vitro or through cognate interaction with resident T cells in vivo. The DCs injected under the skin migrate to regional lymph nodes and interact with tumor-specific T cell precursors. Effector cells are released into the peripheral circulation and migrate into tissues where they encounter and destroy antigen-expressing cells (e.g., tumor)

(Fig. 12.12). Trial design focused on immunologic responses to antigen-pulsed DC vaccines in a heterogeneous group NSCLC patients treated surgically, medically, and with multimodality approaches.

Any patient with histologically confirmed stage I–IIIB NSCLC was eligible, irrespective of prior therapy. Subjects would be immunized twice, 1 month apart. Blood was drawn prior to and serially following immunization out to 1 year. Safety parameters were continually monitored. The primary endpoint was the rate of immune induction by IFN-gamma ELISPOT in individual patients immunized with prime and boost vaccine 1 month apart. Comparative analysis between subjects would determine relative importance of tumor burden (surgically resected vs. measurable persistent disease) and effect of prior radiation or chemotherapy on immune induction. Data would be analyzed in context of host factors that may influence vaccine efficacy, including immune regulatory elements responsible for variable rates of induction. In context, immediate goals and longitudinal objectives were dependent on the reliability of immune induction, and momentum would be built on this definable metric. Anecdotal clinical outcomes would be noted.

12.4.3.1 Formulation and Dosing

Vaccines were prepared according to FDA guidelines for cellular therapies. Patients underwent a 2 h leukapheresis procedure to harvest mononuclear cells in numbers adequate for vaccine production. Autologous dendritic cells were generated from peripheral blood monocyte culture in growth factor-enriched culture medium. Two different DC preparations were sequentially tested on a similar immunization schedule [86]. In the first series of 18 patients, DC vaccines were matured in vitro after antigen pulsing using a cocktail of bioactive factors. The second series of 18 subjects received immature DC vaccines.

Tumor Antigens. All vaccines were prepared with antigen derived from the NSCLC tumor cell line TC1650. This line overexpresses CEA, Her2/neu, WT1, survivin, and NY-ESO-1, which promised at least one shared antigen with over 95 % of NSCLC. A master cell bank comprised of tumor cell line confirmed free of contaminants and adventitial virus was established as a renewable source of antigen.

Final DC Vaccine. Based on literature suggesting that apoptotic bodies offered a more highly immunogenic alternative to simple necrotic cell debris, cells were apoptosed with UV irradiation prior to lethal irradiation. Vaccines were produced over 8 days. The final vaccine product (autologous DCs pulsed ex vivo with processed TC1650) was aliquoted for two immunizations (prime and boost) plus several test vials for sterility testing and quality assurance. 24 h after the cryopreservation, a test vial was thawed and tested for endotoxin and for bacterial and fungal testing with extended culture. After minimum 2-week sterility testing, the vaccines were released for injection. Each subject received two sequential intradermal injections of 10^8 pulsed DCs in the thigh 1 month apart. Subjects were monitored clinically for adverse events.

12.4.3.2 Results

36 individuals with definitively treated stage I–IIIB NSCLC were accrued and immunized with one of the two DC vaccine preparations (matured and immature DCs). The dominant adverse event noted was local wheal and flare reaction at the site of injection 24–48 h following immunization. There were no serious adverse events related to the experimental therapy. Immunological response was measured by IFN-γ ELISPOT, comparing relative number of antigen-reactive T cells from pre-vaccine to serial timepoints postimmunization. Measurable immunological responses by IFN-gamma ELISPOT assay were noted in 67 % of subjects and were irrespective of disease stage or prior therapy.

Rates of induction were independent of phenotypic maturation state of DCs at the time of delivery, and both preparations showed rates comparable to other cancer vaccines in the literature. Immune induction inversely correlated with relative numbers of circulating regulatory T cells at the time of immunization, and there was no apparent increase in regulatory T cells in any subject following immunization. Numbers are too small to draw conclusions about therapeutic benefit, although anecdotal survival, especially in those with advanced-stage disease, is more favorable than would be predicted based on historical controls.

12.4.4 Modified DC Vaccine 1650-G

Rationale and Trial Design. Believing efficacy would depend more on the ability to induce an immunological response than on any specific vaccine formulation or adjuvant a simplified derivative of DC vaccines, 1650-G, was produced [87]. This vaccine combines the processed antigen component of a DC vaccine (tumor cell line 1650) with the recombinant GM-CSF as an immune adjuvant. GM-CSF, known to stimulate antigen uptake and presentation in vivo, would be used in lieu of antigen loading of autologous DCs ex vivo; the antigen profile of the allogeneic tumor cell line 1650 would continue to confer multivalent coverage; the use of similar antigen, immunization schedule, and monitoring facilitated comparison to previously tested DC vaccines that would be used as a benchmark for immunological activity. In contrast to DC vaccines, 1650-G would be an economical and transportable alternative with which to pursue advanced phase investigation.

The initial feasibility trial was an open-label nonrandomized multi-site investigation in patients with stage I/II NSCLC and no evidence of disease following surgical resection. A prime vaccine and a single boost were given 1 month apart, similar to the prescribed schedule for autologous DC vaccines. Each immunization delivered 1.0×10^8 processed 1650 tumor cells plus 100 μg GM-CSF in 0.6 ml volumes; vaccine was injected intradermally at two locations in the thigh (0.3 ml/injection, 0.6 ml total); opposite thighs were used for prime and boost vaccine. Immunologic response by IFN-γ ELISPOT was the primary endpoint. Consistent with literature and prior experience, immune responses were expected in only a percentage of study patients.

Rate of immune induction relative to previously tested DC vaccines was the principal metric of vaccine potency; immunologic comparability of 1650-G to DC vaccines would provide a foundation for further studies. Establishing infrastructure for vaccine collaborative group and testing the potential of the vaccine to be transported and delivered to cancer patients in community cancer clinics also fulfilled an important objective of research.

12.4.4.1 Formulation and Dosing

Vaccines are batch produced from a master cell bank. Each dose is comprised of 10^8 processed 1650 cells (apoptosed and lethally irradiated) plus 100 μg of clinical grade GM-CSF in 0.6 ml sterile saline. Vials of prepared vaccine are stored in the gas phase of liquid nitrogen until delivery. Test vials were subject to sterility testing as previously described.

12.4.4.2 Results

Eleven individuals received two serial immunizations. The dominant adverse event was self-limited injection site reaction, and there were no serious unanticipated adverse events. Immune response measured by ELISPOT was seen in 6/11 of immunized patients, which is comparable to the more resource-intensive DC vaccine (Fig. 12.13). The observed biological activity coupled with ease of production, reduced cost, and portability make 1650-G an attractive candidate for randomized clinical investigation and subsequent clinical implementation [87].

12.4.5 Randomized Trial of Second-Line Immuno-Chemotherapy for Advanced NSCLC

12.4.5.1 Rationale and Trial Design

Compelling insights into the immune-potentiating effects of docetaxel are especially relevant to patients with advanced

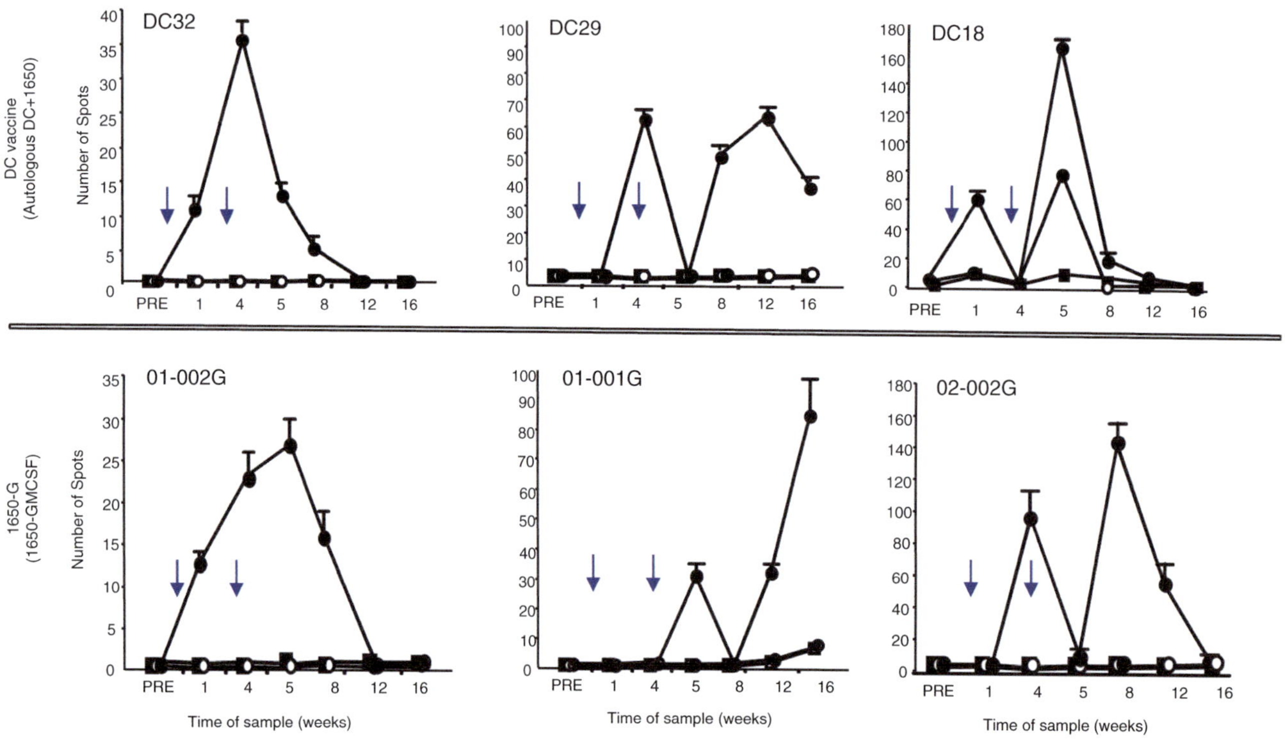

Fig. 12.13 IFN-γ ELISPOT – DC vaccine compared to 1650-G vaccine. Representative immunologic responses are shown from individuals participating in a DC vaccine study (*top*) and patients receiving vaccine 1650-G (*bottom*). Both vaccines use the processed 1650 cell line as a source of antigen. Immunization schedule was the same in both studies. *Graphs* show measurements of lymphocytes ("spots") from available timepoints (pre-vaccine to 16 weeks post) responding to (•)1650-pulsed autologous DCs, (▪) DCs alone, or (○) lymphocytes alone. Arrows indicate time of vaccine delivery. Comparable rates of immune induction and patterns of response across the study population indicate similarities that overshadow differences in immune adjuvant similarities in the kinetics indicate that either approach has potential for therapeutic benefit. These data are the basis for advanced phase investigation using the simplified derivative of DC vaccines: 1650-G

NSCLC [88, 89]. The primary objective is to show that the immune system can be mobilized for therapeutic benefit in a population with predictable outcomes from conventional chemotherapy.

12.4.5.2 Study Description

Open-label 2:1 randomized trial to assess therapeutic efficacy of 1650-G and concurrent docetaxel (same treatment cycle) as second-line therapy for progressive stage IIIB or IV NSCLC not amenable to curative surgical or radiotherapy. A minimum study number of 120 patients and a maximum of 174 patients is based on an integrated phase II/III trial design. Patients are to be enrolled across eight sites in the Commonwealth of Kentucky from outpatient clinics, through self-referral from the community, or referral from a primary treating physician. Chemotherapy (docetaxel) and procedures related to standard of care are the same in both study arms. All subjects would undergo four treatment cycles; each treatment cycle is 3 weeks. Vaccines (experimental arm) are administered day 1 of each cycle and docetaxel given day 5 of each cycle (Fig. 12.14).

Endpoints. The study specifically examines differences in outcomes between experimental and control arms. Primary endpoints include time to progression (TTP), survival, and immune-related response criteria (irRC). This latter measure includes allowance for moderate increases in tumor burden to accommodate protracted immune-mediated responses and inflammatory changes. Consistent with literature and prior experience with this vaccine, 50–70 % of individuals would be expected to show immune response by IFN-γ ELISPOT following immunization. A secondary hypothesis is that clinical response will favor the group with immunological response. Correlative studies are designed to address the most understandable reasons for therapeutic success or treatment failure.

12.4.6 Perspectives

DC vaccines have potential for therapeutic efficacy in NSCLC but are costly and resource intensive. 1650-G is an immunologically comparable alternative. Beyond the

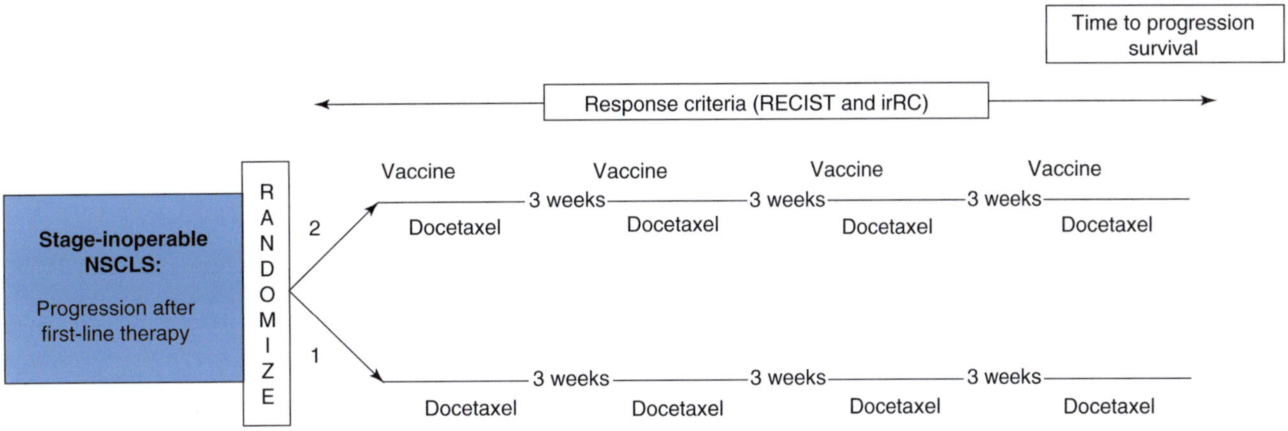

Fig. 12.14 Trial schema vaccine 1650-G: randomized trial of second-line immuno-chemotherapy (SLIC) for advanced NSCLC

obvious appeal of low cost, 1650-G is portable, uniform, and multivalent [87].

Although complexity is not a known requisite for efficacy, the simplicity of vaccine 1650-G has generated skepticism about its therapeutic potential. There are differing opinions on whole-cell vaccines but no feature that precludes efficacy.

In pursuing efficacy, this vaccine shares a common set of hurdles of cancer vaccines. The most well-recognized biological obstacles to optimal potential include a corrupted tumor microenvironment containing regulatory T cells and aberrantly matured myeloid cells, a tumor-specific T cell repertoire that is prone to immunologic exhaustion and senescence, and highly mutable tumor targets capable of antigen loss and immune evasion. Clinical factors that continue to impact development and implementation include non-standardized assays and uncertain relevance of immune monitoring, protracted time courses for therapeutic endpoints, and a lack of correlative biomarkers for assessment of clinical efficacy.

12.5 Renal Cell Carcinoma: Vaccines Targeting Its Vasculature[4]

Renal cell carcinoma (RCC) remains a significant health concern since many patients present with metastatic disease at initial diagnosis. RCC tumors are typically highly vascularized due to dysregulated angiogenesis, resulting in leaky, chaotic blood vessels that serve to limit immune effector cell access to the tumor that may in part be responsible for the modest clinical success noted for cancer immunotherapeutic approaches. Current first-line therapeutics in the advanced-stage disease setting include antiangiogenic small molecule drugs that have yielded high objective clinical response rates, although these tend to be transient in nature, with most patients ultimately becoming drug refractory.

The implementation of gene-based therapeutic vaccines targeting the tumor vasculature is a promising treatment option that may extend disease-free intervals and overall patient survival, either as a stand-alone therapy or in combination with existing treatment options. Such molecular therapies range from the delivery of *ex vivo* gene-modified antigen-presenting cells to the direct injection of recombinant viral vaccines.

12.5.1 Conventional Therapy

Renal cell carcinoma (RCC) accounts for approximately 3 % of all cancers in adults, with metastases identified in 20–30 % of patients at the time of initial diagnosis. Metastatic RCC, if left untreated, has a 5-year disease-free survival rate of only 2–11 % [90]. Following nephrectomy, conventional treatments with standard chemotherapeutic agents, hormones, and radiotherapy have exhibited minimal success. This has prompted extensive evaluation of alternate treatment strategies, including immunotherapies, in the adjuvant and advanced-stage disease settings.

12.5.2 Tumor Vasculature in the TME

Solid tumors of various tissue types, including renal, ovarian, and lung, are typically highly vascularized. Blood and lymphatic vessels in the tumor microenvironment (TME) support cancer progression by (i) delivering oxygen and nutrients, (ii) providing a conduit by which primary tumors can metastasize, (iii) recruiting/supporting cancer stem cells and vascular cell precursors that promote tumor neovascularization,

[4]Molecular immunotherapeutics and vaccines for renal cell carcinoma and its vasculature by *Nina Chi Sabins, Jennifer L. Taylor, Devin B. Lowe and Walter J. Storkus* in Molecular Vaccines – From Prophylaxis to Therapy, Volume 1, Springer-Verlag Wien, 2013, Ed. Matthias Giese.

and (iv) recruiting immune regulatory cell populations (Treg cells) that limit protective antitumor immune responses.

The vasculature in the TME is typically characterized as "abnormal," here defined as tortuous, irregular networks of blood vessels with highly unstable and permeable capillaries branching from the main vessel bed. Instability in the tumor vasculature increases interstitial pressure within the tumor, preventing the delivery of tumoricidal drugs and immune effector cells into the TME [91].

Tumor Vascular Endothelial Cells (VECs). Tumor VEC exhibit differential gene expression when compared to VEC isolated from healthy tissue, with such transcripts believed to underlie tumor blood vessel destabilization [92]. Silencing these genes using siRNA approaches may block VEC migration and vascular tube formation [93], thus supporting tumor VEC as a highly relevant therapeutic target. Another characteristic of the tumor vasculature is the aberrant mural cell coverage of the blood vessels. VEC recruit platelet-derived growth factor receptor (PDGFR)-β-expressing mural cells by secreting PDGF [94].

Mural cells support VEC survival and differentiation and can be subclassified into smooth muscle cell and pericyte populations. Normal mature pericytes have been found to play a major role in vessel stabilization, maturation, remodeling, and repair. Tumor pericytes are typically immature and loosely attached to the capillary and may even be absent in some areas, leading to vessel destabilization. Such pericytes have been characterized phenotypically by overexpression of SMA, RGS5, and tumor endothelial marker-1 (TEM1) in a range of tumor models [95].

12.5.2.1 Immune Dysfunction in the TME

Solid tumors are frequently hypoxic resulting in increased expression of hypoxia-induced factors (HIFs) and impaired effector T cell and dendritic cell (DC) function. Upregulated HIF expression also leads to increased VEGF expression, which can attenuate DC differentiation and increase STAT3 activation via VEGFR2-mediated signaling, thus promoting the intrinsic expression of immunosuppressive factors including IL-10 and TGF-β in these regulatory antigen-presenting cells. In many cancer patients, type 1 pro-inflammatory responses required for tumor destruction are inhibited or functionally dysregulated by the suppressive influence of Treg or myeloid-derived suppressor cells (MDSC) and/or by type 2 inflammatory molecules.

Furthermore, type 1 tumor-specific T cells may become functionally exhausted and undergo premature (apoptotic) death due to chronic stimulation by cognate tumor antigens in cancer-bearing patients [96]. Such immune evasion tactics assumed by the tumor serve to limit the protective host immunological responses and allow for tumor survival and progression.

12.5.3 Immune Targeting of RCC

Optimism for the use of biologic response modifiers and vaccines has been fueled by past reports which indicate that, like melanoma, RCC progression and regression may be controlled immunologically [97]. Notably, a minor but significant frequency of RCC patients exhibit apparent spontaneous tumor regression, and patients on chronic immunosuppression regimens to retain kidney allografts exhibit increased risk of developing RCC. Furthermore, the magnitude of tumor-infiltrating lymphocytes (TILs) has been suggested to represent a prognostic indicator for patient survival [98]. In this regard, type 1 TILs (i.e., those producing IFN-γ and capable of mediating the cytolytic function) appear to represent the primary immunologic mediators of objective clinical responses.

Although administration of high-dose interleukin-2 (IL-2; aka T cell growth factor) has yielded durable complete responses in a minority of treated patients with metastatic RCC, severe toxicities have also been observed for this approach [99], suggesting the need to identify more specific/focused immunotherapy approaches.

12.5.3.1 Antiangiogenic Small Molecule Drugs

Judah Folkman presented the idea of angiogenesis as a therapeutic target in cancer [100]. His theory spurred the development of several antiangiogenic therapies including monoclonal antibodies reactive against angiogenic growth factors (and their cognate receptors) and small molecule inhibitors of proangiogenic receptor tyrosine kinases. Indeed in 2005, it was suggested that normalization of the tumor vasculature could be achieved via administration of antiangiogenic agents as a novel cancer therapy. This approach coordinately allowed for the improved delivery of co-applied chemotherapeutic agents into the TME.

Bevacizumab. The humanized monoclonal antibody bevacizumab (Avastin) has been shown to induce a transient normalization of the tumor vasculature in treated patients, which when coupled with chemotherapy promoted enhanced antitumor effects [101]. Targeting soluble VEGF increases the preponderance of PDGF in the TME, thus inducing pericyte recruitment and activation and capillary stabilization. Huang et al. recently reported that at a given dose of anti-VEGFR2 antibody, the tumor vasculature became normalized in mice. Furthermore, this treatment reprogrammed the TME to be more pro-inflammatory and increasingly receptive to T effector cell infiltration [102]. Alternatively, pharmacological agents, such as sunitinib, targeting VEGF receptors (i.e., VEGFR1-3), as well as other proangiogenic tyrosine kinase receptors (i.e., PDGFRβ), can also inhibit dysregulated angiogenesis leading to a temporary normalization of the vasculature.

Tyrosine Kinase Inhibitors (TKIs). Due to the highly vascularized nature of RCC, several clinical trials have utilized tyrosine kinase inhibitors (TKIs) that antagonize angiogenesis as a means to treat this disease. One such inhibitor is sunitinib malate [103], which has exhibited pronounced (albeit transient) efficacy in phase I/II clinical trials and is approved as a first-line treatment for patients with RCC. However, a phase III trial showed that while progression-free survival early on was higher in patients receiving sunitinib (11 months) compared to interferon treatment (5 months), the overall survival benefit associated with this approach was not dramatically different between the two groups (26.4 months vs. 21.8 months).

Sunitinib. Although sunitinib was initially developed as an angiostatic agent, recent reports suggest that this TKI actually "normalizes" the tumor vasculature by selective pruning of immature and fragile vessels, leaving the more differentiated vessels intact with mature pericyte coverage. This normalization event leads to a decrease in interstitial pressure and improved delivery of chemotherapeutic drugs and effector T cells into the TME [104].

This corresponds with results from a study by Ganss et al. showing that inflammation of the TME induced by local radiotherapy, in conjunction with adoptive transfer of tumor-specific cells, can induce microvasculature remodeling toward a phenotype resembling normal tissue [105]. The normalized endothelium exhibited increased expression of type 1 chemokines CXCL9 and CXCL10 as well as their cognate receptor CXCR3. CXCL10 is an endogenous angiogenic inhibitor that acts as a chemoattractant for type 1 T cells and has been shown to induce apoptosis in human CXCR3b$^+$ endothelial cells but not tumor cells [106].

Additionally, patients treated with sunitinib exhibit reductions in MDSC and Treg populations and normalized type 1 T cell responses in vitro. Murine tumor models suggest that sunitinib suppresses STAT3 activation and boosts the efficacy of immunotherapy by promoting tumor-specific effector T cells while also suppressing MDSC and Treg in vivo [107]. Sunitinib treatment has been shown to skew expression of chemokines and their receptors toward a type 1 profile [42] as well as increased expression of VCAM1 and CXCL9 (MIG) with increased IFN-γ producing T cells within the TME and tumor-draining lymph nodes (TDLN) implying this TKI may represent a potent immune adjuvant.

12.5.4 Current Therapeutic Vaccines for RCC

Autologous tumor cell vaccines have been modified by either co-administration with, or genetically modified to express, inflammatory cytokines including GM-CSF, IFN-γ, and IL-2. Another tumor vaccine formulation is represented by RCC antigen-presenting cell (APC) fusion hybrids, which generate hybrid APCs that are capable of expressing RCC gene products and presenting their derivative peptide epitopes to T cells [108].

Viral-Based Delivery Systems. An alternative approach to cellular-based vaccines (i.e., modified tumor cells, APC, T cells) is genetic vaccination using recombinant viral-based delivery systems. Various reports have shown virus-based vaccinations possess therapeutic advantages over protein antigen-/adjuvant-based approaches, presumably due to the intrinsic pro-inflammatory properties of viruses (via activation of Toll-like receptors (TLR) expressed by APC) and their ability to infect professional APC, allowing for ectopic expression of the vaccine antigen within patient DC [109, 110]. Additionally, high-titer recombinant viruses are easy to produce, and when compared to cell-based therapies that require costly time-consuming methods due to their patient-specific nature, viral vectors can be administered to any given patient as an off-the-shelf treatment modality.

Vaccinia Virus Ankara. The recombinant modified vaccinia virus Ankara (MVA) encoding RCC antigen 5T4, TroVax, has been tested in several clinical trials. Initial trials in RCC patients showed some objective clinical responses after administration of the TroVax vaccine [111, 112]; however, in phase III trials employing TroVax with or without cytokines (IFN-γ and IL-2) in combination with sunitinib, no significant difference in survival between the experimental and control groups could be demonstrated [113]. A second MVA vaccine was developed containing the recombinant MUC1 and IL-2 transgenes, administered with or without cytokines. Although some RCC patients exhibited anti-MUC1 T cell responses, treatment with this vaccine formulation did not result in objective clinical responses based on RECIST criteria [114].

Pulsed DCs. Another approach involves DC pulsed or transfected with RCC-derived total mRNA (encoding the complete repertoire of RCC-associated antigens) [115]. More recently, a direct intradermal injection of mRNA-based vaccine encoding MUC1, CEA, Her-2/neu, telomerase, survivin, and MAGE-A1 has been evaluated in a phase I/II clinical trial involving 30 RCC patients.

A general summary of therapeutic vaccines targeting molecularly defined RCC-associated antigens is provided in Table 12.10. In general, these approaches have proven immunogenic, with post-vaccine type 1 T cell responses often being associated with improved clinical outcomes.

Table 12.10 Clinical vaccines incorporating molecularly defined RCC-associated antigens

Vaccine format	Vaccine targeted antigen	Trial phase	Number of RCC patients treated	Vaccine immunogenicity	Clinical outcomes	References
Polypeptide vaccine +/– IL-2 or IFN-α	Selection of 4 defined TAA peptides from panel based on patient in vitro responses pretreatment	I	10	8/10 patients with positive DTH response to vaccine; 2/10 patients with increased type 1 T cell response to peptides post-vaccine	6 SD	[117]
AutoDC + MUC1 peptide + PADRE peptide + IL-2	MUC1	I	20	10/20 patients with type 1 T cell response to peptides	1 CR, 2 PR, 5 SD, 2 MR; T cell responses correlated to OCR	[118]
MKC1106-PP gene prime/peptide boost	PRAME, PSMA	I	2	2/2 patients with type 1 T cell response to peptides	2/2 with SD > 11 months	[119]
CA-IX (G250) peptide + IFA	CA-IX	I	23	5/10 evaluable patients with type 1 CD8+ T cell response to peptide	3 PR; 6 SD	[120]
Mature AutoDC + CA-IX (G250) peptides	CA-IX	I	6	No specific immunity to CA-IX	No OCR	[121]
Tumor antigen RNA + GM-CSF	MUC1, CEA, HER2/Neu, telomerase, survivin, MAGE-A1	I/II	30	8/10 evaluable patients with type 1 T cell response to vaccine peptides	16 SD; 1 PR	[116]
Telomerase peptide + Montanide adjuvant	Telomerase	I/II	4	Not described, progressor tumor in 1 patient was an MHC I loss variant	No OCR	[122]
AutoDC + telomerase peptide	Telomerase	I/II	10	2/8 evaluable patients with DTH response; CTL responses only in 3 patients with OCR	1 SD, 2 MR correlates with strongest T cell IFN-γ response to peptide	[123]
Mutant VHL peptide + Montanide adjuvant	Mutant VHL	I/II	6	4/5 evaluable patients with CD8+ T cell responses to antigen	No OCR, extended OS if patients responded to vaccination	[124]
IM901 + GM-CSF +/– CY	9 natural MHC I presented TAA (PLIN2, APOL1 (2),CCND1, GUCY1A3, PRUNE2, MET, MUC1, RGS5) + 1 natural MHC II presented TAA (MMP7) peptides	I + II	96	64–74 % of evaluable patients displayed CD8+ T cell responses to 1 or more vaccine peptides	Better OS observed if patients made immune response to multiple peptides	[125]
TG4010 (rVaccinia virus) +/– IFN-α/IL-2	MUC1	II	37	6/28 and 6/23 evaluable patients made CD4+ and CD8+ T cell responses to vaccine, respectively; immune responders with longer OS	6/20 patients with SD for more than 6 months	[114]

MVA-5T4 (TroVax; modified vaccinia Ankara) +/– sunitinib, IL-2 or IFN-α	5T4	III	288	56 % of evaluable patients developed anti-5T4 antibody responses post-vaccine; T cell responses not evaluated	Magnitude of antibody response was associated with longer OS, greatest impact for smaller tumors	[111–113, 126, 127]
IMA901 +/– sunitinib	9 natural MHC I presented TAA (PLIN2, APOL1 (2),CCND1, GUCY1A3, PRUNE2, MET, MUC1, RGS5) + 1 natural MHC II presented TAA (MMP7) peptides	III	330	In progress, results expected in 2014	In progress, results expected in 2014	In progress

Abbreviations: AlloDC allogeneic dendritic cells, *APOL1* APOlipoprotein L1 antigen, *AutoDC* autologous dendritic cells, *CA-IX* carbonic anhydrase-IX antigen (also known as G250), *CCND1* cyclin D1 antigen, *CEA* carcinoembryonic antigen, *CR* complete response, *CTL* cytotoxic T lymphocyte, *CY* cyclophosphamide, *DTH* delayed-type hypersensitivity, *GUCY1A3* guanylate cyclase soluble subunit alpha-3 antigen, *HER2* human epidermal growth factor receptor 2 (also known as Neu), *IFA* incomplete Freund's adjuvant, *MAGE-A1* melanoma-associated antigen 1, *MET* c-MET proto-oncogene antigen (also known as hepatocyte growth factor receptor), *MHC* major histocompatibility complex, *MMP7* matrix metalloproteinase 7 antigen, *MR* mixed response, *MUC1* mucin-1 antigen, *OCR* objective clinical response, *OS* overall survival, *PADRE* pan-DR presented epitope, *PR* partial response, *PRAME* preferentially expressed antigen in MElanoma, *PRUNE2* protein prune homolog 2 antigen, *PSMA* prostate-specific membrane antigen, *RGS5* regulator of G-protein signaling 5 antigen, *SD* stabilization of disease, *TAA* tumor-associated antigen, *VHL* von Hippel–Lindau protein, *5T4* trophoblast glycoprotein antigen (also known as TPBG)

12.5.4.1 Genetic Vaccines Encoding Tumor Antigens

Genetic aberrations can potentially develop within the evolving and heterogeneous RCC lesion over many months to years under immune selective pressure [128]. Vaccines based on whole tumor cells, tumor-APC hybrids, and/or tumor-derived mRNA or cDNA, tumor antigens derived from mutated, or overexpressed proteins have thus far underperformed as therapeutic agents. These vaccine formulations may merely reinforce an existing, yet failing, immune repertoire given the immune dominance of certain tumor antigens over others and to immune evasion paradigms assumed by the heterogeneous tumor mass. Competition by a myriad peptide epitopes for loading on to major histocompatibility complex (MHC) molecules expressed by (cross-presenting) APCs in vivo could also limit effective immune activation against a broad range of otherwise therapeutic tumor antigen targets.

Recently, several groups [129, 130] have shown that while treatment with antiangiogenic agents may lead to the transient normalization of the tumor vasculature and to at least transient tumor regression, ultimately, upon treatment cessation, the tumors often recur and may even exhibit more aggressive behavior with regard to their invasiveness and metastatic potential. Since these drugs only limit angiogenesis (i.e., via receptor tyrosine kinase (RTK) signaling antagonism) rather than eradicating the vasculature outright, it is likely that tumor-associated vascular cells ultimately adapt to a state of drug resistance.

A possible means to circumvent this problem is to specifically instigate immune targeting of tumor pericytes and/or vascular endothelial cells to provide a durable policing force capable of preferentially destroying/regulating tumor-associated stromal cells while sparing the vasculature in normal, tumor-uninvolved organs in the patient. By focusing type 1 immune responses in the tumor vascular niche, one may also activate the TME (i.e., modulating its cytokine milieu and pattern/level/activation state of adhesion molecules expressed) leading to the enhanced recruitment and (poly)functionality of anti-RCC T effector cells.

Rosenberg's group has recently shown that T cells engineered to express a chimeric antigen receptor (CAR) specific for VEGFR2, which is overexpressed in the vasculature of many solid cancers, including RCC, were able to limit the growth of five different types of established, vascularized tumors in mice and to coordinately induce VEGFR2-specific host T cell responses [131]. This treatment strategy is currently under investigation in phase I trials for RCC as well as melanoma patients. It has also been shown that treatment with fibroblasts genetically altered to express endostatin, another molecule critical for tumor angiogenesis, leads to reduced tumor burden with increased infiltration of $CD4^+$, $CD8^+$, and CD49b/VLA-4^+ lymphocytes in a metastatic RCC mouse model when combined with rIL-2 administration, indicating an additive immunomodulatory effect of the vaccine [127].

Current genetic immunization strategies for RCC have been limited to those using recombinant vaccinia viruses encoding tumor antigens, which have thus far met with moderate clinical success. Unfortunately, vaccinia vectors can only be applied once or twice due to the rapid host development of neutralizing antibodies that serve to limit the booster capacity of further administrations of this modality.

Given the ability of lentivirus to transduce endogenous DC in vivo in the absence of evoking neutralizing antiviral immunity [132] and therefore the potential of providing reiterated dosing to patients, a lentiviral-based vaccine was designed to promote specific immune targeting of the tumor vasculature and, more specifically, vascular pericytes.

Pericytes isolated from human and mouse RCC tumors differentially overexpress a cohort of antigens (compared to homologous cells in the normal kidney), including delta-like 1 homolog (DLK1). Therapeutic DLK1 peptide- and (lentiviral) gene-based vaccines were both observed to be immunogenic and effective in regulating the growth of RENCA (RCC) tumors in vivo. Effectively treated RCC tumors displayed vascular normalization based on reduced vascular leak and tissue hypoxia and were highly infiltrated by $CD8^+$ TIL in the perivascular space. Residual pericytes in the TME were tightly approximated to blood vessels and were deficient in expression of DLK1, supportive of vaccine-induced immunoselection of mature mural cell populations in vivo.

12.5.5 Existing Vaccine Platforms May Be Suboptimal

Current single-modality treatments for RCC, either immune targeting of cancer cells or antiangiogenic pharmacological agents, have thus far yielded limited clinical success. While functional tumor-specific T cells may be activated by vaccination, these cells typically do not effectively traffic into tumor lesions exhibiting an unstable vasculature, given the lack of recruitment signals and high interstitial pressures that serve as a physical barrier to lymphocytic extravasation. The transient vascular normalization seen in tumors treated with antiangiogenic treatments may circumvent the limitation of T cell trafficking if used in combination with vaccine-based therapies.

Vaccines promoting immune targeting of cancer cells can select for resistant (i.e., antigen or MHC loss) variants, leading to the maintenance of occult disease or the progression of tumors that are "invisible" to the adaptive immune system. The antiangiogenic action mediated by a vascular antigen-specific $CD8^+$ T cell repertoire would be

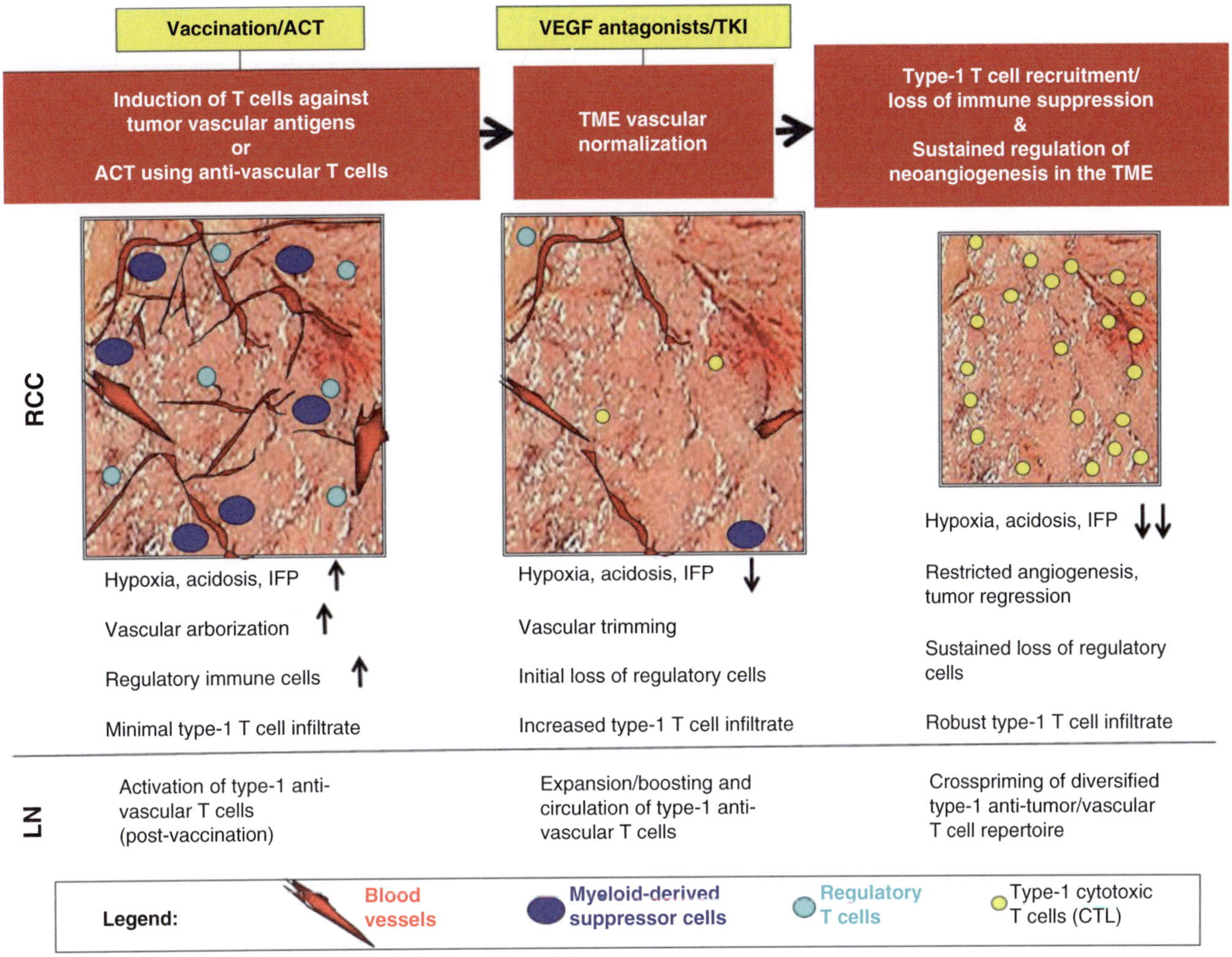

Fig. 12.15 Paradigm for the improved therapeutic benefit of combination vaccines targeting the RCC blood vasculature. Untreated RCC tumor (*left panel*) is populated by regulatory immune cells (myeloid-derived suppressor cells [*MDSC*] and regulatory T cells [Treg]) with minimal type 1 T effector cells present. An unstable, disorganized vasculature in the progressor lesion leads to hypoxia, acidosis, and high interstitial fluid pressure (*IFP*). Active vaccination against tumor vascular antigens and subsequent activation of specific T cells in the vaccine-draining lymph node (*LN*), or the adoptive transfer of vascular antigen-specific T cells (i.e., adoptive cell therapy; ACT) lead to circulating levels of type 1 T effector cells that are inefficient in trafficking into RCC tumors. Staggered co-treatment with antiangiogenic drugs such VEGF antagonists or TKI acts to at least transiently normalize the tumor vasculature, leading to reduced hypoxia/acidosis/IFP, as well as to remove regulatory cell populations (*middle panel*), allowing for the increased recruitment and effector function of type 1 vaccine-induced or ACT T cells (*right panel*). Subsequent immune-mediated eradication of tumor cells and the presentation of tumor (and alternate stromal antigens) by locoregional DC populations may lead to the cross-priming of a diversified repertoire of therapeutic type 1 T cells in tumor-draining lymph nodes, resulting in extended clinical benefit (*right panel*)

anticipated to delete specific vascular cell populations and therefore complement the specific inhibition of receptor signaling that is hallmark of alternative pharmacological antiangiogenic treatment modalities such as anti-VEGF antibodies (i.e., bevacizumab) and small molecule tyrosine kinase inhibitors (i.e., sunitinib).

Frequently, vascularized tumors treated with these agents rapidly become drug refractory due to their adoption of compensatory growth/progression pathways. Given such limitations, molecular vaccines targeting vascular stromal antigens could represent a logical second-line approach in the many cases of developed resistance to bevacizumab, sunitinib, or similar antiangiogenic drugs. These vaccines may also represent effective co-first-line therapeutic agents (Fig. 12.15), since the specific activation, recruitment, and function of antitumor stroma-associated antigen T effector cells in the TME would be anticipated to be improved by the co-administration of antiangiogenic TKI that reduce suppressor cell populations (most notably in RCC patients) and the activation of a pro-inflammatory TME in vivo.

12.5.6 Adoptive Cell Therapy (ACT)

Treatment with genetically modified recombinant T cell receptor (TCR) has recently been shown to promote cancer regression in hematological malignancies [133]. Implementing a similar strategy, tumor antigen-specific T cells can be isolated from RCC tumor-infiltrating lymphocytes (TIL) in vitro, with RCC antigen-specific TCRs subsequently isolated, cloned, and transduced into patient T cells to confer antitumor specificity. Once expanded ex vivo, such antitumor effector cells may be adoptively transferred as a therapeutic agent.

Additionally, given the recent success in treatments using adoptive transfer of T cells genetically engineered to express CARs, there has been increasing interest in exploiting this strategy in the setting of solid tumors. For instance, clinical trials are underway to test the safety and efficacy of T cells engineered to express carcinoembryonic antigen (CEA)-reactive CARs in metastatic colon carcinoma and folate receptor-alpha (FR-α)-reactive CARs in advanced-stage ovarian cancer. In a phase 1 clinical trial for RCC patients, many individuals receiving T cells genetically engineered to express a CAR directed against carbonic anhydrase-IX (CA-IX; aka G250) RCC-associated protein developed corollary anti-G250 antibody responses and T cell-mediated immunity [134].

References

1. Ostrand-Rosenberg, S.: Immune surveillance: a balance between protumor and antitumor immunity. Curr. Opin. Genet. Dev. **18**, 11–18 (2008). doi:10.1016/j.gde.2007.12.007
2. Vajdic, C.M., van Leeuwen, M.T.: Cancer incidence and risk factors after solid organ transplantation. Int. J. Cancer. J. Int. du Cancer **125**, 1747–1754 (2009). doi:10.1002/ijc.24439
3. Kapoor, A.: Malignancy in kidney transplant recipients. Drugs **68**(Suppl 1), 11–19 (2008)
4. Schreiber, R.D., Old, L.J., Smyth, M.J.: Cancer immunoediting: integrating immunity's roles in cancer suppression and promotion. Science **331**, 1565–1570 (2011). doi:10.1126/science.1203486
5. Hanahan, D., Coussens, L.M.: Accessories to the crime: functions of cells recruited to the tumor microenvironment. Cancer Cell **21**, 309–322 (2012). doi:10.1016/j.ccr.2012.02.022
6. Lluis, J.M., Buricchi, F., Chiarugi, P., Morales, A., Fernandez-Checa, J.C.: Dual role of mitochondrial reactive oxygen species in hypoxia signaling: activation of nuclear factor-{kappa}B via c-SRC and oxidant-dependent cell death. Cancer Res. **67**, 7368–7377 (2007). doi:10.1158/0008-5472.CAN-07-0515
7. Conlon, P.J., Miller, S.D., Claman, H.N.: The induction of tolerance to DNFB contact sensitivity by using hapten-modified lymphoid cells. III. Effects of hapten concentration on the ability of MLS-disparate cells to induce rapid unresponsiveness. J. Immunol. **125**, 807–813 (1980)
8. Greene, M.I., Benacerraf, B.: Studies on hapten specific T cell immunity and suppression. Immunol. Rev. **50**, 163–186 (1980)
9. van der Bruggen, P., et al.: A gene encoding an antigen recognized by cytolytic T lymphocytes on a human melanoma. Science **254**, 1643–1647 (1991)
10. Cheever, M.A., et al.: The prioritization of cancer antigens: a national cancer institute pilot project for the acceleration of translational research. Clin. Cancer Res **15**, 5323–5337 (2009). doi:10.1158/1078-0432.CCR-09-0737
11. Schumacher, T.N., Schreiber, R.D.: Neoantigens in cancer immunotherapy. Science **348**, 69–74 (2015). doi:10.1126/science.aaa4971
12. Aswaq, M., Richards, V., McFadden, S.: Immunologic response to autologous cancer vaccine. Arch. Surg. **89**, 485–487 (1964)
13. Snyder, A., Chan, T.A.: Immunogenic peptide discovery in cancer genomes. Curr. Opin. Genet. Dev. **30C**, 7–16 (2015). doi:10.1016/j.gde.2014.12.003
14. Hacohen, N., Fritsch, E.F., Carter, T.A., Lander, E.S., Wu, C.J.: Getting personal with neoantigen-based therapeutic cancer vaccines. Cancer Immunol. Res. **1**, 11–15 (2013). doi:10.1158/2326-6066.CIR-13-0022
15. Carreno, B.M., et al.: A dendritic cell vaccine increases the breadth and diversity of melanoma neoantigen-specific T cells. Science (2015). doi:10.1126/science.aaa3828
16. van Rooij, N., et al.: Tumor exome analysis reveals neoantigen-specific T-cell reactivity in an ipilimumab-responsive melanoma. J. Clin. Oncol. **31**, e439–e442 (2013). doi:10.1200/JCO.2012.47.7521
17. Leach, D.R., Krummel, M.F., Allison, J.P.: Enhancement of antitumor immunity by CTLA-4 blockade. Science **271**, 1734–1736 (1996)
18. van den Eertwegh, A.J., et al.: Combined immunotherapy with granulocyte-macrophage colony-stimulating factor-transduced allogeneic prostate cancer cells and ipilimumab in patients with metastatic castration-resistant prostate cancer: a phase 1 dose-escalation trial. Lancet Oncol. **13**, 509–517 (2012). doi:10.1016/S1470-2045(12)70007-4
19. Hodi, F.S., et al.: Improved survival with ipilimumab in patients with metastatic melanoma. N. Engl. J. Med. **363**, 711–723 (2010). doi:10.1056/NEJMoa1003466
20. Prieto, P.A., et al.: CTLA-4 blockade with ipilimumab: long-term follow-up of 177 patients with metastatic melanoma. Clin. Cancer Res. **18**, 2039–2047 (2012). doi:10.1158/1078-0432.CCR-11-1823
21. Topalian, S.L., et al.: Safety, activity, and immune correlates of anti-PD-1 antibody in cancer. N. Engl. J. Med. **366**, 2443–2454 (2012). doi:10.1056/NEJMoa1200690
22. Butte, M.J., Keir, M.E., Phamduy, T.B., Sharpe, A.H., Freeman, G.J.: Programmed death-1 ligand 1 interacts specifically with the B7-1 costimulatory molecule to inhibit T cell responses. Immunity **27**, 111–122 (2007). doi:10.1016/j.immuni.2007.05.016
23. Emens, L.A.: Chemoimmunotherapy. Cancer J. **16**, 295–303 (2010)
24. Sistigu, A., et al.: Immunomodulatory effects of cyclophosphamide and implementations for vaccine design. Semin. Immunopathol. **33**, 369–383 (2011)
25. Zitvogel, L., et al.: Immunogenic tumor cell death for optimal anticancer therapy: the calreticulin exposure pathway. Clin. Cancer Res. **16**, 3100–3104 (2010)
26. Aymeric, L., et al.: Tumor cell death and ATP release prime dendritic cells and efficient anticancer immunity. Cancer Res. **70**, 855–858 (2010)
27. Ramakrishnan, R., et al.: Chemotherapy enhances tumor cell susceptibility to CTL-mediated killing during cancer immunotherapy in mice. J. Clin. Invest. **120**, 1111–1124 (2010)
28. Liu, J.Y., et al.: Single administration of low dose cyclophosphamide augments the antitumor effect of dendritic cell vaccine. Cancer Immunol. Immunother. **56**, 1597–1604 (2007)
29. Lutsiak, M.E., et al.: Inhibition of CD4(+)25+ T regulatory cell function implicated in enhanced immune response by low-dose cyclophosphamide. Blood **105**, 2862–2868 (2005)

30. Ge, Y., et al.: Metronomic cyclophosphamide treatment in metastasized breast cancer patients: immunological effects and clinical outcome. Cancer Immunol. Immunother. **61**, 353–362 (2012)
31. Emens, L.A., et al.: Timed sequential treatment with cyclophosphamide, doxorubicin, and an allogeneic granulocyte-macrophage colony-stimulating factor-secreting breast tumor vaccine: a chemotherapy dose-ranging factorial study of safety and immune activation. J. Clin. Oncol. **27**, 5911–5918 (2009)
32. Holtl, L., et al.: Allogeneic dendritic cell vaccination against metastatic renal cell carcinoma with or without cyclophosphamide. Cancer Immunol. Immunother. **54**, 663–670 (2005)
33. Ghiringhelli, F., et al.: Metronomic cyclophosphamide regimen selectively depletes CD4+ CD25+ regulatory T cells and restores T and NK effector functions in end stage cancer patients. Cancer Immunol. Immunother. **56**, 641–648 (2007)
34. Ellebaek, E., et al.: Metastatic melanoma patients treated with dendritic cell vaccination, interleukin-2 and metronomic cyclophosphamide: results from a phase II trial. Cancer Immunol. Immunother. **61**, 1791–1804 (2012)
35. Kyte, J.A., et al.: Telomerase peptide vaccination combined with temozolomide: a clinical trial in stage IV melanoma patients. Clin. Cancer Res. **17**, 4568–4580 (2011)
36. Harrop, R., et al.: Vaccination of colorectal cancer patients with TroVax given alongside chemotherapy (5-fluorouracil, leukovorin and irinotecan) is safe and induces potent immune responses. Cancer Immunol. Immunother. **57**, 977–986 (2008)
37. Nistico, P., et al.: Chemotherapy enhances vaccine-induced antitumor immunity in melanoma patients. Int. J. Cancer **124**, 130–139 (2009)
38. Quoix, E., et al.: Therapeutic vaccination with TG4010 and first-line chemotherapy in advanced non-small-cell lung cancer: a controlled phase 2B trial. Lancet Oncol. **12**, 1125–1133 (2011)
39. Obeid, M., et al.: Calreticulin exposure dictates the immunogenicity of cancer cell death. Nat. Med. **13**, 54–61 (2007)
40. Chakraborty, M., et al.: External beam radiation of tumors alters phenotype of tumor cells to render them susceptible to vaccine-mediated T-cell killing. Cancer Res. **64**, 4328–4337 (2004)
41. Formenti, S.C., Demaria, S.: Systemic effects of local radiotherapy. Lancet Oncol. **10**, 718–726 (2009)
42. Butts, C., et al.: Updated survival analysis in patients with stage IIIB or IV non-small-cell lung cancer receiving BLP25 liposome vaccine (L-BLP25): phase IIB randomized, multicenter, open-label trial. J. Cancer Res. Clin. Oncol. **137**, 1337–1342 (2011)
43. Gulley, J.L., et al.: Combining a recombinant cancer vaccine with standard definitive radiotherapy in patients with localized prostate cancer. Clin. Cancer Res. **11**, 3353–3362 (2005)
44. Coppin, C., et al.: Targeted therapy for advanced renal cell cancer (RCC): a Cochrane systematic review of published randomised trials. BJU Int. **108**, 1556–1563 (2011)
45. Bhatia, S., Thompson, J.A.: Systemic therapy for metastatic melanoma in 2012: dawn of a new era. J. Natl. Compr. Canc. Netw. **10**, 403–412 (2012)
46. Blank, C.U., Hooijkaas, A.I., Haanen, J.B., Schumacher, T.N.: Combination of targeted therapy and immunotherapy in melanoma. Cancer Immunol. Immunother. **60**, 1359–1371 (2011)
47. Comin-Anduix, B., et al.: The oncogenic BRAF kinase inhibitor PLX4032/RG7204 does not affect the viability or function of human lymphocytes across a wide range of concentrations. Clin. Cancer Res. **16**, 6040–6048 (2010)
48. Boni, A., et al.: Selective BRAFV600E inhibition enhances T-cell recognition of melanoma without affecting lymphocyte function. Cancer Res. **70**, 5213–5219 (2010)
49. Schwartzentruber, D.J., et al.: gp100 peptide vaccine and interleukin-2 in patients with advanced melanoma. N. Engl. J. Med. **364**, 2119–2127 (2011)
50. Weber, J.S., et al.: Ipilimumab increases activated T cells and enhances humoral immunity in patients with advanced melanoma. J. Immunother. **35**, 89–97 (2012)
51. Hodi, F.S., et al.: Improved survival with ipilimumab in patients with metastatic melanoma. N. Engl. J. Med. **363**, 711–723 (2010)
52. Prieto, P.A., et al.: CTLA-4 blockade with ipilimumab: long-term follow-up of 177 patients with metastatic melanoma. Clin. Cancer Res. **18**, 2039–2047 (2012)
53. Cooper, M.A., et al.: Human natural killer cells: a unique innate immunoregulatory role for the CD56(bright) subset. Blood **97**, 3146–3151 (2001)
54. Gauvrit, A., et al.: Measles virus induces oncolysis of mesothelioma cells and allows dendritic cells to cross-prime tumor-specific CD8 response. Cancer Res **68**, 4882–4892 (2008). 68/12/4882 [pii]. doi:10.1158/0008-5472.CAN-07-6265
55. Breitbach, C.J., et al.: Intravenous delivery of a multi-mechanistic cancer-targeted oncolytic poxvirus in humans. Nature **477**, 99–102 (2011). doi:10.1038/nature10358
56. Zamarin, D., Palese, P.: Oncolytic Newcastle disease virus for cancer therapy: old challenges and new directions. Future Microbiol. **7**, 347–367 (2012). doi:10.2217/fmb.12.4
57. Liu, J., Wennier, S., McFadden, G.: The immunoregulatory properties of oncolytic myxoma virus and their implications in therapeutics. Microbes Infect **12**, 1144–1152 (2010). doi:10.1016/j.micinf.2010.08.012
58. Maatta, A.M., et al.: Evaluation of cancer virotherapy with attenuated replicative Semliki forest virus in different rodent tumor models. Int. J. Cancer **121**, 863–870 (2007). doi:10.1002/ijc.22758
59. Rommelaere, J., et al.: Oncolytic parvoviruses as cancer therapeutics. Cytokine Growth Factor Rev. **21**, 185–195 (2010). doi:10.1016/j.cytogfr.2010.02.011
60. Di Piazza, M., et al.: Cytosolic activation of cathepsins mediates parvovirus H-1-induced killing of cisplatin and TRAIL-resistant glioma cells. J. Virol. **81**, 4186–4198 (2007). JVI.02601-06 [pii]. doi:10.1128/JVI.02601-06
61. Angelova, A.L., et al.: Oncolytic rat parvovirus H-1PV, a candidate for the treatment of human lymphoma: in vitro and in vivo studies. Mol. Ther. **17**, 1164–1172 (2009), mt200978 [pii]. doi:10.1038/mt.2009.78
62. Rommelaere, J., Cornelis, J.J.: Antineoplastic activity of parvoviruses. J. Virol. Methods **33**, 233–251 (1991)
63. Raykov, Z., et al.: Combined oncolytic and vaccination activities of parvovirus H-1 in a metastatic tumor model. Oncol. Rep. **17**, 1493–1499 (2007)
64. Grekova, S.P., Raykov, Z., Zawatzky, R., Rommelaere, J., Koch, U.: Activation of a glioma-specific immune response by oncolytic parvovirus Minute Virus of Mice infection. Cancer Gene Ther. **19**, 468–475 (2012). doi:10.1038/cgt.2012.20
65. Moehler, M.H., et al.: Parvovirus H-1-induced tumor cell death enhances human immune response in vitro via increased phagocytosis, maturation, and cross-presentation by dendritic cells. Hum. Gene Ther. **16**, 996–1005 (2005). doi:10.1089/hum.2005.16.996
66. Moehler, M., et al.: Oncolytic parvovirus H1 induces release of heat-shock protein HSP72 in susceptible human tumor cells but may not affect primary immune cells. Cancer Gene Ther. **10**, 477–480 (2003). doi:10.1038/sj.cgt.7700591
67. Moehler, M., et al.: Activation of the human immune system by chemotherapeutic or targeted agents combined with the oncolytic parvovirus H-1. BMC Cancer **11**, 464 (2011). doi:10.1186/1471-2407-11-464
68. Bhat, R., Dempe, S., Dinsart, C., Rommelaere, J.: Enhancement of NK cell antitumor responses using an oncolytic parvovirus. Int. J. Cancer J. Int. du Cancer **128**, 908–919 (2011). doi:10.1002/ijc.25415
69. Morales, O., et al.: Activation of a helper and not regulatory human CD4+ T cell response by oncolytic H-1 parvovirus. PLoS One **7**, e32197 (2012)

70. Raykov, Z., et al.: B1 lymphocytes and myeloid dendritic cells in lymphoid organs are preferential extratumoral sites of parvovirus minute virus of mice prototype strain expression. J. Virol. **79**, 3517–3524 (2005), 79/6/3517 [pii]. doi:10.1128/JVI.79.6.3517-3524.2005
71. Olijslagers, S., et al.: Potentiation of a recombinant oncolytic parvovirus by expression of Apoptin. Cancer Gene Ther. **8**, 958–965 (2001). doi:10.1038/sj.cgt.7700392
72. Giese, N.A., et al.: Suppression of metastatic hemangiosarcoma by a parvovirus MVMp vector transducing the IP-10 chemokine into immunocompetent mice. Cancer Gene Ther. **9**, 432–442 (2002). doi:10.1038/sj.cgt.7700457
73. Wetzel, K., et al.: MCP-3 (CCL7) delivered by parvovirus MVMp reduces tumorigenicity of mouse melanoma cells through activation of T lymphocytes and NK cells. Int. J. Cancer **120**, 1364–1371 (2007). doi:10.1002/ijc.22421
74. Haag, A., et al.: Highly efficient transduction and expression of cytokine genes in human tumor cells by means of autonomous parvovirus vectors; generation of antitumor responses in recipient mice. Hum. Gene Ther. **11**, 597–609 (2000). doi:10.1089/10430340050015789
75. Enderlin, M., et al.: TNF-alpha and the IFN-gamma-inducible protein 10 (IP-10/CXCL-10) delivered by parvoviral vectors act in synergy to induce antitumor effects in mouse glioblastoma. Cancer Gene. Ther. **16**, 149–160 (2009), cgt200862 [pii]. doi:10.1038/cgt.2008.62
76. Raykov, Z., Grekova, S., Leuchs, B., Aprahamian, M., Rommelaere, J.: Arming parvoviruses with CpG motifs to improve their oncosuppressive capacity. Int. J. Cancer **122**, 2880–2884 (2008). doi:10.1002/ijc.23472
77. Tarver, T.: Cancer facts & figures 2012. American Cancer Society (ACS). J. Consumer Health Internet **16**, 366–367 (2012)
78. Howlader N, et al. (eds).: SEER cancer statistics review, 1975–2009 (Vintage 2009 Populations). National Cancer Institute, Bethesda. http://seer.cancer.gov/csr/1975_2009_pops09/. Based on November 2011 SEER data submission, posted to the SEER web site, Apr 2012
79. Hirschowitz, E.A., Hiestand, D.M., Yannelli, J.R.: Vaccines for lung cancer. J. Thorac. Oncol. **1**, 93–104 (2006)
80. Palucka, K., Banchereau, J.: Cancer immunotherapy via dendritic cells. Nat. Rev. Cancer **12**, 265–277 (2012). doi:10.1038/nrc3258
81. Cranmer, L.D., Trevor, K.T., Hersh, E.M.: Clinical applications of dendritic cell vaccination in the treatment of cancer. Cancer Immunol. Immunother. **CII 53**, 275–306 (2004). doi:10.1007/s00262-003-0432-5
82. Keenan, B.P., Jaffee, E.M.: Whole cell vaccines – past progress and future strategies. Semin. Oncol. **39**, 276–286 (2012). doi:10.1053/j.seminoncol.2012.02.007
83. Keilholz, U., et al.: Immunologic monitoring of cancer vaccine therapy: results of a workshop sponsored by the Society for Biological Therapy. J. Immunother. **25**, 97–138 (2002)
84. Wolchok, J.D., et al.: Guidelines for the evaluation of immune therapy activity in solid tumors: immune-related response criteria. Clin. Cancer Res. **15**, 7412–7420 (2009). doi:10.1158/1078-0432.CCR-09-1624
85. Disis, M.L.: Immunologic biomarkers as correlates of clinical response to cancer immunotherapy. Cancer Immunol. Immunother. **CII 60**, 433–442 (2011). doi:10.1007/s00262-010-0960-8
86. Hirschowitz, E.A., Foody, T., Hidalgo, G.E., Yannelli, J.R.: Immunization of NSCLC patients with antigen-pulsed immature autologous dendritic cells. Lung Cancer **57**, 365–372 (2007). doi:10.1016/j.lungcan.2007.04.002
87. Hirschowitz, E.A., et al.: Pilot study of 1650-G: a simplified cellular vaccine for lung cancer. J. Thorac. Oncol. **6**, 169–173 (2011). doi:10.1097/JTO.0b013e3181fb5c22
88. Garnett, C.T., Schlom, J., Hodge, J.W.: Combination of docetaxel and recombinant vaccine enhances T-cell responses and antitumor activity: effects of docetaxel on immune enhancement. Clin. Cancer Res. **14**, 3536–3544 (2008). doi:10.1158/1078-0432.CCR-07-4025
89. Kodumudi, K.N., et al.: A novel chemoimmunomodulating property of docetaxel: suppression of myeloid-derived suppressor cells in tumor bearers. Clin. Cancer Res. **16**, 4583–4594 (2010). doi:10.1158/1078-0432.CCR-10-0733
90. Rohrmann, K., et al.: Immunotherapy in metastatic renal cell carcinoma. World J. Urol. **23**, 196–201 (2005)
91. Lizee, G., Radvanyi, L.G., Overwijk, W.W., Hwu, P.: Improving antitumor immune responses by circumventing immunoregulatory cells and mechanisms. Clin. Cancer Res. **12**, 4794–4803 (2006)
92. Gerhardt, H., Semb, H.: Pericytes: gatekeepers in tumour cell metastasis? J. Mol. Med. **86**, 135–144 (2008)
93. Lu, C., et al.: Gene alterations identified by expression profiling in tumor-associated endothelial cells from invasive ovarian carcinoma. Cancer Res. **67**, 1757–1768 (2007)
94. Hellberg, C., Ostman, A., Heldin, C.H.: PDGF and vessel maturation. Recent Results Cancer Res. **180**, 103–114 (2009)
95. Heath, V.L., Bicknell, R.: Anticancer strategies involving the vasculature. Nat. Rev. Clin. Oncol. **6**, 395–404 (2009)
96. Jain, R.K.: Normalization of tumor vasculature: an emerging concept in antiangiogenic therapy. Science **307**, 58–62 (2005)
97. Kolbeck, P.C., Kaveggia, F.F., Johansson, S.L., Grune, M.T., Taylor, R.J.: The relationships among tumor-infiltrating lymphocytes, histopathologic findings, and long-term clinical follow-up in renal cell carcinoma. Mod. Pathol. **5**, 420–425 (1992)
98. Kondo, T., et al.: Favorable prognosis of renal cell carcinoma with increased expression of chemokines associated with a Th1-type immune response. Cancer Sci. **97**, 780–786 (2006)
99. Biswas, S., Eisen, T.: Immunotherapeutic strategies in kidney cancer – when TKIs are not enough. Nat. Rev. Clin. Oncol. **6**, 478–487 (2009)
100. Folkman, J.: Role of angiogenesis in tumor growth and metastasis. Semin. Oncol. **29**, 15–18 (2002)
101. Ma, J., Waxman, D.J.: Combination of antiangiogenesis with chemotherapy for more effective cancer treatment. Mol. Cancer Ther. **7**, 3670–3684 (2008)
102. Huang, Y., et al.: Vascular normalizing doses of antiangiogenic treatment reprogram the immunosuppressive tumor microenvironment and enhance immunotherapy. Proc. Natl. Acad. Sci. U. S. A. **109**, 17561–17566 (2012)
103. Faivre, S., Demetri, G., Sargent, W., Raymond, E.: Molecular basis for sunitinib efficacy and future clinical development. Nat. Rev. Drug Discov. **6**, 734–745 (2007)
104. Zhou, Q., Guo, P., Gallo, J.M.: Impact of angiogenesis inhibition by sunitinib on tumor distribution of temozolomide. Clin. Cancer Res. **14**, 1540–1549 (2008)
105. Ganss, R., Ryschich, E., Klar, E., Arnold, B., Hammerling, G.J.: Combination of T-cell therapy and trigger of inflammation induces remodeling of the vasculature and tumor eradication. Cancer Res. **62**, 1462–1470 (2002)
106. Feldman, E.D., et al.: Interferon gamma-inducible protein 10 selectively inhibits proliferation and induces apoptosis in endothelial cells. Ann. Surg. Oncol. **13**, 125–133 (2006)
107. Ozao-Choy, J., et al.: The novel role of tyrosine kinase inhibitor in the reversal of immune suppression and modulation of tumor microenvironment for immune-based cancer therapies. Cancer Res. **69**, 2514–2522 (2009)
108. Avigan, D.E., et al.: Phase I/II study of vaccination with electrofused allogeneic dendritic cells/autologous tumor-derived cells in patients with stage IV renal cell carcinoma. J. Immunother. **30**, 749–761 (2007)

109. Kass, E., et al.: Induction of protective host immunity to carcinoembryonic antigen (CEA), a self-antigen in CEA transgenic mice, by immunizing with a recombinant vaccinia-CEA virus. Cancer Res. **59**, 676–683 (1999)
110. Yang, S., Tsang, K.Y., Schlom, J.: Induction of higher-avidity human CTLs by vector-mediated enhanced costimulation of antigen-presenting cells. Clin. Cancer Res. **11**, 5603–5615 (2005)
111. Amato, R.J., et al.: Vaccination of renal cell cancer patients with modified vaccinia ankara delivering tumor antigen 5T4 (TroVax) administered with interleukin 2: a phase II trial. Clin. Cancer Res. **14**, 7504–7510 (2008)
112. Amato, R.J., et al.: Vaccination of renal cell cancer patients with modified vaccinia Ankara delivering the tumor antigen 5T4 (TroVax) alone or administered in combination with interferon-alpha (IFN-alpha): a phase 2 trial. J. Immunother. **32**, 765–772 (2009)
113. Amato, R.J., et al.: Vaccination of metastatic renal cancer patients with MVA-5T4: a randomized, double-blind, placebo-controlled phase III study. Clin. Cancer Res. **16**, 5539–5547 (2010)
114. Oudard, S., et al.: A phase II study of the cancer vaccine TG4010 alone and in combination with cytokines in patients with metastatic renal clear-cell carcinoma: clinical and immunological findings. Cancer Immunol. Immunother. **60**, 261–271 (2011)
115. Geiger, C., Regn, S., Weinzierl, A., Noessner, E., Schendel, D.J.: A generic RNA-pulsed dendritic cell vaccine strategy for renal cell carcinoma. J. Transl. Med. **3**, 29 (2005)
116. Rittig, S.M., et al.: Intradermal vaccinations with RNA coding for TAA generate CD8+ and CD4+ immune responses and induce clinical benefit in vaccinated patients. Mol. Ther. **19**, 990–999 (2011)
117. Suekane, S., et al.: Phase I trial of personalized peptide vaccination for cytokine-refractory metastatic renal cell carcinoma patients. Cancer Sci. **98**, 1965–1968 (2007)
118. Wierecky, J., et al.: Immunologic and clinical responses after vaccinations with peptide-pulsed dendritic cells in metastatic renal cancer patients. Cancer Res. **66**, 5910–5918 (2006)
119. Weber, J.S., et al.: A phase 1 study of a vaccine targeting preferentially expressed antigen in melanoma and prostate-specific membrane antigen in patients with advanced solid tumors. J. Immunother. **34**, 556–567 (2011)
120. Uemura, H., et al.: A phase I trial of vaccination of CA9-derived peptides for HLA-A24-positive patients with cytokine-refractory metastatic renal cell carcinoma. Clin. Cancer Res. **12**, 1768–1775 (2006)
121. Bleumer, I., et al.: Preliminary analysis of patients with progressive renal cell carcinoma vaccinated with CA9-peptide-pulsed mature dendritic cells. J. Immunother. **30**, 116–122 (2007)
122. Yasukawa, M., Ochi, T., Fujiwara, H.: Relapse of renal cell carcinoma with disappearance of HLA class I following hTERT peptide vaccination. Ann. Oncol. **21**, 2122–2124 (2010)
123. Märten, A., et al.: Telomerase-pulsed dendritic cells: preclinical results and outcome of a clinical phase I/II trial in patients with metastatic renal cell carcinoma. Ger. Med. Sci. **4**, Doc02 (2006)
124. Rahma, O.E., et al.: A pilot clinical trial testing mutant von Hippel-Lindau peptide as a novel immune therapy in metastatic renal cell carcinoma. J. Transl. Med. **8**, 8 (2010)
125. Walter, S., et al.: Multipeptide immune response to cancer vaccine IMA901 after single-dose cyclophosphamide associates with longer patient survival. Nat. Med. **18**, 1254–1261 (2012)
126. Harrop, R., et al.: MVA-5T4-induced immune responses are an early marker of efficacy in renal cancer patients. Cancer Immunol. Immunother. **60**, 829–837 (2011)
127. Harrop, R., et al.: Analysis of pre-treatment markers predictive of treatment benefit for the therapeutic cancer vaccine MVA-5T4 (TroVax). Cancer Immunol. Immunother. **61**, 2283–2294 (2012)
128. Khong, H.T., Restifo, N.P.: Natural selection of tumor variants in the generation of "tumor escape" phenotypes. Nat. Immunol. **3**, 999–1005 (2002)
129. Ebos, J.M., et al.: Accelerated metastasis after short-term treatment with a potent inhibitor of tumor angiogenesis. Cancer Cell **15**, 232–239 (2009)
130. Paez-Ribes, M., et al.: Antiangiogenic therapy elicits malignant progression of tumors to increased local invasion and distant metastasis. Cancer Cell **15**, 220–231 (2009)
131. Chinnasamy, D., et al.: Gene therapy using genetically modified lymphocytes targeting VEGFR-2 inhibits the growth of vascularized syngenic tumors in mice. J. Clin. Invest. **120**, 3953–3968 (2010)
132. He, Y., Zhang, J., Donahue, C., Falo Jr., L.D.: Skin-derived dendritic cells induce potent CD8+ T cell immunity in recombinant lentivector-mediated genetic immunization. Immunity **24**, 643–656 (2006)
133. Morgan, R.A., et al.: Cancer regression in patients after transfer of genetically engineered lymphocytes. Science **314**, 126–129 (2006)
134. Lamers, C.H., et al.: Immune responses to transgene and retroviral vector in patients treated with *ex vivo*-engineered T cells. Blood **117**, 72–82 (2011)
135. O'Brien, M.A., et al.: Local tumour ablative therapies: opportunities for maximising immune engagement and activation. Biochim. Biophys. Acta **1846**(2), 510–523 (2014)

Noninfectious Noncancer (NINC) Vaccines

13

Contents

13.1 Indications for Innovative NINC Vaccines

When in 2012 the author of this textbook invited international vaccine experts to contribute to "Molecular Vaccines – From Prophylaxis to Therapy," he used as working title "NINC vaccines" (*non**in*fectious and *non**c*ancer) for sub-summarizing all vaccine developments which did not fall into the classification of infectious and cancer vaccines and meet very various indications as presented in Fig. 13.1 Meanwhile the term NINC vaccines becomes more and more popular in the scientific world simply by collecting all vaccines against other targets than pathogens and cancer.

13.1.1 Immunogenicity of Drug Molecules

The handicap of most drug molecules like nicotine, cocaine, or ethanol is that they are too small that the immune system typically ignores them. These molecules are non-immunogenic. To overcome that, drug molecules are conjugated to a protein carrier (hapten) to facilitate antigen presentation and the induction of T cell help. Natural microbial haptens like tetanus toxoid or diphtheria toxoid are generally powerful immunogens with the disadvantage to induce an antibody response against the carrier. Booster immunizations are limited, and the carrier will be neutralized. Synthetic hapten carriers can circumvent this bottleneck [1].

In case of alcohol, an immunization against this addiction is not possible. The ethanol molecule is so small that it cannot be successfully attached to any available hapten protein. Figure 13.2 illustrates the conjugation of nicotine to a synthetic carrier.

How the hapten–antigen complex activates the adaptive immunity remains unclear. Studies by Palm and Medzhitov demonstrate that the induction of antibodies is TLR independent [2]. Nevertheless, T and B cell responses induced are primarily hapten specific, rather than protein specific. Happened antigens use alternative innate pathway to adaptive immunity.

M. Giese, *Introduction to Molecular Vaccinology*, DOI 10.1007/978-3-319-25832-4_13

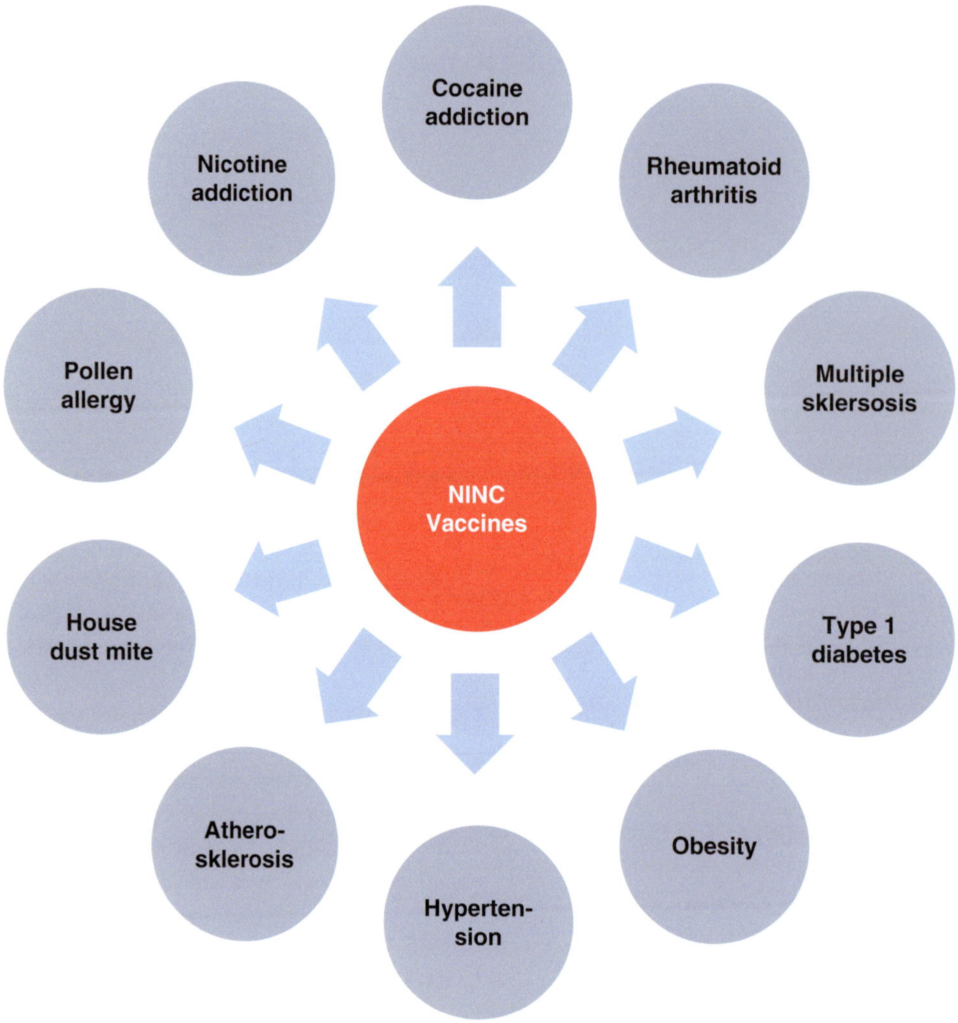

Fig. 13.1 NINC vaccines are experimentally developed against autoimmune diseases (such as type 1 diabetes, multiple sclerosis, rheumatoid arthritis), allergies (pollen, house dust mite), drug addiction (nicotine, cocaine), and other diseases (obesity, hypertension, atherosclerosis). Thereby, NINC vaccines follow the same immunological principles as classical vaccines do: they introduce a small amount of the foreign substance into the body, provoking the immune system to create antibodies that block the pharmacological effects of the drug the next time it appears

13.1.2 Antigen-Specific Immunotherapy Targeting CD4+ T Cells

Autoimmunity or allergies can be combatted by antigen-specific vaccines targeting T cells. The antigen against which the body produces (auto-) antibodies will be administered in escalating doses. This vaccination strategy focuses to reinstate a long-lasting immunological tolerance to the targeted (self) antigen. Naturally occurring CD4+ regulatory T cells play a central role in this approach. They suppress immune responses of other cells and prevent excessive reactions. It has been shown that regulatory T cells can be induced by specific antigen vaccination [3]. Peptide-induced cells are FoxP3(−) and secret IL-10 upon stimulation.

IL-10 blocks NF-κB activity and downregulates the expression of Th1 cytokines, MHC class II antigens, and co-stimulatory molecules on macrophages and prevents autoimmunity (see Chap. 2).

Chronic stimulation of regulatory CD4+ T cells by peptide administration in a dose-dependent manner results in transcriptional changes as demonstrated by genome analysis [4]. The expressed transcriptional factors c-Maf and NFIL3 and the co-stimulatory molecules, LAG-3, TIGIT, PD-1, and TIM-3, contribute to progressive suppression of inflammatory T cell function and consequently suppression of inflammatory cytokines. On the other hand, these transcriptional changes support the secretion of IL-10.

As discussed earlier, many factors influence the success of each vaccination strategy. Also the outcome of the antigen-specific immunotherapy targeting CD4+ T cells and the prevention of immunopathological adverse events depend on the nature of the antigen, protein versus peptide, self versus nonself antigen, doses, route of administration, frequency of administration, and the choice of adjuvant.

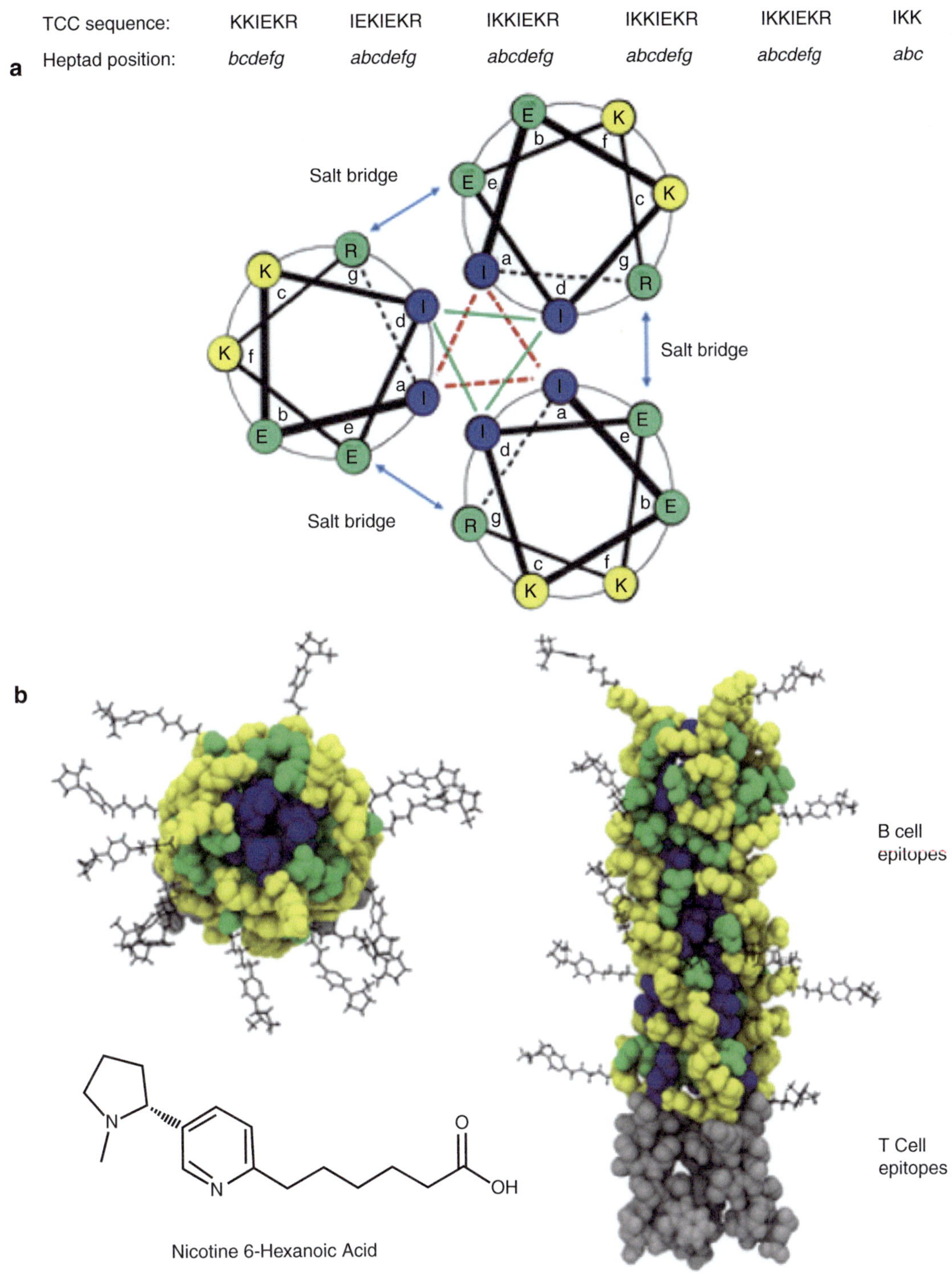

Fig. 13.2 Structure of the trimeric coiled-coil protein. (**a**) The amino acid sequence of each amphipathic peptide is comprised of 5 heptad repeats containing isoleucine at the "a" and "d" positions to form the hydrophobic interior of the trimer and lysine, arginine, and glutamic acid at the remaining positions. The carboxyl sequences of the CD4+ T cell epitope are not represented. The position of each residue within the heptad repeat following self-assembly of the trimeric protein is represented by the three helical wheel projections. Forty-eight lysine residues (*yellow*) are solvent exposed and available for hapten conjugation. Isoleucines (*blue*) comprise the hydrophobic core, and arginine and glutamic acid residues (*green*) form salt bridges that stabilize the trimeric structure. (**b**) Homology model of the TCCnic peptide with rendered atoms represented by space-filling Van der Waals radii. The model on the left is a view down the symmetrical axis of the trimer, whereas the right hand model is a longitudinal view. The C-terminal portion contains CD4+ T cell epitopes (*gray spheres*) required for B cell help. Nicotine-6-hexanoic acid haptens (*black bonds*) were manually added to the ε-amino group of 12 randomly chosen lysine residues using the molefacture plug-in from the Visual Molecular Dynamics software package (Credit: Miller et al. [1])

13.2 Type I Allergy: Edible Vaccines Against Pollinosis and House Dust Mite[1]

13.2.1 The Two Major Allergic Diseases in Japan

In industrial countries, 30–40 % of the population suffers from some kind of IgE-mediated type I allergic disease such as asthma, allergic rhinitis, conjunctivitis, and atopic dermatitis [5]. Japanese cedar (*Cryptomeria japonica*, Cry j) pollinosis is the most predominant seasonal allergic disease in Japan and is caused by pollen spread over most areas of Japan in early spring from February to April. Epidemiological studies indicate that about 27 % of the Japanese population is afflicted with this allergic disease [6].

Furthermore, more than half of the general population has circulating IgE specific for cedar pollen allergens. The number of patients with *Cryptomeria* pollinosis and the economic cost associated with it is expected to increase steadily, resulting in a strong social demand for the development of a reliable and effective way of controlling this pollinosis.

House dust mite (HDM) is also a major source of inhalant allergens which cause chronic allergic disease such as bronchial asthma in as much as 10 % of the population in many parts of the world. About 45–80 % of patients with allergic asthma are sensitized to allergens in HDM, especially *Dermatophagoides farinae* (Der f) and *D. pteronyssinus* (Der p) [7]. Thus, these patients suffer from allergic symptoms or reactions in response to HDM and/or have elevated allergen-specific serum IgE, suggesting that HDM allergens are crucial for the development of bronchial asthma [8].

13.2.2 Allergic Pathogens

Cedar Pollen. Two major allergens of Japanese cedar pollen, Cry j 1 and Cry j 2, have been isolated and characterized. More than 90 % of patients with Japanese cedar pollinosis have IgE specific to both [9]. Cry j 1 is a basic glycoprotein pectate lyase with an apparent molecular mass of 41–45 kDa and a pI of 8.9–9.2. Cry j 2 is also a basic protein with polygalacturonate activity and a molecular mass of 37 kDa and pI of 8.6–8.8; they are specifically localized in the cell walls of papilla and amyloplasts in cedar pollen, respectively. Both Cry j 1 and Cry j 2 have several isoforms that differ in primary structure and result from posttranslational modifications. The nucleotide sequences of Cry j 1 and Cry j 2 cDNAs have been determined and their amino acid sequences deduced [10].

House Dust Mite. Those derived from HDM are some of the most common indoor allergens associated with bronchial asthma, rhinitis, and atopic dermatitis. HDM is responsible for more than 70 % of childhood bronchial asthma cases, and to date, more than 20 HDM allergens have been identified and characterized [8]. The major HDM allergens are classified into group 1 (Der f 1 and Der p 1; molecular mass, 25 kDa) and group 2 (Der f 2 and Der p 2; molecular mass, 14 kDa). Sera from 50 to 70 % of mite-sensitive patients are reactive to either or both of these allergens.

Group 1 Allergen. Group 1 allergen is a heat labile acidic glycoprotein and is mainly found in HDM feces. This protein has papain-like cysteine protease activity that is involved in the pathogenesis of allergy through cleavage of CD23 and CD25 from the surface of immune cells. Group 1 allergen is synthesized as an enzymatically inactive pro-group 1 protein which is then processed into the more allergenic mature and enzymatically active proteins of 222 (Der p 1) and 223 (Der f 1) amino acids which share 82 % sequence homology [11]. IgE binding to group I allergens is highly dependent on their tertiary structure.

Group 2 Allergens. Group 2 allergens comprise 129 amino acid residues and share 87 % homology [12]. More than 80 % of mite-allergic patients are sensitized against group 2 allergens, which are present at high concentrations in mite feces [13]. Although the biological function of group 2 allergens is not known, they show similarities in sequence, size, and distribution of cysteine residues to a family of epididymal proteins [14].

13.2.3 Conventional Therapy

Allergic diseases are characterized by allergen-specific IgE production and the activation of effector cells including eosinophils, mast cells, and basophils. These events are regulated by Th2 cells, which preferentially produce IL-4, IL-5, and IL-13. Therefore, allergic diseases have been defined as inadequate peripheral regulation of allergen-specific T cells.

Treatment strategies for these allergic diseases generally involve pharmacotherapy using antihistamines, corticosteroids,

[1] Rice seed-based allergy vaccines: induction of allergen-specific oral tolerance against cedar pollen and house dust mite allergies by *Fumio Takaiwa and Takachika Hiroi* in Molecular Vaccines – From Prophylaxis to Therapy, Volume 2, Springer-Verlag Wien, 2013, Ed. Matthias Giese.

etc. However, although these approaches reduce clinical symptoms by blocking the release of critical mediators of allergic reactions or by inhibiting allergic inflammation, they are not curative and sometimes induce impaired performance as a result of side effects.

Desensitization. It is well established that allergen-specific immunotherapy is the only way to modulate these immune reactions, bringing about effects that persist for many years without the need for further treatment and which reduce the risk of development of sensitization to further allergens or development of asthma in children with rhinitis [15]. Conventional allergen-specific immunotherapy has been practiced for almost a century. Success can be achieved by repeated subcutaneous injections of increasing doses of native allergen extracts over a period of at least 3–5 years for induction of immune tolerance (desensitization).

This treatment is sometimes accompanied by severe side effects, such as anaphylaxis caused by capture of the allergen together with specific anti-allergen IgE on the surface of mast cells and basophils. Recently, sublingual immunotherapy has been developed and has provided a safer and more beneficial route [16]. The basic principle of allergen-specific immunotherapy is to induce immune tolerance to allergens through multiple cellular and molecular mechanisms [17] leading to reduction in inflammatory cell recruitment and activation and in mediator secretion. The induction of a tolerant state in peripheral T cells represents an essential step in allergen-specific immunotherapy [18].

Peripheral T cell tolerance is characterized mainly by the generation of allergen-specific regulatory T cells (Tregs) (Foxp3$^+$ CD4$^+$CD25$^+$, induced Foxp3$^+$CD4$^+$, Tr1, and Th3) leading to suppressed T cell proliferation and Th1 and Th2 cytokine responses against allergen. This is accompanied by a significant increase in allergen-specific IgG4 and IgG1 subclasses of IgG antibody and in IgA and a decrease in IgE in the late stage of disease. Figure 13.3 illustrates the mechanisms of pollen allergy.

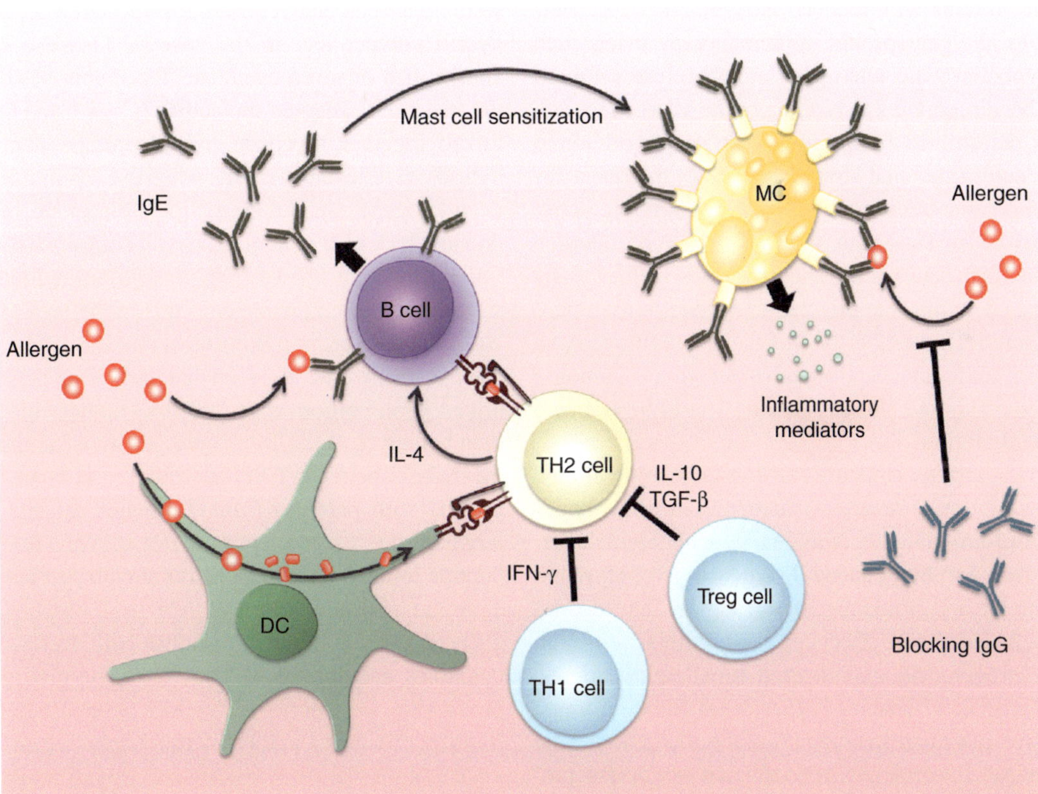

Fig. 13.3 Allergic sensitization. Allergen is taken up via epithelial surfaces such as the skin or the mucosa of airways and gut. Dendritic cells (DC) phagocytose and process allergens into peptides which in turn are presented on MHC class II and induce generation of TH2 cells. This process can be inhibited by IFN-γ secreting TH1 cells or regulatory T cells (Treg) secreting IL-10 and/or TGF-β. TH2 cells produce IL-4 which promotes class switch of allergen-specific B cells to IgE. IgE antibodies bind to FcεRI receptors on mast cells and upon allergen re-encounter induce release of inflammatory mediators such as histamine. Presence of high levels of blocking IgG can inhibit allergen binding to mast cell surface IgE (From: Scheiblhofer et al. [114])

13.2.4 Development of Vaccine for Allergic Disease

Safer and noninvasive oral immunotherapy has long been desired as an alternative to the conventional subcutaneous application. Modified allergens with reduced IgE binding activity (low allergenicity) represent the most promising and elegant approach to circumvent the risk of anaphylactic reactions in allergen-specific immunotherapy. To address these requirements, rice seed-based oral allergy vaccines have been recently developed, containing modified recombinant allergens with reduced or no allergenicity, or allergen-derived T cell epitope peptides. These oral vaccines are a simple, safe, and cost-effective form of immunotherapy.

13.2.4.1 Hypoallergenic Tolerogens with Reduced Allergenicity

To create hypoallergenic tolerogens, natural allergen extracts used for induction of immune tolerance (desensitization), which can bind to specific IgE on mast cells and basophils and lead to anaphylactic side effects, need to be replaced by recombinant proteins with reduced allergenicity [19]. New approaches to allergen-specific immunotherapy using such modified hypoallergenic tolerogens are therefore required [20]. It has been reported that binding of the allergen to specific IgE is determined by a continuous stretch of amino acids or by conformational structures; hence, the quest for ideal hypoallergenic tolerogens with low IgE binding activity has involved investigating the reassembly of allergen fragments to form various mosaic structures, achieved by means such as deletion, site-directed mutagenesis, fragmentation, oligomeric formation, or molecular shuffling. As a result, amino acids and peptides involved in IgE binding would be removed, and allergen folding would be changed by sequence alteration.

In particular, tertiary structure can be significantly altered by mutation of cysteine residue(s) disrupting disulfide bond-dependent conformation. Recombinant hypoallergenic allergen derivatives exhibit reduced IgE reactivity but retain T cell reactivity and immunogenicity; hence, they do not induce IgE-mediated side effects even when relatively high doses of tolerogen are administered to allergic patients. Reduced allergenicity enables higher doses to be administered, which results in greater efficacy of the allergen-specific immunotherapy. Interestingly, recombinant oligomers preserve IgE reactivity but lose allergenic activity because of altered presentation of IgE epitopes.

The efficacy of recombinant hypoallergenic allergen derivatives of the major birch pollen allergen Bet v 1 has been confirmed in clinical trials (currently at phase III) with allergic patients [21]. The production of allergen-specific IgG antibodies (especially IgG4) with blocking activities that inhibit not only allergen-induced release of inflammatory mediators from mast cells and basophils but also IgE-facilitated antigen presentation to T cells has been shown to be induced by subcutaneous and sublingual immunotherapy.

13.2.4.2 T Cell Epitope Peptide as a Minimum Tolerogen

Allergens are recognized by T cell receptors (TCRs) and major histocompatibility complex (MHC)-II through interaction with their T cell epitope. Immunotherapy using T cell epitope peptide is an attractive approach for safe allergen-specific immunotherapy because it does not contain an IgE cross-linking epitope that could induce anaphylaxis [22]. However, T cell epitopes derived from allergens, which are recognized by specific T cells, vary according to MHC-II class haplotypes. This is a serious obstacle in the development of peptide immunotherapy that takes advantage of T cell epitope peptides. To overcome this problem, artificial hybrid epitope peptides composed of the complete T cell epitope repertoires derived from one or a few allergens have been created.

Several major T cell epitopes from many allergy patients were identified and chosen for inclusion in the artificial hybrid polypeptide. In the case of Japanese cedar pollen allergy, five or seven candidate T cell epitopes derived from the two major allergen molecules (Cry j 1 and Cry j 2) were linked together to create hybrid epitope peptides. These hybrids have several benefits when used as immunotherapeutic tolerogens, since they exhibit little or no IgE reactivity due to a lack of B cell epitopes and conformational changes. For example, the hybrid 7Crp peptide (seven linked epitopes) showed no binding to specific IgE in the sera of 48 patients with Japanese cedar pollinosis symptoms [23].

It is interesting to note that the 7Crp peptide induced T cell proliferation with 100-fold higher immunogenicity than a mixture of the T cell epitopes used for construction of the hybrid peptide. Clinical trials have been mainly performed with peptides from the major cat and bee venom allergens Fel d 1 and Api m 1, respectively. It is known that peptide immunotherapy performed with peptides from Fel d 1 or the phospholipase A2 Api m 1 induced a Tr1-type allergen-specific immune response with decreased Th2-type cytokines and increased IL-10 and allergen-specific IgG4 production. Low doses of peptides have also been shown to improve clinical symptoms without inducing adverse events.

13.2.5 Seed-Based Oral Vaccine

Seed provides a suitable production platform for recombinant allergy vaccines and, when orally administered, acts as a delivery vehicle to gut-associated lymphoid tissue (GALT), including Peyer's patches (PPs) and a large cluster of lymphoid follicles of the mucosal immune tissues. The production of vaccines in seed offers several advantages, including no requirement for cold transportation and storage, needle-free administration, no risk of contamination with human pathogens, low cost, and a production process that can easily be scaled up as required [24].

For practical use of plant-made oral allergy vaccines, the continuous administration of high-dose tolerogen required for induction of immune tolerance (desensitization) means that high and consistent expression is critical for efficacy. To maximize yield in this system, the transferred genes encoding these tolerogens will need to be synthesized using codons optimized for expression in seed [25]. Furthermore, because accumulation of recombinant proteins is also largely dependent on intracellular localization, it is important to target them stably and at high concentration to suitable locations by means of intracellular targeting signals. In the case of seeds, a signal peptide for targeting the secretory pathway and a sorting signal to target protein bodies (PBs) are mandatory for stable accumulation of product. Strong tissue-specific promoters rather than constitutive promoters are preferable for high-level expression of antigens in the desired tissue.

Endosperm-Specific Promoter. For expression of antigens in transgenic rice seed, strong endosperm-specific promoters, such as those for major storage protein glutelin (GluB), 26 kDa globulin, or 10 and 16 kDa prolamin, have been used for expression in rice endosperm [26]. Using these promoters, target gene products were highly accumulated as distinctly detectable proteins in CBB-stained SDS-PAGE gels, accounting for 4–6 % of total seed proteins (3–5 mg/g dry seeds).

Thus far, using this system, hybrid T cell epitope peptides (7Crp) from Japanese cedar pollen allergens Cry j 1 and Cry j 2 and their structurally disrupted full length forms, subunit antigen from major mite allergen Der p 1 and a modified mite allergen Der f 2, in which Cys residues implicated in disulfide bonds were mutated to Ser (Ala), were all found to be highly accumulated in the endosperm of transgenic rice [27]. They were deposited predominantly in ER-derived PBs or in the unique ER-derived compartment, the Der f body.

These recombinant proteins are consistently inherited over several subsequent generations without silencing. Furthermore, these antigens remain stable without loss of immunogenicity even when the seed is stored at ambient temperature for several years.

13.2.5.1 Delivery to GALT as Oral Seed-Based Allergy Vaccine

Oral delivery of plant-based antigens induces not only mucosal but also systemic immune responses. Repeated oral administration is inclined to induce immune tolerance to the fed antigen rather than sensitization, especially when the antigen is deposited in particulate PBs as the storage organelle of the seed. PBs of <10 nm are principally taken up by M cells in the follicle-associated epithelium of PPs in GALT of the small intestine and then presented to antigen-presenting cells (APCs) such as dendritic cells (DCs) in adjacent mucosal T cell areas [28]. Moreover, there is a possibility that DCs in the lamina propria (LP) extend their dendrites into the lumen and sample PBs.

The GALT contains an organized macro-architecture of zones of B and T lymphocytes that respond to antigens presented by DCs, which can induce memory B and T cells. There are at least three subsets of DCs with distinct tissue distribution in PPs. $CD11b^+$ DCs are present in the subepithelial domain (SED) regions, $CD8^+$ DCs in the T cell-rich interfollicular region (IFR), and double-negative $CD4^-CD8\alpha^-$ DCs in both SED and IFRs (Fig. 13.4).

IL-10-producing immature DCs contribute to immunologic tolerance through inducing Tr1 regulatory cells. It should be noted that GALT is the preferential site for peripheral induction of $Foxp3^+$ natural Tregs (Fig. 13.5). $CD103^+$ DCs of the LP of small intestine (mucosal DCs) are particularly competent at inducing $Foxp3^+$ T cells via TGF-β and retinoic acid (RA) (Fig. 13.5). Plasmacytoid DCs (pDCs) presenting dietary antigens are responsible for induction of oral tolerance and immune suppression (Fig. 13.5).

It has been demonstrated that to achieve the same level of efficacy, orally delivered mucosal immunotherapy requires >100- to 1000-fold as much antigen as subcutaneous injection [29]. This is because the purified antigen is degraded by digestive enzymes in the gastrointestinal tract and by exposure to the harsh environment in the stomach before arrival at the mucosal immune cells in the GALT. By contrast, when orally delivered via cereal seeds such as rice grains, bioencapsulation of antigen by the double barrier of PBs and cell wall characteristic of plant cells has the advantage of protecting the antigen from proteolysis [30].

Gastrointestinal Enzyme Digestion. This is not the case when the antigen is delivered by other plant vegetative cells. It should be noted that PBs derived from the ER are more resistant to gastrointestinal enzyme digestion than those in protein storage vacuoles (PSVs), as shown by comparing digestibility and immune tolerance-inducing capacity between ER-derived PB (PB-I) and PSV (PB-II)-localized antigens [31]. This physical difference may be related to the polymerized or aggregated arrangement of antigen formed with cysteine-rich prolamins observed in ER-derived PBs. In fact, when transgenic rice seeds containing several allergen derivatives deposited in ER-derived PB or PSV are fed to mice, PB-I-localized allergen derivatives manifest greater resistance to enzymatic digestion than PB-II-localized or synthesized naked forms. The dose of PB-I-localized T cell epitope required for suppression of allergen-specific IgE levels in mice was about 20-fold and threefold lower than the amounts required of synthetic peptide and PB-II-localized form, respectively.

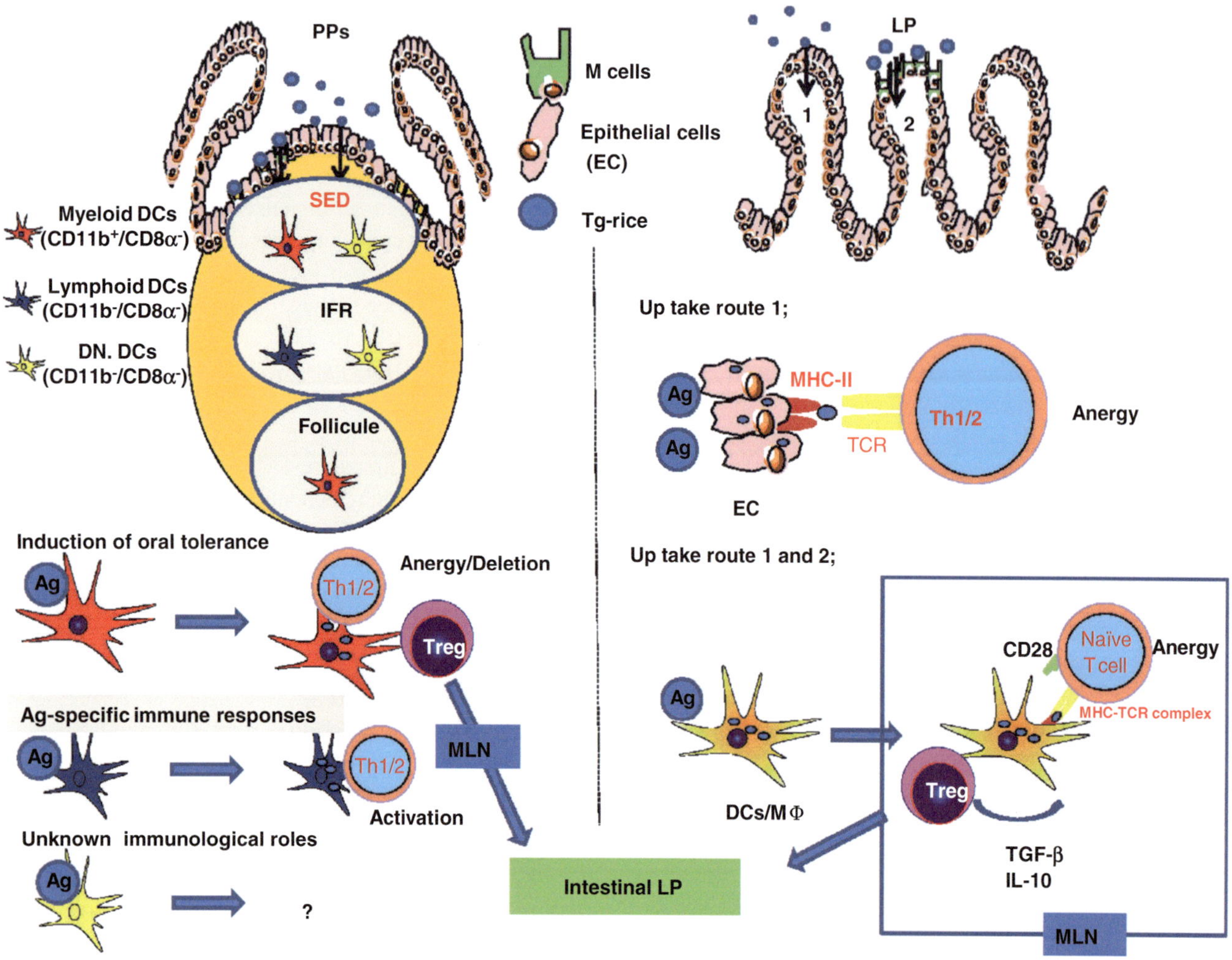

Fig. 13.4 Fed allergens are taken to the mucosal immune system in Peyer's patches and intestinal lamina propria. Antigens fed by oral vaccination cross M cells of both Peyer's patches (PPs) and intestinal epithelial cells in the lamina propria (LP). Antigens are processed and presented on MHC-II molecules by CD11b⁺ CD8α⁻ myeloid DCs in PPs to induce oral tolerance but not CD11b⁻ CD8α⁺ lymphoid DCs. DC/macrophage (Mϕ)-cached antigens in intestinal LP are also processed and presented on MHC-II molecules and thereafter carried to the mesenteric lymph node (MLN) as an attending lymph node in the intestinal mucosa. Moreover, antigens are also processed and directly presented on MHC molecules by intestinal epithelial cells to induce oral tolerance in intestinal LP. *SED* subepithelial domain, *IFR* interfollicular region

Rice Cooking. The rice-based allergy vaccine is heat stable and can thus tolerate storage at room temperature for several years and boiling in the process of rice cooking. It has been confirmed that steamed or cooked transgenic rice retains its efficacy for inducing oral immune tolerance. In fact, extracts from the treated seeds can still elicit T cell proliferative activity even after autoclaving for 20 min.

13.2.5.2 Induction of Immune Tolerance in GALT

The immunological mechanism implicated in tolerance induction is dependent on the frequency, duration, and dose of antigen administered. Repeated low-dose administration of antigen favors tolerance driven by Tregs, whereas high doses favor anergy or cell deletion-driven tolerance of the kind thought to be responsible for the induction of tolerance as a quiescent immune state [32]. It has been shown that for oral tolerance, Fas (CD95)-dependent apoptosis is responsible for the deletion of effector T cells [33] (Fig. 13.6a).

Anergy. T-lymphocyte anergy occurs through TCR ligation in the absence of co-stimulatory signals and is prevented by cognate interaction between CD80/86 (B7) on APCs and CD28 (CTLA-4) on effector T cells (Fig. 13.6b). CTLA-4 is known to play a pivotal role in controlling the suppressive functions of Tregs. The interactions of co-stimulatory

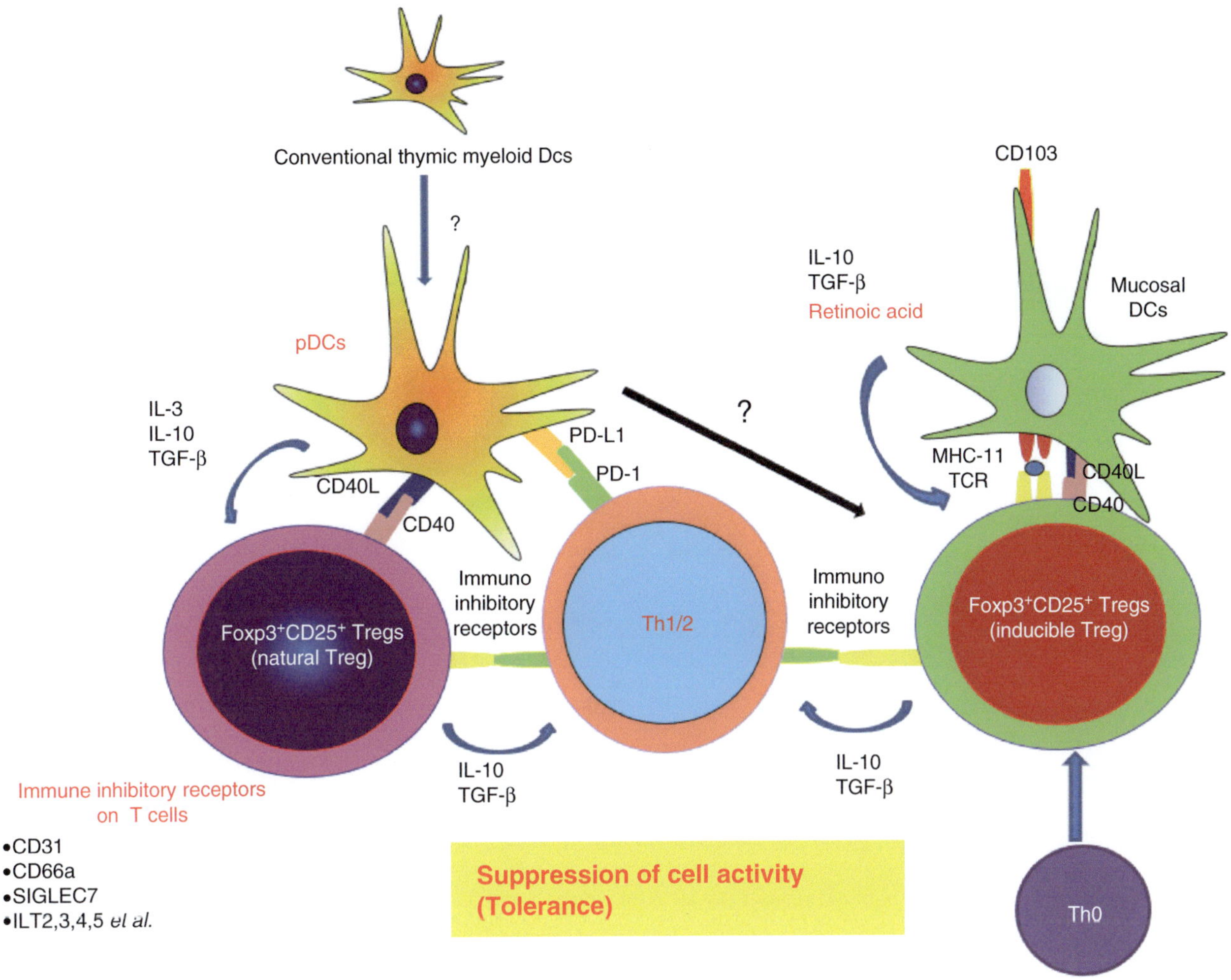

Fig. 13.5 Two subsets of $Foxp3^+$ $CD25^+$ $CD4^+$ Tregs for the induction of antigen-specific tolerance. Plasmacytoid dendritic cells (pDCs) derived from conventional thymic myeloid DCs produce IL-10 and TGF-β and induce more IL-10-producing natural regulatory T cells (Tregs), contributing to the suppression of immune responses. The environment of the gut mucosa is particularly permissive for the generation of inducible Tregs. $CD103^+$ DCs excel in converting $CD4^+$ naive T cells into $Foxp3^+$ inducible Tregs in the absence of TGF-β, under the production of the vitamin A metabolite retinoic acid in small intestinal lamina propria

molecules play a key role in the regulation of T cell activation and tolerance [34]. Participation of other B7 and CD28 family members as co-stimulation factors involved in immune regulation has also been discovered (Fig. 13.6b).

By contrast, orally administered low-dose antigen can induce active suppression by induction of inhibitory immune responses mediated by Treg cells. These cells include naturally occurring $Foxp3^+CD4^+$ $CD25^+$ Treg cells and antigen-inducible Tregs comprising $Foxp3^+$ inducible $CD4^+$ cells, IL-10-producing Tr1 cells, TGF-β-producing Th3 cells, and regulatory $CD8^+$ T cells [35]. Naturally occurring Tregs are generated in the thymus, whereas induced Treg cells are generated in the periphery from naive T cells.

It has been shown that peripheral conversion of $CD4^+$ T cells to Tregs occurs primarily in GALT, because the gut is an entry site for numerous antigens such as foods and commensal bacteria. Differentiation of naive $CD4^+$ T cells to IL-10-producing Tr1 cells is mediated by IL-27 produced by the Treg-modified DCs in the presence of TGF-β and IL-6. Generation of $Foxp3^+$ inducible Treg cells is induced by TGF-β and RA produced by intestinal $CD103^+$ DCs in gut LP. RA has been characterized as a key regulator of the TGF-β-dependent immune response. IL-6 inhibits TGF-β-induced Foxp3 induction, resulting in Th17 cells, while RA can counteract this inhibition [36]. Suppression of Thl and Th17 cell response by Tregs is involved in prevention of inflammation.

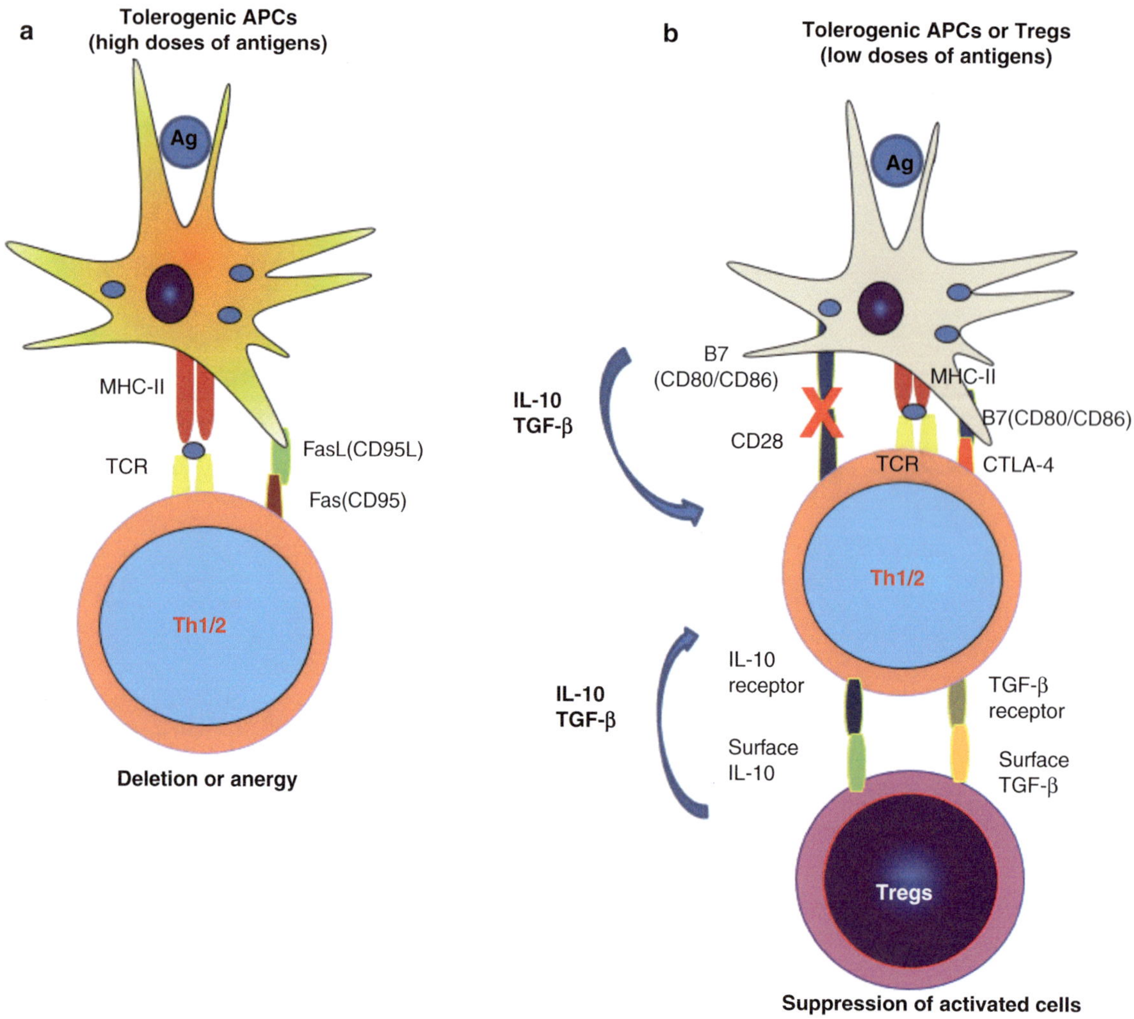

Fig. 13.6 Immunological mechanism implicated in immune tolerance is dependent on the dose of antigen. The generation of an immune response requires ligation of the T cell receptor (TCR) with peptide–MHC-II complexes whether with high dose of antigen or low dose without regulatory T cells (Tregs). (**a**) In oral tolerance induction by high-dose antigen, inhibitory ligations (Fas-Fas-L) lead to immune regulatory responses such as deletion and anergy of allergen-specific CD4+ Th2 cells. (**b**) In oral tolerance induction by repeated low dose of antigen, Tregs and/or tolerogenic antigen-presenting cells (APCs) are elicited. Ligation of cell surface T cell suppressive cytokines IL-10 and TGF-β by Tregs suppresses immune responses, which are maintained by production of soluble forms of these cytokines. Tolerogenic APCs lead to suppression of antigen-specific immune responses in the absence of B7-CD28 ligation

13.2.6 Efficacy of Rice-Based Allergy Vaccines

In a mouse model of Japanese cedar pollinosis, oral administration of the dominant T cell epitope of Cry j 2 inhibited specific T cell responses in Cry j 2-sensitized mice [37]. Sneezing frequency, as a measurable clinical symptom, was decreased not only by systemic injection but also by oral administration of the dominant T cell epitope of Cry j 2 [38]. The efficacy of oral transgenic rice seed that accumulated the major mouse T cell epitopes derived from Cry j 1 and Cry j 2 as fusion proteins with soybean seed protein glycinin was then examined by oral feeding [39] (Fig. 13.7a).

When systemically challenged with total protein of cedar pollens after daily administration for 4 weeks, the production of allergen-specific serum IgE and IgG antibodies was inhibited, when compared with mice fed with non-transgenic rice seeds (Fig. 13.7b). Both allergen-specific CD4+ T cell proliferative responses and levels of Th2 cytokines such as IL-4, IL-5, and IL-13 were inhibited (Fig. 13.7c). Histamine release from mast cells and sneezing, as measures of clinical symptoms of allergy, were also suppressed (Fig. 13.7d, e).

These results showed that a rice-based oral vaccine expressing T cell epitope peptides can induce oral tolerance against cedar pollen allergens and alleviate clinical symptoms prophylactically.

Based on this evidence, transgenic rice seed accumulating 7Crp peptide composed of human major T cell epitopes from Cry j 1 and Cry j 2 has been developed as a rice-based

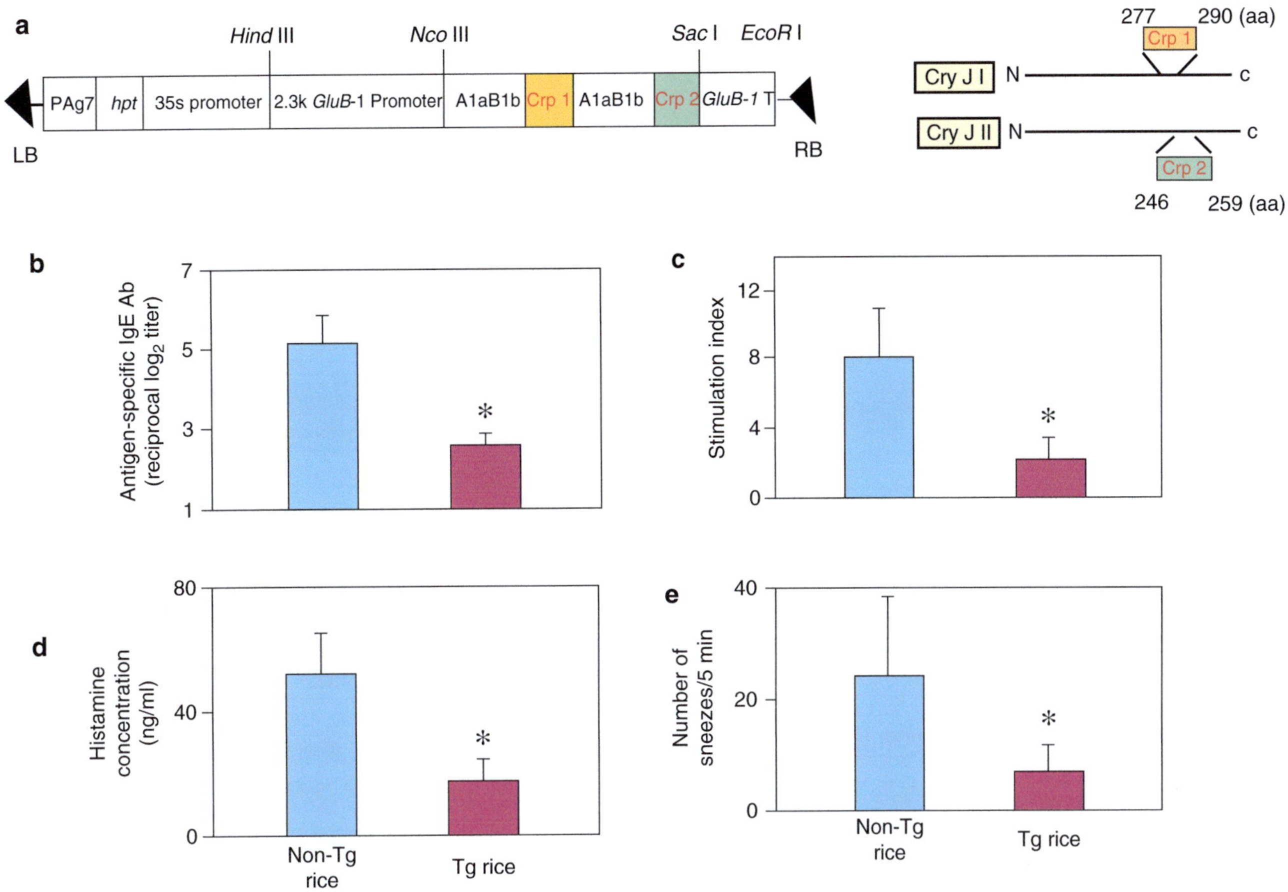

Fig. 13.7 Transgenic rice expressing T cell epitopes for Cry j 1 and Cry j 2 induces oral tolerance by inhibiting Th2-mediated IgE responses. Schematic representation of the transformation plasmid and the two selected major T cell epitopes of Cry j 1 and Cry j 2 (Crp 1 and Crp 2, respectively) (**a**). Inhibition of allergen-specific serum IgE (**b**) and CD4+ T cell responses (**c**) by oral administration of transgenic (Tg) rice seeds. Serum histamine levels (**d**) and the number of sneezes (**e**) were inhibited in the group of mice fed with Tg rice seeds. Data are expressed as mean ± SD. *, $p<0.01$ for the group of mice fed with Tg rice seeds (*blue*) in comparison with the group of mice fed with non-Tg rice seeds (*magenta*)

peptide vaccine for cedar pollen allergy in humans [40]. The 7Crp peptide was highly accumulated in transgenic rice seed (about 3 mg/g dry seed) and was deposited in ER-derived PBs suitable for delivery to GALT. To examine its safety, chronic toxicity and reproductive toxicity were examined by feeding transgenic rice seeds to monkeys and rats; no adverse effects were detected [41].

For HDM allergy, transgenic rice grains have been generated with accumulated mature Der p 1, from a Der p 1 fragment (p45-145) which covers most human and mice major T cell epitopes, and Der f 2 derivatives with reduced IgE reactivity resulting from disrupted intramolecular disulfide bonds [42]. The plant-derived Der p 1 was posttranslationally modified with a high-mannose-type glycan structure. Glycosylated Der p 1 displayed reduced IgE binding capacity in comparison with its unglycosylated counterpart (Fig. 13.8a).

Results. When mite allergen transgenic rice seeds containing the Der p 1 fragment (p45-145) were fed to mice that were subsequently immunized with recombinant Der p 1, allergen-specific CD4+ T cell proliferation (Fig. 13.8b) and production of allergen-specific IgE and IgG (Fig. 13.8c) were suppressed compared to mice fed non-transgenic rice seeds. Production of Th2 cytokines IL-4, IL-5, and IL-13 was also significantly diminished by oral vaccination of transgenic rice seeds (Fig. 13.8d). As measureable clinical symptoms, development of allergic airway inflammation by infiltration of eosinophils and lymphocytes into the airway (Fig. 13.8e) and bronchial hyperresponsiveness (Fig. 13.8f) were also inhibited by prophylactic vaccination with transgenic rice seeds.

When transgenic rice seeds containing Der f 2 derivatives were fed to mice, immune tolerance against Der f 2 antigen was induced in a similar way to other allergens. Interestingly, the inhibition of Der f 2-specific IgE and IgG production indicated that the efficacy of these derivatives was related to the resistance of Der f 2-containing PBs to digestive enzymes in the gastrointestinal tract.

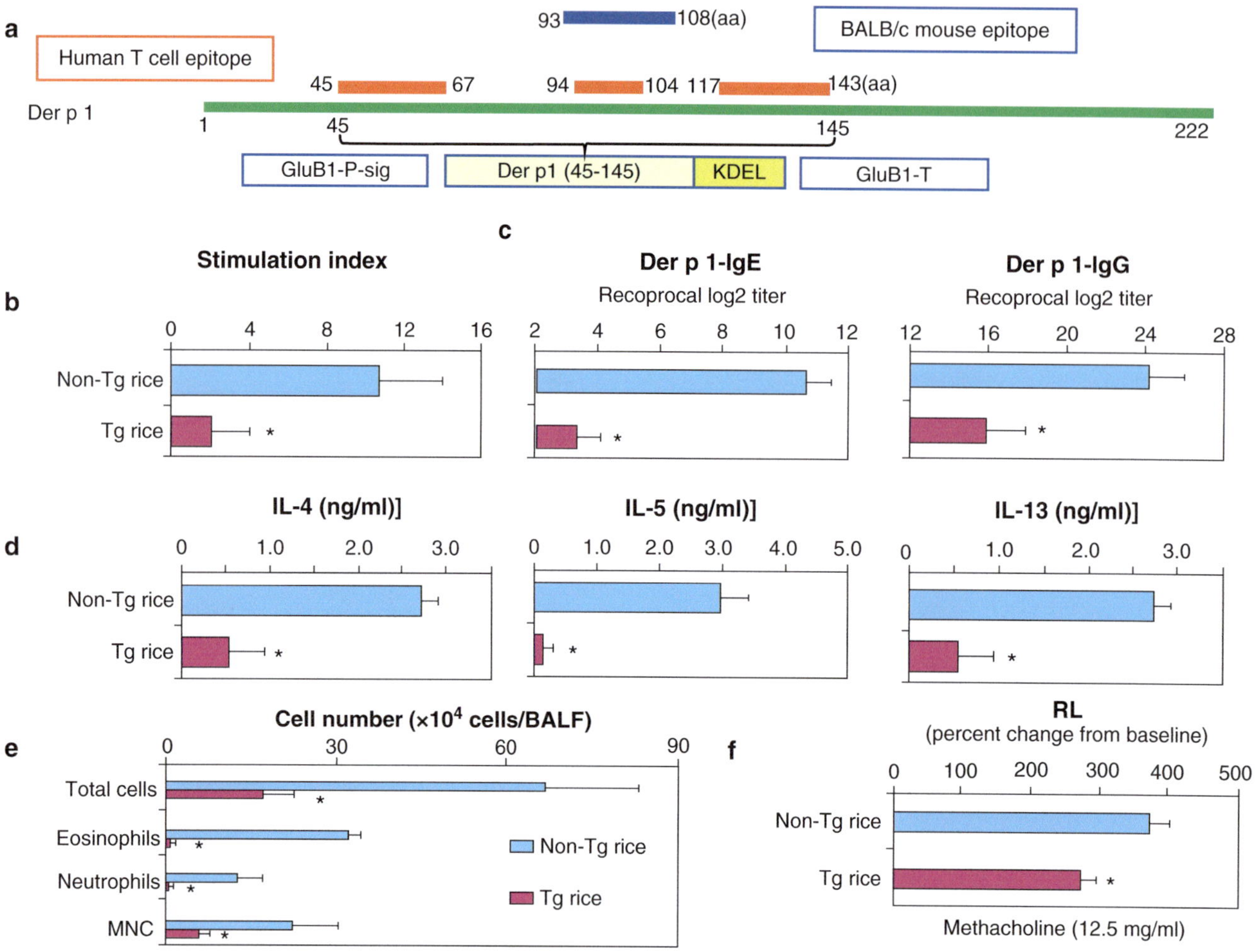

Fig. 13.8 Transgenic rice expressing T cell epitopes for Der p 1 induces oral tolerance by inhibiting Der p 1-specific immune responses. Schematic representation of the transformation plasmid and the selected major T cell epitope of Der p 1 (**a**). Splenic CD4$^+$ T cells prepared from negative control mice (data not shown), mice fed non-transgenic (Tg) rice (*magenta*), or mice fed Tg rice (*blue*) were cultured with irradiated normal splenocytes and allergen for 7 days and proliferative (stimulation) index measured (**b**). Oral administration of Tg rice seeds led to inhibition of allergen-specific (**b**) CD4$^+$ T cell proliferative responses and (**c**) serum IgE and IgG titers. Concentration of cytokines (IL-4, IL-5, and IL-13) released into the culture supernatant was assayed (**d**). Inhibition of allergen-induced inflammatory cell infiltration by prophylactic oral vaccination with Der p 1-Tg rice. The total number of cells and the number of eosinophils, neutrophils, and mononuclear cells (MNC) in the bronchoalveolar lavage fluid (BALF) was measured (**e**). Bronchial hyperresponsiveness to aerosolized methacholine (MCh) was measured 24 h after the second allergen challenge (**f**). Data are expressed as mean ± SD. *, $p<0.01$ for the group of mice fed with Tg rice seeds in comparison with the group of mice fed with non-Tg rice seeds

13.2.7 Perspectives

Production of vaccine antigens must conform with the specific guidelines and regulations for pharmaceutical products under conditions of good manufacturing practice (GMP) [43]. It is, therefore, necessary to develop reliable processing steps (purification) for each product. To date, plant-made vaccine candidates for parenteral delivery entering clinical trials have been mainly developed using transient expression systems by viral and *Agrobacterium* vectors. The downstream processing stage of production is generally expensive, representing up to 80 % of overall production costs.

Validation. It is important to note that direct oral vaccination using products of transgenic crops without any further processing is highly advantageous in terms of stability and efficient delivery to GALT, and as crop seeds containing antigen can be considered as oral formulations with a natural coating, they are appropriate vehicles for mucosal delivery. One possible obstacle will be validation of plant production systems for making a commercial pharmaceutical reagent. In addition, there are likely to be variations in accumulation of product due to physiological differences in biological systems.

Daily Oral Consumption. Closed molecular farming facilities (closed glasshouses) with strictly controlled environmental conditions would be ideal and are recommended to reduce variation of product concentration in targeted tissue as well as to prevent outcrossing. However, in the case of allergy vaccines, very large quantities of seeds will be required for

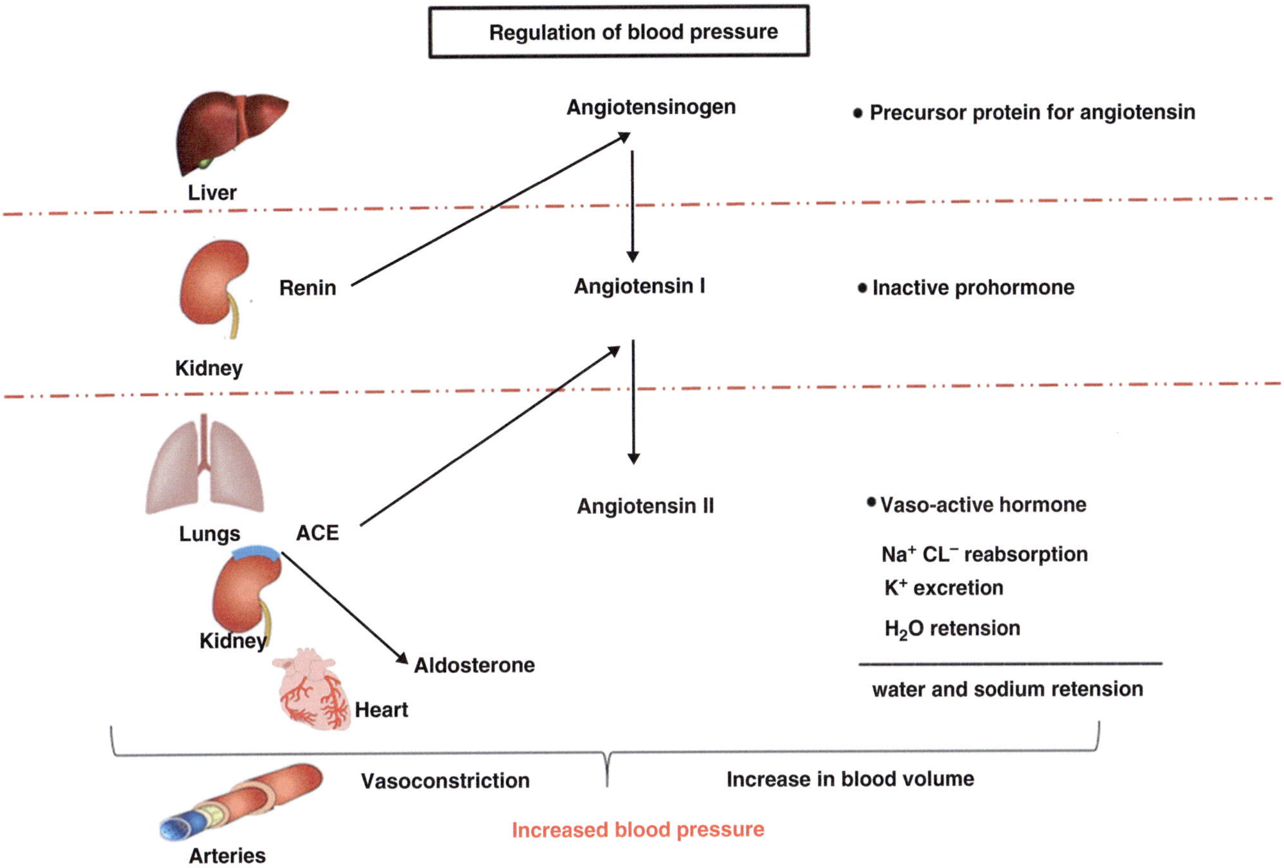

Fig. 13.9 The renin–angiotensin system (RAS) or the renin–angiotensin–aldosterone system (RAAS) is a hormone system that regulates blood pressure and fluid balance. Shortly: when blood volume is low, the kidneys secrete renin directly into circulation. Renin converts angiotensinogen released by the liver to angiotensin I. Angiotensin I is subsequently converted to angiotensin II by the liver enzyme angiotensin converting enzyme (ACE). Angiotensin II is a potent vasoactive peptide that causes blood vessels to constrict, resulting in increased blood pressure. Angiotensin II also stimulates the secretion of the hormone aldosterone from the adrenal cortex. Aldosterone induces the tubules of the kidneys to increase the reabsorption of sodium and water into the blood that will increase the volume of fluid in the body. This reabsorption also increases blood pressure (Figure by M. Giese Heidelberg/Germany)

commercialization. For example, daily oral consumption of cooked transgenic rice (about 70 g) for a minimum of 3 months and continuing for a number of years may be required for desensitization against cedar pollen allergens. Such transgenic rice will have to be produced for about 20 million patients afflicted with Japanese cedar pollinosis.

13.3 Hypertension and Vaccines[2]

13.3.1 Disease

Hypertension is a chronic medical condition characterized by elevation of blood pressure in the arterial system. Although hypertension is usually asymptomatic, it is a potent risk factor for cardiovascular diseases, such as stroke, myocardial infarction, heart failure, and end-stage renal disease.

It has been estimated that approximately 26.4 % of the adult population in the world had hypertension in 2000 [44]. The prevalence is projected to reach a value of 29.2 % by the year 2025. This is surprising, when we consider that a large number of new and effective antihypertensive agents have become widely available in recent years and the choice of drug classes available has increased dramatically during the past 30 years. Figure 13.9 gives an overview on the complex regulatory network of blood pressure.

Hypertension Paradox. The fact that prevalence of hypertension and its complications continues to increase in spite of many important advances in our knowledge of hypertension pathophysiology and treatment has been called the "hypertension paradox" [45].

One of the causes of this paradox is the problem of low rates of treatment and control of high blood pressure, which is often caused by low adherence to drug therapy. One of the countries with the greatest success rates for hypertension

[2]Vaccines for hypertension and atherosclerosis by *Hiroyuki Sasamura, Tasuhiko Azegami, and Hiroshi Itoh* in Molecular Vaccines – From Prophylaxis to Therapy, Volume 2, Springer-Verlag Wien, 2013, Ed. Matthias Giese.

control is the United States; even so, recent data indicate that approximately 20 % of Americans with hypertension are unaware of their condition, 28 % are not receiving therapy, and approximately half do not have their blood pressure controlled to recommended levels [46]. The data for other countries are generally much lower. For these reasons, new strategies to deal with the growing epidemic of hypertension are required.

13.3.2 Conventional Therapy

Systemic blood pressure is determined by the product of cardiac output and total peripheral resistance. Both cardiac output and total peripheral resistance are finely controlled by multiple mechanisms involving the kidney, the endocrine system, the central nervous system, and the vasculature. One of the important endocrine regulators of blood pressure is the renin–angiotensin system (RAS) [47].

Renin and Angiotensinogen. Renin is a proteolytic enzyme that is synthesized in the juxtaglomerular apparatus (JGA) of the kidney and stored in intracellular granules. During states of low blood pressure, renin is secreted from the JGA cells and enters the circulation. Angiotensinogen, which is the physiological substrate of renin, is a glycoprotein that is synthesized in the liver and enters the blood stream.

Angiotensin I. After proteolytic cleavage by renin, a 10-amino acid peptide (angiotensin I) is formed. This is then converted to the 8-peptide angiotensin II after interaction with angiotensin converting enzyme (ACE) which is located primarily in endothelial cells.

Angiotensin II. Angiotensin II acts on multiple target organs, including the vasculature, heart, kidney, adrenal, and central nervous system. The effects to increase blood pressure are mediated almost exclusively by the G-protein-coupled angiotensin type 1 (AT1) receptor. In contrast, the AT2 receptor has predominantly antagonistic effects to the AT1 receptor and may act to decrease blood pressure.

RAS. The importance of the RAS in blood pressure control has been confirmed by the efficacy of RAS inhibitors not only for the control of blood pressure but also for the reduction of hypertensive complications, including cardiovascular disease and stroke [48]. Although many other regulatory systems other than the RAS contribute importantly to the pathophysiology of hypertension, the importance of RAS derives from the fact that inhibition of RAS is a safe and effective method to decrease hypertension in humans. It is therefore easy to understand why the RAS is the main target for attempts to produce effective vaccines for hypertension (Fig. 13.10).

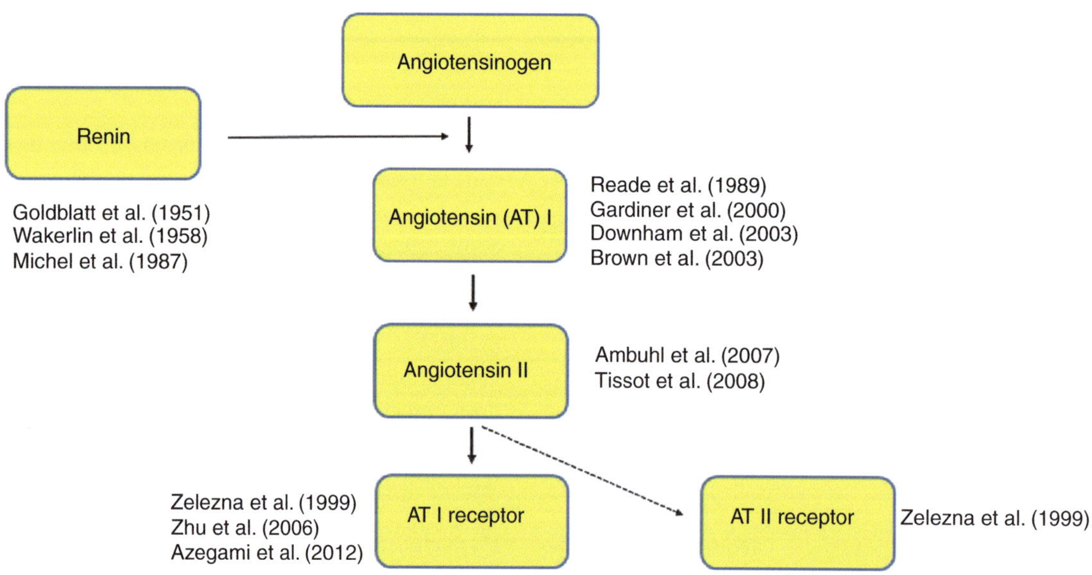

Fig. 13.10 Overview of the renin–angiotensin system and major targets (*yellow*) for hypertension vaccines, published from 1951 to 2012

13.3.3 Development of Vaccine for Hypertension

13.3.3.1 Heterologous Renin Vaccine

The first clinical study to attempt immunization against the RAS for the treatment of hypertension was reported by Goldblatt et al. in 1951 [49]. In this study, the authors injected heterologous (hog) renin into patients with severe hypertension and examined the effects on antirennin titers and blood pressures. Their paper describes the results in 8 patients, who were given between 7 and 66 injections (28,000–142,000 units) of hog renin over a period of 3.5–33 weeks. Almost all patients developed detectable increases in serum antirennin antibodies. However, no significant decrease in blood pressure was detectable in these patients, and the authors concluded that this could be because the renin administered was of hog origin and not human. Since there is species specificity in the actions of renin, the production of antibodies to heterologous renin may not affect the actions of native human renin.

Nephritis. Further studies were performed using animal models. In 1987, Michel et al. reported the results of using pure human renin to immunize marmosets [50]. Three subcutaneous injections of 30 μg each of pure renin protein resulted in a high titer of renin antibodies.

Furthermore, blood pressure was significantly reduced from 125 ± 13 to 87 ± 8 mmHg, together with significant decreases in plasma renin activity and plasma aldosterone. However, the authors found that the marmosets also developed immunological renal disease, characterized by the presence of immunoglobulin and macrophage infiltration co-localizing with renin in the kidney [48]. Similarly, when spontaneously hypertensive rats (SHRs) were immunized with purified mouse submandibular renin, the systolic blood pressure was significantly decreased; however, the authors again found that the kidneys of renin-immunized SHR showed a chronic autoimmune interstitial nephritis associated with the renin-producing JGA cells of the kidney [51].

These experiments on renin immunization were performed using the whole renin protein as the immunogen. It has been suggested that the large size of renin may have facilitated the development of autoimmune disease and the fact that renin production occurs at only one anatomic site may have resulted in localized accumulation of antibodies [52].

13.3.3.2 PMD3117 Vaccine

Consequently, the target for vaccination against the RAS shifted to the angiotensin peptide itself. After performing preliminary studies in rats and humans, Brown et al. performed a clinical randomized double-blind placebo-controlled study of a vaccine against angiotensin I (PMD3117) in patients with essential hypertension. In their protocol, patients were given either 3 doses of 100 μg of peptide equivalent vaccine at 21-day intervals, or 4 doses at 14-day intervals, and blood pressure changes were estimated as the differences in the pre- and postvaccination rise in 24 h ambulatory blood pressure after 2 weeks of withdrawal of ACE inhibitors or ARB between the active vaccine and placebo. Although the authors found significant changes in plasma renin and urine aldosterone, they did not detect a significant difference in blood pressure between the active vaccine- and placebo-treated groups [53].

13.3.3.3 CYT006-AngQb Vaccine

The next important breakthrough for angiotensin II vaccines was the development of new virus-like particle (VLP) technology. The VLPs are macromolecular assemblies formed from bacteriophage coat protein monomers, which spontaneously assemble in a capsid structure. The angiotensin peptide was fused at its N-terminus to a CGG spacer sequence and conjugated to VLP. Using this vaccine (AngQb), Ambuhl et al. examined the effects of subcutaneous administration of angiotensin II vaccine first in a rat model (SHR) and then in healthy human volunteers [54].

Next, Tissot et al. performed a multicenter, double-blind, placebo-controlled phase IIa trial of the efficacy of the AngQb vaccine in 72 patients with mild to moderate hypertension. Patients were randomized to receive either 100 μg vaccine, 300 μg vaccine, or placebo, at weeks 0 and 4, and 12. 24 h ambulatory blood pressure was measured before treatment and at week 14. When the mean ambulatory daytime blood pressures were compared, the authors found a significant decrease of 9 mmHg in the systolic blood pressure ($p = 0.015$), with a similar trend for diastolic blood pressure (4 mmHg reduction, $p = 0.064$) in the 300 μg group. Furthermore, the 300 μg vaccine reduced the early morning blood pressure surge compared with placebo (25 mmHg reduction in systolic blood pressure ($p < 0.0001$) and 13 mmHg reduction in diastolic blood pressure ($p = 0.0035$)) [55] (Fig. 13.11). A significant increase in mild, transient reactions at the injection site was found, and a total of 10 participants reported mild, transient influenza-like symptoms. The study by Tissot et al. can be considered a landmark study, because it was the first study to show that vaccination can reduce blood pressure in humans.

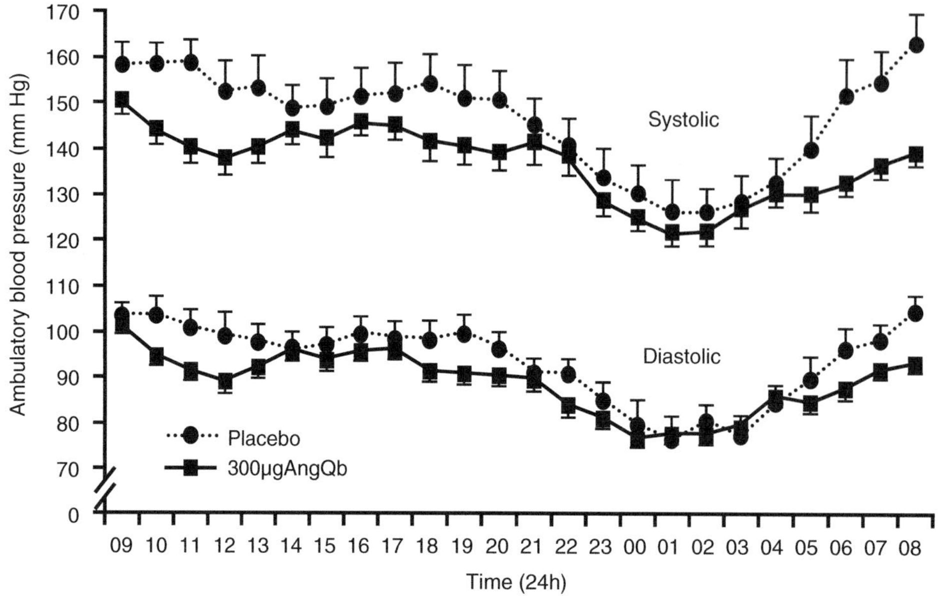

Fig. 13.11 Effects of injection with angiotensin II vaccine (AngQb) or placebo on 24 h ambulatory blood pressure profiles in patients with mild-to-moderate hypertension (From Tissot et al. [55] with permission)

13.3.3.4 AT1 Receptor Vaccine

Several groups have focused on the angiotensin type 1 (AT1 receptor) as a potential future target for the development of vaccines for hypertension and hypertensive complications [56]. One of the theoretical advantages of the AT1 receptor vaccine over the angiotensin II vaccine is that direct inhibition at the receptor level may result in more complete suppression of the RAS and enhanced effectiveness of the vaccine. Furthermore, unlike the angiotensin II vaccine which blocks the action of angiotensin II at both AT1 and AT2 receptors, specific blockade of the AT1 receptor does not affect the actions of angiotensin II at the AT2 receptor, and this may be an advantage for organ protection.

The group of Itoh synthesized a seven-amino acid peptide sequence corresponding to amino acids 181–187 in the second extracellular loop of rat AT1a receptor (AFHYESR) first described by Zhu et al. [57] and conjugated it to the carrier protein Keyhole Limpet Hemocyanin (KLH) (Fig. 13.12). In preliminary experiments, the effects of 1, 3, and 6 injections of vaccine on blood pressure and AT1 receptor antibody titers in the spontaneously hypertensive rat, a rodent model of essential hypertension [5], were compared. A single injection of the AT1 vaccine caused increased antibody titers, but these levels were significantly lower than the titers produced by 3 or 6 injections. In contrast, both 3 and 6 injections of AT1 vaccine produced comparable increases in AT1 antibody titers and significant decreases in the blood pressure.

Also the effects of the AT1 receptor vaccine on the development of renal injury, using the NO (nitric oxide) synthase inhibitor L-NAME, were investigated. Previous studies have shown that the use of L-NAME results in renal injury, including proteinuria and glomerular and renal vascular injury [58]. Rats, however, given 3 injections of the AT1 receptor vaccines had a significant suppression of proteinuria after L-NAME administration. Moreover, histological indicators of renal injury were significantly suppressed in the AT1 receptor vaccine group, similar to the results found in rats treated continuously with the ARB candesartan, suggesting that vaccination against the RAS may be effective not only for the attenuation of hypertension but also for the prevention of hypertensive renal injury.

13.3.4 Perspectives

The study by Tissot et al. demonstrated the proof of concept that patients with hypertension could be treated by vaccination against a vasoactive substance. Three injections of angiotensin vaccine resulted in an increase of antibody titers

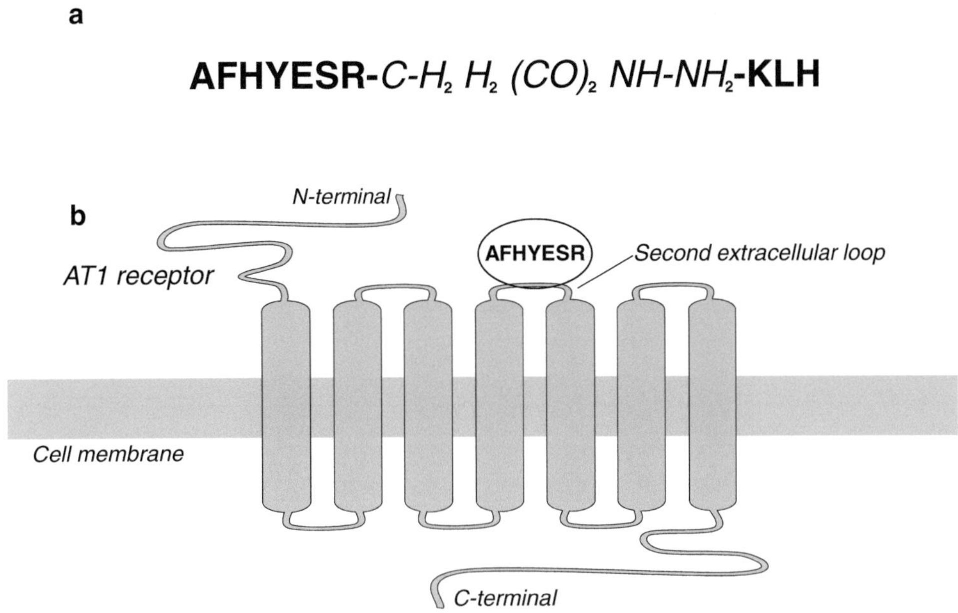

Fig. 13.12 (**a**) Structure of the KLH-conjugated AT1 receptor peptide sequence used in our studies on hypertension and atherosclerosis. (**b**) Structure of angiotensin type 1 (AT1) receptor and localization of the peptide sequence in the second extracellular loop of the receptor

over several months with an average half-life of about 4 months after the third injection. This half-life could be compatible with a treatment regimen of several injections per year. Such treatment could be very attractive for increasing adherence to hypertension therapy, which currently requires daily and life-long medication.

Although these results are encouraging, there are many caveats when considering the vaccine approach as a strategy for the treatment of hypertension. First, multiple antihypertensive agents are already available; therefore, it is possible to question the importance of the development of hypertension vaccines. On the other hand, the fact that the prevalence of hypertension and hypertensive complications is increasing despite the availability of these medications suggests that new approaches to hypertension treatment should be considered and the risk/benefit of the vaccine approach compared to other strategies.

Safety Issues. An important concern is that the effects of vaccine therapy may be irreversible and result in hypotension, particularly during states of salt and volume depletion, where an active RAS contributes to survival. Other important safety issues including the potential for developing stimulatory as well as inhibitory antibodies, as well as the risk of developing autoimmune disease, was reported in the renin-immunized animal models.

Although no major adverse effects related to vaccination were reported in the study by Tissot et al., local injection site-related erythema was found in all groups including the placebo group. It is possible that such local reactions could be avoided by using alternative vaccination routes (e.g., by oral or nasal vaccines). Because hypertension itself is asymptomatic, it is important that vaccines for hypertension should have minimal side effects, if they are to be developed for routine clinical use.

13.4 Atherosclerosis and Vaccines[3]

13.4.1 Disease

Atherosclerosis is predominantly a disease of the medium to large arteries and is characterized by the presence of lipid-containing plaques in the vessel wall, eventually resulting in luminal narrowing and susceptibility to plaque rupture and lumen thrombosis. Atherosclerosis is directly responsible for the major syndromes of cardiovascular disease, including stroke, angina pectoris, myocardial infarction, aneurysmal

[3]Vaccines for hypertension and atherosclerosis by *Hiroyuki Sasamura, Tasuhiko Azegami and Hiroshi Itoh* in Molecular Vaccines – From Prophylaxis to Therapy, Volume 2, Springer-Verlag Wien, 2013, Ed. Matthias Giese.

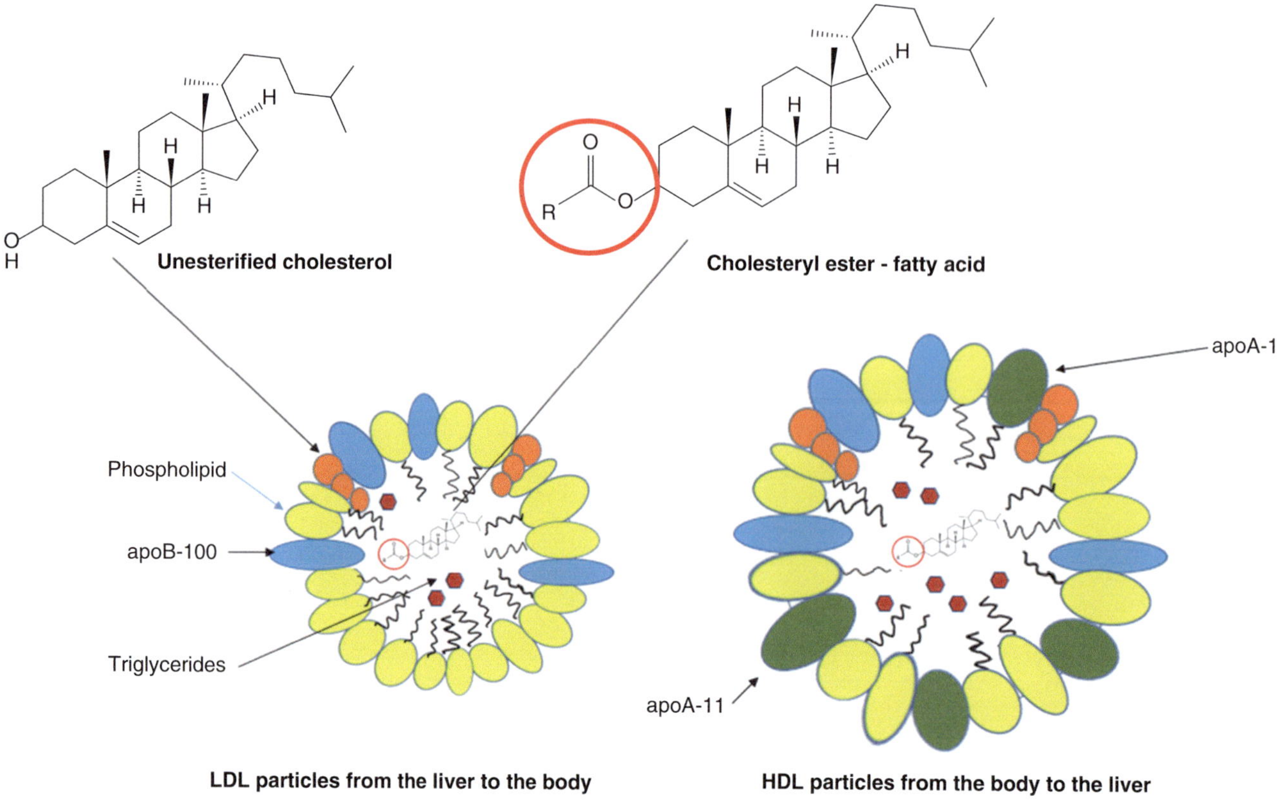

Fig. 13.13 Cholesterol is an essential structural component of all animal (not plant or bacterial) cell membranes and therefore biosynthesized by all cells. Cholesterol is only slightly soluble in water and transported in blood inside lipoproteins, low-density lipoproteins (LDL). LDL particles are the major blood cholesterol and cholesteryl ester carriers. Apolipoprotein B-100 (apoB) is the primary apolipoprotein of LDL and ligand for activation of the LDL receptor. LDLs carry cholesterol from the liver to the cells in the body, whereas high-density lipoproteins (HDL) carry the cholesterol back to the liver. HDL contains "A-1" and "A-11" lipoproteins. ApoA proteins promote inter alia fat efflux from tissues to the liver. HDL molecules are larger than LDL molecules (Figure by M. Giese Heidelberg/Germany)

disease, and peripheral artery disease, and is therefore a major cause of morbidity and mortality throughout the world.

Risk Factors. Multiple risk factors are known to increase the susceptibility to atherosclerosis. One of the most important is age, and atherosclerosis in some form is known to occur as part of the aging process. However, increased risk is also associated with hypercholesterolemia, hypertension, diabetes, obesity, and male gender.

13.4.2 Conventional Therapy

Although the association of atherosclerosis with high cholesterol levels has been well recognized, recent studies have shown that atherosclerosis is essentially a chronic inflammatory disease, mediated by a complex interaction between the endothelial cells and smooth muscle cells of the vessel wall with multiple immunomodulatory cells [59].

Oxidized LDL. Cholesterol is transported in the bloodstream in association with a family of apolipoproteins to form lipoproteins. An important lipoprotein for the pathogenesis of atherosclerosis is the low-density lipoprotein (LDL), which can accumulate in the arterial intima, where it is susceptible to oxidative modification into oxidized LDL. Oxidized LDL is known to cause damage to arterial walls and triggers a complex series of reactions resulting in inflammation and immune cell activation in the vessel wall (Fig. 13.13).

Foam Cells. Important components of the immune response to oxidized LDL-associated vascular wall injury include macrophages, monocytes, leukocytes, dendritic cells, and T cells. In particular, the macrophages ingest the oxidized LDL and turn into foam cells, enlarging in size until they eventually rupture, and cause further deposition of oxidized LDL, resulting in a vicious cycle with further recruitment of immunomodulatory cells (Fig. 13.14).

The inflammatory process occurring in the arteries results in the activation of multiple cytokines, growth factors, and other vasoactive compounds. These contribute to smooth muscle cell proliferation and invasion, deposition of collagen and other extracellular matrix proteins, and formation of the fibrous cap which can rupture and cause thrombosis.

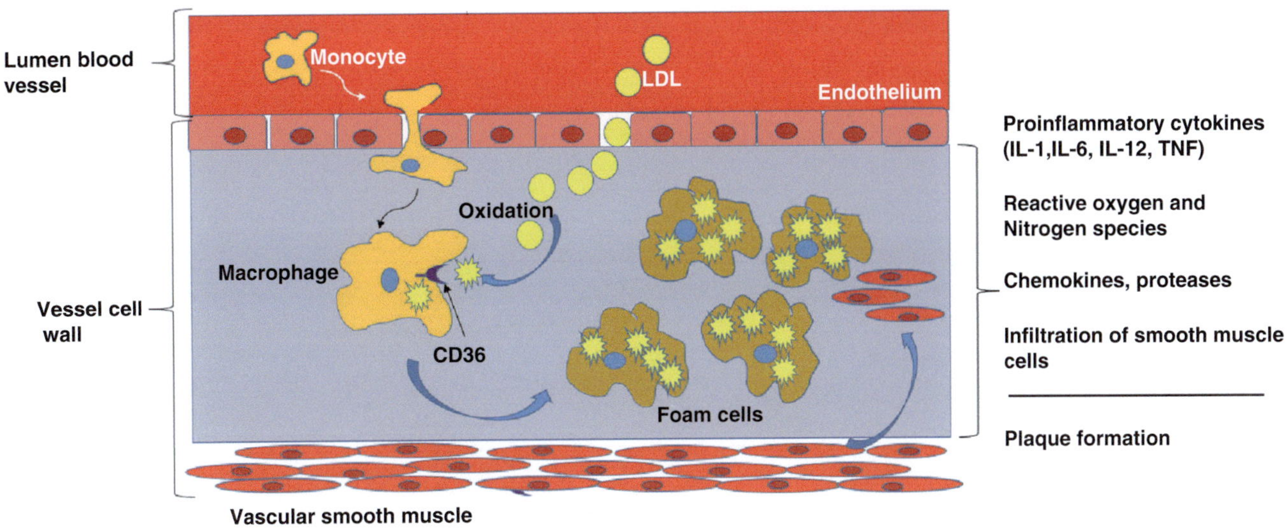

Fig. 13.14 Low-density lipoprotein (LDL) carrying cholesterol has long been recognized in the development of atherosclerosis. Modified LDL, such as oxidized LDL (oxLDL), provokes inflammation and infiltrates into the cell wall. Hereupon monocytes migrate into the cell wall to uptake oxLDL through their scavenger receptors (CD36). Because macrophages are unable to degrade LDL, cholesterol intracellulary accumulates and leads to the formation of foam cells (cholesterol-laden macrophages). Accumulated cholesterol can activate the inflammasome, leading to the release of pro-inflammatory cytokines, reactive oxygen and nitrogen species, chemokines, proteases, and other molecules. Modified LDL particles can also bind to TLRs (TLR1, TLR2, TLR4) and thus activate the expression of specific pro-inflammatory genes (Figure by M. Giese Heidelberg/ Germany)

Current therapy of atherosclerosis starts with non-pharmaceutical interventions aimed at changing lifestyles. These are aimed at reducing the risk factors for atherosclerosis development and include changes such as dietary modifications, cessation of smoking, weight control, and increased exercise.

The pharmaceutical intervention for which there is the greatest clinical evidence for both primary and secondary prevention is the use of HMG-CoA reductase inhibitors (statins), which reduce serum cholesterol levels by inhibiting the pathway of cholesterol production in the liver. Other agents for which there is evidence for secondary prevention of cardiovascular events include nicotinic acid (niacin) and antiplatelet agents. Furthermore, treatment with RAS inhibitors may have a beneficial effect beyond their antihypertensive effect.

13.4.3 Vaccines for Atherosclerosis

Similar to vaccines for hypertension, the history of development of vaccines for atherosclerosis has a long history. Although vaccines for hypertension have focused predominantly on the RAS, in the case of vaccines for atherosclerosis, multiple targets in different cells have become candidates for atherosclerosis vaccine and immunomodulatory treatments (Fig. 13.15).

13.4.3.1 LDL Vaccines

One of the earliest approaches for inhibition of atherosclerosis was the use of immunization with beta-lipoprotein reported by Gero et al. in 1959 [60]. Subsequent studies examined the effects of immunization with LDL and its derivatives. Palinski et al. examined the effects of immunization of hypercholesterolemic rabbits with malondialdehyde-modified LDL and found a significant reduction in the extent of atherosclerotic lesions [61]. Ameli et al. reported a similar effect using immunization with homologous LDL, with a smaller (nonsignificant) effect using oxidized LDL [62]. These results have been replicated in other studies [63].

ApoB-100 is the main protein component of LDL, and oxidation of LDL results in degradation of apoB into smaller fragments which are further modified by reactive aldehydes. It has been suggested by Nilsson et al. that vaccines based on apoB peptide antigens may be an important candidate for the development of vaccines for atherosclerosis [64]. Fredrikson et al. examined the effects of immunization with apoB-100 peptide sequences on the development of atherosclerotic lesions in hypercholesterolemic mice and found a 60 % reduction in atherosclerosis [65]. Interestingly, it was later shown that an anti-atherogenic effect could be found in the absence of an increase in peptide-specific IgG, suggesting the contribution of cellular immune responses in the atheroprotective effect [66].

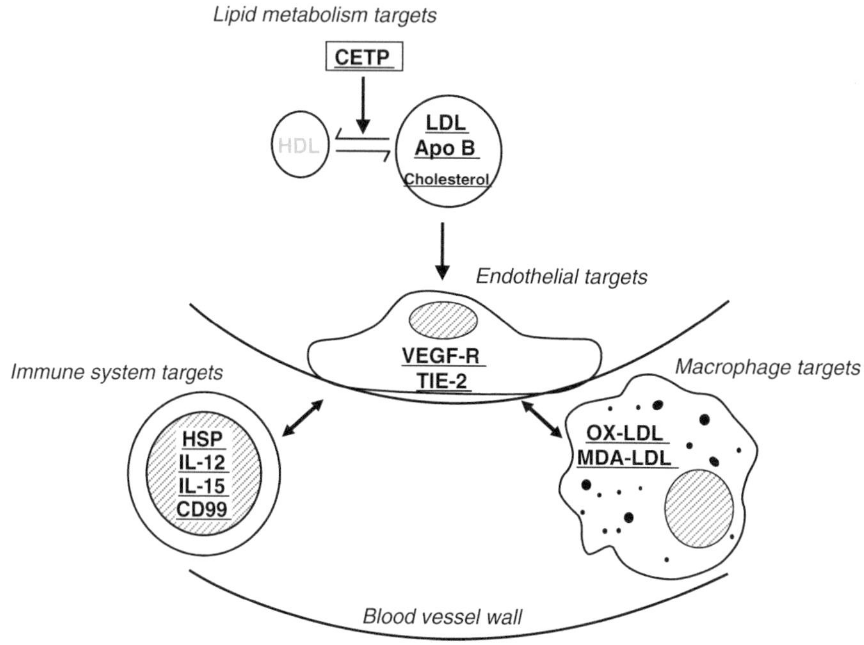

Fig. 13.15 Simplified overview of major targets for atherosclerosis vaccines/immune therapy (vaccine targets are *underlined*)

13.4.3.2 CETP Vaccine

Another approach has been the development of vaccines against cholesteryl ester transfer protein, which is involved in the regulation of the balance of HDL and LDL [67]. Rittershaus et al. immunized rabbits with a peptide containing a region of CETP known to be required for neutral lipid transfer function. They found that HDL levels were increased and LDL levels decreased in the vaccinated rabbits fed with a high cholesterol diet. They also found a 39.6 % reduction in the aortic atherosclerotic area [68]. In a phase I human trial, the same group found that 8 out of 15 subjects (53 %) developed anti-CETP antibodies after two injections, without major side effects. A subsequent phase 2 clinical trial on patients with low HDL levels confirmed that the vaccine was well tolerated and produced anti-CETP antibodies in greater than 90 % of patients and that the % increase in HDL was correlated with the peak antibody titer.

DNA and DC Vaccines. Newer approaches for the development of vaccines for atherosclerosis include the use of DNA vaccines and dendritic cell-based strategies. In the study by Mao et al., hypercholesterolemic rabbits were immunized intramuscularly with plasmids containing an epitope of CETP C-terminal fragment, as well as immunomodulatory CpG sequences, and a marked (80 %) reduction in atherosclerotic plaque lesions was found [69]. Beneficial results have also been reported for DNA vaccination strategies targeting cytokines and growth factors such as IL-15 [70], CD99 [71], TIE2 [72], and VEGFR-2 [73]. Another experimental approach is the use of dendritic cells to induce a specific humoral immune response. Favorable results have been reported for dendritic cells pulsed with oxidized LDL [74] or apoB-100 [75].

The group of Itoh has recently examined the effects of vaccination against the AT1 receptor on the development of atherosclerosis in ApoE-deficient mice fed with a high-fat and high-salt diet. Preliminary results suggest that the use of this vaccine targeting the AT1 receptor not only results in decrease in the Sudan Red-positive atherosclerotic area in the aorta in this model but also an attenuation of albuminuria. Previous studies from other laboratories have suggested that RAS inhibition with drugs can attenuate atherosclerosis by multiple mechanisms, including decreased vascular pro-inflammatory response, decreased retention of atherosclerotic lipoproteins, and increased lipid release [76].

Mucosal Immunization. Also the use of oral and nasal mucosal immunization strategies, as a method to induce tolerance and immune unresponsiveness to proatherogenic antigens, was investigated. One of the most studied are heat shock proteins (HSPs), which are thought to be involved in proatherogenic immune-mediated responses. Harats et al. and Maron et al. examined the effects of oral or nasal immunization with HSP 65 in mouse models, and both groups found an attenuation of atherosclerosis [77, 78]. Similarly, van Puijvelde et al. reported that oral administration of HSP60 or a HSP60 peptide to atherosclerotic mice resulted in induction of oral tolerance and a significant reduction in the atherosclerotic plaque size [79]. On the other hand, Yuan et al. reported that intranasal immunization of a DNA vaccine directed toward CETP resulted in a significant anti-CETP IgG response which lasted for 28 weeks and a significant decrease in atherogenesis [80, 81].

In a small-scale clinical study, Bourinbaiar et al. examined the effects of administration of a tablet containing pooled antigens derived from pig adipose tissue to 13 volunteers over 3 months [82]. They reported an increase in HDL-C levels in 12 out of 13 patients and a significant reduction in waist, midarm, and thigh circumferences.

13.4.4 Perspectives

The major challenge in developing a vaccine against atherosclerosis for widespread clinical use is the difficulty of performing clinical studies of sufficient length and in sufficient numbers of patients to enable conclusions about the safety and efficacy of the vaccine treatment.

In the case of hypertension, it is possible to design a clinical protocol with a time scale of weeks or months. In contrast, the development of atherosclerosis occurs over years or even decades, and accurate assessment of atherosclerosis may require expensive and invasive methods such as angiography or intravascular ultrasound. The use of biomarkers as surrogate markers is one way to circumvent this problem, but their predictive ability for hard endpoint markers is still limited at present.

13.5 Obesity Treatment and Vaccines[4]

13.5.1 Disease

Obesity is defined as a medical condition characterized by accumulation of excess body fat to the extent that it may have adverse effects on health [83].

The body mass index (BMI), calculated by the ratio of weight (kg) for the square of height (m^2), is a measurement tool routinely used in the clinic to diagnose overweight and obesity, which in spite of providing no information concerning body fat distribution, with few exceptions, correlates well with the percentage of body fat. Body mass index defines people as normal weight if their BMI is between 18.5 and 24.9 kg/m^2, overweight if their BMI is between 25 and 29.9 kg/m^2, and obese when it is greater than 30 kg/m [84].

Obesity is most often the result of a combination of excessive food energy intake and a lack of physical activity in genetically predisposed individuals. Only a limited number of cases are due primarily to monogenetic causes; endocrine disorders, such as Cushing syndrome and hypothyroidism; or previous use of drugs that cause weight gain.

Chronic Disease. Obesity is a chronic disease, as evidenced by the high likelihood of weight regain after weight loss attained by medical therapies, and therefore, there is a need for a long-term approach to the disease [85]. However, clinicians have few tools to fight obesity. Diet and exercise are still the cornerstones for obesity treatment, and current anti-obesity drugs achieve only relative short-term weight loss and are often followed by weight regain.

The available weight loss treatments include different combinations of diet, exercise, behavioral modification, and pharmacotherapy. Many diets with different macronutrient composition have demonstrated efficacy in weight loss, and even though there is currently no evidence that clearly supports a superiority of a single dietary approach above the other diets used for weight loss, the degree of adherence to the prescribed calorie reduction appears to be the most important determinant of success. Physical activity is also a valuable aid for weight loss; however, it is even more important for weight maintenance once weight loss is achieved.

13.5.2 Conventional Therapy

Pharmacotherapy for obesity includes drugs that can either suppress appetite or alter nutrient absorption, with the purpose of inducing weight loss.

These drugs generally are capable to induce 5–10 % weight loss, the minimum requirement for a drug to be approved for weight loss by the regulatory authorities such as the Food and Drug Administration (FDA) and the European Medicines Agency (EMA). In addition to weight reduction, these drugs should provide a good safety profile and beneficial actions on several cardiovascular risk factors [86]. Even when there is only a modest weight loss and the patient does not reach a normal body weight, these are able to confer health benefits to the patient and improvement of obesity comorbidities. Weight loss in people suffering from obesity is associated to a reduction in low-density lipoprotein cholesterol, total cholesterol, and blood pressure, with decreased risk of development of type 2 diabetes, and may be beneficial for cardiovascular disease in the long-term.

Appetite Suppressant Drugs. At the present, there are two anti-obesity drug classes available in the market approved by the FDA, appetite suppressors and the lipase inhibitor orlistat, of which the former is the only drug authorized by EMA and marketed in Europe. Appetite suppressant drugs include the central nervous system stimulants, such as phentermine, phendimetrazine, and diethylpropion. Phentermine is the

[4]Anti-ghrelin therapeutic vaccine a novel approach for obesity treatment by *Sara Andrade, Marcos Carreira, Felipe F. Casanueva, Polly Roy, and Mariana P. Monteiro* in Molecular Vaccines – From Prophylaxis to Therapy, Volume 2, Springer-Verlag Wien, 2013, Ed. Matthias Giese.

most widely used drug for weight loss, owing to the fact of being in the US market for decades and to its low cost. Phentermine hydrochloride is a noradrenergic sympathetic amine approved for the short-term treatment of obesity. Phentermine belongs to a class of drugs that stimulate the central nervous system and conveys a response of "fight or flight" which blocks the feeding drive and induces anorexia. The most common side effects associated with phentermine include insomnia, irritability, and increase in blood pressure. Sibutramine and rimonabant are another two appetite suppressant drugs that were recently withdrawn from the market due to safety concerns, after suspension being recommended due to cardiovascular and psychiatric side effects, respectively.

Orlistat. Orlistat is a lipase inhibitor that prevents hydrolysis of dietary triglycerides and consequently prevents the absorption of dietary fat that is excreted unaltered by the gastrointestinal tract. The drug is widely available and approved for long-term use; nevertheless, it produces only a modest weight loss and is associated with high rates of gastrointestinal side effects, such as steatorrhea, fecal incontinence, and flatulence [87].

Topiramate. The FDA has recently approved two new drugs that will be available in the market in near future, which are lorcaserin, a selective 5-hydroxytryptamine receptor 2c agonist [88], and a combination of phentermine and topiramate [89]. Topiramate is a sulfamate-substituted monosaccharide marketed since 1996 and formerly approved by the FDA for seizure disorders and prevention of migraine headaches. Topiramate, among other drugs for which previous clinical trials data suggested that could promote weight loss as a side effect of their therapeutic usage, was used off-label as adjuvant therapy in obesity treatment, along with the antidepressives, fluoxetine, sertraline, and bupropion, and the antidiabetic drug, metformin [90].

Bariatric Surgery. For morbid obesity, the surgical approach, termed bariatric surgery, is the only therapy that provides sustainable weight reduction [91]. In 1992, the National Institutes of Health Consensus Development Conference, in a position statement, affirmed the superiority of surgical over nonsurgical approaches in this condition. Bariatric surgery is reserved for patients in whom medical weight loss treatments are known to fail and have not shown long-term effectiveness, namely, in patients with BMI > 40 kg/m^2 or >35 kg/m^2 associated with high-risk comorbid conditions.

In severe obesity, surgical treatments, by decreasing the risk for development of new obesity-associated comorbidities and improving the existing ones, are also more cost-effective at producing and maintaining weight loss. Obesity surgery provides a significant risk reduction for development of new health-related conditions, namely, cardiovascular, cancer, endocrine (including diabetes mellitus and hypertension), respiratory, musculoskeletal, infectious, psychiatric, and mental disorders.

Weight loss, after bariatric surgery, usually results in improvement or resolution of multiple medical conditions that eliminates the use of medications and absenteeism from work in patients who were previously morbidly obese. When compared to matched controls, the patients submitted to surgery display a significant reduction in health-care use rates and total direct health-care costs. Bariatric surgery also significantly decreases overall 5-year mortality rate, with a reduction in the relative risk of death of 89 % compared to controls.

13.5.3 Regulation of Food Intake and Energy Homeostasis

The physiological systems that regulate energy homeostasis include brain centers, such as the hypothalamus, brainstem, and reward centers in the limbic system, which regulate food intake and energy expenditure through the secretion of neuropeptides. These centers are modulated by neural and hormonal signals coming from the periphery. Hormones synthesized by the adipose tissue, like leptin, reflect the long-term nutritional status of the body and are able to influence long-term body weight regulation, while gastrointestinal hormones, like ghrelin, peptide tyrosine tyrosine (PYY), and glucagon-like peptide 1 (GLP-1) among several other hormones, modulate these pathways acutely and are able to regulate food intake and energy expenditure [92] (Fig. 13.16).

ARC and PVN. In the hypothalamus, the most important food intake-regulating nuclei are located, the arcuate (ARC) and the paraventricular nuclei (PVN). The ARC of the basal hypothalamus receives signals from the periphery and plays an integrative role in appetite regulation. The ARC projects second-order neurons to the PVN, which is involved in the regulation of visceral efferent activity. In the ARC, there are two well-characterized neuronal populations involved, one appetite stimulating that co-expresses neuropeptide Y and Agouti-related protein (NPY/AgRP) and another appetite inhibiting that co-expresses proopiomelanocortin and cocaine- and amphetamine-regulated transcript (POMC/CART) [93] (Fig. 13.17).

13.5.4 Ghrelin

Ghrelin is a gastrointestinal hormone that promotes food intake and decreases energy expenditure [94]. Ghrelin is

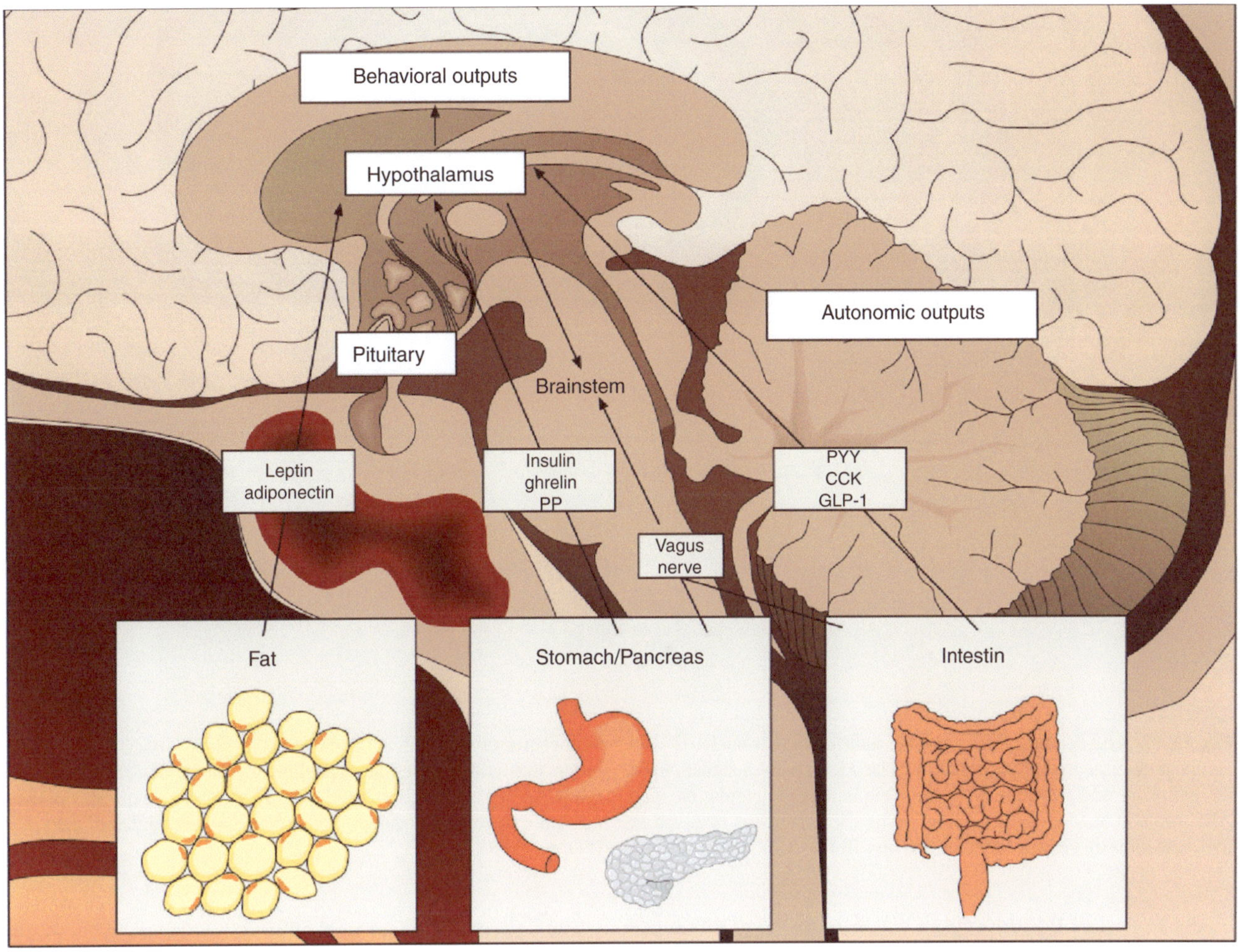

Fig. 13.16 The physiological systems that regulate energy homeostasis. Brain centers, such as the hypothalamus, brainstem, and reward centers in the limbic system, which regulate food intake and energy expenditure through the secretion of neuropeptides. These centers are modulated by neural and hormonal signals coming from the periphery. Hormones synthesized by the adipose tissue, like leptin, and gastrointestinal hormones, like ghrelin, peptide tyrosine tyrosine (PYY), and glucagon-like peptide 1 (GLP-1), modulate these pathways and are able to regulate food intake and energy expenditure

produced predominantly in the gastric fundus [95] and conveys orexigenic signals to the hypothalamus [96].

Ghrelin acts in the ARC of the basal hypothalamus, stimulating the production and release of NPY and suppressing POMC [97]. NPY is the most potent signal in the central nervous system that stimulates food intake and decreases energy expenditure, while POMC is a precursor protein that through proteolytic cleavage originates various peptides, among which α-MSH that decreases appetite and increases energy expenditure [98].

Ghrelin plasma levels rise before meals and are suppressed after food intake [99] in lean but not in obese patients [100]. There is a negative correlation between fasting ghrelin levels and body mass index. Fasting serum ghrelin levels are usually lower in obese subjects compared with controls, and fasting plasma levels rise after diet-induced weight loss [101] and in patients with nervous anorexia. Therefore, with the exception of patients with Prader–Willi syndrome, ghrelin does not seem to play a causative role in obesity in general, and its decreased concentrations are believed to represent a physiological adaptation to the positive energy balance.

Recent studies suggest that weight loss attained after bariatric surgery is also due to endocrine effects of the surgery, which are able to interfere with appetite pathways by suppressing the rise in ghrelin levels that is usually observed after caloric deprivation [102].

13.5.5 Rational for an Anti-ghrelin Vaccine

In view of the fact that ghrelin is the only orexigenic hormone identified so far, it has been considered a promising target in the development of new treatments for obesity.

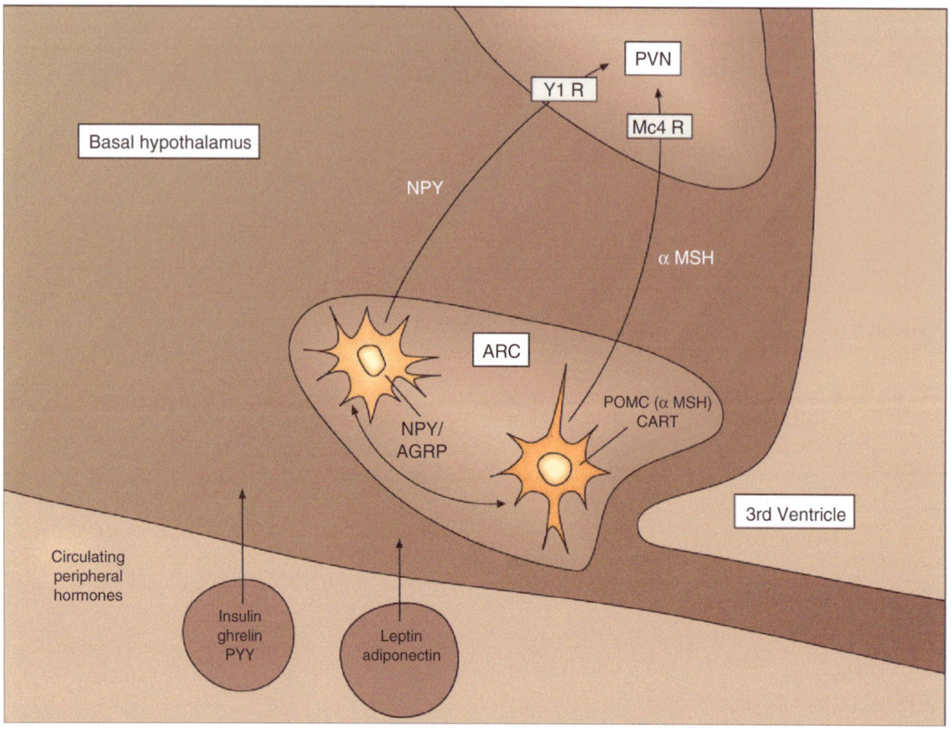

Fig. 13.17 The arcuate (ARC) and the paraventricular nuclei (PVN) are located in the basal hypothalamus. The ARC receives signals from the periphery and plays an integrative role in appetite regulation. The ARC projects second-order neurons to the PVN, which is involved in the regulation of visceral efferent activity. In the ARC, there are two well-characterized neuronal populations involved – one appetite stimulating that co-expresses neuropeptide Y and Agouti-related protein (NPY/AgRP) and another appetite inhibiting that co-expresses proopiomelanocortin and cocaine- and amphetamine-regulated transcript (POMC/CART)

As a proof of this concept, it was demonstrated that inoculation of monoclonal anti-ghrelin antibodies in mice inhibited acute ghrelin-mediated orexigenic effects, but it were unable to change long-term food intake [103]. More recently, another study suggested that the use of a mixture of monoclonal antibodies targeting different haptens but not the antibodies individually promotes not only an increase in energy expenditure but also reduced deprivation-induced food intake [104]. Ghrelin receptor antagonists, GSH-R1, demonstrated improved glucose tolerance, suppressed appetite, and promoted weight loss [105], thus confirming the potential of ghrelin blocking as a potential treatment target for obesity. The suppression of endogenous ghrelin bioactivity with anti-ghrelin vaccines using keyhole limpet hemocyanin (KLH) as carrier protein or bovine serum albumin (BSA) was also tested in mice and pigs, respectively. These vaccines were able to induce the development of antibodies against the active form of ghrelin and also to decrease body weight gain and fat mass [106].

13.5.5.1 Anti-ghrelin Vaccine Using Virus-Like Particles

Virus-like particles (VLPs) have been used as immunogenic molecules in several recombinant vaccines in the last few years in order to induce the production of specific antibodies against endogenous molecules with a preponderant role in chronic diseases, such as the anti-angiotensin vaccine developed for arterial hypertension treatment.

The main goal of this study was to develop an effective anti-ghrelin vaccine using a chemical conjugate of active ghrelin with protein tubules of NS1 of the Bluetongue Virus (BTV). Although this protein is not part of the viral capsid, NS1 tubules possess the same immunogenic characteristics as classical VLPs [107].

13.5.6 Feasibility Study

Male adult C57BL6/J mice, normal weight and with diet-induced obesity mice (DIO) ($n = 18$/group), were randomized into three weight-matched groups ($n = 6$/group). Normal weight mice had unrestricted access to tap water and regular rat chow and DIO mice to a hypercaloric diet with 60 % of fat, after weaning and until a week before the first immunization study when food was switched to regular rat chow.

Mice received three intraperitoneal (i.p.) injections with two-week intervals, containing 500 μl of 75 μg of immunoconjugate, 75 μg of NS1 protein alone or PBS. A dose chosen after performing a dose-finding study in which the 75 μg dose of the immunoconjugate has demonstrated to be adequate in inducing the development of anti-ghrelin antibodies and reduce food intake.

After the immunizations, energy expenditure was accessed by indirect calorimetry. For that mice were individually placed in a small grid cage to limit locomotor activity, which was placed into a sealed chamber containing a sodium hydroxide recipient to adsorb carbon dioxide. The lid of the chamber was sealed and pierced by a volumetric pipette to measure the volume of oxygen consumed. The time elapsed until 1 ml was consumed was registered and repeated until 5 concordant values were obtained. The energy expenditure was then calculated considering that 4.82 kcal is the average energy released per liter of O_2 consumed.

Anti-ghrelin antibodies titer was determined two weeks after each immunization. Plasma levels of active ghrelin, leptin, insulin, growth hormone, and IGF- and TNF-α were determined by ELISA using specific commercial kits according to the manufacturer instructions.

Two weeks after the third immunization, mice were sacrificed, and the stomach fundus and the hypothalamus were recovered and immediately frozen by immersion in liquid nitrogen to evaluate ghrelin, neuropeptide Y (NPY), and proopiomelanocortin (POMC) expression.

13.5.7 Safety and Efficacy of the Vaccine

Normal weight mice treated with the immunoconjugate displayed a significant decrease in daily food intake (0.44 g NS1-Ghr vs. 0.14 g PBS vs. 0.16 g NS1, $p<0.001$) (Fig. 13.18). In addition, after the first two inoculations, there was also an acute decrease in food intake in the group of mice that received the immunoconjugate when compared to the PBS control, corresponding to 95.3 % and 94.8 % of the PBS control, respectively, although without reaching statistical significance. There were no significant differences in body weight gain between the different groups of mice during the study span (3.83 g ± 0.40 g NS1-Ghr vs. 5.00 g ± 0.26 g PBS vs. 5.33 g ± 0.49 g NS1, p = NS) [108].

Diet-Induced Obesity (DIO). In DIO mice, after changing from the hypercaloric to the standard diet, there was an increase in daily food intake followed by rapid stabilization. DIO mice inoculated with the immunoconjugate did not display a significant decrease in cumulative food intake when compared to controls (147.64 ± 2.46 g NS1-Ghr, 147.80 ± 5.89 g NS1, 150.37 ± 3.65 g PBS, p = NS), although there was a significant decrease of food intake in 24 h immediately after each inoculation of the immunoconjugate, corresponding to 66.16 % ($p=0.036$), 82.22 % ($p=0.008$), and 50.09 % ($p=0.039$) of the food intake of the PBS group, after the three inoculations, respectively. DIO mice body weight decreased in response to the change from the hypercaloric to the standard diet (13.84 % compared to baseline), although after the inoculations, there were no significant differences in body weight among the different experimental groups (32.17 ± 0.872 g NS1-Ghr vs. 31.33 ± 1.282 g NS1 vs. 31.83 ± 0.833 g PBS, p = NS) [108].

Normal weight mice inoculated with the immunoconjugate developed specific anti-ghrelin antibodies, with increasing titers after each inoculation, reaching a maximum of 1265 ± 492 2 weeks after the last inoculation. The control groups that received either NS1 protein alone or PBS presented basal titers of 332 ± 114 and 324 ± 143, $p=0.035$, respectively, which were maintained throughout the study and were not altered by the immunizations, which suggests nonspecific bindings related to the detection method. DIO mice inoculated with the immunoconjugate also developed specific anti-ghrelin antibodies in increasing titers until reaching a maximum after the third inoculation in contrast with control groups that maintained their basal titers (2680 ± 1197 NS1-Ghr, 458 ± 31 NS1, and 257 ± 78 PBS group, respectively, $p=0.03$) [108].

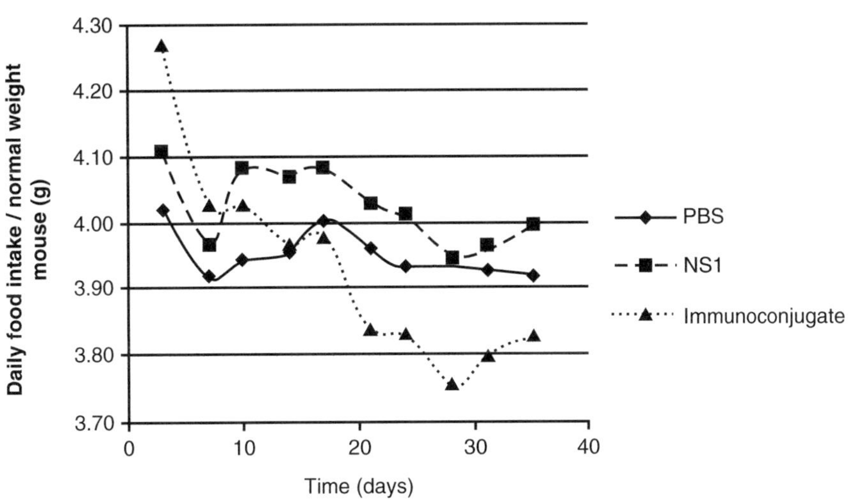

Fig. 13.18 Normal weight mice treated with the immunoconjugate displayed a significant decrease in daily food intake when compared to control mice (0.44 g NS1-Ghr vs. 0.14 g PBS vs. 0.16 g NS1, $p<0.001$)

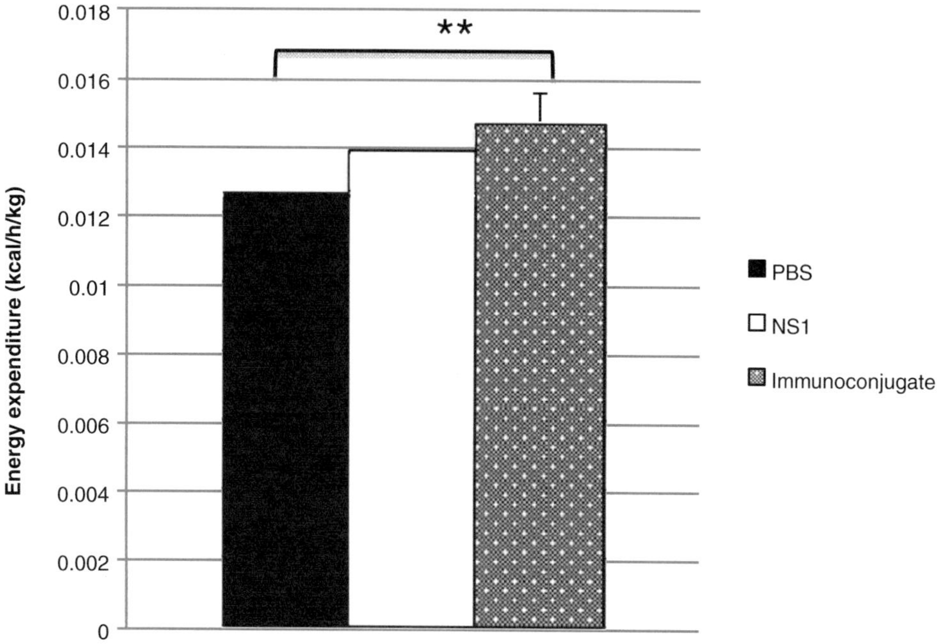

Fig. 13.19 Energy expenditure was significantly higher in normal weight mice inoculated with immunoconjugate when compared with controls (0.0146 ± 0.001 kcal/h/kg NS1-Ghr, 0.0138 ± 0.001 kcal/h/kg NS1, 0.0129 ± 0.001 kcal/h/kg PBS, $p = 0.038$)

Energy expenditure was significantly higher in normal weight mice inoculated with immunoconjugate when compared with controls (0.0146 ± 0.001 kcal/h/kg NS1-Ghr, 0.0138 ± 0.001 kcal/h/kg NS1, 0.0129 ± 0.001 kcal/h/kg PBS, $p = 0.038$) (Fig. 13.19). DIO mice inoculated with the immunoconjugate also showed higher energy expenditure when compared to the control groups (0.0207 ± 0.01 kcal/h/kg NS1-Ghr, 0.0140 ± 0.002 kcal/h/kg NS1, 0.0159 ± 0.002 kcal/h/kg PBS; $p = 0.044$, NS1-Ghr vs. PBS and $p = 0.008$, NS1-Ghr vs. NS1) [108].

Fasting plasma levels of active ghrelin were significantly higher in normal weight mice that received the immunoconjugate (361.3 ± 79.9 pg/ml) when compared to control groups (186.9 ± 14.8 pg/ml NS1 and 114.1 ± 27.9 pg/ml PBS, $p = 0.009$). DIO mice inoculated with the immunoconjugate also presented higher levels of fasting plasma ghrelin than the controls (429.63 ± 179.27 pg/NS1-Ghr, 147.29 ± 53.17 pg/ml NS1, 105.88 ± 27.76 pg/ml PBS, p = NS) although not statistically significant. There were no significant differences in plasma levels of leptin, insulin, glucose, growth hormone, IGF-1, or TNF-α between the groups. ELISA confirmed the presence of circulating immune complexes of ghrelin–anti-ghrelin antibodies in the plasma of normal weight mice inoculated with the immunoconjugate. There was also a positive correlation between ghrelin plasma levels and the titer of circulating immune complexes ($r = 0.846$) (Fig. 13.20).

Search for immunoglobulin deposits in the kidney by immunohistochemistry failed to reveal any evidence of deposited immune complexes on the glomerular basement membranes.

Gene Expression. In normal weight mice, there was no significant difference in ghrelin expression in the gastric fundus between the three experimental groups of mice (0.94 ± 0.17 NS1-Ghr, 1.79 ± 0.35 NS1, 1.00 ± 0.30 PBS, p = NS). There was also no significant difference in NPY expression in the basal hypothalamus between the study groups (1.32 ± 0.17 NS1-Ghr, 0.94 ± 0.10 NS1, 1.00 ± 0.20 PBS, p = NS). In contrast, POMC mRNA expression was significantly lower in mice inoculated with the immunoconjugate when compared to controls (0.20 ± 0.17 NS1-Ghr, 0.93 ± 0.17 NS1, 1.00 ± 0.10 PBS, $p < 0.05$). In DIO mice the expression of ghrelin after normalization for GADPH expression in stomach cells was also not significantly different among the different study groups (1.27 ± 0.30 NS1-Ghr, 0.38 ± 0.13 NS1, 1.00 ± 0.12 PBS, p = NS). However, DIO mice inoculated with the immunoconjugate had a lower expression of NPY in the basal hypothalamus when compared to control groups (0.59 ± 0.09 NS1-Ghr, 1.03 ± 0.12 NS1, 1.00 ± 0.13 for PBS, $p < 0.05$). The expression of POMC in the basal hypothalamus was not significantly different between the different groups in study (1.04 ± 0.14 NS1-Ghr, 1.32 ± 0.25 NS1, 1.00 ± 0.12 PBS, p = NS) [108].

13.5.8 Perspectives

Since ghrelin is the only orexigenic hormone identified so far, it has been pointed as a promising treatment target for obesity [109]. Several research groups have previously attempted ghrelin neutralization. Passive transfer of

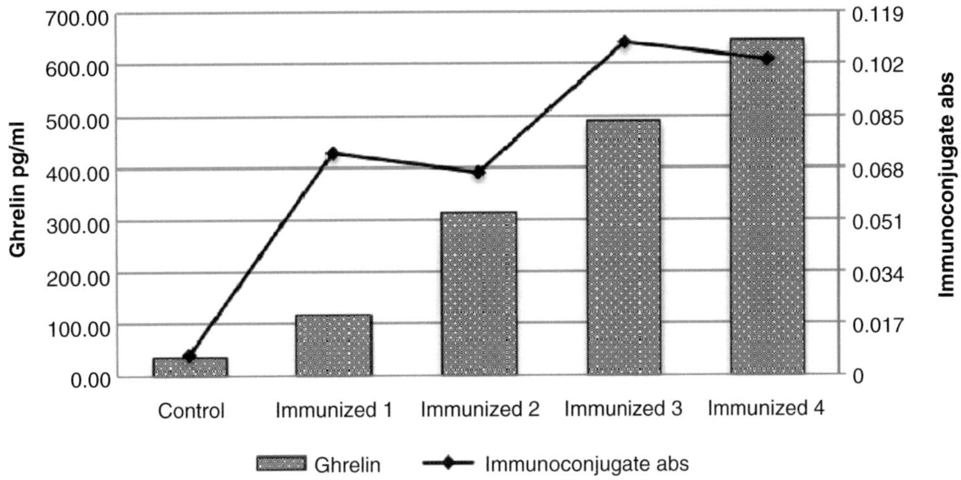

Fig. 13.20 Circulating ghrelin–anti-ghrelin immune complex titers and plasma ghrelin levels. The presence of circulating immune complexes of ghrelin–anti-ghrelin antibodies in the plasma of normal weight mice inoculated with the immunoconjugate was confirmed by ELISA. There was also a positive correlation between ghrelin plasma levels and the titer of circulating immune complexes ($r=0.846$)

monoclonal anti-ghrelin antibodies was unable to change long-term food intake in mice [103]. Antibodies targeted to hydrolyze the octanoyl moiety of ghrelin to form desacyl ghrelin, which has no biological activity, resulted in increased metabolic rate and suppressed 6 h re-feeding after 24 h of food deprivation in mice, but this approach would imply the need of periodic antibody administration [110].

Ghrelin receptor antagonists have also been tested, and GSH-R1a decreased food intake and body weight and improved glucose tolerance due to increased glucose-dependent insulin secretion [105]. Anti-ghrelin vaccines using KLH or BSA as immunogenic substances decreased body weight gain by decreasing feed efficiency in rats and food intake and body weight in pigs [106].

The ability of the VPL vaccine to trigger an immune response was tested in normal weight and DIO male mice that developed increasing titers of specific anti-ghrelin antibodies, confirming the hypothesis that a vaccine consisting of immunoconjugate only is able to trigger an immune response without the need of adjuvants. Furthermore, antibody titers attained after the immunization protocol were not very high, when compared to antibody titers after common infectious diseases, which is also reassuring in safety concerns, since complete neutralization of ghrelin was not the purpose of an anti-ghrelin vaccination strategy for obesity treatment as ghrelin also intervenes in several key biological processes besides appetite regulation, such as growth hormone secretion and gastrointestinal and cardiovascular functions [109].

Vaccinated mice showed significantly higher energy expenditure than the animals of the groups that received either NS1 protein alone or PBS. Higher energy expenditure usually translates into greater ease of weight loss and maintenance. Ghrelin is known to suppress energy metabolism, and ghrelin replacement partially reverses the reduction in body weight and body fat in gastrectomized mice [111]. Ghrelin has been shown to have a long-term effect on energy homeostasis by increasing the respiratory quotient, through decreasing utilization of fat as energy [96]. In addition, ghrelin knockout mice compared to wild-type mice present no change in food intake but have a decreased respiratory quotient when fed with high-fat diet, suggesting that endogenous ghrelin plays a more prominent role in determining the type of metabolic substrate that is used for maintenance of energy balance, than in the regulation of food intake [112].

In vaccinated normal weight mice, there were no significant differences in the genetic expression of NPY gene in the basal hypothalamus in comparison to control mice. However, in vaccinated DIO mice, there was a significant decrease of NPY gene expression in the basal hypothalamus compared with controls reflecting a decrease in central orexigenic signals [113]. The expression of POMC in the basal hypothalamus was significantly lower in vaccinated normal weight animals compared to controls that could represent a compensatory mechanism to the decreased peripheral orexigenic signals in order to prevent the reduction in feeding threshold of normal weight mice, which could also explain why these findings only occurred in the normal weight mice but not on DIO mice.

Ghrelin is a growth hormone secretagogue, and ghrelin neutralization could induce alterations in GH/IGF-1 axis. Since this vaccine appears to have no effect in GH and IGF-1 levels, this suggests that the vaccine is unlikely to cause endocrine adverse effects on the growth hormone axis.

References

1. Miller, K.D., Roque, R., Clegg, C.H.: Novel anti-nicotine vaccine using a trimeric coiled-coil hapten carrier. PLoS One **9**, e114366 (2014). doi:10.1371/journal.pone.0114366
2. Palm, N.W., Medzhitov, R.: Immunostimulatory activity of haptenated proteins. Proc. Natl. Acad. Sci. U. S. A. **106**, 4782–4787 (2009). doi:10.1073/pnas.0809403105
3. Nicolson, K.S., et al.: Antigen-induced IL-10+ regulatory T cells are independent of CD25+ regulatory cells for their growth, differentiation, and function. J. Immunol. **176**, 5329–5337 (2006)
4. Burton, B.R., et al.: Sequential transcriptional changes dictate safe and effective antigen-specific immunotherapy. Nat. Commun. **5**, 4741 (2014). doi:10.1038/ncomms5741
5. Gerth van Wok, R.: Allergy: a global problem. Allergy **57**, 1097–1110 (2002)
6. Okamoto, Y., et al.: Present situation of cedar pollinosis in Japan and its immune responses. Allergol. Int. **58**, 155–162 (2009)
7. Tovey, E.R., Chapman, M.D., Platts-Mills, T.A.: Mite faces are a major source of house dust allergens. Nature **289**, 592–593 (1981)
8. Thomas, W.R., et al.: Characterization and immunobiology of house dust mite allergens. Int. Arch. Allegy Immunol. **129**, 1–18 (2002)
9. Hashimoto, M., et al.: Sensitivity to two major allergens (Cry J 1 and Cry J 2) in patients with Japanese cedar (Cryptomeria japonica) pollinosis. Clin. Exp. Allergy **25**, 848–852 (1995)
10. Namba, M., et al.: Molecular cloning of the second allergen, Cry J II, from Japanese cedar pollen. FEBS Lett. **353**, 124–128 (1994)
11. Dilworth, R.J., Chua, K.Y., Thomas, W.R.: Sequence analysis of cDNA coding for a major house dust mite allergen, Der f I. Clin. Exp. Allergy **21**, 25–32 (1991)
12. Thomas, W.R., Smith, W.: House-dust-mite allergens. Allergy **53**, 821–832 (1998)
13. Park, G.M., et al.: Localization of a major allergen, Der p 2, in the gut and faecal pellets of Dermatophagoides pteronyssinus. Clin. Exp. Allergy **30**, 1293–1297 (2000)
14. Thomas, W.R., Chua, K.Y.: The major mite allergen Der p 2 – a secretion of the male mite reproductive tract? Clin. Exp. Allergy **25**, 667–669 (1995)
15. Frew, A.J.: Immunotherapy of allergic diseases. J. Allergy Clin. Immunol. **111**, S712–S719 (2003)
16. Moingeon, P., et al.: Immune mechanisms of allergen-specific sublingual immunotherapy. Allergy **61**, 151–165 (2006)
17. Larche, M., Akids, C.A., Valenta, R.: Immunological mechanisms of allergen-specific immunotherapy. Nat. Rev. Immunol. **6**, 761–766 (2006)
18. Akdis, M., Akids, C.A.: Mechanisms of allergen-specific immunotherapy. J. Allergy Clin. Immunol. **119**, 780–791 (2007)
19. Linhart, B., Valenta, R.: Molecular design of allergy vaccines. Curr. Opin. Immunol. **17**, 646–655 (2005)
20. Valenta, R., et al.: From allergen genes to allergy vaccines. Ann. Rev. Immunol. **28**, 211–241 (2010)
21. Gronlund, H., Gafvelin, G.: Recombinant Bet v 1 vaccine for treatment of allergy to birch pollen. Hum. Vaccin. **6**, 970–977 (2010)
22. Larche, M.: Peptide immunotherapy for allergic diseases. Allergy **62**, 325–331 (2007)
23. Hirahara, K., et al.: Preclinical evaluation of an immunotherapeutic peptide comprising 7 T cell determinants of Cry J 1 and Cry J 2, the major Japanese cedar pollen allergens. J. Allergy Clin. Immunol. **108**, 94–100 (2001)
24. Nochi, T., et al.: Rice-based mucosal vaccine as a global strategy for cold-chain- and needle-free vaccination. Proc. Natl. Acad. Sci. U. S. A. **104**, 10986–10991 (2007)
25. Lau, O.S., Sun, S.S.M.: Plant seeds as bioreactors for recombinant protein production. Biotechnol. Adv. **27**, 1015–1022 (2009)
26. Takaiwa, F., et al.: Endosperm tissue is good production platform for artificial recombinant proteins in transgenic rice. Plant Biotech. J. **5**, 84–92 (2007)
27. Yang, L., et al.: Expression of hypoallergenic Der f 2 derivatives with altered intramolecular disulphide bonds induces the formation of novel ER-derived protein bodies in transgenic rice seeds. J. Exp. Bot. **63**, 2947–2959 (2012)
28. Kunisawa, J., Kurashima, Y., Kiyono, H.: Gut-associated lymphoid tissues for the development of oral vaccines. Adv. Drug Deliv. Rev. **64**, 523–530 (2012)
29. Streatfiled, S.J.: Mucosal immunization using recombinant plant-based oral vaccines. Methods **38**, 150–157 (2006)
30. Takaiwa, F.: Seed-based oral vaccines as allergen-specific immunotherapy. Hum. Vaccin. **7**, 357–366 (2011)
31. Takagi, H., et al.: Rice seed ER-derived protein body as an efficient delivery vehicle for oral tolerogenic peptides. Peptides **31**, 421–425 (2010)
32. Burks, A.W., Laubach, S., Jones, S.M.: Oral tolerance, food allergy, and immunotherapy: implications for future treatment. J. Allergy Clin. Immunol. **121**, 1344–1350 (2008)
33. Appeman, L.J., Boussiotis, V.A.: T cell anergy and co-stimulation. Immuno. Rev. **192**, 161–180 (2003)
34. Greenwald, R.J., Freeman, G.J., Sharpe, A.H.: B7 family revised. Annu. Rev. Immunol. **23**, 515–548 (2005)
35. Ozdemir, C., Akids, M., Akids, C.A.: T regulatory cells and their counterparts: masters of immune regulation. Clin. Exper. Allergy **39**, 626–639 (2009)
36. Bettelli, E., et al.: Reciprocal developmental pathways for generation of pathogenic effector Th17 and regulatory T cells. Nature **441**, 235–238 (2006)
37. Hirahara, K., et al.: Oral administration of a dominant T cell determinant peptide inhibits allergen-specific TH1 and TH2 cell response in Cry J 2-primed mice. J. Allergy Clin. Immunol. **102**, 961–967 (1998)
38. Murasugi, T., et al.: Oral administration of a T cell epitope inhibits symptoms and reactions of allergic rhinitis in Japanese cedar pollen allergen-sensitized mice. Eur. J. Pharm. **510**, 143–148 (2005)
39. Takagi, H., et al.: A rice-based edible vaccine expressing multiple epitopes induces oral tolerance for inhibition of Th2-mediated IgE response. Proc. Natl. Acad. Sci. U. S. A. **102**, 17525–17530 (2005)
40. Takagi, H., et al.: Oral immunotherapy against a pollen allergy using a seed-based peptide vaccine. Plant Biotech. J. **3**, 521–533 (2005)
41. Domon, E., et al.: 26-week oral safety study in macaques for transgenic rice containing major human T cell epitope peptides from Japanese cedar pollen allergens. Agric. Food Chem. **57**, 5633–5638 (2009)
42. Suzuki, K., et al.: Prevention of allergic asthma by vaccination with transgenic rice seed expressing mite allergen: induction of allergen-specific oral tolerance without bystander suppression. Plant Biotech. J. **9**, 982–990 (2011)
43. Fisher, R., et al.: GMP issues for recombinant plant-derived pharmaceutical proteins. Biotechnol. Adv. **30**, 434–439 (2012)
44. Kearney, P.M., et al.: Global burden of hypertension: analysis of worldwide data. Lancet **365**, 217–223 (2005)
45. Chobanian, A.V.: Shattuck Lecture. The hypertension paradox–more uncontrolled disease despite improved therapy. N. Engl. J. Med. **361**, 878–887 (2009)
46. Egan, B.M., Zhao, Y., Axon, R.N.: US trends in prevalence, awareness, treatment, and control of hypertension, 1988–2008. JAMA **303**, 2043–2050 (2010)
47. Nguyen Dinh Cat, A., Touyz, R.M.: A new look at the renin-angiotensin system–focusing on the vascular system. Peptides **32**, 2141–2150 (2011)
48. Weber, M.: Achieving blood pressure goals: should angiotensin II receptor blockers become first-line treatment in hypertension? J. Hypertens. Suppl. **27**, S9–S14 (2009)
49. Goldblatt, H., Haas, E., Lamfrom, H.: Antirenin in man and animals. Trans. Assoc. Am. Physicians **64**, 122–125 (1951)

50. Michel, J.B., et al.: Active immunization against renin in normotensive marmoset. Proc. Natl. Acad. Sci. U. S. A. **84**, 4346–4350 (1987)
51. Michel, J.B., et al.: Physiological and immunopathological consequences of active immunization of spontaneously hypertensive and normotensive rats against murine renin. Circulation **81**, 1899–1910 (1990)
52. Gradman, A.H., Pinto, R.: Vaccination: a novel strategy for inhibiting the renin-angiotensin-aldosterone system. Curr. Hypertens. Rep. **10**, 473–479 (2008)
53. Brown, M.J., et al.: Randomized double-blind placebo-controlled study of an angiotensin immunotherapeutic vaccine (PMD3117) in hypertensive subjects. Clin. Sci. (Lond.) **107**, 167–173 (2004)
54. Ambuhl, P.M., et al.: A vaccine for hypertension based on virus-like particles: preclinical efficacy and phase I safety and immunogenicity. J. Hypertens. **25**, 63–72 (2007)
55. Tissot, A.C., et al.: Effect of immunisation against angiotensin II with CYT006-AngQb on ambulatory blood pressure: a double-blind, randomised, placebo-controlled phase IIa study. Lancet **371**, 821–827 (2008)
56. Azegami, T., Sasamura, H., Hayashi, K., Itoh, H.: Vaccination against the angiotensin type 1 receptor for the prevention of L-NAME-induced nephropathy. Hypertens. Res. **35**, 492–499 (2012)
57. Zhu, F., et al.: Target organ protection from a novel angiotensin II receptor (AT1) vaccine ATR12181 in spontaneously hypertensive rats. Cell. Mol. Immunol. **3**, 107–114 (2006)
58. Ishiguro, K., Sasamura, H., Sakamaki, Y., Itoh, H., Saruta, T.: Developmental activity of the renin-angiotensin system during the "critical period" modulates later L-NAME-induced hypertension and renal injury. Hypertens. Res. **30**, 63–75 (2007)
59. Libby, P.: Inflammation in atherosclerosis. Nature **420**, 868–874 (2002)
60. Gero, S., et al.: Inhibition of cholesterol atherosclerosis by immunisation with beta-lipoprotein. Lancet **2**, 6–7 (1959)
61. Palinski, W., Miller, E., Witztum, J.L.: Immunization of low density lipoprotein (LDL) receptor-deficient rabbits with homologous malondialdehyde-modified LDL reduces atherogenesis. Proc. Natl. Acad. Sci. U. S. A. **92**, 821–825 (1995)
62. Ameli, S., et al.: Effect of immunization with homologous LDL and oxidized LDL on early atherosclerosis in hypercholesterolemic rabbits. Arterioscler. Thromb. Vasc. Biol. **16**, 1074–1079 (1996)
63. de Jager, S.C., Kuiper, J.: Vaccination strategies in atherosclerosis. Thromb. Haemost. **106**, 796–803 (2011)
64. Nilsson, J., Fredrikson, G.N., Bjorkbacka, H., Chyu, K.Y., Shah, P.K.: Vaccines modulating lipoprotein autoimmunity as a possible future therapy for cardiovascular disease. J. Intern. Med. **266**, 221–231 (2009)
65. Fredrikson, G.N., et al.: Inhibition of atherosclerosis in apoE-null mice by immunization with apoB-100 peptide sequences. Arterioscler. Thromb. Vasc. Biol. **23**, 879–884 (2003)
66. Fredrikson, G.N., Bjorkbacka, H., Soderberg, I., Ljungcrantz, I., Nilsson, J.: Treatment with apo B peptide vaccines inhibits atherosclerosis in human apo B-100 transgenic mice without inducing an increase in peptide-specific antibodies. J. Intern. Med. **264**, 563–570 (2008)
67. Ryan, U.S., Rittershaus, C.W.: Vaccines for the prevention of cardiovascular disease. Vascul. Pharmacol. **45**, 253–257 (2006)
68. Rittershaus, C.W., et al.: Vaccine-induced antibodies inhibit CETP activity in vivo and reduce aortic lesions in a rabbit model of atherosclerosis. Arterioscler. Thromb. Vasc. Biol. **20**, 2106–2112 (2000)
69. Mao, D., et al.: Intramuscular immunization with a DNA vaccine encoding a 26-amino acid CETP epitope displayed by HBc protein and containing CpG DNA inhibits atherosclerosis in a rabbit model of atherosclerosis. Vaccine **24**, 4942–4950 (2006)
70. van Es, T., et al.: IL-15 aggravates atherosclerotic lesion development in LDL receptor deficient mice. Vaccine **29**, 976–983 (2011)
71. van Wanrooij, E.J., et al.: Vaccination against CD99 inhibits atherogenesis in low-density lipoprotein receptor-deficient mice. Cardiovasc. Res. **78**, 590–596 (2008)
72. Hauer, A.D., et al.: Vaccination against TIE2 reduces atherosclerosis. Atherosclerosis **204**, 365–371 (2009)
73. Petrovan, R.J., Kaplan, C.D., Reisfeld, R.A., Curtiss, L.K.: DNA vaccination against VEGF receptor 2 reduces atherosclerosis in LDL receptor-deficient mice. Arterioscler. Thromb. Vasc. Biol. **27**, 1095–1100 (2007)
74. Habets, K.L., et al.: Vaccination using oxidized low-density lipoprotein-pulsed dendritic cells reduces atherosclerosis in LDL receptor-deficient mice. Cardiovasc. Res. **85**, 622–630 (2010)
75. Hermansson, A., et al.: Immunotherapy with tolerogenic apolipoprotein B-100-loaded dendritic cells attenuates atherosclerosis in hypercholesterolemic mice. Circulation **123**, 1083–1091 (2011)
76. Hayashi, K., Sasamura, H., Azegami, T., Itoh, H.: Regression of atherosclerosis in apolipoprotein E-deficient mice is feasible using high-dose angiotensin receptor blocker, candesartan. J. Atheroscler. Thromb. **19**, 736–746 (2012)
77. Harats, D., Yacov, N., Gilburd, B., Shoenfeld, Y., George, J.: Oral tolerance with heat shock protein 65 attenuates Mycobacterium tuberculosis-induced and high-fat-diet-driven atherosclerotic lesions. J. Am. Coll. Cardiol. **40**, 1333–1338 (2002)
78. Maron, R., et al.: Mucosal administration of heat shock protein-65 decreases atherosclerosis and inflammation in aortic arch of low-density lipoprotein receptor-deficient mice. Circulation **106**, 1708–1715 (2002)
79. van Puijvelde, G.H., et al.: Induction of oral tolerance to HSP60 or an HSP60-peptide activates T cell regulation and reduces atherosclerosis. Arterioscler. Thromb. Vasc. Biol. **27**, 2677–2683 (2007)
80. Yuan, X., et al.: Intranasal immunization with chitosan/pCETP nanoparticles inhibits atherosclerosis in a rabbit model of atherosclerosis. Vaccine **26**, 3727–3734 (2008)
81. Jun, L., et al.: Effects of nasal immunization of multi-target preventive vaccines on atherosclerosis. Vaccine **30**, 1029–1037 (2012)
82. Bourinbaiar, A.S., Jirathitikal, V.: Effect of oral immunization with pooled antigens derived from adipose tissue on atherosclerosis and obesity indices. Vaccine **28**, 2763–2768 (2010)
83. WHO: Obesity and overweight fact sheet N°311. http://www.who.int/mediacentre/factsheets/fs311/en/print.html (2006). Accessed 3 July 2009
84. Clinical Guidelines on the Identification, Evaluation, and Treatment of Overweight and Obesity in Adults–the Evidence Report. National Institutes of Health. Obesity Res. **6**(Suppl 2), 51S–209S (1998)
85. Bray, G.A.: Lifestyle and pharmacological approaches to weight loss: efficacy and safety. J. Clin. Endocrinol. Metab. **93**, S81–S88 (2008). jc.2008-1294 [pii]. doi:10.1210/jc.2008-1294
86. Fujioka, K.: Management of obesity as a chronic disease: nonpharmacologic, pharmacologic, and surgical options. Obes. Res. **10**(Suppl 2), 116S–123S (2002). doi:10.1038/oby.2002.204
87. Rucker, D., Padwal, R., Li, S.K., Curioni, C., Lau, D.C.: Long term pharmacotherapy for obesity and overweight: updated meta-analysis. BMJ **335**, 1194–1199 (2007). bmj.39385.413113.25 [pii]. doi:10.1136/bmj.39385.413113.25
88. Bays, H.E.: Lorcaserin: drug profile and illustrative model of the regulatory challenges of weight-loss drug development. Expert Rev. Cardiovasc. Ther. **9**, 265–277 (2011). doi:10.1586/erc.10.22
89. Bays, H.E., Gadde, K.M.: Phentermine/topiramate for weight reduction and treatment of adverse metabolic consequences in obesity. Drugs Today (Barc.) **47**, 903–914 (2011). 1718738 [pii]. doi:10.1358/dot.2011.47.12.1718738
90. Snow, V., Barry, P., Fitterman, N., Qaseem, A., Weiss, K.: Pharmacologic and surgical management of obesity in primary care: a clinical practice guideline from the American College of Physicians. Ann. Intern. Med. **142**, 525–531 (2005). 142/7/525 [pii]

91. Bult, M.J., van Dalen, T., Muller, A.F.: Surgical treatment of obesity. Eur. J. Endocrinol. **158**, 135–145 (2008). 158/2/135 [pii]. doi:10.1530/EJE-07-0145
92. Field, B.C., Chaudhri, O.B., Bloom, S.R.: Obesity treatment: novel peripheral targets. Br. J. Clin. Pharmacol. **68**, 830–843 (2009). BCP3522 [pii]. doi:10.1111/j.1365-2125.2009.03522.x
93. Schwartz, M.W., Woods, S.C., Porte Jr., D., Seeley, R.J., Baskin, D.G.: Central nervous system control of food intake. Nature **404**, 661–671 (2000). doi:10.1038/35007534
94. De Vriese, C., Delporte, C.: Ghrelin: a new peptide regulating growth hormone release and food intake. Int. J. Biochem. Cell Biol. **40**, 1420–1424 (2008). S1357-2725(07)00138-0 [pii]. doi:10.1016/j.biocel.2007.04.020
95. Kojima, M., et al.: Ghrelin is a growth-hormone-releasing acylated peptide from stomach. Nature **402**, 656–660 (1999). doi:10.1038/45230
96. Tschop, M., Smiley, D.L., Heiman, M.L.: Ghrelin induces adiposity in rodents. Nature **407**, 908–913 (2000). doi:10.1038/35038090
97. Cone, R.D., et al.: The arcuate nucleus as a conduit for diverse signals relevant to energy homeostasis. Int. J. Obes. Relat. Metab. Disord. **25**(Suppl 5), S63–S67 (2001). doi:10.1038/sj.ijo.0801913
98. Millington, G.W.: The role of proopiomelanocortin (POMC) neurones in feeding behaviour. Nutr. Metab. (Lond.) **4**, 18 (2007). 1743-7075-4-18 [pii]. doi:10.1186/1743-7075-4-18
99. Cummings, D.E., et al.: Plasma ghrelin levels after diet-induced weight loss or gastric bypass surgery. N. Engl. J. Med. **346**, 1623–1630 (2002). doi:10.1056/NEJMoa012908346/21/1623
100. English, P.J., Ghatei, M.A., Malik, I.A., Bloom, S.R., Wilding, J.P.: Food fails to suppress ghrelin levels in obese humans. J. Clin. Endocrinol. Metab. **87**, 2984 (2002)
101. Hansen, T.K., et al.: Weight loss increases circulating levels of ghrelin in human obesity. Clin. Endocrinol. (Oxf.) **56**, 203–206 (2002). 1456 [pii]
102. Monteiro, M.P., et al.: Increase in ghrelin levels after weight loss in obese Zucker rats is prevented by gastric banding. Obes. Surg. **17**, 1599–1607 (2007). doi:10.1007/s11695-007-9324-7
103. Lu, S.C., et al.: An acyl-ghrelin-specific neutralizing antibody inhibits the acute ghrelin-mediated orexigenic effects in mice. Mol. Pharmacol. **75**, 901–907 (2009). mol.108.052852 [pii]. doi:10.1124/mol.108.052852
104. Zakhari, J.S., Zorrilla, E.P., Zhou, B., Mayorov, A.V., Janda, K.D.: Oligoclonal antibody targeting ghrelin increases energy expenditure and reduces food intake in fasted mice. Mol. Pharm. **9**, 281–289 (2012). doi:10.1021/mp200376c
105. Esler, W.P., et al.: Small-molecule ghrelin receptor antagonists improve glucose tolerance, suppress appetite, and promote weight loss. Endocrinology **148**, 5175–5185 (2007). en.2007-0239 [pii]. doi:10.1210/en.2007-0239
106. Vizcarra, J.A., Kirby, J.D., Kim, S.K., Galyean, M.L.: Active immunization against ghrelin decreases weight gain and alters plasma concentrations of growth hormone in growing pigs. Domest. Anim. Endocrinol. **33**, 176–189 (2007) S0739-7240(06)00112-3 [pii]. doi:10.1016/j.domaniend.2006.05.005
107. Ghosh, M.K., Borca, M.V., Roy, P.: Virus-derived tubular structure displaying foreign sequences on the surface elicit CD4+ Th cell and protective humoral responses. Virology **302**, 383–392 (2002). S004268220291648X [pii]
108. Andrade, S., Carreira, M., Ribeiro, A.: Development of an anti-ghrelin vaccine for obesity treatment. Endocr. Rev. **32,** P2-305 (2011). (The Endocrine Society)
109. Kojima, M., Kangawa, K.: Ghrelin: structure and function. Physiol. Rev. **85**, 495–522 (2005). 85/2/495 [pii]. doi:10.1152/physrev.00012.2004
110. Mayorov, A.V., et al.: Catalytic antibody degradation of ghrelin increases whole-body metabolic rate and reduces refeeding in fasting mice. Proc. Natl. Acad. Sci. U. S. A. **105**, 17487–17492 (2008). doi:10.1073/pnas.0711808105
111. Dornonville de la Cour, C., et al.: Ghrelin treatment reverses the reduction in weight gain and body fat in gastrectomised mice. Gut. **54**, 907–913 (2005). doi:10.1136/gut.2004.058578
112. Wortley, K.E., et al. Genetic deletion of ghrelin does not decrease food intake but influences metabolic fuel preference. Proc. Natl. Acad. Sci. U. S. A. **101**, 8227–8232 (2004) doi:10.1073/pnas.04027631010402763101
113. Kalra, S.P., Dube, M.G., Sahu, A., Phelps, C.P., Kalra, P.S.: Neuropeptide Y secretion increases in the paraventricular nucleus in association with increased appetite for food. Proc. Natl. Acad. Sci. U. S. A. **88**, 10931–10935 (1991)
114. Scheiblhofer, S., Thalhamer, J., Weiss, R.: Novel vaccines for Type I allergy. In: Giese, M. (ed.) Molecular vaccines – from prophylaxis to therapy, vol. 2. Springer, Wien (2013)

Index

M. Giese, *Introduction to Molecular Vaccinology*, DOI 10.1007/978-3-319-25832-4

MIX
Papier aus verantwortungsvollen Quellen
Paper from responsible sources
FSC® C105338

If you have any concerns about our products,
you can contact us on
ProductSafety@springernature.com

In case Publisher is established outside the EU,
the EU authorized representative is:
Springer Nature Customer Service Center GmbH
Europaplatz 3, 69115 Heidelberg, Germany

Printed by Libri Plureos GmbH
in Hamburg, Germany